MANUAL OF Pulmonary Function Testing

MANUAL OF Pulmonary Function Testing

Gregg L. Ruppel, MEd, RRT, RPFT

Director
Pulmonary Function Laboratory
St. Louis University Health Sciences Center
St. Louis, Missouri

SEVENTH EDITION

with 116 illustrations

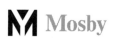 Mosby

St. Louis   Baltimore   Boston   Carlsbad   Chicago   Minneapolis   New York   Philadelphia   Portland
London   Milan   Sydney   Tokyo   Toronto

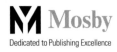

Dedicated to Publishing Excellence

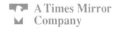

A Times Mirror
Company

Publisher: Don E. Ladig
Editor: Janet Russell
Project Manager: Linda McKinley
Production Editor: Jennifer Furey
Designer: Renée Duenow
Cover Design: David A. Scott
Manufacturing Manager: Linda Ierardi
Cover photo © Scott Camazine, Science Source/Photo Researchers

SEVENTH EDITION
Copyright © 1998 by Mosby, Inc.

Previous editions copyrighted 1994

Printed in the United States of America
Composition by Graphic World, Inc.
Lithography/color film by Graphic World, Inc.
Printing/binding by R.R. Donnelley and Sons, Inc.

Mosby, Inc.
11830 Westline Industrial Drive
St. Louis, Missouri 63146

Library of Congress Cataloging in Publication Data

Ruppel, Gregg, 1948–
    Manual of pulmonary function testing / Gregg L. Ruppel. — 7th ed.
        p.   cm.
    Includes bibliographical references and index.
    ISBN 0–8151–2299–3
    1. Pulmonary function tests—Handbooks, manuals, etc.   I. Title.
    [DNLM: 1. Respiratory Function Tests.   2. Respiratory Function
Tests—examination questions.   WB 284 R946m 1997]
RC734.P84R86   1997
616.2'4075—dc21
DNLM/DLC
for Library of Congress
                                                                97–26485
                                                                CIP

98 99 00 01 02 / 9 8 7 6 5 4 3 2

To Carol, for her patience and encouragement

Preface

THE PRIMARY FUNCTIONS of the lung are oxygenation of mixed venous blood and removal of carbon dioxide. Gas exchange depends on the integrity of the entire cardiopulmonary system, including airways, pulmonary blood vessels, alveoli, respiratory muscles, and respiratory control mechanisms. A few pulmonary function tests assess individual parts of the cardiopulmonary system. However, most lung function tests measure the status of the lungs' components in an overlapping way.

This seventh edition describes many common pulmonary function tests, their techniques, and the pathophysiology that may be evaluated by each test. Spirometry, lung volume measurements, diffusing capacity, and blood gas analysis are discussed as the basic tests of lung function. Also included are chapters on ventilation and ventilatory control and cardiopulmonary exercise tests. Chapter 8 covers bronchial challenge, metabolic measurements, pediatric pulmonary function testing, disability determination, and preoperative evaluation. Pulmonary function testing equipment and quality assurance are addressed in separate chapters.

This seventh edition elaborates on material presented in the first six editions. Changes to this edition reflect suggestions of the users of previous editions. New to this edition is a preliminary chapter describing the indications for performing various categories of pulmonary function tests. This chapter attempts to lend perspective to why specific tests may be needed. Learning objectives have been added at the start of each chapter. Each test section includes criteria for acceptability and interpretive strategies. The criteria are organized to help those performing pulmonary function tests adhere to recognized standards. These criteria are based largely on the most recent recommendations of the American Thoracic Society and the clinical practice guidelines of the American Association for Respiratory Care. The interpretive strategies are presented as a series of questions that can be used as a starting point for test interpretation. The chapter on pulmonary function equipment has been expanded to include some new technologies such as portable peak flow meters and bedside blood gas analyzers. Chapter 10 addresses calibration, quality control, quality assurance, and safety issues. It includes the current equipment recommendations of the American Thoracic Society, as well as safety guidelines from the Centers for Disease Control and Prevention. Case studies are included in most chapters as examples of the performance and interpretation of specific tests.

As in previous editions, each chapter includes self-assessment questions. The questions in this edition are new, and answers may be found in Appendix A. A selected bibliography at the end of each chapter is arranged according to topics within the chapter, including standards and guidelines. As in previous editions, reference equations, nomograms, and sources for reference values are found in the appendixes, along with information on the use of reference values. Sample calculations for lung volumes, plethysmography, diffusion, and exercise tests are also included in the appendixes.

This manual is intended to serve as a text for students of pulmonary function testing and as a reference for technologists and physicians. Because of the variety of methods and equipment used in pulmonary function evaluation, some tests are discussed in general terms. For this reason, readers are encouraged to use the selected bibliographies provided. The presentation of indications, pathophysiology, and clinical significance of various tests presumes a basic understanding of cardiopulmonary anatomy and physiology. Again, readers are urged to refer to the General References included in the Selected Bibliography to refresh their background knowledge of lung function. The terminology used is that of the American College of Chest Physicians–American Thoracic Society Joint Committee on Pulmonary Nomenclature. In some instances test names reflect common usage that does not follow the ACCP-ATS recommendations.

Gregg L. Ruppel, MEd, RRT, RPFT

Acknowledgments

My thanks to Drs. William Kistner, John Winter, and James Wiant for their encouragement in the development of the original text. My special thanks to Drs. Roger Secker-Walker, Susan Marshall, and Gerald Dolan for comments and constructive criticisms in the preparation of the revised editions. Special thanks also go to Ronald Gilmore and Jack Tandy for their contributions to the illustrations in previous editions. A note of thanks also to Thomas Anderson, MEd, RRT; David Shelledy, MA, RRT; Patricia Dent, BS, MS, RPT; and Barbara Disborough, MA, RRT for their reviews of and suggestions for the fourth edition. Louis Metzger, RPFT; Donald Barker, BS, PA, RPFT; David Hoover, RRT, RPFT; Randall Krohn; James Kemp, MD; Alan Hibbett, RPFT; and Michael Snow, RPFT all provided guidance and suggestions for the fifth edition. Cesar Keller, MD, and Deborah Stanger, RD, provided insight for case studies for the sixth edition. Robert Brown, RRT, RPFT, and Deborah White, RRT, RPFT suggested significant changes for the seventh edition.

My appreciation for illustrations provided goes to the following companies:

Abbott Critical Care Systems
Biochem International
Warren E. Collins, Inc.
HealthScan Products, Inc.
Jones Medical Instrument Co.
Marquette Medical Systems
Medical Graphics, Inc.
Nonin Medical, Inc.

Novametrix Medical Systems, Inc.
Pulmonary Data Service Instrumentation
Radiometer America
Hans Rudolph, Inc.
SensorMedics Corp.
Spirometrics, Inc.
Vitalograph Medical Instrumentation

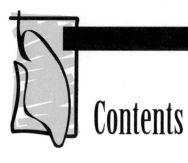

Contents

MANUAL OF Pulmonary Function Testing

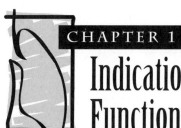

CHAPTER 1
Indications for Pulmonary Function Testing

OBJECTIVES

After studying this chapter and reviewing its tables, you should be able to do the following:

1 Categorize pulmonary function tests according to specific purposes

2 List indications for spirometry, lung volumes, diffusing capacity, blood gases, and exercise or metabolic testing

3 Identify diseases that commonly require pulmonary function assessment

4 Describe patient preparation and assessment before testing

5 Relate pulmonary history information to the indications for testing

THIS CHAPTER PROVIDES AN OVERVIEW of pulmonary function testing. Common pulmonary function tests are introduced, and the indications for each test are discussed. Diseases that commonly require pulmonary function tests are described, and guidelines regarding patient preparation and assessment are presented. Adequate patient preparation, physical assessment, and pulmonary history help the tests provide answers to clinical questions. The importance of patient instruction in obtaining valid data is discussed. These topics are developed more fully in subsequent chapters.

Pulmonary Function Tests

Many different tests are used to evaluate lung function. These tests can be divided into categories based on which aspect of lung function they measure (Table 1-1). Although each of these tests can be performed alone, two or more are often done together. Determining which tests to do depends on the clinical question to be answered. This question may be explicit, such as "Does the patient have **asthma?**" or less obvious, such as "Does this patient, who needs abdominal surgery, have any pulmonary disease that might complicate the procedure?" In either case, indications for specific tests are useful (Table 1-2).

AIRWAY FUNCTION

The most basic test of pulmonary function is the vital capacity (VC) test. This test simply measures the largest volume of air that can be moved into or out of the lungs. In the mid-1800s, John Hutchinson developed a simple water-sealed **spirometer** that allowed measurement of VC. Hutchinson popularized the concept of using VC to assess lung function. He observed that VC was related to the standing height of the subject. He also developed tables to estimate the expected VC for a healthy subject. The VC was usually graphed on chart paper, which allowed subdivisions of the VC to be identified (see Chapter 2).

Forced vital capacity (FVC) is a refinement of the simple VC test. During the 1930s Alvan Barach observed that patients with asthma or **emphysema** exhaled more slowly than healthy subjects. He noted that airflow out of the lungs was important in detecting **obstruction** of the airways. Barach used a rotating chart drum (**kymograph**) to display VC changes. He even evaluated the effects of **bronchodilator** medications using the forced expiratory spirogram.

Around 1950, Gaensler began using a microswitch in conjunction with a water-sealed spirometer to time FVC. He concluded that healthy subjects consistently exhaled approximately

1

| **TABLE 1-1** | Categories of Pulmonary Function Tests |

A. Airway function
  1. Simple spirometry
     a. VC, expiratory reserve volume (ERV), inspiratory capacity (IC)
  2. Forced vital capacity maneuver
     a. FVC, FEV_1, FEF, PEF
        (1) Prebronchodilator and postbronchodilator
        (2) Prebronchochallenge and postbronchochallenge
     b. MEFV curves, $\dot{V}_{max_x}$
        (1) Prebronchodilator and postbronchodilator
        (2) Prebronchochallenge and postbronchochallenge
  3. Maximal voluntary ventilation (MVV)
  4. Maximal inspiratory/expiratory pressures (MIP/MEP)
  5. Airway resistance (Raw) and Compliance (C_1)
B. Lung volumes and ventilation
  1. Functional residual capacity (FRC)
     a. Open-circuit (N_2 washout)
     b. Closed-circuit/rebreathing (He dilution)
     c. Thoracic gas volume (VTG)
  2. Total lung capacity (TLC), residual volume (RV), RV/TLC ratio
  3. Minute ventilation, alveolar ventilation, and dead space
  4. Distribution of ventilation
     a. Multiple-breath N_2
     b. He equilibration
     c. Single-breath techniques
C. Diffusing capacity tests
  1. Single-breath (breath holding)
  2. Steady state
  3. Other techniques
D. Blood gases and gas exchange tests
  1. Blood gas analysis and blood oximetry
     a. Shunt studies
  2. Pulse oximetry
  3. Capnography
E. Cardiopulmonary exercise tests
  1. Simple noninvasive tests
  2. Tests with exhaled gas analyses
  3. Tests with blood gas analyses
F. Metabolic measurements
  1. Resting energy expenditure (REE)
  2. Substrate utilization

80% of their FVC in 1 second, and almost all of the FVC in 3 seconds. He used the forced expired volume in the first second (FEV_1) to assess **airway obstruction.** In 1955 Leuallen and Fowler demonstrated a graphic method used to assess airflow. They measured airflow between the 25% and 75% points on a forced expiratory spirogram. This measure was described as the maximal midexpiratory flow rate (MMFR). This and other measurements were used to describe airflow from both healthy and airflow-obstructed patients. To standardize terminology, the MMFR is now referred to as the forced expiratory flow 25%-75% ($FEF_{25\%-75\%}$).

In addition to displaying FVC as a volume-time spirogram, it can also be represented by plotting airflow against volume. In the late 1950s, Robert Hyatt and others began using the flow-volume display to assess airway function. The tracing was termed the maximal expiratory flow volume (MEFV) curve. By combining it with an inspiratory maneuver, a closed loop was displayed. This figure was called the **flow-volume loop** (see Chapter 2).

Peak expiratory flow (PEF) is measured using either a flow-sensing spirometer or a **peak flow meter.** In the 1960s Wright popularized the use of peak flow to monitor asthmatic patients. Peak

TABLE 1-2   Indications for Spirometry

Spirometry may be indicated to:

A. Detect the presence or absence of lung disease
   1. History of pulmonary symptoms
      a. Dyspnea, wheezing
      b. Cough, phlegm production
      c. Chest pain, orthopnea
   2. Physical indicators
      a. Decreased breath sounds
      b. Chest wall abnormalities
   3. Abnormal laboratory findings
      a. Chest x-ray study
      b. Blood gases

B. Quantify the extent of known disease on lung function
   1. Pulmonary disease
      a. Chronic obstructive pulmonary disease
      b. Asthma
      c. Cystic fibrosis
      d. Interstitial diseases
   2. Cardiac disease (congestive heart failure)
   3. Neuromuscular disease (Guillain-Barré syndrome)

C. Measure effects of occupational or environmental exposure
   1. Smoking
   2. Working in hazardous or dusty environments

D. Determine beneficial or negative effects of therapy
   1. Bronchodilators or steroids
   2. Cardiac drugs (antiarrhythmics, diuretics)
   3. Lung resection, reduction, or transplant
   4. Pulmonary rehabilitation

E. Assess risk for surgical procedures
   1. Lung resection (lobectomy, pneumonectomy)
   2. Thoracic procedures (sternotomy)
   3. Abdominal procedures

F. Evaluate disability or impairment
   1. Social Security or other compensation programs
   2. Legal or insurance evaluations

flow can be readily assessed from the flow-volume loop as well. Recently, portable peak flow meters that allow monitoring at home, as well as in the hospital or clinic, have been developed.

The FVC and its components, along with flow-volume loops and peak flow, are all used to measure response to bronchodilator medications (see Chapter 2). Tests are repeated before and after inhalation of a bronchodilator, and the percentage of change is calculated. The same tests may be used to assess airway response after a challenge to the airways. This challenge may be in the form of an inhaled agent (e.g., **methacholine**) or a physical agent (e.g., exercise). In either case, airflow is assessed before and after the challenge. During bronchodilator studies, the percentage of change after challenge is calculated (see Chapter 8).

Maximal voluntary ventilation (MVV) was described as early as 1941. It was originally called the maximal breathing capacity by Cournand and Richards. In the MVV test, the patient breathes rapidly and deeply for 12 to 15 seconds. The volume of air exchanged is expressed in liters per minute. The MVV gives an estimate of the peak ventilation available to meet physiologic demands.

Measurement of respiratory muscle strength is accomplished by assessing maximal inspiratory pressure (MIP) and maximal expiratory pressure (MEP). This can be done using either a pressure **transducer** or a simple aneroid **manometer.** MIP and MEP are important adjuncts to forced expiratory spirometry for monitoring both obstruction and **restrictive disease.**

Airway resistance (Raw) measurements date back to the development of the body **plethysmograph** in the early 1950s. Julius Comroe, Arthur Dubois, and others perfected a technique that provided estimates of **alveolar** pressure. The patient sat in an airtight box called a plethysmograph (see Chapter 9). The plethysmograph calculated pressure drop across the airways related to flow at the mouth (see Chapter 2). This technique is still widely used. The same equipment can also be used to measure thoracic gas volume (VTG).

Lung **compliance** is measured by passing a small balloon into the esophagus to measure pleural pressure. Pleural pressure can then be related to volume changes to estimate the distensibility of the lung (see Chapter 2). Other less invasive techniques are available but are not widely used.

LUNG VOLUMES AND VENTILATION

Measurement of lung volumes dates back to the early 1800s, well before Hutchinson's development of spirometry. Various techniques have been used to estimate the volume of gas remaining in the lung after a complete exhalation. Davy used a hydrogen dilution technique to estimate residual air. This technique was later improved by Meneely and Kaltreider using helium (He) instead of hydrogen. Around the same time, Darling, Cournand, and Richards began using oxygen breathing to wash nitrogen (N_2) out of the lungs. The collection and analysis of the volume of N_2 exhaled allowed the functional residual capacity (FRC) to be estimated. Using simple spirometry and FRC determinations allows total lung capacity (TLC) and residual volume (RV) to be calculated. As previously discussed, the other commonly used method for measuring lung volumes uses the body plethysmograph. Estimation of lung volumes from chest radiographs is possible but is not widely used.

Closed-circuit (He dilution) and open-circuit (N_2 washout) techniques are both widely used to measure FRC. Besides determining lung volumes, each technique provides useful information about distribution of ventilation within the lungs. The pattern of N_2 washout can be displayed graphically. The time required for He to equilibrate during **rebreathing** provides a similar index of the evenness of ventilation. In the early 1950s and 1960s, a single-breath N_2-washout technique was developed by Fowler. This method plotted N_2 concentration in expired air after a single breath of 100% oxygen. The single-breath N_2 washout provided information about gas distribution in the lungs. It also allowed estimates of the lung volume at which airway closure occurred when the subject exhaled completely (see Chapter 3).

Measurement of resting ventilation requires only a simple gas metering device and a means of collecting expired air. Portable computerized spirometers allow **minute ventilation, tidal volume** (VT), and breathing rate to be readily measured in almost any setting. Determination of **alveolar ventilation** or **dead space** (wasted ventilation) requires measurement of arterial partial pressure of carbon dioxide ($PaCO_2$) in addition to total ventilation. Alternately, the partial pressure of carbon dioxide (PCO_2) can be estimated from expired CO_2. The availability of blood gas analyzers and exhaled CO_2 analyzers makes these measurements routine.

DIFFUSING CAPACITY TESTS

The basis for the modern single-breath **diffusing capacity** (DL_{co}) test was described by August and Marie Krogh in 1911. They showed that small but measurable differences existed between inspired and expired gas containing **carbon monoxide** (CO). This change could be related to the uptake of gas across the lung. Although they used the method to test a series of patients, they did not employ the single-breath technique for clinical purposes. Around 1950 Forrester and his colleagues revisited the method. They developed it as a tool to measure the gas exchange capacity of the lung. About the same time, Filley and others were promoting other techniques using CO to measure diffusing capacity. Most of these techniques allowed patients to breathe normally, rather than hold their breath. These methods are called steady-state techniques. Each method has certain limitations. However, the single-breath technique is the most widely used and standardized in the United States.

BLOOD GASES AND GAS EXCHANGE TESTS

Measurement of gases (O_2 and CO_2) in the blood began with volumetric methods used since the early 1900s. In 1957 Sanz introduced the glass **electrode** to measure **pH** of fluids potentiometrically. In 1958 Severinghaus added an outer jacket containing a **bicarbonate buffer** to the glass electrode. The electrode-buffer was separated from the blood being analyzed by a membrane that was permeable to CO_2. This allowed the pressure of CO_2 in the blood to be measured as a pH change in the electrode. In 1956 Leland Clark covered a platinum electrode with a polypropylene membrane. When a voltage was applied to the electrode, O_2 was reduced at the platinum **cathode** in proportion to its partial pressure. These three electrodes (pH, P_{CO_2}, and partial pressure of oxygen [P_{O_2}]) are the basis of modern blood gas analyzers. Today, blood gas analysis is available using portable instruments with miniature electrodes. Electrodes to measure **electrolytes** (K^+, Na^+, Cl^-) are also included in some blood gas analyzer systems.

Blood **oximetry** was developed during World War II to monitor the effects of exposure to high-altitude flight. During the 1960s spectrophotometric analyzers that could measure the total **hemoglobin (Hb)**, along with oxyhemoglobin and **carboxyhemoglobin (COHb)** levels were perfected. Blood oximetry testing has been combined with blood gas analysis so that both can be accomplished with a single instrument. **Pulse oximetry** was developed in the 1970s as a result of efforts to monitor cardiac rate by using a light beam to sense pulsatile blood flow. It was quickly discovered that not only could the pulse be sensed, but changes in light **absorption** could be used to estimate arterial oxygen saturation.

Capnography, or monitoring of exhaled carbon dioxide, was developed in conjunction with the **infrared** gas analyzer. This sensitive and rapidly responding analyzer allows exhaled CO_2 to be monitored continuously. Most critical care units, operating rooms, and emergency departments use some combination of blood gas analysis, pulse oximetry, and capnography for patient monitoring. Blood gas analysis is an integral part of routine pulmonary function testing because it is the definitive test of the basic functions of the lung.

CARDIOPULMONARY EXERCISE TESTS

The simplest types of exercise tests are those in which the subject performs work and only noninvasive measurements are made. Such measurements include heart rate and rhythm monitoring using an electrocardiogram. Other simple, noninvasive measurements are blood pressure and respiratory rate monitoring. Analysis of exhaled gas is noninvasive, but the patient does have to breathe through a **mouthpiece** or mask. Ventilation and V_T can be estimated by collecting the exhaled air. Analysis of expired gases permits **oxygen consumption** and **CO_2 production** to be measured, along with several derived variables. When invasive measures (blood gas analysis, arterial catheters, pulmonary artery catheters) are used, the entire range of physiologic variables that affect exercise can be monitored. Computers allow sophisticated measurements to be made rapidly while the subject continues to exercise (**breath-by-breath** gas analysis).

METABOLIC MEASUREMENTS

Measurement of energy expenditure and caloric requirements dates to the early 1900s. Basal metabolic rate **(BMR)** was measured by allowing a subject to rebreathe from a volume spirometer containing added oxygen. An estimate of energy expenditure could be derived by plotting the rate at which oxygen was consumed. A similar approach is taken today, except that oxygen consumption and carbon dioxide production are monitored using gas analyzers. Resting energy expenditure **(REE)** has replaced BMR as the primary variable related to metabolic needs. Although BMR was used to detect disorders that affected **metabolism**, REE is used to manage critically ill patients whose caloric requirements may be impossible to estimate.

Indications for Pulmonary Function Testing

Each category of pulmonary function testing includes specific reasons why each test may be necessary. These reasons for testing are called indications. Some pulmonary function tests have well-defined indications. The same indications that apply to one type of test (e.g. spirometry) may apply to other categories as well.

SPIROMETRY

Spirometry is the pulmonary function test performed most often because it is indicated in many situations (see Table 1-2). Spirometry is often performed as a screening procedure. It may be the first test to indicate the presence of pulmonary disease. However, spirometry alone may not be sufficient to completely define the extent of disease, response to therapy, preoperative risk, or level of impairment. Spirometry must be performed correctly because of the serious impact its results can have on the patient's life.

LUNG VOLUMES

Lung volume determination usually includes the VC and its subdivisions, along with the FRC. From these two basic measurements the remaining lung volumes and capacities can be calculated (see Chapters 2 and 3). Lung volumes are almost always measured in conjunction with spirometry, although the indications for them are distinct (Table 1-3). The most common reason for measuring lung volumes is to identify restrictive lung disease. A reduced VC suggests **restriction,** particularly if airflow is normal. Measurement of FRC and determination of the TLC are necessary to confirm restriction. If TLC is reduced, restriction is present. The severity of the restrictive process is determined by the extent of reduction of the TLC. TLC and its components can be determined by several different methods. For patients with obstructive lung diseases (chronic obstructive pulmonary disease [**COPD**], asthma), lung volumes measured by body plethysmography may be indicated (see Chapter 3).

DIFFUSING CAPACITY

Diffusing capacity is measured by having the patient inhale a low concentration of CO and a **tracer** gas to determine gas exchange within the lungs (DL_{CO}). Several methods of evaluating the uptake of CO from the lungs are available, but the single-breath technique ($DL_{CO}SB$) is most commonly used. This method is also called the breath-hold technique because CO transfer is measured during 10 seconds of breath holding. DL_{CO} is usually measured in conjunction with spirometry and lung volumes. Although most pulmonary and cardiovascular diseases reduce DL_{CO} (Table 1-4), it may be increased in some cases (see Chapter 5). DL_{CO} testing is commonly used to monitor diseases caused by dust. These are conditions in which lung tissue is infiltrated by substances such as asbestos that disrupt the normal structure of the gas exchange units. DL_{CO} testing is also used to evaluate pulmonary involvement in systemic diseases such as rheumatoid arthritis. DL_{CO} measurements are often included in the evaluation of patients with obstructive lung disease.

BLOOD GASES

Blood gas analysis is often done in conjunction with pulmonary function studies. Blood is drawn from a peripheral artery without being exposed to air (i.e., anaerobically). The radial artery is often used for a single arterial puncture or indwelling catheter. Blood gas analysis includes measurement of hydrogen ion activity (pH), along with the PCO_2 and PO_2. The same specimen may be used for blood oximetry to measure total Hb, oxyhemoglobin saturation (**O_2Hb**), carboxyhemoglobin (COHb), and methemoglobin (**MetHb**).

Blood gas analysis is the ideal measure of pulmonary function because it assesses the two primary functions of the lung (oxygenation and CO_2 removal). Evaluation of any pulmonary disorder might be considered a reason for performing blood gas analysis. Very specific indications for blood gas analysis are widely used (Table 1-5). Blood gas analysis is most commonly used to determine the need for supplemental oxygen and to manage patients who require ventilatory support. Some pulmonary function measurements require blood gas analysis as an integral part of the test (i.e., **shunt** or dead space studies). Blood gas analysis is invasive; noninvasive measurements of oxygenation or gas exchange are often preferred if they are safer or less costly. Many noninvasive techniques (e.g., pulse oximetry) rely on blood gas analysis to verify their validity (see Chapter 6).

TABLE 1-3   Indications for Lung Volume Determination

Lung volume determinations may be indicated to:
A. Diagnose or assess the severity of restrictive lung disease (reduced TLC)
B. Differentiate between obstructive and restrictive disease patterns
C. Assess response to therapy
  1. Bronchodilators, steroids
  2. Lung transplantation, resection, reduction
  3. Radiation or chemotherapy
D. Make preoperative assessments of patients with compromised lung function
E. Determine or evaluate disability
F. Assess gas trapping by comparison of plethysmographic lung volumes with gas dilution lung volumes
G. Standardize other lung function measures (i.e., specific conductance)

TABLE 1-4   Indications for DL_{CO}

Diffusing capacity (DL_{CO}) measurements may be indicated to:
A. Evaluate or follow the progress of parenchymal lung diseases
    1. Dusts (asbestos, silica, metals)
    2. Organic agents (allergic alveolitis)
    3. Drugs (amiodarone, bleomycin)
B. Evaluate pulmonary involvement in systemic diseases
    1. Rheumatoid arthritis
    2. Sarcoidosis
    3. Systemic lupus erythematosus (SLE)
    4. Systemic sclerosis
    5. Mixed connective tissue disease
C. Evaluate obstructive lung disease
    1. Follow the progression of disease
        a. Emphysema
        b. Cystic fibrosis
    2. Differentiate types of obstruction
        a. Emphysema
        b. Chronic bronchitis
        c. Asthma
    3. Predict arterial desaturation during exercise in COPD
D. Evaluate cardiovascular diseases
    1. Primary pulmonary hypertension
    2. Acute or recurrent pulmonary thromboembolism
    3. Pulmonary edema and congestive heart failure
E. Quantify disability associated with interstitial lung disease
F. Evaluate pulmonary hemorrhage, polycythemia, or left-to-right shunts (increased DL_{CO})

TABLE 1-5   Indications for Blood Gas Analysis

Blood gas analysis and/or blood oximetry may be indicated to:
A. Evaluate adequacy of lung function
    1. Ventilation
        a. Pa_{CO_2}
    2. Acid-base status
        a. pH
        b. Pa_{CO_2}
    3. Oxygenation and oxygen-carrying capacity
        a. Pa_{O_2}
        b. Total Hb, O_2Hb, COHb, MetHb
    4. Intrapulmonary shunt
    5. V_D/V_T ratio
B. Determine need for supplemental oxygen (for clinical or reimbursement purposes)
    1. Presence or severity of resting hypoxemia
    2. Exercise desaturation
    3. Nocturnal desaturation
    4. Adequacy of oxygen prescription
C. Monitor ventilatory support
    1. Assess or follow respiratory failure
    2. Adjust therapy to improve oxygenation (PEEP, CPAP, pressure support)
D. Document the severity or progression of known pulmonary disease
E. Provide data to correct or corroborate other pulmonary function measurements
    1. Correct DL_{CO} measurements (Hb and COHb)
    2. Determine accuracy of pulse oximetry, transcutaneous monitors, or indwelling blood gas devices

PEEP, Positive end-expiratory pressure; *CPAP,* continuous positive airway pressure.

TABLE 1-6   Indications for Exercise Testing

Exercise testing may be indicated to:
A. Determine the level of cardiorespiratory fitness
B. Document or diagnose exercise limitation as a result of fatigue, dyspnea, or pain
   1. Cardiovascular diseases
      a. Myocardial ischemia or dyskinesis
      b. Cardiomyopathy
      c. Congestive heart failure
      d. Peripheral vascular disease
   2. Pulmonary diseases
      a. Airway obstruction or hyperreactivity
      b. Interstitial lung disease
      c. Pulmonary vascular disease
   3. Mixed cardiovascular, pulmonary, or unknown etiologies
C. Evaluate adequacy of arterial oxyhemoglobin saturation
   1. Exercise desaturation/hypoxemia
   2. Oxygen prescription
   3. Right-to-left shunt
D. Assess preoperative risk, particularly lung resection or reduction
E. Assess disability, particularly related to occupational lung disease
F. Evaluate therapeutic interventions such as heart or lung transplantation

EXERCISE TESTS

Physical exercise stresses the heart, lungs, and the pulmonary and peripheral circulatory systems. Exercise testing allows simultaneous evaluation of the cellular, cardiovascular, and ventilatory systems. Cardiopulmonary exercise tests can be used to determine the level of fitness or extent of **dysfunction.** Appropriately designed tests can determine the role of cardiac or pulmonary involvement. Understanding the physiologic basis for the patient's inability to exercise is key to offering effective therapy. Table 1-6 lists some indications for exercise tests.

Equipment used to measure oxygen consumption and CO_2 production during exercise can also measure resting metabolic rates. This allows estimates of caloric needs in patients who are critically ill. Indications for performing studies of REE are detailed in Chapter 8.

Patterns of Impaired Pulmonary Function

Patients are usually referred to the pulmonary function laboratory to evaluate signs or symptoms of lung disease. In some instances, the clinician may wish to exclude a specific diagnosis such as asthma. Indications for different categories of pulmonary function tests have been described previously. Sometimes, patients display patterns during testing that are consistent with a specific diagnosis. This section presents an overview of some commonly encountered forms of impaired pulmonary function.

OBSTRUCTIVE AIRWAY DISEASES

An obstructive airway disease is one in which airflow into or out of the lungs is reduced. This simple definition includes a variety of pathologic conditions. Some of these conditions are closely related regarding how they cause airway obstruction. For example, mucus hypersecretion is a component of **chronic bronchitis,** asthma, and **cystic fibrosis** (CF), even though their causes are quite distinct.

Chronic Obstructive Pulmonary Disease

The term *COPD* is often used to describe long-standing airway obstruction caused by emphysema, chronic bronchitis, or asthma. These three conditions may be present alone or in combination (Fig. 1-1). **Bronchiectasis** is also sometimes considered a component of COPD. COPD is characterized by **dyspnea** at rest or with exertion, often accompanied by a productive cough. Delineation of the

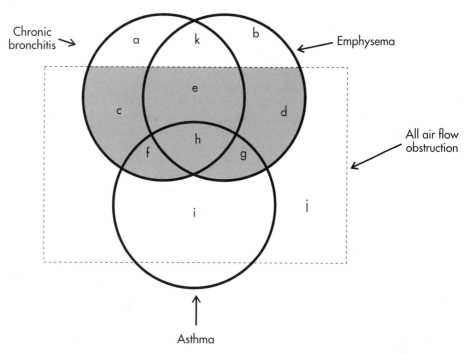

FIG. 1-1 *A nonproportional diagram depicting the relationship between various components of COPD.* Emphysema, chronic bronchitis, and asthma overlap to varying degrees *(shaded areas)*. There is also overlap between chronic obstruction in small airways and all airway obstructive diseases *(large dashed square)*. *a,* Patients with chronic bronchitis but no airflow obstruction; *b,* patients with anatomic changes related to emphysema, but no obstruction; *c,* patients with chronic cough and airflow obstruction; *d,* patients with emphysema and obstruction as demonstrated by spirometry; *e,* combined chronic bronchitis and emphysema, commonly occurring in the same subject as a result of cigarette smoking; *f,* combined chronic bronchitis and asthma; *g,* combined emphysema and asthma; *h,* combined asthma, chronic bronchitis, and emphysema; *i,* patients with asthma manifested by reversible obstruction (spirometry or peak flow); *j,* other forms of airway obstruction, including cystic fibrosis, bronchiolitis obliterans, or upper airway abnormalities (e.g., vocal cord dysfunction) are not considered part of COPD; *k,* subjects with cough and morphologic evidence of emphysema, but no obstruction. (Modified from American Thoracic Society: Standards for the diagnosis and care of patients with chronic obstructive pulmonary disease, *Am J Respir Crit Care Med* 152:S77-S120, 1995.)

type of obstruction depends on the history, physical examination, and pulmonary function studies. Unfortunately, the term *COPD* is used to describe the clinical findings of dyspnea or cough without attention to the actual cause. This may lead to inappropriate therapy. Other similar terms include chronic obstructive lung disease (COLD) and chronic airway obstruction (CAO).

Emphysema
Emphysema means "air trapping" and is defined morphologically. The air spaces distal to the terminal bronchioles are abnormally increased in size. The walls of the alveoli undergo destructive changes. This destruction results in overinflation of lung units. If the process mainly involves the respiratory bronchioles the emphysema is termed *centrilobular.* If the alveoli are also involved, the term *panlobular emphysema* is used to describe the pattern. These distinctions require examination of lung tissue either by biopsy or at postmortem. Because this is often impractical, emphysema is suspected when there is airway obstruction with air trapping. Physical assessment, chest x-ray studies, and pulmonary function studies are the primary diagnostic tools.

Emphysema is caused primarily by cigarette smoking. Repeated inflammation of the respiratory bronchioles results in tissue destruction. As the disease advances, more and more alveolar walls are destroyed. Loss of elastic tissue results in airway collapse and **hyperinflation.** Some emphysema is caused by the absence of a protective enzyme, α_1**-antitrypsin.** The lack of this enzyme is caused by a genetic defect. α_1-Antitrypsin inhibits proteases in the blood from attacking healthy tissue. Deficiency of α_1-antitrypsin causes gradual destruction of alveolar walls resulting in panlobular emphysema. Chronic exposure to environmental pollutants can also contribute to the development of emphysema. The natural aging of the lung also causes some changes that resemble the disease entity. The natural decline of elastic recoil in the lung reduces maximal airflow and increases lung volume as we age. Surgical removal of lung tissue sometimes causes the remaining lung to overinflate.

The main symptom of emphysema is breathlessness, either at rest or with exertion. **Hypoxemia** may contribute to this dyspnea, particularly in advanced emphysema. However, the destruction of alveolar walls also causes loss of the capillary bed. Ventilation-perfusion matching may be relatively well preserved in patients with emphysema. As a result, oxygen levels may be only slightly decreased. This type of patient is sometimes called the pink puffer. As the disease advances, the loss of alveolar surface causes a decreased ability to oxygenate mixed venous blood. DL_{CO} is reduced. The patient becomes increasingly breathless, particularly with exertion. This dyspnea can cause problems with nutrition, and patients are often below their ideal body weight. As noted, symptoms of chronic bronchitis and asthma may be present as well.

The chest x-ray film of a patient with emphysema shows flattened diaphragms and increased air spaces. The lung fields appear hyperlucent (dark) with little vascularity. The heart appears to be hanging from the great vessels. The physical appearance of the chest confirms what is shown radiographically. The chest wall is immobile with the shoulders elevated. The diameter of the chest is increased anteroposteriorly (i.e., so-called barrel chest). There is little **diaphragmatic** excursion during inspiration. Intercostal retractions may be prominent. Accessory muscles (neck and shoulders) are used to lift the chest wall. Breath sounds are distant or absent. Patients may need to support the arms and shoulders to catch their breath. Breathing is often done through pursed lips to alleviate the sensation of dyspnea.

Chronic bronchitis

Chronic bronchitis is diagnosed by clinical findings. It is present when there is excessive mucus production, with a productive cough on most days, for at least 3 months for 2 years or more. The diagnosis is made by excluding other diseases that also result in excess mucus production. These include cystic fibrosis, **tuberculosis,** abscess, tumors, or bronchiectasis.

Chronic bronchitis, like emphysema, is caused primarily by cigarette smoking. It may also result from chronic exposure to environmental pollutants. Chronic bronchitis causes the mucus glands lining the airways to hypertrophy and increase in number. There is also chronic inflammation of the bronchial wall with infiltration of leukocytes and lymphocytes. The number of ciliated epithelial cells decreases. This causes impairment of mucus flow in the airways. Similar changes occur in respiratory bronchioles. Excessive mucus and poor clearance make the patient susceptible to repeated infections. Some patients who have chronic bronchitis caused by cigarette smoking experience a decrease in cough and mucus production after smoking cessation. Some airway changes, however, usually persist.

Chronic cough is the defining symptom of chronic bronchitis. Some patients do not consider cough abnormal and refer to it as "smoker's cough" or "morning cough." In addition to cough, chronic bronchitis may produce dyspnea, particularly with exertion. Blood gas abnormalities usually accompany chronic bronchitis. Ventilation-perfusion mismatching causes hypoxemia. If hypoxemia persists, the patient may develop secondary polycythemia. **Cyanosis** may be present due to the combination of arterial **desaturation** and increased Hb levels. Chronic hypoxemia may also lead to right-sided heart failure (i.e., **cor pulmonale**). Advanced chronic bronchitis is also often accompanied by **hypercapnia.**

Unlike the emphysema patient, the patient with chronic bronchitis may show few clinical signs of underlying disease. Body weight may be normal or increased with minimal changes to the chest wall. Patients with bronchitis may appear normal except for cough and dyspnea. The chest x-ray film in chronic bronchitis differs markedly from that in emphysema. The congested airways are easily visible. The heart may appear enlarged with the pulmonary vessels prominent. The diaphragms may appear normal or flattened, depending on the degree of hyperinflation present. If there is right-sided heart failure, swelling (**edema**) of the lower extremities is often present.

Pulmonary infections can seriously aggravate chronic bronchitis. The appearance of the sputum produced can help predict worsening function. If it is normally white, a change to discolored sputum indicates the beginning of an infection. This may be accompanied by worsened hypoxemia and shortness of breath. Early treatment can potentially reverse an otherwise serious complication. Failure to manage the chest infection can result in severe hypoxemia and hypercapnia, with exacerbation of right-sided heart failure. Acute respiratory failure superimposed on chronic failure is the most common cause of death in patients with COPD.

Bronchiectasis

Bronchiectasis is pathologic dilatation of the bronchi. It results from destruction of the bronchial walls by severe, repeated infections. The terms *saccular, cystic,* and *tubular* are used to describe the appearance of the bronchi. Most bronchiectasis involves prolonged episodes of infection. Bronchiectasis is common in CF, as well as following bronchial obstruction by a tumor or foreign body. When the entire bronchial tree is involved, the disease is assumed to be inherited or caused by developmental abnormalities.

The main clinical feature of bronchiectasis is a very productive cough. The sputum is usually purulent and foul-smelling. **Hemoptysis** is also common. Frequent bronchopulmonary infections lead to gas exchange abnormalities similar to chronic bronchitis. Right-sided heart failure follows advancement of the disease. Chest x-ray studies, bronchograms, and computed tomography (CT) scans are used to identify the type and extent of the disease.

Treatment of bronchiectasis includes vigorous bronchial hygiene. Regular antibiotic therapy is used to manage the repeated infections. **Bronchoscopy** and surgical **resection** are sometimes required to manage localized areas of infection. Patients with recurrent hemoptysis may require resection of the offending lobe.

Management of chronic obstructive pulmonary disease

COPD often includes components of emphysema and chronic bronchitis (see Fig. 1-1). This association most likely is due to the common risk factor of cigarette smoking. **Hyperreactive** airways disease (asthma) may also be present. Reversibility of obstruction, however, is usually less than in uncomplicated asthma. Bronchiectasis and bronchiolitis are also commonly found in patients with COPD.

Treatment of COPD begins with smoking cessation and avoiding irritants that inflame the airways. Other measures aimed at keeping the airways open are also important. Inhaled bronchodilators, especially β-agonists, are commonly used. Combinations of **β-adrenergic** and **anticholinergic** bronchodilators, together with inhaled **corticosteroids** provide relief to many patients with COPD. This is often the case, even when there is little improvement in air-flow assessed by spirometry. Some patients require oral steroids (e.g., Prednisone) to manage chronic inflammation. Antibiotics are commonly used at the first sign of respiratory infections. Digitalis and **diuretics** are most often prescribed for the management of right-sided heart failure.

In addition to pharmacologic management, breathing retraining, bronchial hygiene measures, and physical reconditioning are important therapeutic modalities. Breathing retraining is especially important for the patient with advanced COPD. Grossly altered pulmonary mechanics favor hyperinflation and use of accessory muscles. Training in the use of the diaphragm for slow, relaxed breathing can significantly improve gas exchange. Pulmonary rehabilitation, particularly physical reconditioning, permits many patients with otherwise debilitating disease to maintain their quality of life.

Supplemental (O_2) therapy is indicated in COPD when the patient's oxygen tension at rest or during exercise is less than 55 mm Hg. Oxygen may also be prescribed when signs of right-sided heart failure (i.e., cor pulmonale) are present. Many patients desaturate only with exertion. Exercise testing is the only reliable method of detecting exertional desaturation. Low-flow O_2 therapy can be implemented by a number of methods, including portable systems. Chronic O_2 supplementation has been shown to improve survival in patients with COPD.

Single-lung transplantation has recently been used for patients with end-stage COPD who are younger than 60 years old. Although **lung transplantation** causes immediate improvement in pulmonary function, it is expensive. The cost of hospitalization and follow-up care may be prohibitive. In addition, lack of donor organs means that many patients with COPD die while awaiting transplantation. The prognosis for those receiving lung transplants is generally good. In some transplant recipients a severe form of airway obstruction **(bronchiolitis obliterans)** has been found to occur in the transplanted lung. The reason for this obstructive process is unclear, but the progression is rapid. Spirometry is used to monitor transplant recipients to detect early changes associated with bronchiolitis obliterans.

Volume reduction surgery has also been used to treat end-stage COPD. In this procedure, lung tissue that is poorly perfused is surgically removed, which allows the remaining lung units to expand with improved ventilation-perfusion matching. This technique works particularly well when there are large areas of trapped gas with little perfusion (bullae). The procedure can be performed on both lungs by **sternotomy,** or unilaterally using a flexible thoracoscope. With both methods, lung volumes are reduced and spirometry and gas exchange improve. Spirometry, lung volumes, and blood gas analysis are used to monitor changes in these patients.

Hyperreactive Airways Disease (Asthma)

Asthma is characterized by reversible airways obstruction. Obstruction is caused by **broncho-spasm,** increased airway secretions, and inflammation of the mucosal lining of the airways. The obstruction is usually easily reversed by inhalation of bronchodilators but may be persistent and severe in some patients. Increased airway responsiveness is related to inhalation of antigens, viral infections, air pollution, or occupational exposure. Asthma can occur at any age but often begins during childhood. Some asthmatic children outgrow the disease, but in others the disease continues into adulthood. In some individuals asthma begins after age 40. There appears to be a hereditary component to asthma; many cases occur in subjects who have a family history of asthma or allergic disorders.

Agents or events that cause an asthmatic episode are called **triggers** (Table 1-7). Antigens such as animal dander, pollens, and dusts are the most common triggers. Other common triggers include exposure to air pollutants, exercise in cold or dry air, occupational exposure to dusts or fumes, and viral upper respiratory infections. Asthma can also be triggered by aspirin or other drugs, by food additives (e.g., metabisulfites), or by emotional upset (e.g., crying, laughing). All of these triggers act on the hyperresponsive airway to produce the symptoms of asthma.

The most common presentation of asthma includes **wheezing,** cough, and shortness of breath. The severity of asthmatic episodes varies, even in the same individual at different times. In many subjects, airway function is relatively normal between intermittent episodes or attacks. Some patients have only cough or chest tightness that subsides spontaneously. However, severe episodes may be life-threatening. In its worst presentation, asthma causes continuous chest tightness and wheezing that may not respond to the usual therapy. Dyspnea and cough can both be extreme, and if unresolved they can progress to respiratory failure.

During an attack there is usually wheezing, noisy breathing, and prolonged expiratory times. If the attack is severe there may be significant air trapping, similar to the pattern seen in patients with emphysema. Accessory muscles of ventilation are used, and breathing may be labored. The most readily available means of assessing the degree of airflow obstruction is by spirometry or by peak flow meter. Similarly, spirometry provides the simplest means of determining the response to

TABLE 1-7 Asthma Triggers

A. Allergic agents
  1. Pollens
  2. Animal dander (proteins)
  3. House dust mites
  4. Molds
B. Nonallergic agents
  1. Viral infections
  2. Exercise
  3. Cold air
  4. Air pollutants (sulfur, nitrogen dioxides)
  5. Cigarette smoke
  6. Drugs (aspirin, beta-blockers)
  7. Food additives
  8. Emotional upset
C. Occupational exposure
  1. Toluene 2,4-diisocyanate (TDI)
  2. Cotton, wood dusts
  3. Grain
  4. Metal salts
  5. Insecticides

bronchodilators. Arterial blood gas testing may be necessary during severe asthmatic episodes. Hypoxemia is commonly present because of ventilation-perfusion mismatching. This usually results in a **respiratory alkalosis,** but evidence of **respiratory acidosis** suggests impending ventilatory failure.

Inhalation challenge tests using methacholine, **histamine,** or cold air are often used to make the diagnosis of hyperreactive airways in subjects who appear normal but have episodic symptoms. Skin testing is also used to demonstrate **sensitivity** to inhaled antigens.

Management of asthma

The first step in asthma management is avoiding known triggers. In some instances this is easily accomplished. However, in the case of air pollution or occupational exposure, avoiding the offending substance may be impossible or expensive. Asthma education usually focuses on helping the affected individual identify and avoid triggers.

Pharmacologic management of asthma is based on bronchodilator therapy. For many patients with mild asthma, two puffs of an adrenergic bronchodilator from a metered-dose inhaler (**MDI**) may be the only treatment required. In severe asthma, β-adrenergic bronchodilators are usually inhaled on a dosing schedule. A wide variety of β-agonists are available, many in oral and inhaled forms. Anticholinergic bronchodilators (i.e., ipratropium bromide) have become widely prescribed for use in conjunction with β-agonists. Ipratropium may be preferred in patients who experience tachycardia or tremor caused by adrenergic drugs. Although most β-agonists have a rapid onset of action (5 to 15 minutes), ipratropium typically takes 30 to 60 minutes for peak effect to occur. **Theophylline** preparations are still widely used in combination with inhaled bronchodilators. Long-acting theophylline drugs (12 to 24 hours) are often prescribed.

Corticosteroids are usually reserved for acute or chronic asthma that responds poorly to conventional bronchodilators. Steroids act primarily as antiinflammatory agents in the airways and may allow adrenergic drugs to bronchodilate more effectively. Because of the adverse side effects of corticosteroids, only patients with severe asthma take them on a continuous basis. Inhaled steroid preparations sometimes eliminate the need for oral forms during chronic therapy. Several different preparations are now available in MDIs.

Cromolyn sodium is used to prophylactically prevent **bronchoconstriction.** It cannot be used for acute episodes, but it may decrease the amount of corticosteroids or bronchodilators necessary. It is available as a nebulized solution, inhaled powder, or MDI.

Perhaps the most significant new tool in the management of asthma is the portable peak flow meter (see "Peak Flow," Chapter 2). This device allows simple monitoring of airway function by the patient at home, as well as by caregivers in a variety of settings. Measurement of peak flow provides objective data to guide both the patient and physician in modifying bronchodilator therapy or seeking early treatment.

Cystic Fibrosis

CF is a disease that primarily affects the mucus producing apparatus of the lungs and pancreas. CF is an inherited disorder, transmitted as an autosomal recessive trait. In Caucasians it occurs in approximately 1 in 2000 live births. CF was once considered a pediatric disease because affected individuals rarely lived to adulthood. Improved detection and aggressive treatment has increased the median survival age well into adulthood.

CF is characterized by malabsorption of food as a result of pancreatic insufficiency and progressive **suppurative** pulmonary disease. In infancy and early childhood, gastrointestinal manifestations seem to predominate. As the child gets older, respiratory complications related to the tenacious mucus production take over. Other organ systems may be involved as well. Children with CF tend to remain chronically infected with respiratory **pathogens,** such as *Staphylococcus aureus* or *Pseudomonas aeruginosa.*

Clinical manifestations of CF include chronic cough and sinusitis, bronchiectasis, and **atelectasis.** Hemoptysis and **pneumothorax** are not uncommon. Chest x-ray studies show changes consistent with bronchiectasis and **honeycombing.** Atelectasis commonly affects entire lobes as a result of mucus impaction. Other complications center around gastrointestinal manifestations (e.g., bowel obstruction and vitamin deficiencies). Most individuals with CF are diagnosed in infancy or early childhood based on elevated sweat chloride levels. However, some young adults are not diagnosed until after age 15. In many instances adolescents or even adults are misdiagnosed as having asthma or related pulmonary diseases. Misdiagnosis usually occurs in individuals who have mild CF with few complications.

Management of Cystic Fibrosis

Removal of the excess mucus produced in CF is the primary focus of management. This usually requires bronchial hygiene measures and pharmacologic intervention. Bronchodilators are used to reverse bronchospasm that commonly accompanies chronic inflammation. A genetically engineered enzyme is now used to reduce mucus viscosity in CF patients. This enzyme (rhDNase) is administered via an aerosol. This reduces the viscosity of secretions and improves airflow. Corticosteroids are used to combat both pulmonary inflammation and bronchial hyperreactivity. Continuous or intermittent antibiotics are also a mainstay of care in the patient with CF. Proper nutrition is similarly very important in managing CF. Pancreatic insufficiency increases the patient's metabolic rate even though nutrients are poorly absorbed in the intestine. Pancreatic enzyme supplements and vitamins are required, particularly in children with CF.

Upper/Large Airway Obstruction

Many obstructive diseases involve the medium or **small airways.** Sometimes airway obstruction occurs in the upper airway (nose, mouth, pharynx) or in the large thoracic airways (trachea, mainstem bronchi). Obstruction can also occur where the upper and lower airways meet at the vocal cords. When obstruction occurs below the vocal cords, the degree of obstruction may vary with changes in thoracic pressure. This occurs because the airways themselves change size as thoracic pressure rises or falls. Obstructive processes above the vocal cords are not influenced by thoracic pressures but may still vary with airflow depending on the type of lesion involved. Regardless of the location of the problem, **large airway obstruction** results in increased work of breathing.

Vocal cord dysfunction or damage can result in significant airway obstruction. The vocal cords are normally held open or abducted during inspiration. When damaged the vocal cords move toward the midline, narrowing the airway opening. This type of obstruction limits flow primarily during inspiration. In some cases, expiratory flow may be reduced as well, but inspiratory flow is typically lower. Common causes of vocal cord dysfunction include laryngeal muscle weakness or mechanical damage as sometimes occurs during intubation of the trachea. Severe infections involving the larynx can leave scar tissue on the vocal cords or supporting structures. Vocal cord dysfunction often mimics asthma. It may become notably worse when ventilation is increased, as happens during exercise. **Neuromuscular** disorders can cause paralysis of the vocal cords, also resulting in variable extrathoracic airway obstruction (see Chapter 2).

Tumors are a common cause of large airway obstruction. Lesions that invade the trachea or mainstem bronchi can significantly diminish airflow. The decrease in flow is directly related to the decrease in cross-sectional area of the airway. If the airway lumen (i.e., the part not obstructed) varies in cross-sectional area with inspiration and expiration, the obstruction is described as variable. During inspiration thoracic pressure decreases and large airways increase their cross-sectional area. During expiration the opposite occurs. If the airway is partially obstructed by a tumor, airflow will be decreased during inspiration and expiration, but more so during expiration. If the tumor reduces the cross-sectional area of the airway but does not vary with the phase of breathing, the obstruction is fixed. In this instance both inspiratory and expiratory flows are reduced approximately equally (see "Flow-Volume Loops," Chapter 2). Tumors in the upper airway may cause variable or fixed obstruction. If an extrathoracic tumor causes the airway cross section to vary with breathing, inspiratory flow is usually reduced.

Neuromuscular disorders that affect the muscles of the upper airway can also affect airway patency. When the muscles of the pharynx or larynx are relaxed (reduced muscle tone), airway collapse may occur during the inspiratory phase of breathing. Any disorder that affects innervation of pharyngeal muscles can cause similar obstructive patterns. Abnormal airflow patterns are sometimes seen in patients who have **obstructive sleep apnea,** although flow measurements cannot predict sleep apnea. **Myasthenia gravis** affects the muscles of respiration, including the muscles of the upper airway. Generalized weakness of these muscles can result in variable extrathoracic obstruction.

Both upper and large airway obstruction commonly result from trauma to the airways. These can occur as the result of motor vehicle accidents or falls. Scarring or stenosis of the trachea may also occur after prolonged endotracheal intubation or tracheostomy. The typical pattern is one of fixed obstruction, although some lesions do vary with the phase of breathing. Granulomatous disease, such as **sarcoidosis** or tuberculosis, can occasionally cause upper airway obstruction. Extrinsic airway compression can also reduce airflow. **Goiters** or **mediastinal** infections are the most common culprits that compress the airways in this way.

Management of Upper or Large Airway Obstruction

Treatment of lesions that produce upper or large airway obstruction is aimed at reversing the offending process. For vocal cord dysfunction, stopping inappropriate therapy (e.g., steroids) is the first step. Speech therapy and breathing retraining have been demonstrated to reduce inspiratory obstruction. In severe cases, a mixture of helium and oxygen (80% He–20% O_2) may be needed to alleviate dyspnea and interrupt the episode. Treatment of neuromuscular disease such as myasthenia gravis often reverses the associated airway obstruction.

Tumors usually require resection. Some **neoplasms** can be managed only by radiation or **chemotherapy.** In either case, spirometry with flow-volume curves (see Chapter 2) is used to assess airway obstruction. Surgical repair of trauma to the upper or large airways directly relieves airway obstruction and reduces work of breathing.

RESTRICTIVE LUNG DISEASE

Restrictive lung disease is characterized by reduction of lung volumes. The VC and TLC are both reduced below the lower limit of normal. Any process that interferes with the bellows action of the lungs or chest wall can cause restriction. Restriction is often associated with (1) **interstitial lung diseases,** including **idiopathic fibrosis,** pneumoconioses, and sarcoidosis; (2) disease of the chest wall and **pleura;** (3) neuromuscular disorders; and (4) congestive heart failure **(CHF).**

Idiopathic Pulmonary Fibrosis

Idiopathic pulmonary fibrosis (IPF) is characterized by alveolar wall inflammation resulting in fibrosis. Vascular changes are usually associated with **pulmonary hypertension.** The patient has increasing exertional dyspnea. On the chest x-ray film, **infiltrates** are visible and advanced IPF shows a honeycombing pattern.

IPF often follows the use of medications such as **bleomycin,** cyclophosphamide, methotrexate, or **amiodarone.** IPF is also associated with a number of autoimmune diseases. Rheumatoid arthritis, systemic **lupus erythematosus** (SLE), and **scleroderma** all produce alveolar wall inflammation and **fibrotic** changes. As each disease progresses, lung volumes are reduced. These reductions in VC and TLC occur as fibrosis causes the lungs to become stiff. Measurement of pulmonary compliance (see Chapter 2) is sometimes helpful in quantifying the effects of the fibrosis. D_{CO} (see Chapter 5) is often reduced due to ventilation-perfusion mismatching. The same process also causes hypoxemia at rest that worsens with exertion.

Management of IPF relies primarily on corticosteroids (Prednisone). Long-term therapy is usually indicated with large initial doses, followed by tapering and then maintenance. Immunosuppressive agents are sometimes used in conjunction with steroids in difficult cases. Pulmonary function studies are routinely used to monitor the patient's progress.

Pneumoconioses

Pneumoconiosis is lung impairment caused by inhalation of dusts. Certain types of dust exposure have been shown to result in pneumoconioses (Table 1-8). Dust particles in the size range between 0.5 and 5.0 µm are considered most dangerous because they are deposited throughout the lung. A carefully taken history (see "Pulmonary History," p. 21), including work

TABLE 1-8 Common Pneumoconioses

Dust	Pneumoconiosis	Occupation
Iron	Siderosis	Welder, miner
Tin	Stannosis	Metal worker
Barium	Baritosis	Miner, metallurgist, ceramics worker
Silica	Silicosis	Sandblaster, brick maker, coal miner
Asbestos	Asbestosis	Brake/clutch manufacturer, shipbuilder, steam fitter, insulator
Talc	Talcosis	Ceramics worker, cosmetics maker
Beryllium	Berylliosis	Alloy maker, electronic tube maker, metal worker
Coal	Coal worker's pneumoconiosis	Coal miner

history, is essential. Most of the pneumoconioses are characterized by pulmonary fibrosis and chest x-ray abnormalities.

Silicosis, caused by inhalation of silica dust, is common. Silica is deposited in the lung and ingested by macrophages. This results in the formation of nodules around bronchioles and blood vessels. As the silicosis advances fibrosis occurs. The patient usually has cough and dyspnea. In addition to restriction shown by pulmonary function studies, some airways may also be obstructed. As nodules increase in size to more than 1 cm, the condition is labeled progressive massive fibrosis (PMF). PMF is usually accompanied by hypoxemia and pulmonary hypertension. Treatment of silicosis is directed at relieving hypoxemia and managing right-sided heart failure.

Asbestosis results from inhalation of asbestos fibers. Asbestos has been commonly used in the manufacture of insulating materials, brake linings, roofing materials, and fire-resistant textiles. As with most pneumoconioses, the risk of developing asbestosis is related to the intensity and duration of exposure. The onset of symptoms is usually delayed for 20 years. Cigarette smoking has been shown to shorten the period between exposure and onset of symptoms. Inhaled asbestos fibers are engulfed by alveolar macrophages. Fibrosis in alveolar walls and around bronchioles develops. The visceral pleura may also show fibrous deposits. Plaques, made up of collagenous connective tissue, are often found on the parietal pleura. The patient experiences dyspnea on exertion. Pulmonary function tests show restriction and impaired **diffusion.** The chest x-ray film may show irregular densities in the lower lung fields, fibrotic changes (honeycombing) and diaphragmatic calcifications. COPD and lung cancer are also common in patients with asbestosis and are related to cigarette smoking. Treatment consists of assessment with pulmonary function tests (especially diffusing capacity) and relief of symptoms.

Coal worker's pneumoconiosis (CWP) is caused by an accumulation of coal dust in the lungs. It should not be confused with **black lung,** which is a legal term used to describe any chronic respiratory disease in a coal miner. Some coal contains silica, but CWP begins with a reaction to an accumulation of dust called a coal macule. These macules are usually found in the upper lobes. The black coal pigment is deposited around the respiratory bronchioles. Diagnosis of CWP is made by history and chest x-ray film interpretation. Onset of symptoms caused by CWP usually occurs in advanced cases. Coal workers often have respiratory symptoms and physiologic findings consistent with COPD. These symptoms may be related more to cigarette smoking than to coal dust exposure. CWP causes fibrosis, restriction on pulmonary function tests, hypoxemia, and pulmonary hypertension. As in the case of other pneumoconioses, treatment is aimed at relief of the symptoms.

Sarcoidosis

Sarcoidosis is a granulomatous disease that affects multiple organ systems. The disease appears most often in the second through fourth decades. It occurs more commonly in African-Americans, especially in women. The granuloma found in sarcoidosis is composed of macrophages, epithelioid cells, and other inflammatory cells. This granulomatous lesion may resolve with little or no structural change, or it may develop fibrosis in the target organ.

Symptoms of sarcoidosis include fatigue, muscle weakness, fever, and weight loss. Other symptoms involve the specific organ system in which the granulomatous changes occur. The lungs and lymph nodes of the mediastinum are involved in most patients who have sarcoidosis. Dyspnea and cough are the most common presenting symptoms. Chest x-ray films usually show enlargement of the **hilar** and mediastinal lymph nodes. Interstitial infiltrates may also be present. Other systems commonly involved in sarcoidosis include the skin, eyes, musculoskeletal system, heart, and central nervous system.

Pulmonary function tests show a pattern of restriction, with relatively normal flows. Diffusing capacity is usually not reduced except when there is advanced fibrosis of lung tissue. Arterial blood gas measurements may be normal, or there may be hypoxemia. Stress testing may show worsened gas exchange. It is not unusual for sarcoidosis in the early stages to show completely normal lung function. Diagnosis of sarcoidosis is sometimes made via clinical findings and chest x-ray examination, but biopsy of affected tissue is often necessary. This may involve mediastinoscopy or fiberoptic bronchoscopy.

Management of sarcoidosis includes medications to treat symptoms such as fever, skin lesions, or arthralgia. Serious complications involving worsening pulmonary function are usually treated with corticosteroids.

DISEASES OF THE CHEST WALL AND PLEURA

Several disorders involving the chest wall or pleura of the lungs result in restrictive patterns on pulmonary function studies. Conditions affecting the thorax include **kyphoscoliosis** and obesity. Pleural diseases include **pleurisy**, pleural **effusions**, and pneumothorax.

Kyphoscoliosis is a condition that involves abnormal curvature of the spine both anteriorly (**kyphosis**) and laterally (**scoliosis**). Patients who have kyphoscoliosis show rib cage distortion that can lead to recurrent infections as well as blood gas abnormalities. Depending of the degree of spinal curvature, the patient may have normal lung function or restriction. Ventilation may be normal. Lung compression usually causes ventilation-perfusion mismatching and hypoxemia. In severe cases there may be hypercapnia and respiratory acidosis. Treatment of the disorder involves prevention of infections and relief of hypoxemia, if present. Surgical correction is necessary in many cases, and pulmonary function studies are used to evaluate patients both preoperatively and postoperatively.

Obesity restricts ventilation, especially when the obesity is severe. Increased mass of the thorax and abdomen interferes with the bellows action of the chest wall. Obesity is also related to a more general syndrome that consists of hypercapnia and hypoxemia, sleep apnea, and decreased respiratory drive. These findings are sometimes called the **obesity-hypoventilation** syndrome. Chronic hypoxemia in this syndrome results in polycythemia, pulmonary hypertension, and cor pulmonale. Not all patients who are obese show the signs of obesity-hypoventilation syndrome. However, pulmonary function studies usually show restriction in proportion to the excess weight. Weight reduction relieves many of the associated symptoms. Respiratory stimulants, tracheostomy, and continuous positive airway pressure (CPAP) are used to manage the obstructive sleep apnea component.

Pleurisy and pleural effusions can each result in restrictive ventilatory patterns. Pleurisy is characterized by deposition of a fibrous **exudate** on the pleural surface. It is associated with other pulmonary diseases such as pneumonia or lung cancer. Pleurisy is often accompanied by chest discomfort or pain, and may precede the development of pleural effusions. Pleural effusion is an abnormal accumulation of fluid in the pleural space. This fluid may be either a **transudate** or an exudate. Transudate occurs when there is an imbalance in the hydrostatic or oncotic pressures, as occurs in CHF. Exudates are associated with infections or with inflammation as in lung carcinoma. Patients with pleural effusions usually have symptoms that relate to the extent of the effusion. Small effusions often go unnoticed. When the effusion is large, there may be atelectasis from compression and associated blood gas changes. Pulmonary function tests show restriction as a result of volume loss. In some cases, there is restriction caused by splinting as a result of pain. Treatment of pleurisy and pleural effusions is directed toward the underlying cause. Large or unresolved pleural effusions often require thoracentesis or chest tube drainage.

Pneumothorax is a condition in which air enters the pleural space. This air leak may be due to a perforation of the lung itself or of the chest wall (e.g., chest trauma). Small pneumothoraces may not cause any symptoms. Large pneumothoraces result in severe dyspnea and chest pain. Physical examination of the patient reveals decreased chest movement on the affected side. Breath sounds are usually absent. A chest x-ray study shows a shift of the mediastinum away from the pneumothorax. Small pneumothoraces usually resolve without treatment as gas is reabsorbed from the pleural space. Large air leaks usually require a chest tube with appropriate drainage to allow lung reexpansion.

Pulmonary function tests are usually contraindicated in the presence of pneumothorax. However, undiagnosed pneumothorax may present a risk if pulmonary function studies are performed. Maneuvers that generate high intrathoracic pressures (i.e., FVC or MVV_x) can aggravate an untreated pneumothorax. The potential for development of a **tension pneumothorax** exists when these maneuvers are performed. In a tension pneumothorax, air enters the pleural space but cannot escape. Increasing pressure compresses the opposite lung, as well as the heart and great vessels. Compression of the mediastinum interferes with venous return to the heart and can cause a rapid drop in blood pressure. A tension pneumothorax can be fatal if not treated immediately. Patients referred for pulmonary function studies who have known or suspected pneumothoraces should be tested very carefully. In many instances the information obtained may not justify the risk to the patient.

NEUROMUSCULAR DISORDERS

Diseases that affect the spinal cord, peripheral nerves, neuromuscular junctions, and the respiratory muscles can all cause a restrictive pattern of pulmonary function. Most of these disorders result in an inability to generate normal respiratory pressures. The VC and TLC are usually reduced. Some chronic neuromuscular disorders are associated with decreased lung compliance. Blood gas abnormalities, particularly hypoxemia, may result if the degree of involvement is severe. Stiff lungs and rapid respiratory rates often result in respiratory alkalosis (**hyperventilation**). Progressive muscle weakness results in **hypoventilation** and respiratory failure.

Diaphragmatic paralysis may be bilateral or unilateral. Bilateral paralysis may be the end stage of various disorders. The most prominent finding is **orthopnea,** or shortness of breath in the supine position. In the upright position, the patient has a marked increase in VC and improvement in gas exchange. Simple spirometry in the supine and sitting positions can demonstrate the functional impairment. Unilateral paralysis usually results from damage to one of the phrenic nerves (e.g., trauma, surgery, or tumor). As with bilateral paralysis, there is a marked change in VC from supine to sitting position. Diagnosis of the affected side may require chest x-ray, examination or fluoroscopy. Reduced inspiratory pressures (see "Maximal Inspiratory Pressure," Chapter 2) may suggest diaphragmatic involvement.

Amyotrophic lateral sclerosis (**ALS**, or Lou Gehrig's disease) affects the anterior horn cells of the spinal cord. Progressive muscle weakness results in a gradual decrease in VC and TLC. Pulmonary function studies are done serially to assess the progression of the disease.

Guillain-Barré syndrome is a progressive disease involving the peripheral nerves. Lower extremity weakness ascends to the upper extremities and face. There may be marked respiratory muscle weakness along with weakness of the pharyngeal and laryngeal muscles. Serial measurements of the VC, MIP, and MEP are used to follow the disease progression.

Myasthenia gravis is an abnormality of neuromuscular transmission. It particularly affects muscles innervated by the bulbar nuclei (i.e., face, lips, throat, neck). The patient with myasthenia gravis has pronounced fatigability of the muscles. Speech and swallowing difficulties can occur with prolonged exercise of the associated muscles. Progression of a myasthenic crisis can be assessed using VC and respiratory pressures. Analysis of the flow-volume curve (see Chapter 2) may be helpful in detecting upper airway obstruction brought on by muscular weakness.

CONGESTIVE HEART FAILURE

CHF is often used synonymously with left **ventricular** failure. Failure of the left ventricle may be caused by systemic hypertension, coronary artery disease, or aortic insufficiency. CHF may also be associated with **cardiomyopathy,** congenital heart defects, and left-to-right shunts. In each case, fluid backs up in the lungs. The pulmonary venous system becomes engorged. Fluid may spill into the alveolar spaces (pulmonary edema) or the pleural space (effusion).

The patient who has CHF usually has shortness of breath on exertion, cough, and fatigue. If coronary artery disease is the cause of CHF there may be chest pain (**angina**) as well. Exertional dyspnea is related to pulmonary venous congestion. The fluid overload in the lungs reduces lung volume and makes the lungs stiff (decreased compliance). Dyspnea is usually worse when the patient is supine (i.e., orthopnea). This orthopnea results from increased pulmonary vascular congestion with increased venous return. Dyspnea brought on by CHF may be difficult to distinguish from other causes (e.g., chronic pulmonary disease). The chest x-ray film usually shows increased pulmonary congestion. The heart (left ventricle) may appear enlarged, particularly if systemic hypertension in the cause.

Treatment of CHF is directed at the underlying cause. The **myocardial** workload can be reduced to relieve systemic hypertension. This is usually accomplished by vasodilator therapy. Reducing fluid retention is also important in managing CHF. Diuretics such as furosemide (Lasix) are commonly used to reduce the **afterload** on the ventricle. Oxygen therapy may also help reduce myocardial workload, especially if there is hypoxemia. If the cause of CHF is an arrhythmia, **antiarrhythmic** agents are typically used. Inotropic agents such as dobutamine may be used to increase myocardial contractility, especially after an acute infarction. Pulmonary function tests, particularly lung volumes and DL_{CO}, may be used to monitor the effects of treatment.

LUNG TRANSPLANTATION

Lung transplantation has evolved as an effective treatment for end-stage lung disease. Lung transplantation has been used for patients with CF, primary pulmonary hypertension, and COPD (Table 1-9). Double-lung transplants are usually performed in patients who have CF, generalized bronchiectasis, or in some types of COPD. Heart-lung transplants have been used for

TABLE 1-9 Indications for Lung Transplantation

Transplant type	Disease state
Heart-lung	Eisenmenger's syndrome, severe cardiac defect
	Pulmonary hypertension, cor pulmonale
	End-stage lung disease, coexisting severe cardiac disease
Double-lung	Cystic fibrosis
	Generalized bronchiectasis
	COPD with severe chronic bronchitis or extensive bullae
Single-lung	Restrictive fibrotic lung disease
	Eisenmenger's syndrome (less severe cardiac anomalies)
	COPD
	Primary pulmonary hypertension

Modified from American Thoracic Society: Lung transplantation, *Am Rev Respir Dis* 147:772-776, 1993.

Eisenmenger's syndrome, pulmonary hypertension with cor pulmonale, and end-stage lung disease coexisting with severe heart disease. Single-lung transplantation has been used effectively in patients with COPD who are younger than approximately 60 years old. Single-lung transplantation offers the benefit that two recipients can share a single donor's organs. Survival rates for lung transplant recipients have steadily improved. Longer survival is mainly due to more potent antirejection drugs (e.g., **cyclosporine**) and better adjunctive therapy. Pulmonary function tests are used to both assess potential transplant candidates and follow them postoperatively.

Preoperative evaluation consists of documentation of the severity of the specific disease process. Spirometry, lung volumes, DL_{CO}, and blood gas analysis are all used to rank the level of dysfunction. The same tests are also used to detect sudden worsening of lung function that might necessitate rapid intervention. Cardiopulmonary exercise testing may be indicated to determine the extent of the physiologic abnormality. For example, a patient with borderline pulmonary hypertension at rest may develop severe hypertension during even mild exertion.

Most transplantation programs list patients as prospective candidates when their pulmonary disease has advanced beyond predefined limits. An extended wait for lung transplantation is a direct result of the shortage of donor organs. Patients are often referred for transplant evaluation when a major decline in their condition is observed. The term *transplant window* has been used to describe the time period during which the patient is sick enough to require transplantation, but healthy enough to have a reasonable chance of success.

Posttransplant follow-up relies heavily on pulmonary function tests. Spirometry has been used extensively to monitor improvements resulting from transplantation. Recipients of double-lung transplants often show lung function values approaching those of normal subjects within a few months. Blood gas changes usually occur immediately after surgery. Single-lung transplant (SLT) recipients show similar **gains.** However, because SLT patients retain a native lung, improvement in pulmonary function is usually less than when both lungs are replaced. Interpretation of spirometry, lung volumes, and blood gases in SLT patients is often complicated by the presence of the transplanted lung along with the native lung.

Besides monitoring improved lung function, pulmonary function tests are used to detect rejection and the development of bronchiolitis obliterans. Rejection may be difficult to distinguish from other pulmonary complications (e.g., pneumonia) in patients who are immunosuppressed. There is some evidence that spirometric changes (FVC, FEV_1, $FEF_{25\%-75\%}$) may signal episodes of acute rejection. Chronic rejection is thought to be associated with the development of bronchiolitis obliterans. This pattern is characterized by the development of severe airflow limitation in the transplanted lung. Spirometry, particularly indices of small airway function, may provide the earliest signs of bronchiolitis obliterans.

Preliminaries to Patient Testing

Several preliminary steps precede any pulmonary function study. These include patient preparation, physical measurements and assessment, brief pulmonary history, and instructions to the patient in the performance of specific test maneuvers. In addition, pulmonary function tests are usually done in an ordered sequence. The testing sequence may be determined by laboratory policy, or it may be adapted for specific needs by the technologist performing the procedure.

PATIENT PREPARATION

Patient preparation for pulmonary function studies consists mainly of instructions given to the subject in advance of the actual test session. These instructions focus on taking or withholding specific medications, refraining from smoking, and other guidelines related to specific tests (e.g., exercise tests, blood gases).

WITHHOLDING MEDICATIONS

Patients referred for evaluation of airflow limitation are often already taking bronchodilators or related drugs. If response to bronchodilator is to be assessed, bronchodilators should be withheld at least 4 to 6 hours before testing. The exact length of time to withhold a bronchodilator is dictated by the onset of action and duration of the drug. Guidelines for withholding specific bronchodilators are presented in detail in Chapter 2 ("Before- and After-Bronchodilator Studies"). It may be impossible for some patients to withhold their bronchodilators. The patient should be instructed to take their bronchodilator when breathing problems require it.

Care should be taken when instructing outpatients about withholding medications. Some patients may be unable to correctly identify all of their medications. Hence, it may be difficult for them to correctly withhold only bronchodilators. Some patients incorrectly withhold all medications. This may cause serious problems for patients who rely on insulin (diabetic patients), antiarrhythmics, or antihypertensives used for high blood pressure. If the patient is uncertain, it may be preferable to not withhold any medications.

SMOKING CESSATION

Patients referred for pulmonary function tests should be asked to refrain from smoking for 24 hours before the test. Smoking cessation is especially important if DL_{CO} tests or arterial blood gas tests are ordered. Smoking has been shown to reduce diffusing capacity. Smoking raises the level of CO in the blood, which also interferes with the measurement of diffusing capacity. Increased CO in the blood (COHb) makes it difficult to interpret O_2 saturation measured by pulse oximetry (see Chapter 6).

OTHER PATIENT PREPARATION ISSUES

Patients referred for pulmonary function tests should probably be advised not to eat a large meal immediately before their appointment. The same is true if the patient will be exercising as part of the evaluation. If the patient is scheduled for a bronchial challenge test (see Chapter 8), special instructions concerning medications to withhold are required. In addition, patients receiving bronchial challenge should not drink beverages that contain caffeine or theobromines (cola drinks) or eat chocolate.

Some patients may require special accommodations for pulmonary function tests to be performed safely and accurately. Patients, or those referring patients, should understand the requirements of the tests requested. Patients who are unable to sit or stand may require additional time or equipment for testing to be completed. Patients who have permanent tracheostomies may also require special devices to allow connection to standard pulmonary function circuits. Patients who do not speak the primary language used in the laboratory may require an interpreter to be present during testing. Each of these special needs can be identified by asking appropriate questions before the patient's appointment.

PHYSICAL MEASUREMENTS

Various physical measurements are required for estimating each patient's expected level of pulmonary function. Age, height, and weight are usually recorded in addition to the patient's sex. Race or ethnic origin should also be recorded. Basic physical assessment of the patient's respiratory status may be needed before and during testing.

The patient's age should be recorded as of the last birthday. Some computerized pulmonary function systems store the patient's birth date and calculate the age. This approach is helpful, especially when the patient returns periodically for follow-up testing. Care should be used when entering this type of data into a computerized system. Data entry errors can result in gross overestimation or underestimation of the subject's expected values.

TABLE 1-10	Physical Assessment During Pulmonary Function Testing

A. Breathing pattern
    1. Is there good chest expansion? Is it symmetric?
    2. Is the breathing rate excessive?
    3. Are there any complaints of chest tightness or chest discomfort?
    4. Are accessory muscles being used for breathing?
    5. Is the patient using pursed lips?
B. Breath sounds (with and without auscultation)
    1. Are there audible breath sounds? Are breath sounds distant or absent?
    2. Is there any wheezing? Over which lung fields?
    3. Is there stridor, especially on inspiration?
    4. Are there any other unusual breath sounds (e.g., crackles, rubs)?
C. Respiratory symptoms
    1. Is there any cyanosis?
    2. Is there obvious shortness of breath (mild, moderate, severe)?
    3. Is the patient coughing? If so, is the cough productive?
    4. Is the patient receiving supplemental oxygen? If so, how much?
    5. What is the patient's oxygen saturation (pulse oximetry reading)?

Standing height, in either inches or centimeters, should be recorded with the patient barefoot or in stocking feet. A wall-mounted ruler allows the patient to stand with the back against the wall and the head close to the ruler. If the patient is unable to stand upright, the arm-span method should be used. Patients who have a history of kyphosis, scoliosis, or related problems should also have height estimated using their **arm span.** Arm span may be measured using a ruler or tape measure at least 4 ft long. The patient should extend the arms horizontally on either side, and the distance from the tip of the middle finger to the center of the vertebrum at the level of the scapula is measured. The measurement is repeated for the opposite side, and the two values obtained are added together. This length may be used in all calculations that require standing height.

The patient's weight in pounds or kilograms should be measured with an accurate scale. Because obesity is related to restrictive lung disease, a measurement of weight is needed to interpret reduced lung volumes. Body weight is used to calculate some reference values. When weight is used to predict an expected value, the patient's ideal body weight should be used. Using actual weight in patients who are obese may lead to elevated expected values. Weight is also used to express oxygen consumption (i.e., ml/kg) for exercise and metabolic measurements. The patient's weight may also be required when lung volumes are determined with the body plethysmograph. Weight is used to estimate body volume in the plethysmograph (see Chapter 3).

PHYSICAL ASSESSMENT

Physical assessment of patients referred for pulmonary function studies may be needed to determine whether the individual can perform the test. Documentation concerning physical assessment of the patient can also assist with interpretation of test results. Physical assessment should focus on breathing pattern, breath sounds (if necessary), and respiratory symptoms (Table 1-10). These can be observed simply and noted as necessary. Commentary regarding the patient's signs or symptoms at the time of the test is a useful adjunct, especially when test performance is less than optimal.

PULMONARY HISTORY

Accurate interpretation of pulmonary function studies—from simple screening spirometry to complete cardiopulmonary evaluation—requires clinical information related to possible pulmonary disorders. An ordered array of questions that can be easily answered by the subject provides the most useful history. The interpreter of pulmonary function studies may have little clinical information other than that obtained at the time of testing. A pulmonary history should be taken routinely before pulmonary function testing and should include the following:

1. Age, sex, standing height, weight, race

2. Current diagnosis or reason for test

3. Family history: Did anyone in your immediate family (mother, father, brother, or sister) ever have the following:
   Tuberculosis
   Emphysema
   Chronic bronchitis
   Asthma
   Hay fever or allergies
   Cancer
   Other lung disorders

4. Personal history: Have you ever had, or been told that you had the following:
   Tuberculosis
   Emphysema
   Chronic bronchitis
   Asthma
   Recurrent lung infections
   Pneumonia or pleurisy
   Allergies or hay fever
   Chest injury (if so, what? _____)
   Chest surgery (if so, what? _____)

5. Occupation: Have you ever worked in the following situations:
   In a mine, quarry, or foundry
   Near gases or fumes (if so, what kind?)
   In a dusty place (if so, what kind?)
   What is or was your occupation? (_____)
   How many years? (_____)

6. Smoking habits: Have you ever smoked the following:
   Cigarettes (_____/day)
   Cigars (_____/day)
   Pipe (_____/day)
   How long? (_____ years)
   Do you still smoke?   Y   N
   Do you live with a smoker?   Y   N

7. Cough: Do you ever cough:
   In the morning   Y   N
   At night   Y   N
   Blood   (when_____)
   Phlegm   (when _____)
       (color _____)
       (volume _____)

8. Dyspnea: Do you get short of breath at the following times:
   At rest   Y   N
   On exertion   (when _____)
   At night   Y   N

9. Subject disposition at time of test
   Dyspneic   Y   N
   Wheezing   Y   N
   Coughing   Y   N
   Cyanotic   Y   N
   Apprehensive   Y   N
   Cooperative   Y   N

10. Current medications (for heart, lung, or blood pressure)
   _____ (Last taken:)
   _____ (Last taken:)

Most of these questions can be answered by "Yes," or "No," or by circling an appropriate response. Space may be provided for comments either by the patient or history taker. Patients who cannot read may be embarrassed when asked to complete a questionnaire. It may be preferable to ask the questions verbally. In instances in which the physician performs the test, such history may be redundant if a medical history is available.

Interpretation of pulmonary function tests is best made if the clinical question asked of the test is considered. The clinician requesting the test should indicate the reason for the test. Examples of clinical questions asked of pulmonary function studies include "Does the patient have airway obstruction?" or "Does the patient have hyperreactive airways?" The pulmonary history, including the reason for the test, should be used to decide what is normal or abnormal. Clinical information as provided by the history is especially important when the patient's pulmonary function tests are borderline. For example, an FEV_1 that is 80% of the expected value would be interpreted differently in a healthy young subject tested as part of a routine physical than it would be in a smoker who complained of increasing dyspnea.

Test Performance and Sequence

Pulmonary function laboratories should have written policies and procedures defining how each test is performed (see Chapter 10). Indications for performing a specific test should be related to the clinical question to be answered or to the patient's diagnosis. Testing protocols that can be modified for individual patients are usually the most cost-effective means of obtaining the required data. When the required tests are determined, the exact sequence of tests can be selected. The sequence in which to perform tests may vary according to patient need and the test method used.

TECHNOLOGIST-ADAPTED PROTOCOLS

As described previously, the basis for deciding appropriate pulmonary function testing is the patient's clinical question. The clinical question is often inappropriately stated as a diagnosis. In fact, many patients are referred for pulmonary function studies to establish a diagnosis. For example, a patient may be referred with a diagnosis listed as "asthma." The clinical question is "Does the patient have asthma?" Pulmonary function studies may be able to answer this question, but the exact tests to be performed may not be defined. In this example, spirometry is indicated. Using an adaptive protocol, the technologist performs spirometry, and based on those results, selects appropriate additional tests (Fig. 1-2). Bronchial challenge tests may be performed if spirometry results are normal. Alternatively, additional tests such as lung volumes or DL_{CO} may be necessary.

The correct sequence for performing tests is important. Many laboratories use a fixed order for component pulmonary function tests. This may include spirometry, followed by lung volumes and DL_{CO}. In some instances the order of tests may need to be altered. The methodology used for some tests has definite effects on the results of subsequent procedures. For example, the multiple-breath N_2 washout test to determine FRC gives the patient 100% O_2 for several minutes. If this test is performed immediately before a DL_{CO} test, the elevated O_2 level in the lungs (as well as in the blood and tissues) may reduce the measured DL_{CO}. Similarly, if the N_2 washout or He dilution methods of FRC determination are repeated, sufficient time should be allowed to wash out residual test gas.

PATIENT INSTRUCTION

Many pulmonary function tests are effort dependent. For valid data to be obtained, patients must be instructed and coached for each maneuver. Instruction and coaching are particularly important for the FVC maneuver. Instruction should include a description of what the patient is expected to do, such as "You will take a deep breath in, and then blow out as hard and as fast as possible." In addition to a description of the test, the maneuver should be demonstrated. This can be accomplished by using a mouthpiece and simulating the maneuver expected of the patient. During the actual test, vocal encouragement should be given so that the patient continues for an appropriate interval. Any problems that occur with the first few efforts should be explained before having the patient attempt the test again. For example, "That was a very good effort, but you stopped before blowing out for 6 seconds. Let's try that again, and keep blowing out until I signal you to relax." This type of feedback is important for patients who may be uncertain of what is expected of them. Patients should be instructed that some maneuvers will be repeated so that their best effort can be obtained. They should be assured that repeating some tests is required and does not reflect a problem on their part.

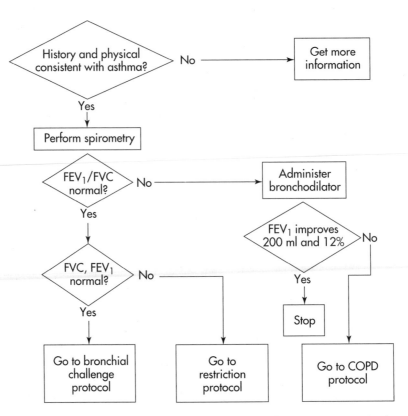

FIG. 1-2 *A protocol-decision diagram, as might be used by a pulmonary function technologist to select appropriate testing.* In this example, a patient with possible asthma is referred for evaluation. The diagram shows routes to appropriate tests based on the results of simple spirometry. It should be noted that if the patient history and physical assessment suggest diagnoses other than hyperreactive airways, more information may be needed.

Patients should also be carefully instructed for tests that require quiet breathing, such as lung volume determinations. Instructions about maintaining a good seal on the mouthpiece and continuing normal breathing can help reduce leaks or interrupted tests. Some maneuvers are very complicated and may be difficult to describe to the patient. The $D_{L_{CO}}$ maneuver and panting in the body plethysmograph each consist of several steps. For these tests, a combination of demonstration and practice may be the most efficient means of instructing the patient.

Even after adequate instruction and demonstration, some patients may be unable to perform certain tests. This may be caused by lack of coordination related to illness or inability to follow even basic instructions. For example, a patient may experience uncontrollable coughing when asked to inspire deeply for an FVC maneuver. If the coughing prevents obtaining valid spirometry results, the fact should be noted in the technologist's comments (see Chapter 10). Suboptimal effort by the patient can usually be detected by poorly reproducible results on effort-dependent tests (e.g., the FVC). Care should be taken that adequate instructions are given and a sufficient number of efforts recorded before deciding that the patient did not give a maximal effort. If the patient cannot continue or refuses to continue a test, the exact reason should be documented in the technologist's comments.

SUMMARY

THIS CHAPTER SERVES AS AN INTRODUCTION to pulmonary function testing. Categories of common pulmonary function tests are listed. This listing should acquaint the reader with the names of various tests, as well as their relationships to one another. Tests are grouped under spirometry, lung volumes, $D_{L_{CO}}$, blood gases and related tests, exercise tests, and metabolic measurements. Within each of these groups are a wide variety of tests and techniques.

Indications for tests are also listed. Many indications overlap. For example, an indication for spirometry may also be an indication for lung volumes, blood gases, or exercise testing. Indications are extremely important because they help the practitioner select appropriate tests. For patients, the clinical question asked of the test must be related to a valid indication for the test.

This chapter also outlines patterns of impaired pulmonary function commonly encountered in the laboratory. This discussion assumes a basic knowledge of respiratory anatomy and physiology. The material presented aims to summarize the underlying pathology involved in common pulmonary diseases. The role of pulmonary function testing is discussed as it relates to diagnosis and assessment of these disease processes.

Patient preparation for pulmonary function studies is covered in a general sense. More detailed information for specific tests is presented in subsequent chapters. Many of the physical measurements and assessments, as well as the pulmonary history, are similar regardless of the tests being performed. Technologist-adapted protocols are described. **Algorithms** for selecting only appropriate tests are becoming increasingly popular. Such tools improve the sensitivity of the tests to answer the clinical question, as well as make tests more cost-effective.

SELF-ASSESSMENT QUESTIONS

1 *Spirometry for the evaluation of pulmonary function was popularized by whom?*
   a. August and Marie Krogh
   b. Alvan Barach
   c. John Severinghaus
   d. John Hutchinson

2 *Which of the following are indications for performing spirometry?*
   I.   Assess the risk of lung resection
   II. Determine the response to bronchodilator therapy
   III. Evaluate the progress of parenchymal lung disease
   IV. Quantify the extent of COPD
   a. I and IV only
   b. II and III only
   c. I, II, and IV
   d. II, III, and IV

3 *The main indication for the measurement of lung volumes is to do which of the following?*
   a. Diagnose or assess the severity of restriction
   b. Evaluate the severity of pulmonary hypertension
   c. Determine the level of cardiopulmonary fitness
   d. Assess the risk of abdominal surgical procedures

4 *DL_{CO} measurements may be indicated to evaluate pulmonary involvement in which of the following systemic diseases?*
   a. Asthma
   b. Sarcoidosis
   c. Exertional hypoxemia
   d. Guillain-Barré

5 *Blood gas analysis is indicated in patients with COPD to do which of the following?*
   a. Monitor airway responsiveness
   b. Determine level of cardiopulmonary fitness
   c. Detect pulmonary hypertension
   d. Assess need for supplementary O_2

6 *Which of the following cause emphysema?*
   I. α_1-Antitrypsin deficiency
   II. Exposure to environmental pollutants
   III. Radiation therapy
   IV. Cigarette smoking
   a. I and II only
   b. III and IV only
   c. I, II, and IV
   d. II, III, and IV

7 *An adult patient complains of chest tightness and cough whenever he jogs in cold weather. These symptoms are consistent with which of the following?*
   a. Cystic fibrosis
   b. Asthma
   c. Pulmonary hypertension
   d. Idiopathic pulmonary fibrosis

8 *Which of the following statements are true concerning tumors in the upper airway?*
   a. There may be variable or fixed obstruction
   b. Fixed obstruction will be present
   c. Variable obstruction will be present
   d. Small airway obstruction will result

9 *Sarcoidosis is a systemic disorder that usually causes which of the following?*
   a. A restrictive ventilatory defect
   b. An obstructive ventilatory defect
   c. Hyperreactive airways
   d. Primary pulmonary hypertension

10 *In which of the following conditions might pulmonary function testing be contraindicated?*
   a. Vocal cord dysfunction
   b. Untreated pneumothorax
   c. Congestive heart failure (CHF)
   d. Bronchiolitis obliterans

11 **Which of the following correctly describe appropriate physical measurements before pulmonary function testing?**

I. Actual body weight should be used to calculate predicted values

II. Standing height should be measured with the patient barefooted

III. Patient with kyphosis should have arm span used instead of height

IV. Age should be recorded to the nearest decade (10 years)

a. I only
b. II and III only
c. I, II, and IV
d. I, II, III, and IV

12 **In addition to explaining the procedure for each pulmonary function test to the patient, the pulmonary function technologist should do which of the following?**

a. Briefly explain the physiologic basis of the test
b. Demonstrate the correct performance of the test maneuver
c. Limit feedback to the patient to reduce the placebo effect
d. Explain the exact number of efforts that will be required for each test

SELECTED BIBLIOGRAPHY

General References

Crapo RO: Pulmonary function testing, *N Engl J Med* 331:25-30, 1994.

Hess D: History of pulmonary function testing, *Respir Care* 34:427-445, 1989.

Spriggs EA: The history of spirometry, *Br J Dis Chest* 72:165-180, 1978.

Indications for Pulmonary Function Testing

American Thoracic Society: Standardization of spirometry: 1994 update, *Am J Respir Crit Care Med* 152:1107-1136, 1995.

American Thoracic Society: Standards for the diagnosis and care of patients with chronic obstructive pulmonary disease, *Am J Respir Crit Care Med* 152:S77-S120, 1995.

American Thoracic Society: Single-breath carbon monoxide diffusing capacity (transfer factor); recommendations for a standard technique—1995 update, *Am J Respir Crit Care Med* 152:2185-2198, 1995.

American Association for Respiratory Care: Clinical practice guidelines: spirometry, *Respir Care* 36:1414-1417, 1991.

American Association for Respiratory Care: Clinical practice guidelines: body plethysmography, *Respir Care* 39:1184-1190, 1994.

American Association for Respiratory Care: Clinical practice guidelines: static lung volumes, *Respir Care* 39:830-836, 1993.

American Association for Respiratory Care: Clinical practice guidelines: assessing response to bronchodilator therapy at the point of care, *Respir Care* 40:1300-1307, 1995.

British Thoracic Society and the Association of Respiratory Technicians and Physiologists: Guidelines for the measurement of respiratory function, *Respir Med* 88:165-194, 1994.

Raffin TA: Indications for arterial blood gas analysis, *Ann Intern Med* 105:390-398, 1986.

Ries AL: Measurement of lung volumes, *Clin Chest Med* 10:177-185, 1989.

Wasserman K, Hansen JE, Sue DY, et al: *Principles of exercise testing and interpretation*, ed 2, Philadelphia, 1994, Lea & Febiger.

Zibrak JD, O'Donnell CR, Marton K: Indications for pulmonary function testing, *Ann Intern Med* 112:763-771, 1990.

Patterns of Impaired Pulmonary Function

American Thoracic Society: Lung transplantation; report of the ATS workshop on lung transplantation, *Am Rev Respir Dis* 147:772-776, 1993.

Bergofsky EH: Respiratory failure in disorders of the thoracic cage, *Am Rev Respir Dis* 119:643-669, 1979.

Burrows B: Airways obstructive diseases: pathogenetic mechanisms and natural histories of the disorders, *Med Clin North Am* 74:547-559, 1990.

Kelly BJ, Luce JM: The diagnosis and management of neuromuscular diseases causing respiratory failure, *Chest* 99:1485-1491, 1991.

Mitchell RS, Petty TL, Schwartz MI: *Synopsis of clinical pulmonary disease,* St Louis, 1989, Mosby.

Murphy DMF, Hall DR, Peterson MR, et al: The effect of diffuse pulmonary fibrosis on lung mechanics, *Bull Eur Physiopathol Respir* 17:27-41, 1981.

National Asthma Education Program: *Expert panel report: guidelines for the diagnosis and management of asthma,* Bethesda, Md, 1991, Department of Health and Human Services (NIH Publication No. 91-3042A).

Nathan SD, Ross DJ, Belman MJ, et al: Bronchiolitis obliterans in single-lung transplant recipients, *Chest* 107:967-972, 1995.

Newman KB, Mason UG, Schmaling KB: Clinical features of vocal cord dysfunction, *Am J Respir Crit Care Med* 152:1382-1386, 1995.

Putnam MT, Wise RA: Myasthenia gravis and upper airway obstruction, *Chest* 109:400-404, 1996.

Snider GL: Emphysema: the first two centuries and beyond, *Am Rev Respir Dis* 146:1615-1623, 1992.

Preliminaries to Patient Testing

American Thoracic Society: Standards for the diagnosis and care of patients with chronic obstructive pulmonary disease, *Am J Respir Crit Care Med* 152:S77-S120, 1995.

Social Security Administration: *A guide to pulmonary function studies under the social security disability program,* US Department of Health and Human Services, SSA Pub. No. 64-055, 1994.

CHAPTER 2

Spirometry and Related Tests

OBJECTIVES

After studying this chapter and reviewing the case studies, you should be able to do the following:

1 Identify airway obstruction using the forced vital capacity and forced expiratory volume (FEV_1)

2 Differentiate between obstruction and restriction as causes of reduced vital capacity

3 Distinguish between large and small airway obstruction by evaluating flow-volume curves

4 Determine whether there is a significant response to bronchodilators

5 Recognize abnormal values for airway resistance and compliance

6 Determine whether spirometry is acceptable and reproducible

THIS CHAPTER BEGINS WITH SIMPLE spirometry testing–measurement of the vital capacity (VC). Then the most widely used pulmonary function tests, those based on the forced vital capacity (FVC) maneuver, are described. Special emphasis is placed on the performance of each test. Criteria for judging the acceptability of test data are provided. Flow-volume curves are described as a special way of presenting spirometric data. Other tests described include peak expiratory flow (PEF), maximal voluntary ventilation (MVV), maximal inspiratory pressure (MIP), minimal expiratory pressure (MEP), airway resistance (Raw), and lung compliance (CL). Bronchodilator studies to determine reversibility of airway obstruction are also presented. For each of these areas, interpretive strategies are suggested using questions that test interpreters might ask. Case studies and self-assessment questions are included at the end of the chapter.

Vital Capacity

DESCRIPTION

VC is the volume of gas measured from a slow, complete expiration after a **maximal inspiration**, without forced or rapid effort (Fig. 2-1). VC is normally recorded in either liters (L) or milliliters (ml), and reported at body temperature, pressure and saturation (BTPS). VC is sometimes referred to as the slow vital capacity, distinguishing it from FVC. Inspiratory capacity (IC) and expiratory reserve volume (ERV) are subdivisions of the VC. IC is the largest volume of gas that can be inspired from the resting expiratory level (see Fig. 2-1). IC is sometimes further divided into the tidal volume (VT) and inspiratory reserve volume (IRV). ERV is the largest volume of gas that can be expired from the resting end-expiratory level (see Fig. 2-1). Both the IC and ERV are recorded in liters or milliliters, corrected to BTPS.

TECHNIQUE

VC is measured by having the subject inspire maximally and then exhale completely into a spirometer. (See Chapter 9 for a complete discussion of spirometers.) The subject is instructed to perform the maneuver slowly and completely. VC can also be measured from **maximal expiration** to maximal inspiration. The spirometer does not need to produce a graphic display if only VC is

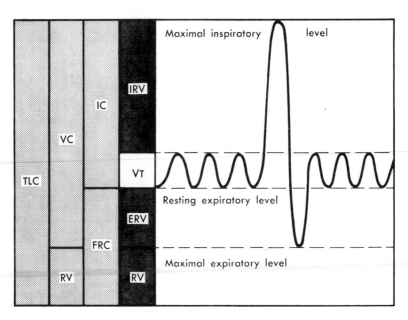

FIG. 2-1 *Lung volumes and capacities.* Diagrammatic representation of various lung compartments based on a typical spirogram. *TLC,* Total lung capacity; *VC,* vital capacity; *RV,* residual volume; *FRC,* functional residual capacity; *IC,* inspiratory capacity; *VT,* tidal volume; *IRV,* inspiratory reserve volume; *ERV,* expiratory reserve volume. *Shaded areas* indicate relationships between the subdivisions and relative sizes as compared with the TLC. The resting expiratory level should be noted because it remains more stable than other identifiable points during repeated measurements, and therefore is used as a starting point for FRC determinations. (Modified from Comroe JH Jr, Forster RE, Dubois AB, et al: *The lung: clinical physiology and pulmonary function tests,* ed 2, St Louis, 1962, Mosby.)

BOX 2-1
CRITERIA FOR ACCEPTABILITY—VITAL CAPACITY

1 End-expiratory volume varies by less than 100 ml for three preceding breaths.

2 Volume plateau observed at maximal inspiration and expiration.

3 Two acceptable VC maneuvers should be obtained; volumes within 200 ml.

4 VC should be within 200 ml of FVC value.

---

to be measured. If subdivisions of VC are to be determined (see Fig. 2-1), some means of recording volume change is required. The graphic display may be a computer screen or a recording device (see Chapter 9). The display allows the technologist to determine that the test is performed correctly (Box 2-1).

Obtaining a valid slow VC is important. The subdivisions of the VC (IC and ERV) are used in the calculation of residual volume (RV) and total lung capacity (TLC). An excessively large VT (i.e., greater than 1.0 L) or an irregular breathing pattern during the VC maneuver may reduce ERV or IC. When either ERV or IC is erroneously reduced, other lung volumes may be incorrectly estimated (see Chapter 3).

IC is measured by having the subject breathe normally for several breaths and then inhale maximally. The volume inspired from the resting expiratory level is measured by the computer or from a spirogram. This is usually done as part of a slow VC maneuver. IC may also be calculated by subtracting the ERV from the VC.

ERV is measured by having the subject breathe normally for several breaths and then exhale maximally. The change in volume from the end-expiratory level to the maximal expiratory level is the ERV. ERV may also be calculated by subtracting the IC from the VC. The **accuracy** of the IC and ERV measurements depends on the stability of the end-expiratory level. Three or more tidal breaths should be recorded before the VC maneuver is performed. The end-expiratory volume should vary by less than 100 ml. If the end-expiratory volume is not consistent, the

ERV may be measured incorrectly (i.e., too large or too small). Even if the end-expiratory level is constant, the V_T usually increases when the subject breathes through a mouthpiece with nose clip in place. This increase in V_T may change the IC or ERV, depending on the subject's breathing pattern. Erroneous estimates of ERV may affect the calculation of RV, as described in Chapter 3.

SIGNIFICANCE AND PATHOPHYSIOLOGY

Normal values for lung function parameters are obtained by studying healthy subjects. The predicted or reference value for a measure such as VC is computed using the following equation:

$$VC = XH - YA - Z$$

where:

$$H = \text{height (cm or inches)}$$
$$A = \text{age (years)}$$
$$X, Y, Z = \text{constants}$$

Predicted values may be read from special tables called nomograms. They may also be calculated by entering the prediction equation into a computer. Normal values for men, women, and children may be found in Appendix B.

VC may vary as much as 20% above or below the predicted normal value in healthy individuals. VC also varies in individuals depending on their body position or the time of day. In adults, VC varies directly with height and inversely with age; tall subjects have larger VCs than short subjects. VC increases up to approximately age 20 and then decreases each year thereafter. It is usually smaller in women than in men because of the difference in body size. Recent evidence indicates that lung volumes may differ significantly according to ethnic origin. Interpretation of lung function should consider the factors of age, height, sex, and national origin. (See "Using Predicted Values" in Appendix B.)

Decreased VC is often caused by loss of distensible lung tissue, as in lung cancer, pulmonary edema, pneumonias, atelectasis, pulmonary vascular congestion, or surgical removal of lung tissue. Other causes of decreased VC include tissue loss, space-occupying lesions, or changes in the lung tissue itself. Tissue loss may result from surgical removal, as in a **lobectomy.** In lung resection the decrease in VC is roughly proportional to the tissue removed. A good example of a space-occupying lesion is a tumor, which directly displaces lung tissue. Fibrotic diseases such as silicosis often change the elastic properties of lung tissue, which usually results in loss of lung volume.

VC may also be reduced in obstructive lung disease (e.g., emphysema). This occurs even when other lung compartments show increased volumes (see "Residual Volume" in Chapter 3). As trapped gas volume increases, VC may become smaller. However, some subjects have well-preserved VC even with increased air trapping.

Some decreases in VC are not caused by lung lesions. VC is often decreased from respiratory center depression or neuromuscular diseases. A low VC may also result from reduction of available thoracic space caused by pleural effusion, pneumothorax, hiatus hernia, or enlargement of the heart. Limited movement of the diaphragm may result from pregnancy, abdominal fluids, or tumors, causing decreased VC. Limitation of chest wall movement from scleroderma, kyphoscoliosis, or pain can also reduce the VC.

When the VC is reduced, additional pulmonary function measurements may be indicated. Forced expiratory maneuvers (see "Forced Vital Capacity," p. 30) can reveal whether the reduced VC is caused by obstruction. Reduced VC without slowing of expiratory flow is a nonspecific finding. Measurement of other lung volumes (see Chapter 3) may be indicated to determine whether a restrictive defect is present.

In adults, VC less than 80% of predicted or less than the 95% confidence limit (see Appendix B) may be considered abnormal. Interpretation of the measured VC in relation to the reference value should consider the clinical question to be answered (Box 2-2). The clinical question is often revealed in the history and physical findings of the subject (see Chapter 1). The terms *mild, moderate,* and *severe* may be used to qualify the extent of reduction of the VC. Although these terms are relative, they should be based on a statistical comparison (i.e., confidence intervals) of the measured VC versus the predicted VC.

Artificially low estimates of the VC may result from poor subject effort. Similarly, inadequate

---

BOX 2-2
INTERPRETIVE STRATEGIES—VITAL CAPACITY

1 Was the test performed acceptably? Is it reproducible?

2 Are reference values correct? Age? Sex? Height? Race?

3 Is VC less than predicted? If so, to what extent? Is it less than the lower limit of normal?

4 How does VC relate to the clinical question to be answered? Is VC correlated to the history and physical findings?

5 Are additional tests indicated? Lung volumes? FVC?

---

patient instruction may affect performance of the test maneuver. These errors may be eliminated by applying appropriate criteria (see Box 2-1). Values for at least three maneuvers should produce acceptable results (see Chapter 10).

IC and ERV are approximately 75% and 25% of the VC, respectively. Changes in IC or ERV usually parallel increases or decreases in the VC. Increased V_T caused by exertion or acid-base disorders may reduce IRV or ERV. This occurs because end-inspiratory and end-expiratory levels (see Fig. 2-1) are altered. A similar pattern is commonly seen when subjects breathe into a spirometer through a mouthpiece with **nose clips** in place. Changes in IC or ERV are of minimal diagnostic significance when considered alone. Reduction of either IC or ERV is consistent with restrictive defects.

Forced Vital Capacity, Forced Expiratory Volume, and Forced Expiratory Flow 25%-75%

DESCRIPTION

FVC is the maximum volume of gas that can be expired when the subject exhales as forcefully and rapidly as possible after a maximal inspiration. This procedure is often referred to as the FVC maneuver. A similar maneuver, beginning at maximal expiration and inspiring as forcefully as possible, is called forced inspiratory vital capacity (FIVC). The FVC and FIVC maneuvers are often performed in sequence to provide a continuous flow-volume loop.

The forced expiratory volume (FEV_T) is the volume of gas expired over a given time interval (T) from the beginning of an FVC maneuver. The time interval is stated as a subscript to FEV. Those intervals in common use are $FEV_{0.5}$, FEV_1, FEV_2, and FEV_3. The FEV_1 measurement is the most widely used. The FVC and FEV_T are both reported in liters corrected to BTPS. $FEV_{T\%}$ is the ratio of FEV_T to FVC expressed as a percentage, where T is the interval from the start of the FVC. The $FEV_{1\%}$(FEV_1/FVC) is by far the most widely used of the various $FEV_{T\%}$ parameters. VC may be used in place of FVC if the VC is significantly larger.

The $FEF_{25\%-75\%}$ is the average flow during the middle 50% of an FVC maneuver. It is usually recorded in liters per second. This test was formerly designated the maximum midexpiratory flow rate (MMFR). Other measures of average flow include the $FEF_{200-1200}$ (the 200 to 1200 ml portion of the FVC), and the $FEF_{75\%-85\%}$. Flows at specific points in the FVC are usually expressed as FEF_X, where the subscript X describes the volume expired. Commonly reported flows are the $FEF_{25\%}$, $FEF_{50\%}$, and $FEF_{75\%}$.

TECHNIQUE

FVC is measured by having the subject, after inspiring maximally, expire as forcefully and rapidly as possible into a spirometer (see Chapter 9). The subject should inspire completely. The inhalation should be rapid but not forced. There should be only a brief pause at maximal inspiration; a prolonged pause (4 to 6 seconds) may decrease flow during the subsequent expiration.

The volume expired may be read directly from a volume-time recording (Fig. 2-2). This method is used by some small portable spirometers. More commonly, the maneuver is displayed on a computer screen. The computer analyzes the signal from the spirometer, then calculates and displays the FVC. A spirometer that produces a printed tracing (either volume-time or flow-

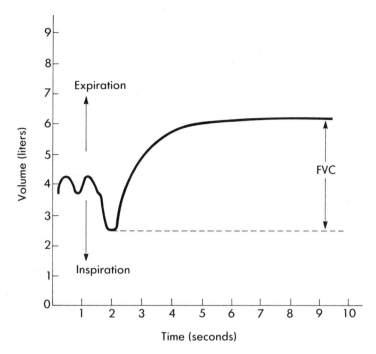

FIG. 2-2 *Forced vital capacity (FVC).* Typical spirogram plotting volume against time as the subject exhales forcefully. In this tracing, expiration causes an upward deflection; in some systems the tracing is inverted. The subject inspires to the maximal inspiratory level *(dashed line)* at which point lung volume is close to TLC. The subject then expires as forcefully and rapidly as possible to the maximal expiratory level, at which point the lungs contain only the RV (see text).

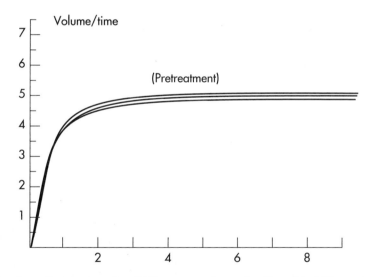

FIG. 2-3 *A volume-time tracing of an FVC maneuver from a healthy subject.* The tracing is computer generated with only the forced expiratory portion of the maneuver displayed. Three FVC efforts are superimposed showing acceptable reproducibility of the maneuvers (see text).

volume) is essential for clinical laboratory purposes to allow visual inspection of the maneuver (Fig. 2-3). Devices providing only numerical data may be helpful for simple screening. Whether used for diagnosis or monitoring, all spirometers should meet the criteria proposed by the American Thoracic Society (see Chapter 10). The FVC maneuver depends on subject effort. Not all subjects may be able to perform it acceptably (Box 2-3).

FEV_1 (and other FEV_T values) may be measured by timing the FVC maneuver over the described intervals. Historically this was done by recording the FVC spirogram on graph paper

---

BOX 2-3
CRITERIA FOR ACCEPTABILITY—FVC MANEUVER

1   Maximal effort; no cough or glottic closure during the first second; no leaks or obstruction of the mouthpiece

2   Good start-of-test; back-extrapolated volume less than 5% of FVC or 150 ml

3   Tracing shows 6 seconds of exhalation or an obvious plateau; no early termination or cut off; or subject cannot or should not continue to exhale

4   Three acceptable spirograms obtained; two largest FVC values within 200 ml; two largest FEV_1 values within 200 ml

---

American Thoracic Society—1994.

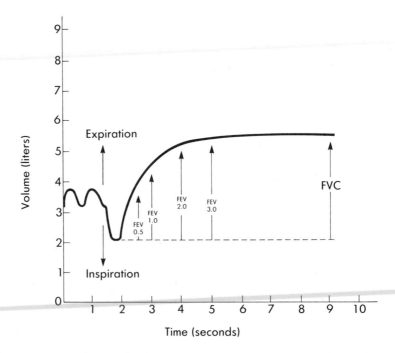

FIG. 2-4 *Determination of FEV_t values from an FVC maneuver.* Various FEV_t values can be measured from the volume-time display of an FVC effort. *Arrows* indicate the FEV at intervals of 0.5, 1, 2, and 3 seconds. The FEV_1 is the most commonly used index of airflow. Precise timing and acceptable start-of-test are required to determine the FEV values accurately (see Box 2-3).

moving at a fixed speed. The FEV for any interval could then be read from the graph as shown in Fig. 2-4. Most modern spirometers time the FVC maneuver by using a computer. The computer then calculates and displays the FEV_1 or other FEV intervals. Accurate measurement of FEV_1 depends on determination of the *start-of-test* (FVC). Computerized spirometers detect the start-of-test as a change in flow or volume above a certain threshold. The computer then stores volume and flow data points in memory and calculates the FEV_1. The spirometer should provide a volume-time display of each maneuver (Fig. 2-5). A graphic representation allows monitoring of patient effort at the beginning of the test.

Some spirometers record both inspiratory and expiratory flows, whereas others record expiratory flow only. If only the expiratory spirogram is presented, assessing the start-of-test may be difficult. Inaccurate FEV values may result if the subject begins the FVC maneuver slowly. Most computerized spirometers correct for a slow start-of-test by *back-extrapolation* (Fig. 2-6). Visualization of the volume-time spirogram is the best means of identifying poor initial effort. Some portable spirometers report the FEV_1 without a spirogram. Such measurements should be used with caution because it may be difficult to determine whether the maneuver was performed acceptably.

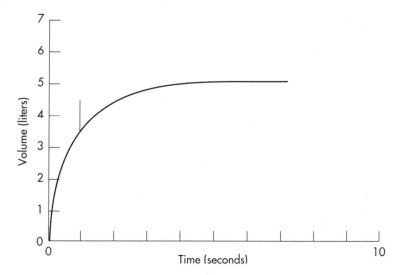

FIG. 2-5 *A volume-time tracing from a healthy subject.* The graph is computer generated and illustrates the FVC maneuver. The computer superimposes a tic mark on the curve to assist in identification of the *FEV₁*.

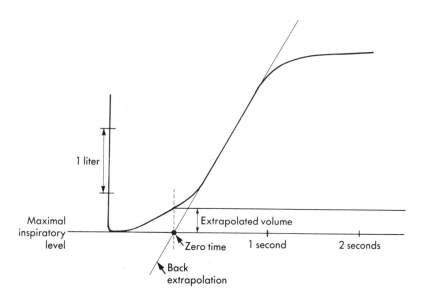

FIG. 2-6 *Back-extrapolation of a volume-time spirogram.* Back-extrapolation is a means of correcting measurements made from a spirogram that does not show a sharp deflection from the maximal inspiratory level. This occurs when a subject does not begin the forced exhalation rapidly enough. A straight line drawn through the steepest part of a volume-time tracing is extended to cross the volume baseline (maximum inspiration). The point of intersection is the back-extrapolated time zero. Timed volumes, such as FEV_1, are measured from this point rather than from the initial deflection from the baseline or from the point of maximal flow. The perpendicular distance from maximal inspiration to the volume-time tracing at time zero defines the back-extrapolated volume. To accurately determine FEV_1, the back-extrapolated volume should be less than 5% of the FVC or less than 150 ml, whichever is greater. FVC efforts with larger extrapolated volumes may be considered unacceptable. These measurements are commonly performed by computer.

The ratio of the FEV_1 to FVC is expressed as follows:

$$FEV_{1\%} = \frac{FEV_1}{FVC} \times 100$$

$FEV_{1\%}$ is also commonly written as FEV_1/FVC. Both ratios are expressed as percentages. FEV_1 and FVC should be the maximal values obtained from at least three acceptable FVC maneuvers. The FEV_1/FVC ratio based on these values may be different than the ratio obtained from any single maneuver. If both VC and FVC maneuvers have been performed, it is preferable to use the largest VC in the calculation. Many computerized spirometers calculate only the ratio obtained from FVC maneuvers.

The $FEF_{25\%-75\%}$ is measured from an FVC maneuver. The time required for the subject to expire the middle 50% of the FVC is divided into 50% of the FVC. To calculate the $FEF_{25\%-75\%}$ manually, a volume-time spirogram is used. The points at which 25% and 75% of the vital capacity have been expired are marked on the curve (Fig. 2-7). A straight line connecting these points can be extended to intersect two timelines 1 second apart. The flow (in liters per second) can then be read directly as the vertical distance between the points of intersection. A computerized measurement of the $FEF_{25\%-75\%}$ requires storage of flow and volume data points for the entire maneuver. Calculation of the average flow over the middle portion of the exhalation is simply 50% of the volume expired divided by the time required to get from the 25% point to the 75% point.

The $FEF_{25\%-75\%}$ depends on the FVC. Large $FEF_{25\%-75\%}$ values may be derived from maneuvers that produce small FVC measurements because the "middle half" of the volume is actually gas expired at the beginning of expiration. This effect may be particularly evident if the subject terminates the FVC maneuver before expiring completely. When the $FEF_{25\%-75\%}$ is used for assessing the response to bronchodilator or bronchial challenge, the effect of changes in the absolute lung volumes should be considered. Measuring the $FEF_{25\%-75\%}$ at the same lung volumes in the comparison tests is called the isovolume technique. Isovolume corrections are usually applied when the FVC changes by more than 10% (indicating a change in TLC or RV). This technique requires that lung volumes (see Chapter 3) be measured in conjunction with flows. The isovolume technique may also be used with other flow measurements that are FVC dependent.

The largest $FEF_{25\%-75\%}$ is not necessarily the value reported. The $FEF_{25\%-75\%}$ is recorded from the maneuver with the largest sum of FVC and FEV_1. Flows must be corrected to BTPS.

Criteria used to judge the acceptability of test results from the FVC maneuver include the following:

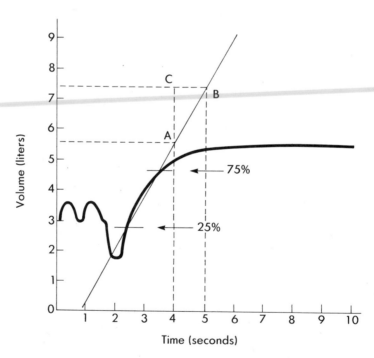

FIG. 2-7 $FEF_{25\%-75\%}$. Short horizontal lines on an FVC spirogram show the points at which 25% and 75% of the FVC have been expired; these points may be determined by multiplying the FVC by 0.25 and 0.75, respectively. A line connecting these points is extended to intersect two timelines 1 second apart, points A and B. The flow rate in liters per second can be read as the vertical distance between the points of intersection (AC)—in this case approximately 2 L/sec. Alternatively, the slope of the line connecting the 25% and 75% points can be determined by dividing half the FVC by the actual time interval between the points. These measurements are usually obtained by computer.

1. The volume-time tracing should show maximal effort with a smooth curve. There should be no coughing or hesitation during the first second. The tracing should show at least 6 seconds of forced effort. An obvious plateau with no volume change (30 ml or less) for at least 1 second should be achieved. Children, adolescents, and some restricted patients may plateau in less than 6 seconds. Subjects with severe obstruction may continue exhalation well past 15 seconds, therefore 6 seconds is simply a minimum. In severe obstruction, very low flows may be observed at the end of expiration. Continuation of the maneuver in these patients will not appreciably change the test results. The FVC maneuver may be stopped if the subject cannot continue for clinical reasons such as excessive coughing or dizziness. Multiple prolonged (longer than 6 seconds) exhalations are seldom necessary.

2. The start-of-test should be abrupt and unhesitating. Each maneuver should have the back-extrapolated volume calculated. FEV_1 and all other flows must be measured after back-extrapolation (see Fig. 2-6). If the volume of back-extrapolation is greater than 5% of the FVC or 150 ml (whichever is greater), the maneuver is unacceptable and should be repeated. The subject should be shown the correct technique for performing the maneuver. Demonstration by the technologist is often helpful.

3. A minimum of three acceptable efforts should be obtained. The test may be repeated any number of times. If reproducible values cannot be obtained after eight attempts, testing may be discontinued. The only criteria for eliminating a test completely is failure to obtain two acceptable maneuvers after at least eight attempts.

4. The two largest FVC and FEV_1 values should be within 200 ml. The second largest value is simply subtracted from the largest value for both FVC and FEV_1. Some clinicians prefer to use 5% as the reproducibility criteria. This may be more appropriate than an absolute volume of 200 ml, particularly in children or those with large FVC values. If the two largest FVC or FEV_1 values are not within 200 ml (or 5%, if that criterion is applied), the maneuver should be repeated. The reproducibility criteria should be applied only after the maneuver has been judged acceptable. Individual spirometric maneuvers should not be rejected solely because they are not reproducible. Bronchospasm or fatigue often affects reproducibility. Interpretation of the test should include comments regarding reproducibility or lack of it.

Data from all acceptable maneuvers should be examined. The largest FVC and the largest FEV_1 should be reported, even if the two values are from different test maneuvers. Flows that depend on the FVC (e.g., the $FEF_{25\%-75\%}$) should be taken from the single best test maneuver. The best test is that maneuver with the largest sum of FVC and FEV_1 (Table 2-1).

A common problem may occur when using these criteria to produce a spirometry report. If a single volume-time or flow-volume tracing is included in the final report, it may not contain the FVC or FEV_1 that appears in the tabular data. It is advisable to maintain recordings, or raw data, for all acceptable maneuvers. Other methods of selecting the best test have been suggested and are sometimes used. PEF may be used to assess subject effort for an FVC maneuver. Selecting the effort with the largest PEF may cause errors if FVC and FEV_1 are not also evaluated.

TABLE 2-1   Comparison of Spirometry Efforts

Test	Trial 1	Trial 2	Trial 3	Best test
FVC (L)	5.20	5.30	5.35*	5.35
FEV_1 (L)	4.41*	4.35	4.36*	4.41
FEV_1/FVC (%)	85	82	82	82
$FEF_{25\%-75\%}$ (L/sec)	3.87	3.92	3.94	3.94
$FEF_{50\%}$ (L/sec)	3.99	3.95	3.41	3.41
$FEF_{25\%}$ (L/sec)	1.97	1.95	1.89	1.89
PEF (L/sec)	8.39	9.44	9.89	9.89

*These values are keys to selecting the best test results. The FEV_1 is taken from trial 1, even though the largest sum of FVC and FEV_1 occurs in trial 3. All FVC-dependent flows (average and instantaneous flows) come from trial 3. It should be noted that the $FEV_{1\%}$ (FEV_1/FVC) is calculated from the FEV_1 of trial 1 and the FVC of trial 3. The maximal expiratory flow-volume curve, if reported, would be the curve from trial 3 as well.

Spirometry may be performed in either the sitting or standing position for adults and children. There is some evidence that FEV may be larger in the standing position in adults and in children younger than 12 years of age. The position used for testing should be indicated on the final report. The use of nose clips is recommended for spirometric measurements that require rebreathing, even if just for a few breaths. Spirometers that record only expiratory flow may require the subject to place the mouthpiece into the mouth after maximal inspiration. If such is the case, nose clips are usually unnecessary. Care should be taken, however, that the subject places the mouthpiece into the mouth before beginning a forced expiration. Failure to do so may result in an undetectable loss of volume. It may be impossible to calculate the volume of back-extrapolation from a tracing that displays only expiratory flow. In either a rebreathing or expiratory flow only spirometer, all mechanical recorders should have pen or paper moving at recording speed when the forced expiration begins. Systems that start pen or paper movement at the same time as exhalation may be unable to accurately record the start-of-test. Such spirometers usually underestimate the FEV_1.

SIGNIFICANCE AND PATHOPHYSIOLOGY

Forced Vital Capacity

See Box 2-4 for interpretive strategies. FVC equals VC in healthy individuals. In subjects without obstruction, FVC and VC should be within 200 ml of each other. FVC and VC may differ if the subject's effort is variable or severe airway obstruction is present. FVC is often lower than VC in subjects with obstructive diseases if forced expiration causes bronchiolar collapse. This pattern is seen in emphysema because of loss of support for the small airways (i.e., airways less than 2 mm in diameter). Large pressure gradients across the walls of the airways during forced expiration collapse the terminal portions of the airways. Gas is trapped in the alveoli and cannot be expired. This causes the FVC to appear smaller than the VC. The FVC can appear larger than the VC if the subject exerts greater effort on the forced maneuver.

FVC can be reduced by mucous plugging and bronchiolar narrowing, as is common in chronic bronchitis, chronic or acute asthma, bronchiectasis, and cystic fibrosis. Reduced FVC is also present in subjects whose trachea or mainstem bronchi are obstructed. Tumors or diseases affecting the patency of the large airways produce this result.

Not all airway-obstructed patients have reduced FVC in relation to their **predicted values.** However, the time required to expire their FVC (forced expiratory time [FET]) is usually prolonged. Healthy subjects can expire their FVC within 4 to 6 seconds. Subjects with severe obstruction (e.g., those with emphysema) may require 20 seconds or more to exhale completely (Fig. 2-8). Accurate measurement of FVC in such individuals may be limited by how long the spirometer can collect exhaled volume. Some spirometers allow only 10 seconds of volume recording. This is usually long enough to diagnose airway obstruction. However, the FVC and $FEV_{1\%}$ may be inaccurate if the subject continues to exhale for a longer time. The American Thoracic Society recommends that spirometers measure FVC for at least 15 seconds (see Chapter 10).

Decreased FVC is also a common feature of restrictive diseases (Fig. 2-9). An FVC less than predicted may result from increased scar tissue as in pulmonary fibrosis. Fibrotic changes often result from inhalation of dust or other toxins that directly damage lung tissue. Fibrosis may also result from the toxic effects of drugs or radiation used in treating lung cancer. Congestion of pulmonary blood vessels, as in pneumonia, pulmonary hypertension, or pulmonary edema, can reduce FVC. Space-occupying lesions (e.g., tumors or pleural effusions) reduce FVC by compressing surrounding lung tissue. Neuromuscular disorders, (e.g., myasthenia gravis) or chest deformities (e.g., scoliosis) limit chest wall movement. Any disease that affects the bellows action of the chest or distensibility of lung tissue itself tends to reduce FVC. Obesity and pregnancy are common causes of reduced FVC because they interfere with movement of the diaphragm and excursion of the chest wall.

Reduced FVC (or VC) is a nonspecific finding. Values lower than 80% of predicted or less than the 95% confidence limit are considered abnormal. (See "Using Normal Values" in Appendix B.) Low FVC may be caused by either obstruction or restriction. Interpretation of the FVC in obstructive diseases requires correlation with flows. Significant differences between the FVC and VC suggests airway collapse. VC may be used to calculate $FEV_{1\%}$ if it is larger than FVC. In restrictive patterns, low FVC may indicate the need to assess other lung volumes, particularly total lung capacity (see Chapter 3). Interpretation of FVC values close to the lower limit of normal depends on the clinical question to be answered. An FVC of 80% of predicted would be interpreted differently in a healthy subject with no symptoms than in a subject with a history of cough or wheezing. An FVC much lower than expected is often accompanied by the complaint of exertional dyspnea.

Forced Expiratory Volume (FEV$_1$)

FEV$_1$ measures the volume expired over a fixed interval, the first second of an FVC maneuver. Although it is considered a measure of flow, FEV$_1$ is reported as a volume. For this reason, it may be reduced in either obstructive or restrictive patterns (see Figs. 2-8 and 2-9). FEV$_1$ values may also be reduced because of poor effort or cooperation by the subject.

An obstructive ventilatory defect is characterized by reduction of maximal airflow at all lung volumes. Flow is limited by airway narrowing during forced expiration. Airway obstruction may be caused by mucus secretion, bronchospasm, and inflammation such as in asthma or bronchitis. Airflow limitation may also result from loss of elastic support for the airways themselves, as in

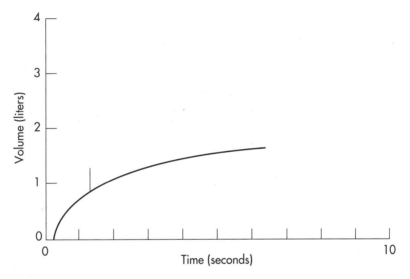

FIG. 2-8 *Computer-generated tracing from a subject with severe airway obstruction.* A tic mark notes the point at which the subject exhaled the *FEV$_1$*. A significant volume is exhaled after the first second, and the tracing does not show an obvious plateau.

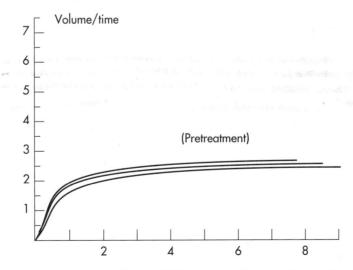

FIG. 2-9 *Computer-generated plot of three FVC maneuvers from a subject with moderately severe restriction.* All three maneuvers show relatively normal flows—most of the FVC is expired in the first second. However, the FVC is much lower than the expected value of 3.5 L for this patient.

emphysema. The earliest changes in obstructive patterns occur in the small airways (i.e., those less than 2 mm). Abnormal flows in small airways may be detected even before FEV_1 decreases. These changes in flows, however, are variable and not specific for small airway disease.

FEV_1, like FVC, may also be decreased in large airway obstruction (trachea and bronchi). Tumors or foreign bodies that limit airflow cause the FEV_1 to be reduced. These defects are easily identified by flow reductions across the entire forced expiration (see "Flow-Volume Curves," p. 40).

FEV_1 and FEV_1/FVC are the most standardized indices of obstructive disease. Reduction of FEV_1 in the presence of a reduced FEV_1/FVC ratio defines an obstructive impairment. The severity of obstructive disease may be gauged by the extent to which FEV_1 is reduced. The ability to work and function in daily life is related to the FEV_1 and FVC. **Morbidity** (likelihood of dying) caused by respiratory disease is similarly related to the degree of obstruction as measured by FEV_1. Subjects with markedly reduced FEV_1 values are much more likely to die from chronic obstructive pulmonary disease (COPD) or lung cancer. Although FEV_1 correlates with prognosis and severity of symptoms in obstructive lung disease, outcomes for individual patients cannot be accurately predicted.

Restrictive processes such as fibrosis, edema, space-occupying lesions, neuromuscular disorders, obesity, and chest wall deformities may all cause FEV_1 to be decreased. Reduction in FEV_1 occurs in much the same way as the reduction in FVC. Unlike the pattern seen in obstructive disease in which FVC is preserved and FEV_1 reduced, in restriction FVC and FEV_1 values are proportionately decreased. Some subjects with moderate or severe restriction have an FEV_1 nearly equal to the FVC. The entire FVC, because it is reduced, is exhaled in the first second. To distinguish between obstructive and restrictive causes of reduced FEV_1 values, the FEV_1/FVC ratio ($FEV_{1\%}$) and other flow measurements are useful. Further definition of obstruction versus restriction may require measurement of lung volumes (e.g., FRC, TLC).

FEV_1 is the most widely used spirometric parameter, particularly for assessment of airway obstruction. FEV_1 is used in conjunction with FVC for simple screening, assessment of response to bronchodilators, inhalation challenge studies, and detection of exercise-induced bronchospasm (see Chapters 7 and 8).

Forced Expiratory Volume ($FEV_{T\%}$)

Commonly reported $FEV_{T\%}$ ratios for healthy young adults are as follows:

$$FEV_{0.5\%} = 50\%\text{-}60\%$$
$$FEV_{1\%} = 75\%\text{-}85\%$$
$$FEV_{2\%} = 90\%\text{-}95\%$$
$$FEV_{3\%} = 95\%\text{-}100\%$$

These ratios may be derived by dividing predicted FEV_t by predicted FVC. Some studies of normal subjects derive equations for the ratio itself. The FEV_1/FVC ratio decreases with increasing age, presumably because of changes in the elastic properties of the lung. Older healthy adults may have FEV_1/FVC ratios in the 65% to 70% range.

Patients with unobstructed airflow can exhale their entire FVC within 4 seconds. Conversely, subjects with obstructive disease have reduced $FEV_{T\%}$ for each interval (i.e., 1 second, 2 seconds, etc.). The FEV_1/FVC ratio is the most important measurement for distinguishing an obstructive impairment. A decreased FEV_1/FVC ratio is the hallmark of obstructive disease. Because the FEV_1/FVC is a ratio, mild or moderate obstructive disease can be identified without reference to absolute predicted values. In young adults, if the ratio is less than 70%, some degree of obstruction is present. In older subjects the normal ratio is slightly lower (see Appendix B for predicted values). The $FEV_{1\%}$ may be as low as 30% in severe obstructive disease.

Diagnosis of an obstructive pattern based on spirometry should focus on three primary variables: FVC, FEV_1, and FEV_1/FVC. Measurements such as $FEF_{25\%\text{-}75\%}$ should be considered only after the presence and severity of obstruction has been determined using the primary variables. If the FEV_1/FVC is borderline abnormal, additional flow measurements may confirm the presence of an obstructive pattern. Care should be taken when interpreting the FEV_1/FVC ratio in subjects who have FVC and FEV_1 values greater than predicted. The FEV_1/FVC ratio may appear to indicate an obstructive pattern because of the variability of the greater than normal FVC and FEV_1 values.

Subjects who have restrictive disease, (e.g., pulmonary fibrosis) often have normal or increased $FEV_{T\%}$ values. Because airflow may be minimally affected in restrictive diseases, FEV_1 and FVC are usually reduced in equal proportion. If the restriction is severe, FEV_1 may approach the FVC value. As a result, $FEV_{1\%}$ appears to be higher than normal. The FEV_1/FVC ratio may be 100% if the FVC is severely reduced. The presence of restrictive disorder may be suggested by a reduced FVC and a normal or increased FEV_1/FVC ratio. Further studies (e.g., measurement of TLC) should be used to confirm the diagnosis of restriction.

Forced Expiratory Flow 25%-75%

$FEF_{25\%-75\%}$ is based on a segment of the FVC that includes flow from medium and small airways. Typical values for healthy young adults average 4 to 5 L/sec. These values decrease with age. $FEF_{25\%-75\%}$ is variable even in normal subjects, with one standard deviation (**SD**) equal to approximately 1 L/sec. Values as low as 65% of those predicted may be statistically within normal limits. This variability requires guarded interpretation of the $FEF_{25\%-75\%}$.

The $FEF_{25\%-75\%}$ is indicative of the status of the medium to small airways. Decreased flows are common in the early stages of obstructive disease. Abnormalities in these measurements, however, are not specific for small airways disease. Although $FEF_{25\%-75\%}$ may suggest changes in the small airways, it should not be used to diagnose small airways disease in individual patients. In the presence of a borderline value for FEV_1/FVC, a low $FEF_{25\%-75\%}$ may help confirm airway obstruction. When FEV_1 and FEV_1/FVC are within normal limits, $FEF_{25\%-75\%}$ should not be graded as to severity. Assessment of $FEF_{25\%-75\%}$ after bronchodilator must consider changes in FVC as well. If FVC increases markedly, $FEF_{25\%-75\%}$ may actually decrease. Isovolume correction (as described previously) can be used to compare $FEF_{25\%-75\%}$ before and after bronchodilator therapy. The inherent variability of $FEF_{25\%-75\%}$ and its dependence on FVC make it less useful than the FEV_1 for assessing bronchodilator response.

Reduced $FEF_{25\%-75\%}$ values are sometimes seen in cases of moderate or severe restrictive patterns. This is assumed to be caused by a decrease in the cross-sectional area of the small airways. $FEF_{25\%-75\%}$ depends somewhat on subject effort because it depends on the FVC exhaled. Subjects who perform the FVC maneuver inadequately often show widely varying midexpiratory flow rates.

Validity of FVC maneuvers depends largely on subject effort and cooperation. Equally important is the instruction and coaching supplied by the technologist. Many subjects need several attempts before performing the maneuver acceptably. Demonstration of proper technique by the technologist helps the subject give maximal effort. Placement of the mouthpiece between the teeth and lips, maximal inspiration, a slight pause, and maximal expiration should all be demonstrated. Emphasis should be placed on the initial burst of air and on continuing expiration for at least 6 seconds. Acceptability of each FVC maneuver should be evaluated according to specific criteria (see Box 2-3). The final report should include comments on the quality of the data obtained (see Chapter 10). These comments may be provided by the technologist, physician, or both.

BOX 2-4
INTERPRETIVE STRATEGIES—FVC MANEUVER

1. Were at least three acceptable spirograms obtained? Are FVC and FEV_1 reproducible (within 200 ml)?
2. Are reference values appropriate? Age? Sex? Height? Race?
3. Is $FEV_{1\%}$ less than predicted? If so, obstruction is present.
   a. Is FVC also reduced? If so, is it caused by obstruction or restriction?
   b. If FVC is less than 80%, lung volumes may be indicated.
   c. Is the obstruction reversible? Bronchodilators may be indicated.
4. Is $FEV_{1\%}$ equal to or greater than expected?
   a. Are FVC and FEV_1 both reduced proportionately? If so, restriction may be present; lung volumes may be indicated.
   b. Are FVC and FEV_1 within normal limits? If so, spirometry is likely normal.
5. Is $FEF_{25\%-75\%}$ less than 65% of predicted? Is $FEV_{1\%}$ or FEV_1 borderline normal? If so, airway obstruction may be present.
6. Are the spirometric findings consistent with the patient history and physical findings? Is bronchial challenge indicated to reveal obstruction?

Validity of the FEV_1 also depends on cooperation and effort. Adequate instruction and demonstration of the FEV maneuver by the technologist is essential. This is true of all the FEV_T parameters commonly recorded because each of these includes the effort-dependent early portion of a forced exhalation. Reproducibility of FEV_1 should be within 200 ml for the two best of at least three acceptable maneuvers. Accurate measurement of FEV_1 requires an acceptable spirometer (see Chapter 10), preferably one that allows inspection of the volume-time curve and back-extrapolation.

Validity of the $FEV_{1\%}$ also depends on subject effort and cooperation. Because the values used to derive the ratio may be taken from separate maneuvers, both FEV_1 and FVC should be reproducible. Poor effort on an FVC test may result in an overestimate of $FEV_{T\%}$. If the subject stops prematurely, the FVC (i.e., denominator of the ratio) will appear smaller than it actually is. The $FEV_{1\%}$ will then appear larger than it actually is. Some clinicians prefer to use the VC to calculate the $FEV_{1\%}$. This may be useful if the VC is significantly larger than FVC because of airway compression.

Patients who have moderate or severe obstruction may require longer than 10 seconds to completely exhale. Although continuing to exhale increases measured FVC, the diagnosis of obstruction can be made with less than complete expiration. In some cases, prolonged effort may be difficult for the subject. The large transpulmonary pressure generated by a forced expiratory maneuver often reduces cardiac output. Subjects may complain of dizziness, seeing "spots," ringing in their ears, or numbness of the extremities. A subject may occasionally faint as a result of the decreased cerebral blood flow. This complication may be serious if it causes the subject to fall, from either a standing or sitting position.

Flow-Volume Curves

DESCRIPTION

The flow-volume curve graphs flow generated during an FVC maneuver against volume change. The FVC may be followed by an FIVC maneuver, plotted similarly. Flow is usually recorded in liters per second and the volume in liters, BTPS. The maximal expiratory flow-volume (MEFV) curve shows flow as the subject exhales from maximal inspiration (TLC) to maximal expiration (RV). The MIFV displays inspiratory flow plotted from RV to TLC. When MEFV and MIFV curves are plotted together, the resulting figure is called a flow-volume (F-V) loop (Fig. 2-10).

TECHNIQUE

The subject performs an FVC maneuver, inspiring fully and then exhaling as rapidly as possible. To complete the loop, the subject inspires as rapidly as possible from the maximal expiratory level back to maximal inspiration. Volume is plotted on the horizontal X axis, and flow is plotted on the vertical Y axis. The F-V loop is usually displayed on a computer screen. It can also be printed or plotted. Expiratory flow is plotted upward. Expired volume is usually plotted from left to right. Air flow should be recorded at 2 L/sec per unit distance on the flow axis. Volume should be recorded at 1 L per unit distance on the volume axis. Scale factors should be at least 5 mm/L/sec for flow and 10 mm/L for volume. These factors are required so that manual measurements can be made from a printed copy of the maneuver.

FVC, as well as PEF and peak inspiratory flow (PIF), can be read directly from the F-V loop. Instantaneous flow at any lung volume can be measured directly from the F-V loop. Maximal flow at 75%, 50%, and 25% of the FVC are commonly reported as the $\dot{V}max_{75}$, $\dot{V}max_{50}$, and $\dot{V}max_{25}$. The subscript in these terms refers to the portion of the FVC remaining. The same flows are also reported as the $FEF_{25\%}$, $FEF_{50\%}$, and $FEF_{75\%}$ with the subscripts referring to the percentage of FVC already exhaled. Most computerized spirometers superimpose timing marks ("tics") on the MEFV curve (see Fig. 2-10). These marks allow FEV_1 (or other FEV_T) values to be read from the F-V loop.

Because flow-volume data are stored by computer, F-V loops can be easily manipulated. Several loops can be compared by superimposing them with contrasting colors. Computer-generated graphs permit bronchodilator or inhalation challenge studies to be presented in a similar manner. A predicted MEFV curve can be plotted using points for PEF and maximal flows at 75%, 50%, and 25% of the FVC. A subject's flow-volume curve can then be superimposed directly over the expected values (Fig. 2-11). Superimposing multiple FVC maneuvers as F-V loops can be used to assess reproducibility of the subject's effort (see Fig. 2-11). Positioning loops side-by-side or superimposing can also help detect decreasing flows with repeated efforts. This pattern may be seen

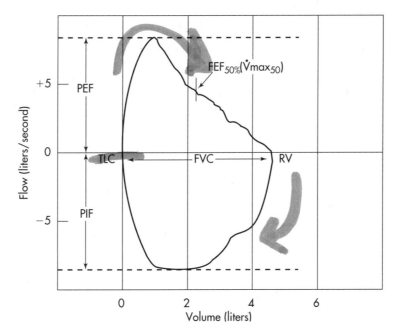

FIG. 2-10 *Flow-volume loop.* A flow-volume recording in which an FVC and an FIVC maneuver are recorded in succession. Flow in liters per second is plotted on the *vertical axis* and volume, in liters, on the *horizontal axis*. The FVC can be read from the tracing as the maximal horizontal deflection along the zero flow line. Peak flows for expiration and inspiration (PEF and PIF) can be read directly from the tracing as the maximal deflections on the flow axis (positive and negative). The instantaneous flow (FEF) at any point in the FVC can also be measured directly. Phenomena, such as small or large airway obstruction, show up as characteristic changes in the maximal flow rates (see Fig. 2-12).

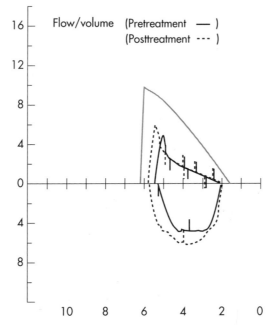

FIG. 2-11 *Computer-generated flow-volume loops.* Flow-volume curves from a subject with combined obstruction and restriction. Multiple F-V loops (in this case before and after bronchodilator therapy) are superimposed by the computer at RV. *Upward tics* on the expiratory limb represent $FEV_{0.5}$, FEV_1, and FEV_3, respectively. *Downward tics* on the expiratory curve represent the $FEF_{25\%}$, $FEF_{50\%}$, and $FEF_{75\%}$, respectively. *Upward tics* on the inspiratory loop represent the $FIF_{50\%}$. The *large gray expiratory curve* is the computer-generated plot of the patient's predicted MEFV. As can be seen from the curves, expiratory flow is decreased at all lung volumes. The subject's FVC (horizontal axis) is also lower than predicted.

because FVC maneuvers can induce bronchospasm. Storing tests in the order performed is recommended. This allows review of the test session and detection of bronchospasm or fatigue.

Reproducible MEFV curves, particularly the PEF, are good indicators of adequate subject effort (Box 2-5). Assessing the start-of-test and determining whether exhalation lasted at least 6 seconds may be difficult when using only the F-V loop. Simultaneous display of flow-volume and volume-time curves is useful (Fig. 2-13). Although computerized systems calculate back-extrapolated volume, a volume-time tracing may be necessary to perform back-extrapolation manually (see Fig. 2-6).

BOX 2-5
CRITERIA FOR ACCEPTABILITY—FLOW-VOLUME LOOP

1   Rapid rise from maximal inspiration to PEF

2   Maximal effort until flow returns to zero baseline; no glottic closure or abrupt end of flow

3   Maximal inspiratory effort with return of volume to point of maximal inspiration (Failure to close loop indicates that effort was not started from maximal inspiration, inspiratory effort was submaximal, or spirometer error.)

4   At least three acceptable loops recorded; superimposed or side-by-side loops should be reproducible, unless bronchospasm occurs

---

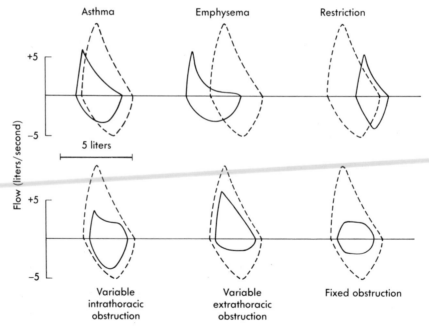

FIG. 2-12 *Normal and abnormal flow-volume loops.* Six curves are shown plotting flow in liters per second against the FVC. In each example, the expected curve is shown by the *dashed lines,* while the curve illustrating the particular disease pattern is superimposed. In patients who have asthma and emphysema, the portion of the expiratory curve from the peak flow to residual volume (RV) is characteristically concave. Both the TLC and RV points are displaced toward higher lung volumes (to the left of the expected curves in this diagram). These patterns are indicative of hyperinflation and/or air trapping. In restrictive patterns the shape of the loop is preserved but the FVC is decreased. The TLC and RV displaced toward lower lung volume (to the right of the expected curves). The bottom three examples depict types of large airway obstruction. Variable intrathoracic obstruction shows reduced flows on expiration despite near-normal flows on inspiration resulting from flow limitation in the large airways during a forced expiration. Variable extrathoracic obstruction shows an opposite pattern. Inspiratory flow is reduced while expiratory flow is relatively normal. Fixed large airway obstruction is characterized by equally reduced inspiratory and expiratory flows. Comparison of the $FEF_{50\%}$ with the $FIF_{50\%}$ may be helpful in differentiating large airway obstructive processes. Because the magnitude of inspiratory flow is effort dependent, low inspiratory flows should be carefully evaluated.

SIGNIFICANCE AND PATHOPHYSIOLOGY

See Box 2-6 for interpretive strategies. Maximal flow at any lung volume during forced expiration or forced inspiration can be easily measured from the F-V loop (Fig. 2-12). Significant decreases in flow or volume are easily detected from a single graphic display. Many clinicians prefer to include the F-V loop or MEFV curve as part of the patient's medical record.

The shape of an MEFV curve from approximately 75% of FVC to maximal expiration is largely independent of subject effort. Flow over this segment is determined by two properties of the lung: elastic recoil and flow resistance. The lung is stretched by maximal inspiration. Elastic recoil determines the pressure applied to gas in the lung during a forced expiration. This pressure is determined by the recoil of the lung and chest wall and, to a certain extent, by the expiratory muscles. Resistance to flow in the airways is the second factor affecting the shape of the flow-volume curve. Flow limitation occurs in the large and medium airways during the early part of a forced expiration. The site of flow limitation migrates "upstream" rapidly during forced expiration. Resistance to flow in small (less than 2 mm) airways is determined primarily by the cross-sectional area. This cross-sectional area can be affected by a number of factors. Destruction of alveolar walls, as in emphysema, reduces support of the small airways. Bronchoconstriction and inflammation directly reduce the lumen of the small airways.

In healthy subjects flow (Vmax) over the effort-independent segment decreases linearly as lung volume decreases. Pressures around airways are balanced by gas pressures in the airways so that flow is limited at an "equal pressure point." As the lung empties, the equal pressure point moves upstream into increasingly smaller airways and continues until small airways begin to close, trapping some gas in the alveoli (the RV). This pattern of airflow limitation in healthy lungs causes the MEFV curve to have a **linear** or slightly concave appearance (see Fig. 2-10).

Flow-Volume Loops in Small Airway Obstruction

Maximal flow is decreased in subjects who have obstruction in small airways, particularly at low lung volumes. The effort-independent segment of the MEFV curve appears more concave or "scooped out" (Fig. 2-13). Values for $Vmax_{50}$ and $Vmax_{25}$ are characteristically decreased. Decreases in $Vmax_{50}$ correlate well with the reduction in $FEF_{25\%-75\%}$ in subjects with small airway obstructive disease.

Because elastic recoil *and* resistance in small airways determine the shape of the MEFV tracing, different lung diseases can cause similar F-V patterns. Emphysema destroys alveoli with loss of elastic tissue and support for small airways. Flow through small airways decreases because of collapse of the unsupported walls. In contrast, bronchitis, asthma, and similar inflammatory processes increase resistance in the small airways. Increased resistance is caused by edema, mucus production, and smooth muscle constriction. Reduction in the cross-sectional area of the small airways reduces flow. Emphysema and chronic bronchitis are often found in the same individual because of their common cause—cigarette smoking. The MEFV curve presents a picture of the extent of obstruction without identifying its cause.

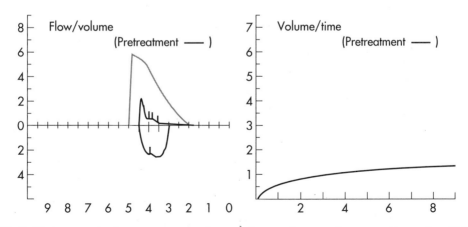

FIG. 2-13 *MEFV and volume-time tracings from a subject with severe obstruction.* The predicted MEFV curve (*gray line*) is superimposed on the patient's best effort (*black line*) for comparison.

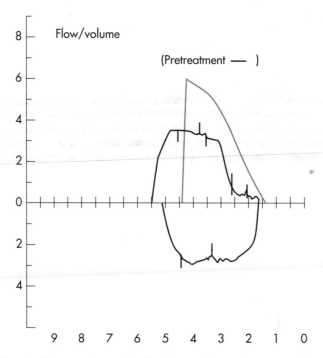

FIG. 2-14 *MEFV tracing from a patient with a fixed upper airway obstruction.* The predicted expiratory curve *(gray line)* is superimposed on the patient's best effort *(black line).* Both the expiratory and inspiratory limbs of the curve show flattening consistent with a fixed obstruction. Note that maximal flow on both limbs is about 3 L/sec, much less than expected in a healthy subject.

Flow-Volume Loops in Large Airway Obstruction

Obstruction of the upper airway, trachea, or mainstem bronchi also shows characteristic patterns. Both expiratory and inspiratory flow may be limited. The F-V loop is extremely useful in diagnosing these large airway abnormalities (Fig. 2-12). Comparison of expiratory and inspiratory flows at 50% of the FVC ($FEF_{50\%}$ and $FIF_{50\%}$, respectively) helps determine the site of obstruction. In healthy subjects the ratio of $FEF_{50\%}$ to $FIF_{50\%}$ is approximately 1.0 or slightly less. Fixed large airway obstruction causes equally reduced flows at 50% of the VC during inspiration and expiration (Fig. 2-14). Obstructive lesions that vary with the phase of breathing also produce characteristic patterns. Variable extrathoracic obstruction usually shows normal expiratory flows but diminished inspiratory flows. The $FEF_{50\%}/FIF_{50\%}$ is greater than 1.0. Because the obstructive process is outside of the thorax, the MEFV portion of the curve appears as it would in a healthy individual. The inspiratory portion of the loop is flattened. Inspiratory flow depends on how much obstruction is present. In variable intrathoracic obstruction, PEF is reduced. Expiratory flow remains constant until the site of flow limitation reaches the smaller airways. This gives the expiratory limb a "squared-off" appearance (see Fig. 2-12). The inspiratory portion of the loop may be completely normal. The $FEF_{50\%}/FIF_{50\%}$ will be much less than 1.0, depending on the severity of obstruction.

Airway obstruction associated with abnormality of the muscular control of the posterior pharynx and larynx sometimes produces a "saw-tooth" pattern visible on the inspiratory and expiratory limbs of the MEFV curve. This pattern is sometimes observed in subjects suspected of having sleep apnea.

Peak inspiratory flow and the pattern of flow during inspiration are largely effort dependent. Poor subject effort may result in inspiratory flow patterns similar to variable extrathoracic obstruction. Instruction by the technologist should emphasize maximal effort during inspiration as well as expiration. If repeated efforts produce reduced inspiratory flows, an obstructive process should be suspected.

Restrictive disease processes may show normal or greater than normal peak flows with linear decreases in flow versus volume. The lung volume displayed on the X axis is decreased. Moderate or severe restriction demonstrates equally reduced flows at all lung volumes. Reduced flows are primarily caused by the decreased cross-sectional area of the small airways at low lung

---

BOX 2-6
INTERPRETIVE STRATEGIES—FLOW-VOLUME LOOP

1 Were at least three acceptable F-V curves obtained? Does the beginning of the expiratory curve show a sharp rise to PEF? If not, suspect patient effort or large airway obstruction.

2 Are the PEF and PIF values consistent? Does PEF or other expiratory flows fall with repeated efforts? If so, suspect hyperreactive airways.

3 Does the expiratory curve from PEF to maximal exhalation appear concave? If so, suspect small airway obstruction.

4 Does either the expiratory or inspiratory portions of the curve show a "squared off" pattern? If so, suspect large airway obstruction. If both, suspect a fixed obstruction.

5 Is the inspiratory curve reproducible? If not, suspect variable effort or fatigue.

6 Does the F-V loop show any other unusual patterns (sudden changes in flow that are reproducible, or "saw-tooth" pattern)?

---

volumes. Simple restriction causes the F-V loop to appear as a miniature of the normal curve (see Fig. 2-12).

Before- and after-bronchodilator F-V loops can be superimposed to measure changes in flow at specific lung volumes. The curves are usually positioned by superimposing at maximal inspiration. This method assumes that any increase in FVC occurs while TLC remains constant. If postbronchodilator lung volume tests are performed, the curves may be superimposed on an absolute volume scale (i.e., isovolume correction). This method shows bronchodilator-induced changes in lung volumes as well as flows. Inhalation challenge studies (see Chapter 8) can be displayed similarly to assess the reduction in flows at specific lung volumes.

Tidal breathing curves or MVV curves can also be superimposed on the F-V loop. The subject's **ventilatory reserve** can be assessed by comparing the areas enclosed under each of the curves. Subjects who have obstructive lung disease may generate F-V loops only slightly larger than their tidal breathing curves. In severe obstruction, flow during tidal breathing may exceed flow during a forced expiration. This is because of dynamic compression of small airways during forced expiration. These patients have limited ventilatory reserve and shortness of breath with exertion.

Peak Expiratory Flow

DESCRIPTION

PEF is the maximum flow attained during an FVC maneuver. When reported in conjunction with other spirometric variables, PEF is expressed in liters per second, BTPS. When performed alone using a peak flow meter, PEF is usually reported in liters per minute, BTPS.

TECHNIQUE

PEF can be easily measured from a flow-volume curve (MEFV). PEF may also be measured by using devices that sense flow directly (see "Flow-Sensing Spirometers," Chapter 9), by using volume displacement spirometers and deriving the rate of volume change. Many portable devices (i.e., peak flow meters) are available to measure maximal flow during forced expiration. Most sense flow as movement of air against a turbine or through an orifice. PEF done in conjunction with spirometry is performed as described for F-V loops.

Measuring PEF with a peak flow meter may be done at the bedside, in the emergency department, in the clinic setting, or at home. In each setting the individual performing the measurement must know how to operate the specific peak flow meter. The maneuver should be demonstrated to the subject. A return demonstration is essential when the subject is being trained to use the peak flow meter at home.

The peak flow meter should be set or zeroed, as required. The subject should sit or (preferably) stand up straight. The subject should inhale maximally; the inhalation should be rapid but not forced. The subject then exhales with maximal effort as soon as the teeth and lips are placed around the mouthpiece. As in the FVC maneuver, a long pause (4 to 6 seconds) at maximal inspiration may decrease the PEF. The expiratory effort only needs to be 1 to 2 seconds to record PEF.

At least three maneuvers should be performed and recorded, along with the order in which the values were obtained. All readings are recorded in order to detect effort-induced bronchospasm. The largest PEF obtained should be reported. The PEF itself is effort dependent and variable. It may be particularly variable in subjects with hyperreactive airways (Box 2-7). There is no widely recognized criteria for reproducibility of PEF efforts.

When PEF is used to monitor asthmatic patients, it is important to establish each person's best PEF (i.e., the largest PEF achieved). Best values can be obtained over 2 to 3 weeks. PEF should be measured twice daily (morning and evening). The personal best is usually observed in the evening after a period of maximum therapy. Daily measurements are then compared with the personal best. The personal best PEF should be reevaluated annually. This allows PEF to be adjusted for growth in children or for progression of disease. PEF should be periodically compared with regular spirometry results (FEV_1).

Portable peak flow meters need to be precise (low variability in the same instrument). **Precision** is more important than accuracy for detecting changes from serial measurements. Peak flow meters should have ranges of 60 to 400 L/min for children and 100 to 850 L/min for adults. Standards for peak flow monitoring devices have been published by the American Thoracic Society (ATS) (see Chapters 9 and 10).

SIGNIFICANCE AND PATHOPHYSIOLOGY

See Box 2-8 for interpretive strategies. The PEF attainable by healthy young adults may exceed 10 L/sec or 600 L/min, BTPS. Even when an accurate **pneumotachometer** is used, the value of PEF measurements may be limited. Peak flow is effort dependent. It primarily measures large airway function. Decreased PEF values should be evaluated for consistent patient effort. PEF values in subjects without hyperreactive airways are usually similar with repeated efforts. Asthmatic subjects often have a pattern of decreasing PEF with repeated trials. Widely varying peak flows without a pattern of induced bronchospasm suggest poor effort or cooperation. However, PEF measurements

---

BOX 2-7
CRITERIA FOR ACCEPTABILITY—PEAK FLOW

1   Subject was standing or sitting up straight.

2   Subject inhaled maximally (rapid, but not forced) and exhaled maximally without holding his or her breath.

3   At least three efforts were performed and recorded in order.

4   Largest PEF obtained is reported.

BOX 2-8
INTERPRETIVE STRATEGIES—PEAK FLOW

1   What is the patient's personal best PEF?

2   Is the current PEF the best of three trials? Was it obtained in the morning or evening? Was it obtained before or after inhaled bronchodilator therapy?

3   Zone system[*]:
    Green   80%-100% of personal best
               Routine treatment can be continued; consider reducing medications
    Yellow   50%-80% of personal best
               Acute exacerbation may be present; temporary increase in medication may be indicated; maintenance therapy may need to be increased
    Red   <50% of personal best
               Bronchodilators should be taken immediately; clinician should be notified if PEF fails to return to yellow or green

[*]National Asthma Education Program, NIH, 1991.

alone are not sufficient to make a diagnosis of asthma. To evaluate fully the associated physiologic impairment, spirometry, lung volumes, diffusing capacity, and airway resistance measurements may be required.

Effort dependence of PEF makes it a good indicator of subject effort during spirometry. Maximal transpulmonary pressures correlate well with maximal PEF. Subjects who exert variable effort during FVC maneuvers are seldom able to reproduce their PEF. Some clinicians use PEF in addition to the FVC and FEV_1 to gauge maximal effort during spirometry. PEF measurements, when performed with a good effort, correlate well with the FEV_1 as measured by spirometry.

Subjects with early small airways obstruction may initially develop high flows during an FVC maneuver. Despite obstruction, these individuals show relatively normal PEF values. When small airway obstruction becomes severe, PEF also decreases. Reduction in PEF is often less than the decrease in $FEF_{50\%}$ or $FEF_{75\%}$ in patients with severe obstruction.

PEF measurements are particularly useful for monitoring asthma patients at home. Daily monitoring of PEF can provide early detection of asthmatic episodes. It can be used to detect day-night patterns (circadian rhythms) related to airway reactivity. PEF monitoring provides objective criteria for treatment. It can help determine specific triggers (e.g., allergens) or workplace exposures that cause symptoms. Daily morning and evening readings are recommended. For patients taking inhaled bronchodilators, PEF may be measured before and after treatment. Significant variation from their personal best or from one reading to the next should be emphasized.

The National Asthma Education Program suggests a "zone" system, based on the individual's personal best or predicted PEF. The zone system uses green, yellow, and red as indicators for maintaining or altering therapy. Green (80% to 100% of the personal best PEF) signals continuation of routine therapy. Yellow (50% to 80% of the personal best PEF) means an acute episode may be starting. Increased medication may be necessary. Red (less than 50% of the personal best PEF) indicates an acute change has occurred. Immediate treatment is required, and the clinician should be notified. This approach dramatically improves the patient's ability to communicate symptomatic changes to the clinician.

Uniformly decreased PEF is often associated with upper airway obstruction but is nonspecific. PEF assessed from F-V loops (along with the PIF) helps define both the severity and site of large airway obstruction.

Maximum Voluntary Ventilation

DESCRIPTION

MVV is the volume of air exhaled in a specific interval during rapid and forced breathing. The maneuver should last at least 12 seconds. It is recorded in liters per minute, BTPS, by extrapolating the volume to 1 minute.

TECHNIQUE

MVV is measured by having the subject breathe deeply and rapidly for a 12- or 15-second interval. The subject should set the rate but breathe as rapidly as possible. The volume breathed should be larger than their VT but less than their VC. The subject should be instructed to move as much air as possible into and out of the spirometer. The technologist should encourage the subject throughout the maneuver.

MVV is continued for at least 12 seconds but no more than 15 seconds. The subject is hyperventilating. Efforts longer than 15 seconds exaggerate the sensation of light-headedness. Even the 12-second interval may produce dizziness or syncope. The test may be performed with the patient in either a sitting or standing position. If done standing, a chair should be available in case of dizziness. Some automated spirometers allow MVV to be terminated before 12 seconds. This accommodates patients who cannot continue because of coughing or light-headedness. If MVV does not last 12 seconds, it should be noted in the technologist's comments (see Chapter 10). At least two MVV maneuvers should be performed. The two largest should be within 10% of each other. The largest value is reported (Box 2-9).

The volume expired is measured by a spirometer. The spirometer must have adequate frequency response over a wide range of flows (see Chapters 9 and 10). Historically, the volume of each breath was read from a volume-time spirogram or from a recording of accumulated volume (Fig. 2-15). Now volume data from each breath are summed by computer for the interval measured. The MVV (for a 12-second test) is calculated as flow in liters per minute, as follows:

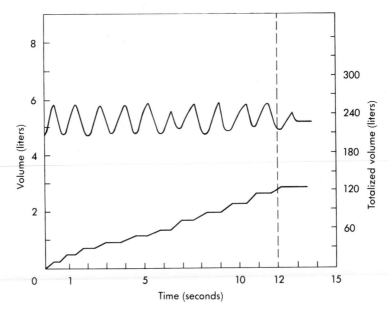

FIG. 2-15 *Maximum voluntary ventilation (MVV).* A composite MVV spirogram on which breath-by-breath volume change and accumulated volume are plotted against time. The *top tracing* shows the actual volume moved during each breath over a 12-second interval. To calculate MVV, the volumes of individual breaths are added and multiplied by a factor of 5 (i.e., 60 seconds/12 seconds = 5). Because the MVV is reported in liters per minute, values for 12 seconds must be extrapolated to 1 minute. The *lower tracing* is computer generated and depicts the accumulated volume, in liters per minute, exhaled during the 12-second maneuver. In this example the volume is approximately 120 L/min, as read from the right-hand scale. Healthy subjects can maintain the same MVV flow throughout the maneuver. Subjects who have pulmonary disease will show decreased absolute values. The MVV may decrease significantly as the maneuver progresses because of respiratory muscle fatigue, increased work of breathing, or because of air trapping.

BOX 2-9
CRITERIA FOR ACCEPTABILITY—MVV

1   Volume-time tracing shows continuous, rhythmic effort, for at least 12 seconds.
2   End-expiratory lung volume is relatively constant.
3   Two acceptable maneuvers obtained; MVV values are within 10%.
4   MVV is approximately equal to $35 \times FEV_1$.

$$MVV = Vol_{12} \times \frac{60}{12}$$

where:

Vol_{12} = volume in liters expired in 12 seconds

60 = factor for extrapolation from seconds to minutes

For other intervals the MVV is calculated similarly. The MVV must be corrected to BTPS.

SIGNIFICANCE AND PATHOPHYSIOLOGY

See Box 2-10 for interpretive strategies. MVV tests the overall function of the respiratory system. It is influenced by airway resistance, respiratory muscles, compliance of the lung or chest wall, and ventilatory control mechanisms. Values in healthy young men average between 150 and 200 L/min. Values are slightly lower in healthy women. MVV decreases with age in both men and women and varies considerably in healthy subjects. Only large reductions in MVV (30% or more) are considered significant.

BOX 2-10
INTERPRETIVE STRATEGIES—MVV

---

1 Was MVV test performed acceptably? At least 12 seconds?

2 Does MVV approximate $FEV_1 \times 35$? If not, suspect subject effort.

3 Is MVV less than 70% of predicted? If so, correlate with obstruction ($FEV_{1\%}$).

4 If no obstruction, look for clinical correlation for reduced MVV. Consider testing maximal respiratory pressures, compliance.

MVV is decreased in subjects with moderate or severe obstructive disease. This may be the result of the increased airway resistance caused by bronchospasm or mucus secretion. Reduction of MVV may also occur because of airway collapse and hyperinflation, as in emphysema. The MVV maneuver exaggerates air trapping and airflow limitation. Volume-time MVV tracings may show a shift if gas trapping occurs during the test. A slight shift is usually noted during the first few breaths even in healthy subjects. The subject adjusts to a lung volume that allows maximal air flow. These first few breaths are usually excluded from the MVV calculation.

The MVV maneuver also places a load on the respiratory muscles. Both inspiratory and expiratory muscles are used in the MVV maneuver. Weakness or decreased endurance of either system may result in low MVV values. Poor coordination of the respiratory muscles caused by a neurologic deficit may also cause a low MVV. Disorders such as paralysis or nerve damage reduce MVV as well.

A markedly reduced MVV correlates with postoperative risk for patients having abdominal or thoracic surgery. Subjects who have low preoperative MVV values show an increased incidence of complications. Reduced strength or endurance of the respiratory muscles may be the factor that allows MVV to predict postoperative problems.

The MVV value may be helpful in estimating ventilation during exercise. Airway-obstructed patients who have an MVV less than 50 L/min often have exercise limitation. Maximal exercise ventilation in healthy subjects is usually less than 70% of their MVV. In airway-obstructed subjects, maximal ventilation during exercise approaches or even exceeds their MVV. This pattern occurs partly because the MVV itself is reduced in obstruction. Highly conditioned healthy subjects may also reach their MVV during maximal exercise (see Chapter 7).

MVV may be normal in subjects who have restrictive pulmonary disease. Diseases that limit lung or chest wall expansion may not interfere significantly with airflow. Subjects who have restrictive disease can compensate by performing the MVV maneuver with low VT and high breathing rates.

The MVV maneuver depends on subject effort and cooperation. Low MVV values may indicate obstruction, muscular weakness, defective ventilatory control, or poor subject performance. Subject effort during the MVV maneuver may be estimated by multiplying their FEV_1 by 35. For example, a subject with an FEV_1 of 2.0 L might be expected to ventilate approximately 70 L/min (35×2.0 L) during the MVV test. If the measured MVV is much less than 70 L/min, poor subject effort may be suspected. If the MVV exceeds 70 L/min by a large volume, the FEV_1 may be erroneous.

Before- and After-Bronchodilator Studies

DESCRIPTION

Spirometry can be performed before and after bronchodilator administration to determine the reversibility of airways obstruction. An $FEV_{1\%}$ less than predicted is a good indication for bronchodilator studies. In most subjects an $FEV_{1\%}$ less than 70% indicates obstruction. In older adults the normal $FEV_{1\%}$ may be slightly less. Subjects whose FEV_1 and FVC are within normal limits may have a low $FEV_{1\%}$. This happens when the FVC is greater than 100% of predicted while the FEV_1 is slightly reduced. Although any pulmonary function parameter may be measured before and after bronchodilator therapy, FEV_1 and specific airway conductance (SGaw) are usually evaluated.

BOX 2-11
USING AN MDI

- Shake the MDI; activate once to prime and check contents. If empty, replace.
- Hold the MDI mouthpiece slightly away from the subject's open mouth;
  or, if a spacer is used
  Place the spacer mouthpiece between the lips, per manufacturer's instructions.
- As the subject inspires slowly from the resting expiratory level, activate the MDI.
- Have the subject continue slowly inhaling to maximal inspiration.
- Have the subject hold the breath for 3 to 5 seconds, followed by a slow exhalation.
- Repeat inhalations as indicated.

TABLE 2-2 **Withholding Medications**

Medication	Time to withhold*
Regular β-agonists	8 hours
Sustained action β-agonists	12 hours
Methylxanthines (theophyllines)	12 hours
Slow-release methylxanthines	24 hours
Atropine-like preparations	8 hours
Cromolyn sodium	8-12 hours
Inhaled steroids	Maintain dosage

*Approximate times; may be adjusted for individual patients.

TECHNIQUE

The patient may take an array of tests, including spirometry, lung volumes, and diffusing capacity (DL_{CO}). Lung volumes should be recorded before bronchodilator administration. This provides a baseline for comparing lung volume changes after bronchodilator therapy. Even though indices of flow (FEV_1, $FEF_{25\%-75\%}$, and SGaw) usually show the greatest change, lung volumes and DL_{CO} may also respond to bronchodilator therapy.

Subjects referred for spirometry testing should withhold routine bronchodilator therapy before the procedure (Table 2-2). Some patients may be unable to manage their symptoms if bronchodilators are withheld. These patients should be instructed to take their bronchodilator medication as needed. In these instances, the time when the medication was last taken should be noted. Some subjects who use bronchodilators shortly before testing (i.e., within 4 hours) still show significant improvement after a repeated dose.

Inhaled bronchodilators can be administered by a metered-dose inhaler (MDI) or a small-volume nebulizer. An MDI provides a reproducible means of administering the bronchodilator. Some subjects are unable to coordinate activation of the MDI with slow, deep inspiration. For these patients use of an aerosol reservoir, or spacer, may provide a more consistent delivery of medication. If the subject is unfamiliar with the MDI, the technologist may need to activate the device (Box 2-11). Small-volume, jet-powered nebulizers may be used to administer more bronchodilator over a longer interval. Nebulizers, if reused, must be carefully disinfected between patients.

β-Adrenergic aerosols, including isoproterenol, metaproterenol, and albuterol, are most commonly used. Each of these drugs has a rapid onset of action, usually within 5 minutes. Maximum bronchodilatation usually takes longer. A minimum interval of 15 minutes between administration and repeat testing is recommended. Even with this delay, peak bronchodilator response may not be observed. Response to atropine-like drugs (ipratropium bromide) may require a delay of 45 to 60 minutes after inhalation.

Bronchodilator administration often causes side effects. The most common side effect of β-agonist use is tachycardia. Increased blood pressure, flushing, dizziness, or light-headedness are not unusual. Monitoring pulse rate and blood pressure is recommended for susceptible patients.

BOX 2-12
INTERPRETIVE STRATEGIES—BRONCHODILATOR STUDIES

1   Are the prebronchodilator and postbronchodilator measurements acceptable? Reproducible within 200 ml? If not, postbronchodilator changes may be erroneous.

2   Is there a 12% or greater improvement in FEV_1 or FVC? Is there also a 200 ml increase? If so, there is a significant improvement.

3   Is there an increase in SGaw (if done) greater than 35%? If so, there is a significant improvement.

4   No significant improvement observed? Trial of bronchodilator therapy may be recommended, if clinically indicated.

This includes subjects with known cardiac arrhythmias or elevated blood pressure. Marked changes in heart rate, rhythm, or blood pressure or symptoms like chest pain indicate a need to stabilize the patient. The referring physician or laboratory medical director should be notified immediately. Management of the patient's symptoms and continuation of testing are the decision of the physician.

Measurements of FEV_1, FVC, $FEF_{25\%-75\%}$, PEF, and SGaw are commonly taken before and after bronchodilator administration. In each case the percentage of change is calculated as follows:

$$\% \text{ Change} = \frac{\text{Postdrug} - \text{Predrug}}{\text{Predrug}} \times 100$$

where:

Postdrug = test parameter after administration

Predrug = test parameter before administration

If the test value improves, the percentage of change will be positive. If the parameter worsens, a negative percentage results. Small prebronchodilator values (e.g., an FEV_1 of 0.5 L) may show large changes even though the improvement is minimal.

FEV_1 is the most commonly used test for quantifying bronchodilator response. If $FEF_{25\%-75\%}$ or flows such as $Vmax_{50}$ are used, they should be isovolume-corrected for changes in the FVC. If FVC increases more than FEV_1 after bronchodilator therapy, $FEV_{1\%}$ may decrease. $FEV_{1\%}$ should not be used to judge bronchodilator response. SGaw may show a marked increase after bronchodilator therapy. Improved conductance may occur despite minimal change in FEV_1 or conventional measures of flow. Spirometry or plethysmography after bronchodilator therapy should meet the usual criteria for acceptability and reproducibility.

SIGNIFICANCE AND PATHOPHYSIOLOGY

See Box 2-12 for interpretive strategies. Reversibility of airway obstruction is considered significant for increases of greater than 12% *and* 200 ml for either the FEV_1 or FVC. If the SGaw is assessed, an increase of 30% to 40% is usually considered significant. Changes in $FEF_{25\%-75\%}$ of 20% to 30% are sometimes considered significant. However, flows that depend on the FVC should be volume-corrected (refer to Case 2B). If not corrected, $FEF_{25\%-75\%}$ may appear to decrease even though FEV_1 and FVC improve.

Diseases involving the bronchial (and bronchiolar) smooth muscle usually improve most from "before" to "after." Increases greater than 50% in the FEV_1 may occur in patients with asthma. Patients with chronic obstructive diseases may show little improvement in flows. Poor bronchodilator response may be related to inadequate deposition of the inhaled drug because of poor inspiratory effort. Some subjects show a paradoxical response to bronchodilator therapy. In these individuals, flows may actually decrease after the bronchodilator therapy. Decreased flows after bronchodilator therapy may also be related to fatigue from multiple FVC efforts. Failure to show a significant improvement after bronchodilator therapy does not exclude a response. Some subjects have a significant response to one drug but little or no response to another. Changes of less than 8% or of less than 150 ml are within the variability of measurement of FEV_1. Such small changes may occur just with testing and are unlikely to be significant.

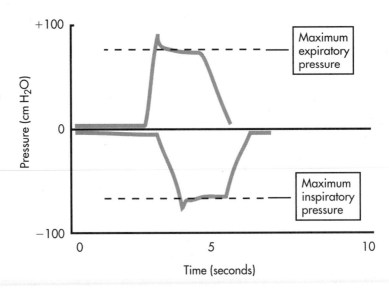

FIG. 2-16 *Maximal inspiratory and maximal expiratory pressures (MIP, MEP).* These tracings plot the respective pressures recorded in cm H_2O against time. Maximal inspiratory pressure shows a downward or negative deflection, whereas maximal inspiratory pressure shows a positive or upward deflection. Each maneuver is conducted with the airway occluded (see text). The occlusion is maintained for a short interval (1 to 3 seconds) and any initial transient tracings are discarded.

Maximal Inspiratory Pressure and Maximal Expiratory Pressure

DESCRIPTION

MIP is the lowest pressure developed during a forceful inspiration against an occluded airway. It is usually measured at maximal expiration and recorded as a negative number in either cm H_2O or mm Hg. MEP is the highest pressure that can be developed during a forceful expiratory effort against an occluded airway. It is usually measured at maximal inspiration and reported as a positive number in either cm H_2O or mm Hg. MIP and MEP are sometimes measured at the resting end-expiratory level (functional residual capacity [FRC]).

TECHNIQUE

The subject is connected to a valve or shutter apparatus, with a flanged mouthpiece and nose clip in place. The airway is occluded by blocking a port in the valve or by closing the shutter. In either system, a small leak is introduced between the occlusion and the subject's mouth. The leak can be created using a large-bore needle or similar small opening. The leak eliminates pressures generated by the cheek muscles by allowing a small amount of gas to enter the oral cavity. This does not significantly change lung volume or the pressure measurement.

Pressure may be measured using a manometer, aneroid-type gauge, or pressure transducer. The pressure-monitoring device should be linear over its range. It should be able to record pressures from −10 to approximately −200 cm H_2O. If a pressure transducer is used, its signal can be directed to a recorder or computer display. If a manometer or aneroid gauge is used, the technologist observes the pressure and records it. Devices that use a "trip" indicator can be misleading. The highest pressure recorded may be a transient tracing that occurs at the very beginning of the maneuver (Fig. 2-16). The technologist should record the plateau pressure that the subject can maintain for 1 to 3 seconds.

For the MIP test, the subject is instructed to expire maximally. Monitoring expiratory flow or having the subject signal helps determine when maximal expiration has been achieved. Then the airway is occluded as described. The subject inspires maximally and maintains the inspiration for 1 to 3 seconds. The first portion of each maneuver is disregarded because it may include transient pressure changes that occur initially (see Fig. 2-16). The most negative value from at least three efforts is recorded.

MEP is recorded similarly. The subject inhales as much as possible, then exhales maximally against the occluded airway for 1 to 3 seconds. Longer efforts should be avoided. Cardiac output

---

BOX 2-13
CRITERIA FOR ACCEPTABILITY—MIP/MEP

1. Pressure tracing (if available) should show 1 to 3 seconds of sustained effort; there should be a pressure plateau after initial transients.
2. Pressure plateau should be observed, 1 to 3 seconds (if manometer is used).
3. At least 3 MIP and 3 MEP maneuvers should be recorded.
4. Best 2 efforts should be within 10% or 10 cm H_2O, whichever is greater.
5. Maximal value for MIP and MEP should be reported.

---

can be reduced by the high thoracic pressures (i.e., **Valsalva maneuvers**) that are sometimes developed. MEP is usually larger than MIP in healthy subjects. The pressure-monitoring device should be able to withstand the higher pressure without damage. The best of at least three MEP efforts is reported. As for MIP, initial pressure transient tracings during the MEP are disregarded. Both MIP and MEP require subject cooperation and effort (Box 2-13). Low values may reflect lack of understanding or insufficient effort.

SIGNIFICANCE AND PATHOPHYSIOLOGY

MIP primarily measures inspiratory muscle *strength*. Healthy adults can generate inspiratory pressures greater than −60 cm H_2O. Decreased MIP is seen in subjects with neuromuscular disease or diseases involving the diaphragm, intercostals, or accessory muscles. MIP may also be decreased in patients with hyperinflation as in emphysema. The diaphragm is flattened by the increased volume of trapped gas in the lungs. The intercostals and accessory muscles may also be compromised by injury to or diseases of the chest wall. Patients with chest wall or spinal deformities (e.g., kyphoscoliosis) may also have reduced inspiratory pressures. MIP is sometimes used to assess subject response to strength training of respiratory muscles. MIP is often used in the assessment of respiratory muscle function in subjects who need ventilatory support.

MEP measures the pressure generated during maximal expiration. It depends on the function of the abdominal muscles and accessory muscles of respiration and the elastic recoil of the lungs and thorax. Healthy adults can generate MEP values more than 80 to 100 cm H_2O. Adult men may develop pressures greater than 200 cm H_2O. MEP may be decreased in neuromuscular disorders, particularly those resulting in generalized muscle weakness. Another common disorder that results in reduction of MEP is high cervical spine fracture. Damage to nerves controlling abdominal and accessory muscles of expiration can dramatically reduce the MEP. However, MIP may be preserved in these patients.

Reduced MEP often accompanies increased RV, as seen in emphysema. A low MEP is associated with inability to cough effectively. Inability to generate an adequate cough may complicate chronic bronchitis, cystic fibrosis, or other diseases that result in excessive mucus secretion.

Accurate measurement of MIP and MEP depends largely on subject effort. The technologist should carefully instruct the subject how to do the maneuver. Low values may result if the subject fails to inhale or exhale completely before the airway is occluded. At least three maximal efforts should be recorded. The best efforts should be reproducible within 10% or 10 cm H_2O, whichever is greater. Widely varying pressures for either MIP or MEP should be assessed carefully before interpretation.

Airway Resistance and Conductance

DESCRIPTION

Airway resistance (Raw) is the pressure difference per unit flow as gas flows into or out of the lungs. Raw is the difference between mouth pressure and alveolar pressure, divided by flow at the mouth. This pressure difference is caused primarily by the friction of gas molecules in contact with the airways. Raw is recorded in centimeters of water per liter per second (cm H_2O/L/sec).

Airway conductance (Gaw) is the flow generated per unit of pressure drop across the airways. It is the reciprocal of Raw (i.e., 1/Raw) and is recorded in liters per second per centimeter of water (L/sec/cm H_2O). Gaw is not commonly reported because it changes with lung volume.

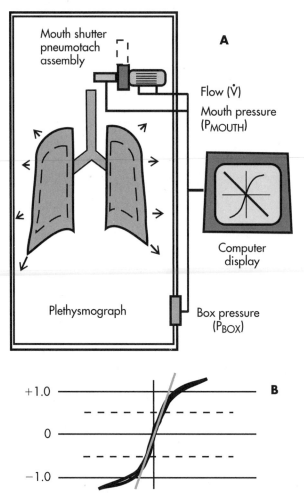

FIG. 2-17 *Measurement of airway resistance (Raw) using the body plethysmograph.* **A,** Diagrammatic representation of the measurement of airway resistance:

$$Raw = \frac{\text{Atmospheric pressure} - \text{Alveolar pressure}}{\text{Flow}}$$

Flow ($\dot{V}$) is measured directly by means of the pneumotachometer. As the subject pants with the shutter open, flow is plotted against box pressure. ($\dot{V}/P_{BOX}$) as an S-shaped curve on the computer display. A shutter occludes the airway momentarily, usually at end-expiration, and a sloping line representing the ratio of mouth pressure to box pressure (P_{MOUTH}/P_{BOX}) is recorded in a manner similar to that used for measurement of VTG (see Chapter 3). In this example the flow tracing (shutter open) and volume tracing (shutter closed) are superimposed. The P_{MOUTH}/P_{BOX} tangent is measured as for the VTG. **B,** The flow tangent is measured from the steep portion of the flow tracing, from −0.5 to +0.5 L/sec. Airway resistance is then calculated as the ratio of these two tangents using appropriate calibration factors (see text and Appendix).

Specific conductance (SGaw) is usually reported and shows the conductance per liter of lung volume. It is reported in liters per second per centimeter of water per liter of lung volume (L/sec/cm H_2O/L).

TECHNIQUE

Raw can be measured as the ratio of alveolar pressure (PA) to air flow ($\dot{V}$). Gas flow at the mouth is measured with a pneumotachometer (see Chapter 9). PA is measured in the body plethysmograph (Fig. 2-17, A). For gas to flow into the lungs during inspiration, PA must fall below atmospheric pressure (mouth pressure). During expiration PA rises above atmospheric pressure. Changes in $\dot{V}$ are plotted against plethysmograph pressure changes. Changes in plethysmograph pressure are proportional to alveolar volume changes. The subject pants with a small VT at a rate

---

BOX 2-14
CRITERIA FOR ACCEPTABILITY—Raw AND SGaw

---

1   Pressure-flow loops should be closed; pressure and flow should be within the calibrated range of the respective transducers.

2   Thermal equilibrium should be established; no drift during recording.

3   Panting frequency should be 1.5 to 3.0 Hz for each maneuver.

4   Raw and SGaw should be calculated for each maneuver; do not average tangents.

5   Mean of three or more acceptable efforts should be reported; individual values should be within 10% of mean.

---

of 1½ to 3 breaths/sec (1.5 to 3 Hz). Shallow, rapid breathing produces an S-shaped pressure-flow curve (Fig. 2-17, *B*). A **tangent** (i.e., the **slope**) is measured from this curve. The tangent passes through zero flow and connects the +0.5 L/sec and −0.5 L/sec flow points. The slope of this line is $\dot{V}/P_{BOX}$. $\dot{V}$ is flow at the mouth and P_{BOX} is plethysmograph pressure.

Immediately after this measurement, a shutter at the mouthpiece is closed and the subject continues panting. Changes in P_{BOX} are then plotted against airway pressure at the mouth (P_{MOUTH}). Because there is no flow into or out of the lungs, P_{MOUTH} equals PA. A second tangent is measured from this curve. The slope of this line is P_A/P_{BOX}, where PA equals alveolar pressure. Computerized plethysmographs usually calculate a "best fit" line to measure the open- and closed-shutter tangents. The technologist should visually inspect all computer-fitted lines. The system should allow the technologist to adjust computer-generated tangents manually.

Raw is then calculated by taking the ratio of these two slopes, as follows:

$$Raw = \frac{P_A/P_{BOX}}{\dot{V}/P_{BOX}} \times \frac{Mouth\ cal}{Flow\ cal}$$

where:

$\dot{V}$ = airflow

P_A = alveolar pressure

P_{BOX} = plethysmographic pressure, measured with the shutter open and closed

Mouth cal = calibration factor for the mouth pressure transducer

Flow cal = calibration factor for the pneumotachometer

Calibration factors for the flow and mouth pressure transducers are included in the previous equation. (See sample calculations in the Appendix F.)

Panting eliminates a number of artifacts from the tracing. Small rapid breaths (2 to 3 per second) reduce thermal drift. Panting helps the subject keep the glottis open. Panting also allows measurements to be made near FRC. The resistances of the mouthpiece and pneumotachometer are subtracted from the subject's Raw.

Conductance (Gaw) can be calculated as the reciprocal of Raw. Specific conductance is calculated by dividing Gaw by the lung volume at which it was measured. Lung volume is measured at the same time, using the plethysmographic method (see Chapter 3). SGaw should be calculated separately for each maneuver because the lung volume at which measurements are made influences Raw and Gaw. After three to five acceptable trials are obtained, calculated Raw and SGaw are averaged. Individual values should be within approximately 10% of the mean (Box 2-14).

Computerized plethysmographs permit thoracic gas volume (VTG), Raw, and SGaw to be measured from a combined maneuver. The subject breathes through the pneumotachometer with the plethysmograph sealed. Tidal breathing is recorded with the subject breathing near FRC. The computer stores this end-expiratory volume as a reference point. Then the subject pants, and the open-shutter slope of $\dot{V}/P_{BOX}$ is recorded. The mouth shutter is then closed and P_{MOUTH}/P_{BOX} is recorded as described previously. The VTG in this maneuver does not equal the FRC because the shutter is closed at a volume different from the FRC. However, the change in volume from the tidal breathing level was stored at the beginning of the maneuver. This volume can be added to or subtracted from the VTG to determine FRC. Most subjects pant above

---

BOX 2-15
INTERPRETIVE STRATEGIES—Raw AND SGaw

1 Were all maneuvers performed acceptably? Pressure-flow curves closed? Thermal equilibrium established?

2 Are individual Raw and SGaw values reproducible? Within 10%?

3 Is Raw greater than 2.4 cm H_2O/L/sec? Is SGaw less than lower limit of normal? If so, suspect obstruction. Correlate with PEF, FEV_1 to distinguish large versus small airway obstruction.

4 If large airway obstruction indicated, check clinical history. Extrathoracic or intrathoracic?

---

their FRC so the VTG in this method is usually slightly greater. The combined maneuver allows VTG, Raw, and SGaw to be determined at the same time. However, optimal panting frequencies are different for VTG and Raw maneuvers. In some subjects the tests may need to be done separately.

Raw and Gaw may be expressed per liter of lung volume as specific resistance and specific conductance (SRaw and SGaw, respectively). Expressing Raw and Gaw in this way allows comparisons to be made between subjects with different lung volumes or in the same subject when lung volume changes.

SIGNIFICANCE AND PATHOPHYSIOLOGY

See Box 2-15 for interpretive strategies. Normal values of Raw in adults range from 0.6 to 2.4 cm H_2O/L/sec. Gaw in healthy adults is between 0.42 and 1.67 L/sec/cm H_2O. SGaw varies in a manner similar to Gaw. SGaw values less than 0.10 to 0.15 L/sec/cm H_2O/L are consistent with airway obstruction. Measurements are standardized at flow rates of ±0.5 L/sec, as described previously.

Raw in healthy adults is divided across the airway as follows:

Nose, mouth, and upper airway $\cong$ 50%

Trachea and bronchi $\cong$ 30%

Small airways $\cong$ 20%

Small airways (less than 2 mm in diameter) contribute only approximately one fifth of the total resistance to flow. Significant obstruction can develop in the small airways with little increase in Raw or decrease in SGaw. Early or mild obstructive processes are not usually identified by abnormal Raw or SGaw. Raw may be increased in an acute asthmatic episode by as much as three times the normal values. Inflammation, mucus secretion, and bronchospasm all increase Raw in the small and medium airways. Raw is increased in advanced emphysema because of airway narrowing and collapse, especially in the bronchioles. Other obstructive diseases (e.g., bronchitis) may cause increases in Raw proportionate to the degree of obstruction in medium and small airways.

Lesions obstructing the larger airways (e.g., tumors, traumatic injuries, or foreign bodies) may cause a significant increase in Raw. Large airway obstruction is often accompanied by increased work of breathing and dyspnea on exertion. Airflow in the trachea and mainstem bronchi is predominately turbulent. Any large airway obstruction can exaggerate this turbulent flow. Breathing low-density gas mixtures (e.g., helium, oxygen) reduces Raw and hence the work of breathing.

Raw is decreased at increased lung volume. The airways (particularly large and medium airways) are distended slightly, and their cross-sectional area increases. For this reason the VTG is always obtained with Raw measurements. Raw and Gaw are often expressed per liter of lung volume. This allows comparison of values in different subjects, or in the same subject after treatment. SGaw is particularly useful for assessing changes in airway caliber after bronchodilator therapy or inhalation challenge. SGaw may change significantly after bronchodilator or inhalation challenge, even though other measures of flow (i.e., FEV_1) vary only slightly. The primary site of airway obstruction (i.e., large versus small airways) may determine which parameters reflect changes in airway caliber.

Raw and SGaw measurements are not influenced by the degree of subject effort. Raw and SGaw measurements may be useful for determining airway status in patients who are unable or unwilling to exert maximum effort. Acceptable panting maneuvers in the plethysmograph require a certain

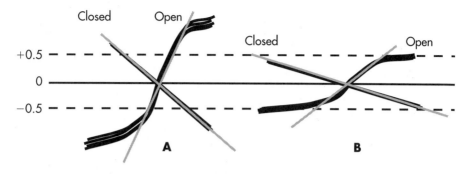

FIG. 2-18 *Airway resistance tracings.* **A,** Tracing from a normal subject. **B,** Tracing from a subject with increased airway resistance caused by obstructive lung disease. Note that the open shutter loop (flow) is flattened because a greater change in alveolar pressure is required to generate flow at the mouth. The closed shutter loop also shows a reduction in mouth pressure (*y* axis) in relation to box pressure (*x* axis). This is consistent with increased lung volume.

degree of subject coordination. Not all subjects may be able to perform these maneuvers. Subjects with severe obstruction may produce pressure-flow curves during panting that are difficult to measure. Such curves may be flat (Fig. 2-18) or show hysteresis. Inspiratory and expiratory flows may produce different resistances, causing the curve to appear as a loop. In these cases, inspiratory flow resistance is usually reported.

In addition to resistance caused by flow through conducting airways, some frictional resistance is caused by the displacement of the lungs, rib cage, and diaphragm. In healthy subjects this tissue resistance is only approximately one fifth of the total resistance, and therefore total pulmonary resistance is approximately 20% greater than the measured Raw.

Pulmonary Compliance

DESCRIPTION

Pulmonary compliance (CL) is volume change per unit of pressure change for the lungs. Lung compliance is recorded in liters (or milliliters) per centimeter of water. Elastic recoil pressure is usually measured with CL. Elastic recoil pressure is the force generated by the lungs, usually at maximal volume. Elastic recoil pressure is reported in centimeters of water.

TECHNIQUE

CL is measured by passing a catheter into the esophagus. The catheter has a 10-cm long balloon near its end. The catheter is inserted through the nose. The patient is then asked to swallow the catheter. The catheter is advanced to midthorax level and connected to a pressure transducer. Proper positioning of the catheter is verified by noting negative pressure deflections on inspiration. If the catheter is advanced too far, the balloon may enter the stomach. This causes positive pressure changes with inspiration. If the balloon is positioned at the level of the heart, cardiac systole may cause an unwanted artifact (Box 2-16).

The pressure transducer is set at zero with a small volume (0.5 to 1.0 ml) of air in the balloon. Pressures are then recorded at different lung volumes. These pressures are plotted to produce a compliance curve (Fig. 2-19). The subject inhales maximally before the test to standardize the measurements. CL increases slightly after a full inspiration. Then the subject inhales again. During this inhalation pressure and volume are measured. Static compliance measurements must be made at zero flow. The subject may hold his or her breath with the glottis open, or flow may be interrupted with a shutter. If a latter technique is used, mouth pressure is subtracted from esophageal pressure to obtain the recoil pressure of the lungs. Similar measurements are recorded during the subsequent expiration.

CL is usually recorded as the slope of the pressure-volume curve from FRC to FRC + 0.5 L (see Fig. 2-19). Because the deep inspiration increases compliance, measurements are usually recorded from the exhalation curve. Maximum static elastic recoil pressure (Pst) is the most negative pressure recorded at maximal inspiration. The optimal method of presenting compliance data is to plot the

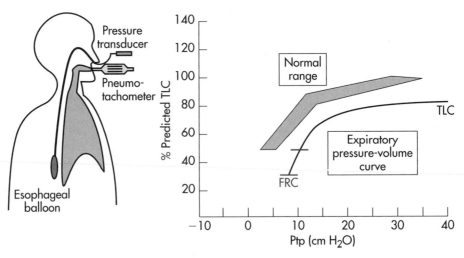

FIG. 2-19 *Measurement of pulmonary compliance (CL) using the esophageal balloon technique.* Determination of CL requires measurement of intrapleural pressure (ΔP) during periods of no flow at various lung volumes. A pressure transducer is connected to an esophageal balloon containing a small amount of air and located in the mid-thorax. The balloon reflects ΔP as the subject inspires to TLC and then expires back to FRC. A pneumotachometer is used to measure gas volumes (ΔV). Static CL is the slope of the line defined by:

$$\frac{\Delta V \text{ (Liters)}}{\Delta P \text{ (cm H}_2\text{O)}}$$

CL is usually recorded from the breathing range of FRC + 500 ml *(horizontal lines)*. Static elastic recoil (Pst) pressure is usually measured at TLC. In the graph shown the expiratory pressure volume is plotted. Transpulmonary pressure (Ptp) is plotted on the X axis and percentage of predicted TLC on the Y axis. The normal range is represented by the *shaded area*. The pressure-volume curve in this example is displaced down and to the right, consistent with lungs that are stiffer than normal.

BOX 2-16
CRITERIA FOR ACCEPTABILITY—LUNG COMPLIANCE

1 Catheter is positioned properly; negative deflection on inspiration; minimal cardiac artifact.

2 At least two inspiratory and expiratory maneuvers are obtained.

3 Compliance and maximal recoil values are reproducible.

---

entire pressure curve (inflation and deflation) versus lung volume. The CL curve can then be plotted along with normal ranges.

Compliance is sometimes measured in patients given positive-pressure mechanical ventilation. The ventilator inflates the lungs-thorax system with a fixed volume. By recording pressure when flow is zero (by occlusion of the exhalation valve), a compliance measurement can be obtained. Pressure may be measured from the ventilator circuit. A more sophisticated technique uses an esophageal balloon like the laboratory method. In each case the volume of gas compressed in the patients lungs is divided by the observed pressure. This compliance measure differs slightly from true CL. It measures the distensibility of the chest wall as well as the lungs. This technique may be influenced by the subject's position or by any contribution from the respiratory muscles.

SIGNIFICANCE AND PATHOPHYSIOLOGY

See Box 2-17 for interpretive strategies. CL measures the distensibility of the lungs. The average CL in a healthy adult is approximately 0.2 L/cm H$_2$O. The lungs are distended in series with the chest wall. The compliance of the thorax (CT) is also approximately 0.2 L/cm

---

BOX 2-17
INTERPRETIVE STRATEGIES—LUNG COMPLIANCE

1   Were the data obtained reproducible? C_L? Pst?

2   Is C_L less than the lower limit of normal? If so, check for clinical correlation. Are lung volumes also reduced?

3   Is C_L greater than upper limit of normal? Check for findings consistent with obstruction (e.g., $FEV_{1\%}$). Is maximal static recoil decreased?

H_2O in healthy subjects. In series, the total compliance (C_{LT}) is calculated using the following equation:

$$\frac{1}{C_L} + \frac{1}{C_T} = \frac{1}{C_{LT}}$$

or substituting the normal values:

$$\frac{1}{0.2} + \frac{1}{0.2} = 10$$

where the reciprocal of 10 is the C_{LT}:

$$\frac{1}{10} = 0.1 \text{ L/cm } H_2O$$

It should be noted that C_{LT} is less than (approximately half) C_L or C_T alone. The elastic forces act in series, counterbalancing the lung tissue and the chest wall. C_L varies with the lung volume at the end-expiratory level (i.e., FRC). To compare the C_L of diseased and normal lungs, the FRC in each case should be known. Plotting the entire C_L curve against lung volume helps relate the two factors.

C_L is decreased in diseases such as edema. Congestion of the pulmonary blood vessels makes the lung stiff. The same is true for diseases in which airways become filled with fluid. Such disorders include atelectasis, pneumonia, or loss of surfactant. Diseases that alter elasticity of lung tissue also lower compliance. Examples include pulmonary fibrosis resulting from silicosis, asbestosis, or sarcoidosis. Decreased C_L may also result when lung volume is reduced as a result of space-occupying lesions such as tumors. When C_L is severely reduced from any cause, symptoms such as dyspnea on exertion are usually present. C_L decreases with age, presumably because of changes in the connective tissues of the lung.

Emphysema is often accompanied by an increase in C_L. Emphysema destroys alveolar septa with loss of elastic tissue. As a result, the **balance** between the lungs and chest wall is upset. The chest wall tends to spring outward. The highly compliant lungs exert less pressure to cause recoil. Hyperinflation results as thoracic volume increases. Subjects with severe air trapping typically have abnormal breathing patterns and markedly increased work of breathing.

Measurement of C_L requires cooperation by the subject. Some subjects may be unable to swallow the esophageal balloon easily. If a mouth shutter is not used to interrupt flow, the subject must hold his or her breath with the glottis open. The C_L and elastic recoil pressure measurements are largely independent of effort, provided the subject is cooperative.

CASE STUDIES

CASE 2A

History

L.L. is a 21-year-old man in good health. He plays college football. His chief complaint is shortness of breath after wind sprints and similar vigorous exercises. He denies any other symptoms, including cough or sputum production. He has never smoked. His grandfather had lung problems, but there is no other history of pulmonary disease involving the family. He states that his brothers and sisters have hay fever. There is no history of exposure to environmental pollutants.

Pulmonary Function Testing

Personal data

Sex: Male
Age: 21 yr
Height: 73 in
Weight: 180 lb

Spirometry and airway resistance

	Before drug	Predicted	% Predicted	After drug	% Predicted	Δ (%)
FVC (L)	6.85	6.04	111	6.73	111	−2
FEV_1 (L)	4.65	4.78	97	5.45	114	17
$FEV_{1\%}$ (%)	70	79	—	81	—	
$FEF_{25\%-75\%}$ (L/sec)	3.9	5	78	4.88	97	25
$\dot{V}max_{50}$ (L/sec)	5.01	6.52	77	6.1	94	22
$\dot{V}max_{25}$ (L/sec)	2.79	3.75	74	3.25	87	16
MVV (L/min)	218	166	131	215	130	−1
Raw (cm H_2O/L/sec)	2.1	0.6-2.4	—	1.6	—	−24
SGaw (L/sec/cm H_2O/L)	0.14	0.10-0.39	—	0.22	—	57

Technologist's Comments

All FVC efforts performed acceptably. All tests meet ATS criteria. Body plethysmograph efforts were reproducible.

Questions

1. Interpret the following:
    a. Prebronchodilator spirometry
    b. Response to bronchodilator
    c. Airway resistance and conductance
2. What is the cause of the patient's symptoms?
3. What other tests might be indicated?
4. What treatment might be recommended based on these findings?

Discussion

1 **Interpretation**

All spirometry efforts before and after bronchodilator therapy were performed acceptably. All body-box maneuvers were acceptable. Spirometry results are within normal limits except for a decrease in the $FEV_{1\%}$. There is a significant increase in the FEV_1, $\dot{V}max_{50}$, $\dot{V}max_{25}$, $FEV_{1\%}$, and $FEF_{25\%-75\%}$ after administration of the bronchodilator. MVV is normal, as are Raw and SGaw. Raw and SGaw also showed significant improvement after bronchodilator therapy.

Impression: Mild obstructive defect with significant response to bronchodilator. Evaluation for exercise-induced bronchospasm may be indicated.

2 **Cause of symptoms**

This subject has normal or slightly above normal values for almost every lung function parameter. The exception is his $FEV_{1\%}$. It is below the expected value, consistent with mild obstruction. Simply evaluating FVC and FEV_1 compared with predicted values might give the impression that he is normal. The $FEV_{1\%}$ indicates that the subject, whose FVC is slightly larger than normal, expired a disproportionately small FEV_1. This pattern of supranormal volumes with lower than normal $FEV_{1\%}$ is sometimes seen in healthy young adults. The slightly decreased values for $FEF_{25\%-75\%}$, $\dot{V}max_{50}$, and $\dot{V}max_{25}$, however, suggest an

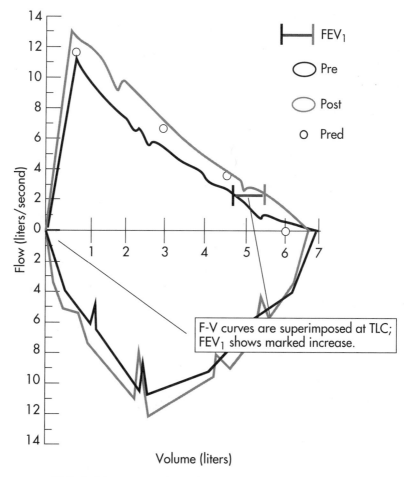

FIG. 2-20 *Case 2A.* Flow volume loops superimposed at TLC.

obstructive process (Fig. 2-20). There is a 17% increase (0.8 L) in FEV_1 after administration of a bronchodilator. This response is significant in view of the subject's complaint of shortness of breath after exercise. He appears to have reversible airway obstruction triggered by exercise.

3   **Other tests**

Further evaluation of L.L. included an exercise test to demonstrate exercise-induced asthma (EIA). After 6 minutes of **treadmill** jogging at 88% of his predicted maximal heart rate, L.L.'s FEV_1 began to fall. Five minutes after stopping the test, his FEV_1 fell to 4.1. Scattered wheezes were heard on auscultation. The obstruction was readily reversed by inhaled bronchodilator. Inhalation-challenge testing was deferred because the obstructive defect was obvious after the exercise test.

4   **Treatment**

The patient was given a regimen of inhaled bronchodilators and cromolyn sodium. He was given a portable peak flow meter to monitor his lung function. He reported marked decrease in symptoms by pretreating himself with the inhaled medication before athletic activities.

CASE 2B ────────────────────────────────

History

R.Z. is a 47-year-old carpenter whose chief complaint is shortness of breath on exertion. His dyspnea, although worse recently, has been present for several years. He smoked 1½ packs of cigarettes a day since age 15 (48 pack/years). He has a cough in the morning. He says that he produces a "small amount of grayish sputum." R.Z.'s father had tuberculosis. A sister had asthma as a child and now as an adult. He denies any extraordinary exposure to environmental dusts or fumes.

Pulmonary Function Testing

Personal data

Sex: Male
Age: 47 yr
Height: 70 in
Weight: 190 lb

Spirometry and airway resistance

	Before drug	Predicted	% Predicted	After drug	% Predicted	% Chg
FVC (L)	4.01	4.97	81	4.49	90	12%
FEV_1 (L)	2.05	3.67	56	2.20	6	7%
$FEV_{1\%}$(%)	51	74	—	49	—	−4%
$FEF_{25\%-75\%}$ (L/sec)	1.2	3.69	33	1.3	35	8%
$\dot{V}max_{50}$ (L/sec)	1.35	5.54	24	2.67	30	24%
$\dot{V}max_{25}$ (L/sec)	0.55	2.58	21	1.02	40	85%
MVV (L/min)	71	136	52	85	63	20%
Raw (cm H_2O/L/sec)	3.1	0.6-2.4	—	2.9	—	−6%
SGaw (L/sec/cm H_2O/L)	0.07	0.1-0.4	—	0.11	—	57%

Technologist's Comments

All tests met ATS criteria. All body plethysmograph efforts were performed acceptably.

Questions

1. Interpret the following:
    a. Prebronchodilator spirometry
    b. Response to bronchodilator
    c. Airway resistance and conductance
2. What is the cause of the patient's symptoms?
3. What other tests might be indicated?
4. What treatment might be recommended based on these findings?

Discussion

1   Interpretation

All spirometry efforts were acceptable. All body-box efforts were reproducible. The subject has a reduced FEV_1, but his FVC is only slightly decreased. $FEF_{25\%-75\%}$ is decreased, as are $\dot{V}max_{50}$ and $\dot{V}max_{25}$. MVV is reduced in proportion to the subject's FEV_1. Raw is greater than the reference value, and SGaw is below the lower limit of normal. Little or no change occurs in FEV_1 after inhaled bronchodilator therapy. FVC improves marginally. SGaw is significantly better after bronchodilator.

Impression: Moderately severe airway obstruction with significant improvement in vital capacity and airway conductance after inhaled bronchodilator.

2   Cause of symptoms

R.Z. is a smoker who has developed moderate airway obstruction. His spirometry results reveal the extent of the obstruction: FEV_1, 56% of predicted; $FEF_{25\%-75\%}$, 33% of predicted; and MVV, 52% of predicted. The FVC is relatively well preserved. It even increases by more than 12% and 200 ml after bronchodilator therapy. The $FEF_{25\%-75\%}$ must always be interpreted cautiously because it is variable even in normal subjects. The 95% confidence limits for this subject include values from 1.45 to 5.93 L/sec. (See Appendix B for predicted values and the standard error of estimate.) His $FEF_{25\%-75\%}$ is well below the lower limit. MVV is reduced as might be expected, almost exactly 35 times his FEV_1. This indicates that the patient made a consistent effort on both the FEV_1 and MVV.

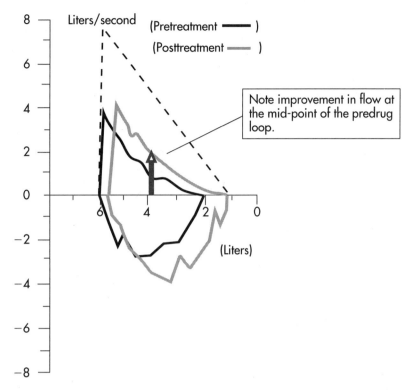

FIG. 2-21 *Case 2B.* Isovolume flow-volume loops. Each loop is plotted at the absolute lung volume at which it was measured. The increase in $FEF_{50\%}$ accurately describes the degree of bronchodilator response.

Raw is above the upper normal limit of 2.4 cm $H_2O/L/sec$. This is consistent with moderate airway obstruction and a productive cough. Specific conductance is low, consistent with increased Raw and increased lung volumes.

FEV_1 does not improve significantly after bronchodilator therapy. The $FEV_{1\%}$ actually decreases as a result of the greater increase in FVC. This pattern is not unusual in patients with obstructive airway disease. Airway resistance falls slightly with inhaled bronchodilator therapy. Most notably, SGaw improves by 57%. The large increase in conductance with only marginal change in flows suggests a shift in lung volumes. Fig. 2-21 shows F-V curves plotted at absolute lung volumes (measured in the body-box). Improvement in flows are evident by noting the curves at any particular lung volume.

Other postbronchodilator changes are also important. MVV improves by 20%. This may be related to a change in lung volume. The $FEF_{25\%-75\%}$ is hardly changed after bronchodilator therapy. This pattern is often seen when the FVC improves. A larger FVC means the time required to exhale the middle half of the breath may be longer. Because the $FEF_{25\%-75\%}$ depends on the FVC, the calculated flow may not improve; it may even go down.

3   **Other tests**

The lung function of this subject is common in both emphysema and chronic bronchitis. Air trapping is consistent with emphysematous changes but may be present in bronchitis and asthma during acute exacerbations. Further evaluation of R.Z. included lung volumes, DL_{CO}, and blood gases. All of these findings were consistent with those from simple spirometry. He had some air trapping, which might explain the improved FVC after bronchodilator therapy. Blood gases and diffusing capacity were relatively normal.

4   **Treatment**

A combination of bronchodilators were used. The patient was also referred to a counselor for smoking cessation and successfully quit smoking. Over 6 months his cough gradually subsided. The patient noted a marked improvement in his dyspnea.

CASE 2C

History

P.W. is a 27-year-old auto mechanic referred to the pulmonary function laboratory by his private physician. His chief complaint is "breathing problems." He describes breathlessness that occurs suddenly and then subsides. He has no other symptoms and no history of lung disease. None of his immediate family has any lung disease. He had smoked a pack of cigarettes a day for the last 10 years. He has no unusual environmental exposure. He claims that gasoline fumes sometimes bring on the episodes of shortness of breath.

Pulmonary Function Tests

Personal data

Sex: Male
Age: 27 yr
Height: 68 in
Weight: 150 lb

Spirometry

	Before drug	Predicted	% Predicted
FVC (L)	3.80	5.15	74
FEV_1 (L)	3.70	4.13	90
$FEV_{1\%}$ (%)	97	80	—
$FEF_{25\%-75\%}$(L/sec)	4.62	4.49	103
$FEF_{50\%}$(L/sec)	4.81	6.01	80
$FEF_{75\%}$(L/sec)	3.12	3.33	94
MVV (L/min)	77	146	53

Respiratory pressures

	Before drug	Predicted	% Predicted
MIP cm H_2O	118	128	92
MEP cm H_2O	57	240	24

Technologist's Comments

All FVC maneuvers were unacceptable; they did not last 6 seconds or plateau. Best FVC values were not within 200 ml. Inspiratory efforts were variable. A total of eight maneuvers were attempted. Respiratory pressure measurements were variable. Patient had difficulty completing all maneuvers.

Questions

1. Interpret the following:
    a. Spirometry
    b. Low value for MEP
    c. Variability of the patient's efforts
2. What is the cause of the patient's symptoms?
3. What other tests might be indicated?
4. What treatment might be recommended based on these findings?

Discussion

1 Interpretation

All spirometry maneuvers and respiratory pressures are unacceptable because of poor patient effort or technical errors. The patient's best effort shows a reduced FVC. The FEV_1 is normal and the $FEV_{1\%}$ is above the expected range. All other flows and the MVV are within normal limits.

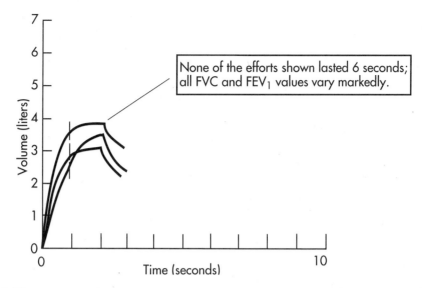

FIG. 2-22 *Case 2C.* Multiple FVC maneuvers are superimposed. None of the recorded efforts are acceptable.

Impression: Spirometry results are inconsistent. The FVC and FEV_1 are not reproducible. Inadequate subject effort or technical errors are present.

2 **Cause of symptoms**

This test shows poor reproducibility, especially for effort-dependent measurements. Fig. 2-22 shows the variability for three FVC maneuvers. The tracings show incomplete exhalations, as well as variability.

The low FVC seems to be consistent with a mild restrictive process. The FEV_1, however, is close to normal. If simple restriction were present, both FVC and FEV_1 would be expected to be reduced similarly. The subject's other flows are normal. Flows that depend on the FVC (e.g., the $FEF_{25\%-75\%}$) might also be in error if the FVC is incorrect. The FEV_1 and MVV do not depend on the FVC. The MVV is much less than 35 times the FEV_1, so the MVV is probably not accurate.

Because of the low MVV, respiratory pressures were measured. MIP appears to be normal but was variable. MEP was also performed variably. The best effort was only 24% of expected. Both MEP and MIP depend largely on patient effort.

Examination of the volume-time spirograms reveals that the subject terminated each FVC maneuver after approximately 2 seconds. The FVC values all varied by more than 200 ml, confirming poor subject cooperation. Lack of reproducibility of the FVC maneuvers is not sufficient reason for discarding the test results. This subject's FVC maneuvers lasted only 2 seconds, despite repeated coaching by the technologist. The efforts did not meet the criteria of continuing for at least 6 seconds or showing an obvious plateau.

The technologist performing the test repeated the FVC maneuver eight times. Only the three best efforts were recorded. Appropriate comments were added at the end of the test data. The poor quality of the data makes it impossible to determine whether the patient's symptoms are real. The patient appears to be malingering; that is, not giving maximal effort on tests that are effort dependent. Poor reproducibility in a subject who is free of symptoms at the time of the test suggests poor effort or lack of cooperation.

3 **Other tests**

Alternative tests that might be attempted should be independent of patient effort. A simple blood gas analysis was performed. The results indicated normal oxygenation and acid-base status. Testing of lung volumes and diffusing capacity was postponed because both of these depend on subject effort and cooperation. A **bronchochallenge** test (see Chapter 8) might have been indicated because the subject had asthma-like symptoms. However, bronchochallenge tests often use spirometry, which this subject was unable or unwilling to perform acceptably.

4 **Treatment**

Before suggesting any treatment, the referring physician contacted the subject's employer to ask about possible environmental hazards that might cause the symptoms. He learned that the subject was facing possible termination for excessive absence from work. The patient's supervisor revealed that the patient claimed to have asthma, which caused his excessive absenteeism.

SUMMARY

THIS CHAPTER HAS DESCRIBED THE most commonly performed pulmonary function study—spirometry. Various spirometry tests have been identified. Techniques for performing the tests and criteria for acceptability have been enumerated. Simple spirometry, F-V loops, and bronchodilator studies have been discussed. Differentiation between obstructive and restrictive disorders was made by explaining the pathophysiologies involved.

Other tests of respiratory mechanics have also been discussed. MVV, maximal respiratory pressures, airway resistance, and pulmonary compliance were related to diagnosis of various lung diseases. Interpretive strategies were presented. These strategies, in the form of questions, provide a systematic approach to understanding the implications of the test results.

Case studies, with representative data and graphics, are included to help relate the tests to real pulmonary disorders. Multiple-choice self-assessment questions and selected references follow.

SELF-ASSESSMENT QUESTIONS

1 *A subject who complains of shortness of breath has an FVC of 2.57 L, but her VC is 2.99 L. These findings suggest which of the following?*
   a. Pulmonary fibrosis
   b. Chest wall abnormality
   c. Emphysema
   d. Fixed upper airway obstruction

2 *A 47-year-old man with a history of cough has the following spirometry results:*

	Measured	Predicted
FVC (L BTPS)	3.85	4.01
FEV_1 (L BTPS)	2.14	3.33

These findings show the presence of which of the following?
   a. Reversible airway obstruction
   b. Moderate obstructive disease
   c. Normal lung function
   d. Incorrectly selected predicted values

3 *A 22-year-old patient with dyspnea performs three spirometry trials:*

	Trial 1	Trial 2	Trial 3
FVC (L BTPS)	4.21	4.44	4.65
FEV_1 (L BTPS)	3.88	3.91	3.93

The pulmonary function technologist should do which of the following?
   a. Report the values from trial 3
   b. Report the largest sum of FVC and FEV_1
   c. Average the data from trials 2 and 3
   d. Perform at least one more maneuver

4 *Why should all values from a series of peak flow measurements be reported?*
   a. PEF may decrease with repeated efforts.
   b. A minimum of 3 values must be averaged.
   c. Peak flow meters do not need to be precise.
   d. Forced exhalation produces a bronchodilator effect.

5 *The shape of the "effort-independent" portion of the expiratory F-V curve is determined by which of the following?*
   I.   Abdominal pressure during forced expiration
   II. Elastic recoil of the lung
   III. Flow resistance in the small airways
   IV. Cross-sectional area of the trachea
   a. I and II only
   b. II and III only
   c. I, III, and IV only
   d. IV only

6 *A patient being evaluated for disability has spirometry performed with the following results reported:*

	Measured	Predicted
FVC (L)	4.00	4.10
FEV_1 (L)	2.00	3.30
MVV (L/min)	105	110

What do these findings indicate?
   a. The patient has moderate obstructive disease.
   b. The patient has restriction.
   c. The patient's FEV_1 is larger than measured.
   d. The patient did not give a good effort on the MVV.

7 A patient with pulmonary fibrosis has a compliance study performed. Which of the following indicate that the esophageal balloon is placed correctly?

   a. No pressure change occurs during inspiration.
   b. Inspiration causes a negative pressure deflection.
   c. Cardiac pulsations are recorded by the pressure transducer.
   d. Only 0.5 ml of air are needed to inflate the catheter balloon.

8 A small leak is introduced into the breathing circuit during the measurement of MIP and MEP to do which of the following?

   a. Allow flow into the alveoli
   b. Prevent artifact caused by the cheek muscles
   c. Zero the pressure measuring apparatus before the maneuver
   d. Stabilize the chest wall during airway occlusion

9 A subject in a plethysmograph has his Raw measured as 2.2 cm H_2O/L/sec at a lung volume of 3.7 L. The calculated SGaw for this patient is which of the following?

   a. 0.59 cm H_2O/L/sec/L
   b. 0.45 cm H_2O/L/sec/L
   c. 0.27 cm H_2O/L/sec/L
   d. 0.12 cm H_2O/L/sec/L

10 Before bronchodilator studies, inhaled β-adrenergic agents should be withheld for how long?

   a. 0.5 to 1.5 hours unless corticosteroids are being used
   b. 8 to 12 hours for regular or long acting preparations
   c. 24 hours for most inhalers
   d. 24 to 48 hours

11 Which of the following is consistent with the flow-volume curve shown above, right?

   a. Normal forced expiratory flow pattern
   b. Variable intrathoracic obstruction
   c. Small airways obstruction
   d. Fixed large airway obstruction

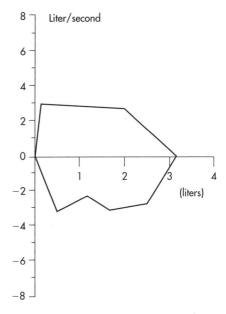

12 A subject has spirometry repeated before and after inhaled bronchodilators. The following data are obtained:

	Predicted	Before drug	After drug
FVC	5.20	4.90	5.30
FEV_1	4.10	3.10	3.30
PEF	9.20	7.77	8.92

Which of the following statements best describes these findings?

   a. There is mild obstruction with significant response to bronchodilators.
   b. There is mild obstruction without significant change after bronchodilator.
   c. There is a paradoxical response to bronchodilators.
   d. Spirometry is within normal limits.

SELECTED BIBLIOGRAPHY

General References

Crapo RO: Pulmonary function testing, *N Engl J Med* 331:25-30, 1994.

Kanner RE, Morris AH (ed): *Clinical pulmonary function testing,* ed 2, Salt Lake City, 1984, Intermountain Thoracic Society.

Forster RE: *The lung: clinical physiology and pulmonary function tests,* ed 3, St Louis, 1986, Mosby.

West JB: *Pulmonary pathophysiology—the essentials,* ed 4, Baltimore, 1992, Williams & Wilkins.

Spirometry

Dillard TA, Hnatiuk OW, McCumber TR: Maximum voluntary ventilation: spirometric determinants in chronic obstructive pulmonary disease patients and normal subjects, *Am Rev Respir Dis* 147:870-875, 1993.

Knudson, RJ, Lebowitz MD: Maximal mid-expiratory flow ($FEF_{25\%-75\%}$): normal limits and assessment of sensitivity, *Am Rev Respir Dis* 117:609, 1978.

Krowka MJ, Enright PL, Rodarte JR, et al: Effect of effort on measurement of forced expiratory volume in one second, *Am Rev Respir Dis* 136:829, 1987.

Leuallen EC, Fowler WS: Maximal midexpiratory flow, *Am Rev Tuberculosis* 72:783, 1955.

Sackner MA, Rao ASV, Birch S, et al: Assessment of time-volume and flow-volume components of forced vital capacity, *Chest* 82:272, 1982.

Smith AA, Gaensler EA: Timing of forced expiratory volume in one second, *Am Rev Respir Dis* 112:882, 1975.

Townsend MC, DuChene AG, Fallat RJ: The effects of underrecording forced expirations on spirometric lung function indexes, *Am Rev Respir Dis* 126:734, 1982.

Peak Expiratory Flow

Cross D, Nelson H: The role of the peak flow meter in the diagnosis and management of asthma, *J Allergy Clin Immunol* 87:120-128, 1991.

Lebowitz MD: The use of peak expiratory flow rate measurements in respiratory disease, *Pediatr Pulmonol* 11:166-174, 1991.

Nowak RM, Pensler MI, Sarkar DD, et al: Comparison of peak expiratory flow and FEV_1: admission criteria for acute bronchial asthma, *Ann Emerg Med* 11:64, 1982.

Before- and After-Bronchodilator Studies

Casaburi R, Adame D, Hong CK: Comparison of albuterol to isoproterenol as a bronchodilator for use in pulmonary function testing, *Chest* 100:1597-1600, 1991.

Dales RE, Spitzer WO, Tousignant P, et al: Clinical interpretation of airway response to a bronchodilator: epidemiologic considerations, *Am Rev Respir Dis* 138:317, 1988.

Guyatt GH, Townsend M, Nogradi S, et al: Acute response to bronchodilator, an imperfect guide for bronchodilator therapy in chronic airflow limitation, *Arch Intern Med* 148:1949, 1988.

Light RW, Conrad SA, George RB: The one best test for evaluating the effects of bronchodilator therapy, *Chest* 72:512, 1977.

Smith HR, Irvin CG, Cherniack RM: The utility of spirometry in the diagnosis of reversible airways obstruction, *Chest* 101:1577-1581, 1992.

Flow-Volume Curves

Acres J, Kryger M: Clinical significance of pulmonary function tests: upper airway obstruction, *Chest* 80:207, 1981.

Bass H: The flow volume loop: normal standards and abnormalities in chronic obstructive pulmonary disease, *Chest* 63:171, 1973.

Chan ED, Irvin CG: The detection of collapsible airways contributing to airflow limitation, *Chest* 107:856-859, 1995.

Haponik EF, Blecker ER, Allen RP, et al: Abnormal inspiratory flow-volume curves in patients with sleep disordered breathing, *Am Rev Respir Dis* 124:571, 1981.

Hyatt RE, Black LF: The flow volume curve, *Am Rev Respir Dis* 107:191, 1973.

Knudson RJ, Slatin RC, Lebowitz MD, et al: The maximal expiratory flow-volume curve: normal standards, variability and effects of age, *Am Rev Respir Dis* 113:587, 1976.

Knudson RJ, Lebowitz MD, Holberg CJ, et al: Changes in the normal maximal expiratory flow-volume curve with growth and aging, *Am Rev Respir Dis* 127:725, 1983.

Miller RD, Hyatt RE: Evaluation of obstructing lesions of the trachea and larynx by flow volume loops, *Am Rev Respir Dis* 108:475, 1973.

Maximal Respiratory Pressures

Arora NS, Rochester DF: Respiratory muscle strength and maximal voluntary ventilation in undernourished patients, *Am Rev Respir Dis* 126:5, 1982.

Black LF, Hyatt RE: Maximal static respiratory pressure in generalized neuromuscular disease, *Am Rev Respir Dis* 103:641, 1971.

Vincken GH, Cosio MG: Maximal static respiratory pressures in adults: normal values and their relationship to determinants of respiratory function, *Bull Eur Physiopathol Respir* 23:435, 1987.

Compliance and Airways Resistance

Baydur A, Behrakis PK, Zin WA, et al: A simple method for assessing the validity of the esophageal balloon technique, *Am Rev Respir Dis* 126:788, 1982.

Behrakis PK, Baydur A, Jaeger MJ, et al: Lung mechanics in sitting and horizontal body positions, *Chest* 83:643, 1983.

Dubois AB, Bothello SV, Comroe JH: A new method for measuring airway resistance in man using a body plethysmograph: values in normal subjects and in patients with respiratory disease, *J Clin Invest* 35:327, 1956.

National Heart and Lung Institute, Division of Lung Diseases: *Procedures for standardized measurements of lung mechanics: principles of body plethysmography,* Bethesda, Md, 1974, National Heart and Lung Institute, pp 1-21.

Standards and Guidelines

American Thoracic Society: Lung function testing: selection of reference values and interpretative strategies, *Am Rev Respir Dis* 144:1202, 1991.

American Thoracic Society: Standardization of spirometry: 1994 update, *Am J Respir Crit Care Med* 152:1107-1136, 1995.

American Association for Respiratory Care: Clinical practice guidelines: spirometry, *Respir Care* 36:1414-1417, 1991.

American Association for Respiratory Care: Clinical practice guidelines: body plethysmography, *Respir Care* 39:1184-1190, 1994.

American Association for Respiratory Care: Clinical practice guidelines: static lung volumes, *Respir Care* 39:830-836, 1993.

American Association for Respiratory Care: Clinical practice guidelines: assessing response to bronchodilator therapy at the point of care, *Respir Care* 40:1300-1307, 1995.

British Thoracic Society and the Association of Respiratory Technicians and Physiologists: Guidelines for the measurement of respiratory function, *Respir Med* 88:165-194, 1994.

National Asthma Education Program: *Expert panel report: guidelines for the diagnosis and management of asthma,* Bethesda, Md, 1991, Department of Health and Human Services (NIH Publication No. 91-3042A).

CHAPTER 3

Lung Volumes and Gas Distribution Tests

OBJECTIVES

After studying this chapter and reviewing its tables and case studies, you should be able to do the following:

1 Describe the measurement of lung volumes using the open- and closed-circuit methods

2 Explain the advantages of measuring lung volumes using the body plethysmograph

3 Calculate residual volume, total lung capacity, and related lung volumes from simple spirometric measures and functional residual capacity

4 Identify uneven distribution of gas in the lungs by either the single- or multiple-breath nitrogen techniques

THIS CHAPTER INTRODUCES THE measurement of lung volumes. Besides the gas that can be exhaled from the lungs (i.e., vital capacity), some gas remains in the lungs at all times. This gas volume must be measured indirectly. Several methods can accomplish this. Each method has advantages and disadvantages. Two of the methods involve having the patient breathe gases not normally present in the lungs: helium (He) (closed-circuit) or 100% oxygen (O_2) (open-circuit). A third method uses the body plethysmograph to measure the volume of thoracic gas (V_{TG}). The open- and closed-circuit techniques can also provide indices of gas distribution in the lungs. The usefulness of these indices has been reduced by the use of nuclear medicine imaging of the lungs, as well as computerized tomography (CT) and magnetic resonance imaging (**MRI**). These imaging techniques provide a direct view of gas distribution in the lungs. Nonetheless, gas distribution indices obtained during lung volume determination are often helpful.

LUNG VOLUMES

Functional Residual Capacity, Residual Volume, Total Lung Capacity, and Residual Volume/Total Lung Capacity Ratio

DESCRIPTION

Functional residual capacity (FRC) is the volume of gas remaining in the lungs at the end of a quiet breath. This point on a simple spirogram is termed the end-expiratory level (see Fig. 2-1). Residual volume (RV) is the volume of gas remaining in the lungs at the end of a maximal expiration (see Fig. 2-1). Total lung capacity (TLC) is the volume of gas contained in the lungs after maximal inspiration. FRC, TLC, and RV are reported in liters or milliliters, corrected to BTPS. The RV/TLC ratio defines the fraction of TLC that cannot be exhaled (RV), expressed as a percentage.

TECHNIQUE

Various methods of measuring lung volumes have been described (Table 3-1). Although some methods estimate TLC directly, FRC is usually measured. RV, which is a component of the FRC, is also measured indirectly. RV cannot be exhaled; it is the volume remaining in the alveoli after the

TABLE 3-1 Methods for Measurement of Lung Volumes

Method	Lung volume	Advantages/disadvantages
Closed-circuit (He dilution; multiple-breath)	FRC	Simple, relatively inexpensive; affected by distribution of ventilation in moderate or severe obstruction; requires IC, ERV to calculate other lung volumes
Open-circuit (multiple-breath N_2 washout)	FRC	Simple, relatively inexpensive; affected by distribution of ventilation in moderate or severe obstruction; requires IC, ERV to calculate other lung volumes
Single-breath N_2 washout	TLC	Calculated from single-breath N_2 distribution test; may underestimate lung volume in the presence of obstruction
Single-breath He dilution	TLC	Calculated as part of DL_{CO} (V_A); may underestimate lung volume in the presence of obstruction
Plethysmograph	V_{TG} (FRC)	Plethysmographic method somewhat complex; not affected by degree of airway obstruction
Chest x-ray	TLC	Requires posterior-anterior and lateral chest films; not accurate in the presence of diffuse, space-occupying diseases

N_2, Nitrogen; *IC*, inspiratory capacity; DL_{CO}, diffusing capacity; V_A, alveolar volume.

airways have closed. FRC is measured and then RV calculated by subtracting expiratory reserve volume (ERV) obtained from simple spirometry. The end-expiratory level is the point in the breathing cycle to which the lungs and chest wall recoil after a quiet breath. This point can be easily identified by watching the tidal breathing pattern using a spirometer. Measurements of FRC are usually started with the subject at the end-expiratory level.

There are two indirect methods of measuring FRC. Each of these methods uses a gas that is not normally present in the lungs. The open-circuit or nitrogen (N_2) washout method uses 100% O_2. The closed-circuit or He dilution technique uses a low concentration of He.

Open-Circuit Method (Multiple-Breath Nitrogen Washout)

The concentration of N_2 in the lungs is presumed to be between 75% and 80%. After the subject has breathed 100% O_2 for several minutes, the N_2 in the lungs can be gradually washed out. Because all N_2 cannot be washed out, the test is usually continued until the alveolar N_2 concentration is approximately 1%. Historically, all exhaled gas was collected in a spirometer or bag that had been flushed with O_2. The concentration of collected N_2 was then measured. The volume that was in the lungs at the end-expiratory level was then computed using the following formula:

$$FRC = \frac{FE N_{2final} \times \text{Expired volume} - N_{2tiss}}{FA N_{2alveolar1} - FA N_{2alveolar2}}$$

where:

$FE N_{2final}$ = fraction of N_2 in volume expired

$FA N_{2alveolar1}$ = fraction of N_2 in alveolar gas initially

$FA N_{2alveolar2}$ = fraction of N_2 in alveolar gas at end (determined from an alveolar sample)

N_{2tiss} = volume of N_2 washed out of blood/tissues

Corrections must be made for N_2 washed out of the blood and tissue. For each minute of O_2 breathing, approximately 30 to 40 ml of N_2 are removed from blood and tissue. Therefore, $N_{2tiss} = 0.04 \times T$ (where T is time of the test). This value was subtracted from the N_2 in the spirometer. Not all of the N_2 in the lungs may be washed out, even after 7 minutes of O_2 breathing. The $FA N_{2alveolar2}$ was measured by taking an alveolar sample near the end of the test. This value was subtracted from alveolar N_2 present at the beginning. The final FRC was then corrected to BTPS (see the Appendix).

To obtain RV, the ERV determined from a slow vital capacity maneuver (see Chapter 2) is subtracted from the FRC:

$$RV = FRC - ERV$$

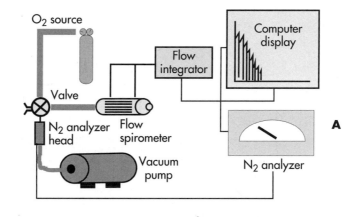

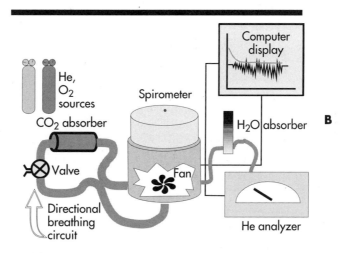

FIG. 3-1 *Open- and closed-circuit FRC systems.* **A,** Open-circuit equipment used for N_2 washout determination of FRC. The subject inspires O_2 from a regulated source and exhales past a rapidly responding N_2 analyzer into a pneumotachometer. Flow and gas concentration are integrated and displayed on a computer screen. FRC is calculated from the total volume of N_2 exhaled and the change in alveolar N_2 from the beginning to the end of the test (see Fig. 3-2 and text). **B,** Closed-circuit equipment used for He dilution FRC determination includes a volume-based spirometer with an He analyzer, CO_2 absorber, and a directional breathing circuit. A fan or blower promotes gas mixing within the rebreathing system. A breathing valve near the mouth allows the subject to be "switched in" to the system after He has been added and the system volume determined. The O_2 source allows the addition of O_2 during the test to replenish that taken up by the subject and to maintain a constant system volume. The CO_2 absorber permits rebreathing without accumulation of CO_2. Water vapor is removed by a chemical absorber before the gas is sampled by the He analyzer. Tidal breathing and the He dilution curve are displayed on the computer.

The method currently used for open-circuit FRC measurement uses a rapid N_2 analyzer in combination with a spirometer to provide a "breath-by-breath" analysis of expired N_2 (Fig. 3-1, *A*). The patient breathes through a mouthpiece-valve system. Precisely at end-expiration, a valve is opened to allow O_2 breathing to begin. Each breath of pure O_2 washes out some of the residual N_2 in the lungs. **Analog signals** proportional to N_2 concentration and volume (or flow) are integrated to derive the exhaled volume of N_2 for each breath. Values for each breath are summed to provide a total volume of N_2 washed out (Fig. 3-2). The test is continued until the N_2 in alveolar gas has been reduced to approximately 1% or for 7 minutes (Box 3-1). FRC is calculated by dividing the volume of N_2 washed out by the difference in N_2 concentration from the beginning to the end of the test. Corrections for N_2 excretion from tissue and blood as well as for BTPS are applied. If a filter is used, its volume should be subtracted from the FRC. A breath-by-breath plot of the %N_2 (or log %N_2) versus volume or number of breaths can be obtained to derive indices of the distribution of ventilation.

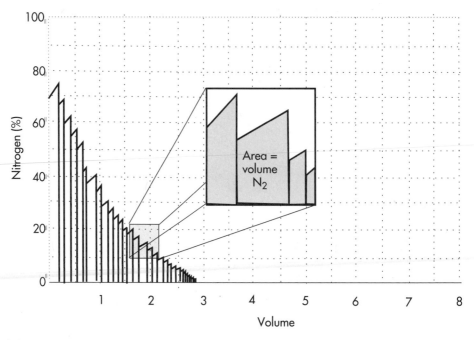

FIG. 3-2 *Open-circuit (N$_2$ washout) determination of FRC.* The concentration (or the log concentration) of N$_2$ is plotted against time or against the volume expired as the subject breathes through a circuit such as that in Fig. 3-1, *A.* The volume of N$_2$ expired with each breath is measured by integrating flow and N$_2$ concentration to determine the area under each curve (see *inset*). The volume of N$_2$ expired for each breath is summed. The test continues until most of the N$_2$ in the lung has been washed out (usually 1.5% or less). FRC is then determined by dividing the volume of N$_2$ expired by the change in alveolar N$_2$ from the beginning to the end of the test, with corrections, as described in the text.

BOX 3-1
CRITERIA FOR ACCEPTABILITY—N$_2$ WASHOUT FRC

1   The washout tracing or display should indicate a continually falling concentration of alveolar N$_2$.

2   The test should be continued until the N$_2$ concentration falls to 1.0%.

3   Washout times should be appropriate for the type of subject tested. Healthy subjects should wash out N$_2$ completely in 3 to 4 minutes.

4   The washout time should be reported. Failure to wash out N$_2$ within 7 minutes should be noted.

5   Multiple measurements should agree within 10%; the average FRC from acceptable trials should be used to calculate lung volumes. At least 15 minutes of room-air breathing should elapse between repeated trials.

Some pulmonary function systems use pneumotachometers that may be sensitive to the composition of expired gas (see Chapter 9). These devices correct for changes in the viscosity of the gas as O$_2$ replaces N$_2$ in the expirate. Such corrections are easily accomplished by software or electronic correction of the analyzer output.

Closed-Circuit Method (Multiple-Breath Helium Dilution)
FRC can also be calculated indirectly by diluting gas in the lungs with an inert gas. A spirometer is filled with a known volume of air, then He is added (Fig. 3-1, *B*). The volume of He is adjusted so that a concentration of approximately 10% is achieved. The exact concentration and volume are measured and recorded before the test is begun. The subject breathes through a valve that allows connection to the rebreathing system. The valve is opened at the end of a quiet breath (i.e., the end-expiratory level). Then the subject rebreathes the gas in the spirometer, with a **carbon dioxide (CO$_2$) absorber** in place, until the concentration of He falls to a stable level (Fig. 3-3). A fan or

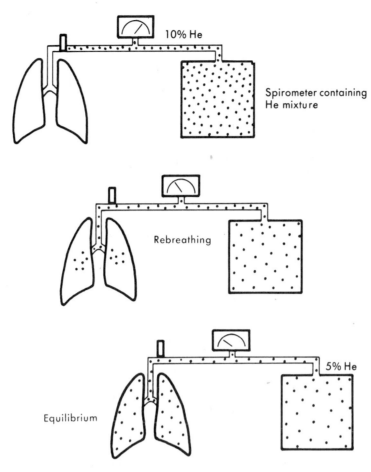

10% He

Spirometer containing
He mixture

Rebreathing

Equilibrium

5% He

FIG. 3-3 *Closed-circuit (He dilution) determination of FRC.* At the beginning of the test the subject's lungs contain no He. The subject then rebreathes a mixture of He and air or O_2 from a system such as that in Fig. 3-1, *B*. He is diluted until equilibrium is reached. The volume of He initially present and its concentration is known, and the volume of the rebreathing system can be calculated. At the end of the test the same volume of He has been diluted in the rebreathing system and the lungs. FRC is derived from the change in He concentration and the known system volume (see text). The patient must be switched from breathing air to the He mixture at the end-expiratory level for accurate measurement of FRC. RV is derived by subtracting the ERV. (Modified from Comroe JH Jr, Forster RE, Dubois AB, et al: *The lung: clinical physiology and pulmonary function tests,* ed 2, St Louis, 1962, Mosby.)

blower mixes the gas within the spirometer system. O_2 is added to the spirometer system to maintain the F_{IO_2} near or above 0.21 and to keep system volume relatively constant.

An older closed-circuit method (i.e., the **bolus** method) added a large volume of O_2 to the spirometer at the beginning of the procedure. The subject then rebreathed and gradually consumed the O_2. Because of the possibility of equilibrium not being attained before the added O_2 was depleted, this method is no longer commonly used.

Equilibration between normal lungs and the rebreathing system takes place in approximately 3 minutes when a 10% He mixture in a system volume of 6 to 8 L is used (Fig. 3-4). The final concentration of He is then recorded. The system volume is computed first. System volume is the volume of the spirometer, breathing circuitry, and valves before the patient is connected. It can be calculated as follows:

$$\text{System volume (L)} = \frac{\text{He}_{\text{added}} \text{ (L)}}{F_{\text{He initial}}}$$

where:

$$\text{He}_{\text{added}} = \text{volume of He placed in the spirometer}$$

$$F_{\text{He initial}} = \%\text{He converted to a fraction (\%He/100)}$$

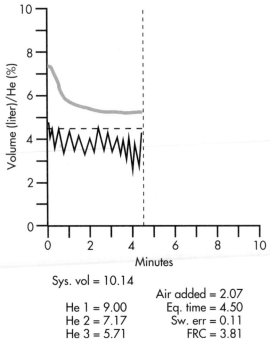

Sys. vol = 10.14

He 1 = 9.00   Air added = 2.07
He 2 = 7.17   Eq. time = 4.50
He 3 = 5.71   Sw. err = 0.11
                           FRC = 3.81

FIG. 3-4 *Computer-generated recording of a closed-circuit FRC determination on a healthy subject.* The upper line on the graph displays concentration of He from the beginning of rebreathing until equilibrium is achieved. The lower line shows the "system volume" of the spirometer and the subject's tidal breathing. A CO_2 absorber removes carbon dioxide produced by the subject, and a computerized valve system replaces O_2 to keep the system volume constant.

When the system volume is known, FRC can be computed as follows:

$$FRC = \frac{(\%He_{initial} - \%He_{final})}{\%He_{final}} \times System\ volume$$

Either percent or **fractional** concentration of He may be used because the term is a ratio.

Some automated systems use a similar method to calculate the system volume; a small amount of He is added to the closed system, followed by a known volume of air. The change in He concentration after the addition of the air is used to determine the system volume. Rebreathing is continued until the He concentration changes by no more than 0.02% over 30 seconds (Box 3-2).

Several corrections are often made to the FRC value obtained by He dilution. A small volume of He dissolves in the subject's blood during the test. As a result, the final He reading is less than it would be due solely to dilution by the subject's FRC. Loss of He to the blood results in a slight increase in the apparent FRC. A volume of 100 ml is usually subtracted from the FRC to correct for this effect. The dead space volume of the breathing valve should also be subtracted from the measured FRC. If a filter is used its volume should also be subtracted.

Most manufacturers provide "switch-in" error correction when the subject begins the test at a point either above or below the actual end-expiratory level (FRC). This type of correction is used for both open- and closed-circuit systems. Depending on the the subject's breathing pattern, a volume difference of several hundred milliliters may result. The effect of the switch-in error may be insignificant, especially with the closed-circuit method. Equilibrium does not occur instantaneously at switch-in. The total volume of spirometer and lungs is constantly changing with tidal breathing, removal of CO_2, and addition of O_2. If the switch-in error is large or the end-expiratory level appears to change during the maneuver, the test may need to be repeated.

In both the open- and closed-circuit techniques, RV is measured indirectly as a subdivision of the FRC. This method is preferred because the resting end-expiratory level depends less on subject effort than maximal inspiration or expiration. The end-expiratory level (and the ERV) must be accurately measured. If tidal breathing is irregular, ERV may be overestimated or underestimated. Subtraction of an ERV value that is too large from the FRC will cause the RV to appear smaller than it actually is. Similarly, a small ERV will produce a larger than actual

---

BOX 3-2
CRITERIA FOR ACCEPTABILITY—He DILUTION FRC

1 A tracing or display of spirometer volume should indicate that no leaks are present (system baseline flat). He concentration should be stable before testing.

2 The rebreathing pattern should be regular. If recorded, successive tidal breaths should show a gradually falling **end-tidal** level as O_2 is consumed. Addition of O_2 should return breathing to close to the system baseline.

3 The test should be continued until the He readings change by less than 0.02% in 30 seconds or until 10 minutes has elapsed.

4 Addition of O_2 should be appropriate for quiet tidal breathing (i.e., 200-400 ml/min).

5 The He equilibration curve, if plotted or displayed should show a smooth and regular fall of He concentration until equilibrium is achieved.

6 Multiple measurements of FRC should agree within 10%; the average of acceptable multiple measurements should be reported.

RV. The subject's tidal breathing pattern must be carefully monitored during the vital capacity (VC) measurement (see Chapter 2).

The accuracy of the open- and closed-circuit techniques depends on all parts of the lung being well ventilated. In subjects who have obstructive disease, some lung units are poorly ventilated. In these patients it is often difficult to wash N_2 out or mix He to a stable level in poorly ventilated parts of the lungs. FRC, RV, and TLC may all be underestimated, usually in proportion to the degree of obstruction. Extending the time of these tests improves their accuracy. However, prolonging the test may not measure completely trapped gas, as found in **bullous** emphysema. Repeated measurements may be indicated to obtain an average value for FRC. With either method there should be an adequate delay between tests. For He dilution, at least 5 minutes should elapse between repeated tests. For N_2 washout, at least 15 minutes of air breathing between tests is recommended.

In either the open- or closed-circuit techniques, a leak will cause erroneous estimates of FRC. Leaks may occur in breathing valves or circuitry or at the subject connection. Some patients have difficulty maintaining an adequate seal at the mouthpiece throughout the test. Failure to properly apply nose clips can also result in a leak. Leaks usually result in an overestimate of lung volume. A leak in an open-circuit system allows room air to enter, increasing the volume of N_2 to be washed out. A leak in a closed-circuit system allows air to dilute the He concentration or He to escape. Each situation causes the test gas concentration to change more than it should. Leaks can usually be identified by inspection of the graphic display or recording (Fig. 3-5). Inaccuracy or malfunction of the gas analyzers in either method are often the cause of errors. Leaks or analyzer problems should be considered whenever FRC values are inconsistent with spirometry results.

Total Lung Capacity and Residual Volume/Total Lung Capacity Ratio

TLC is calculated combining other lung volume measurements. The two most common are as follows:

$$TLC = RV + VC$$

$$TLC = FRC + IC$$

Each method requires accurate measurement of the subdivisions of the VC. TLC can also be calculated using single-breath techniques (i.e., single-breath He dilution or single-breath N_2 washout). Single-breath measurements of lung volumes are usually done as part of other tests, such as the DL_{CO} (diffusing capacity) (see Chapter 5). Single-breath lung volume determinations correlate well with multiple-breath techniques in healthy subjects. However, single-breath lung volume determinations tend to underestimate true values in moderate to severe obstruction. TLC can also be estimated from chest x-ray examination.

The RV/TLC ratio is calculated by dividing the RV by the TLC. This ratio is expressed as a percentage. Either **ATPS** or BTPS values may be used in the ratio, but both RV and TLC must be expressed in the same units.

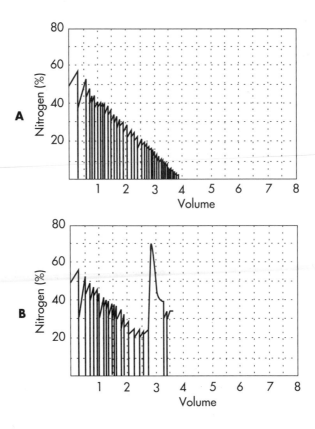

FIG. 3-5 *Open-circuit* N_2 *washout tracings.* **A,** A computer-generated recording of an N_2 washout test in a healthy subject. The tracings show a continuous decrease in end-tidal N_2 concentration with successive breaths. The test is continued until the N_2 concentration falls to less than 1%. **B,** A similar plot of N_2 washout from a healthy subject, but in this instance a leak develops during the test. Leaks may occur if the patient does not maintain a tight seal at the mouthpiece. Leaks are usually easy to detect because room air enters the system and indicates an abrupt increase in N_2 concentration.

The FRC, RV, and TLC should be reported at BTPS. Barrier filters may be used during lung volume determinations, particularly in rebreathing systems. If a filter is used, its volume must be subtracted from the lung volume measured. Sample calculations of both the open- and closed-circuit techniques can be found in Appendix F.

SIGNIFICANCE AND PATHOPHYSIOLOGY

See Box 3-3 for interpretive strategies. FRC varies with body size, with change in body position, and with time of day (i.e., diurnal variation). As with other lung volumes, normal FRC may be affected by racial or ethnic background. Equations for calculating expected FRC are found in Appendix B.

Increased FRC is considered pathologic. FRC values greater than approximately 120% of predicted values represent air trapping. Air trapping may result from emphysematous changes or from obstruction caused by asthma or bronchitis (see Chapter 1). Compensation for surgical removal of lung tissue or thoracic deformity can also cause increased FRC. Elevated FRC usually results in muscular and mechanical inefficiency. As lung volume increases, the chest wall and lungs themselves become "stiffer." This causes an increase in the work of breathing. FRC can increase dynamically; patients with airway obstruction may increase their end-expiratory lung volume **(EELV)** during exercise (see Chapter 7). This change in lung volume with increased ventilatory demand often results in a sensation of breathlessness.

Increased RV indicates that despite maximal expiratory effort, the lungs still contain an abnormally large volume of gas. Elevated RV may occur during an acute asthmatic episode but is usually reversible. Increased RV is characteristic of emphysema and bronchial obstruction; both may cause chronic air trapping. RV and FRC usually increase together. As RV becomes larger, more ventilation is needed to adequately exchange O_2 and CO_2 in the lung. This requires an increase in

```
BOX 3-3
INTERPRETIVE STRATEGIES—He DILUTION FRC
```

1   Was the FRC determination performed acceptably? Were multiple trials performed? If so, were they within 10%?

2   Was the VC maneuver acceptable? Were the ERV and inspiratory capacity (IC) measurements within 5% or 60 ml?

3   Were other lung volumes calculated appropriately (TLC, RV)?

4   Are the reference values appropriate? Age, height, sex, race?

5   Is the TLC less than the lower limit of normal? If so, restriction is present. Are other lung volumes (FRC, RV) reduced in similar proportion?

6   Is the TLC greater than the upper limit of normal? If so, suspect hyperinflation.

7   Is the RV/TLC ratio greater than predicted (≈35%)? Is the TLC normal or increased? If both are true, suspect air trapping.

8   Are lung volumes consistent with spirometric findings in regard to obstruction or restriction? Are they consistent with the history and physical findings?

9   Are additional tests indicated (plethysmographic lung volumes)?

TABLE 3-2   Comparative Lung Volumes for a Healthy Adult Man and Subjects with Air Trapping, Hyperinflation, and Restriction

Value	Normal	Air trapping	Hyperinflation	Restriction
VC (L)	4.80	3.00	4.80	3.00
FRC (L)	2.40	3.60	3.60	1.50
RV (L)	1.20	3.00	3.00	0.75
TLC (L)	6.00	6.00	7.80	3.75
RV/TLC (%)	20	50	38	20

tidal volume, respiratory rate, or both. Because of altered pressure-volume characteristics of the lung, work of breathing is also increased. Subjects with increased RV often display gas exchange abnormalities such as hypoxemia or CO_2 retention.

FRC, RV, and TLC are typically decreased in restrictive diseases (see Chapter 1). Decreased lung volumes are seen in interstitial diseases associated with extensive fibrosis (e.g., sarcoidosis, asbestosis, and complicated silicosis). Restrictive disorders affecting the chest wall include kyphoscoliosis, neuromuscular disorders, and obesity. Diseases that impair the diaphragm often result in reduced lung volumes, particularly TLC. Lung volumes may also be decreased in diseases that occlude many alveoli, such as pneumonia. Congestive heart failure causes pulmonary congestion, which can also reduce the lung volume. Any disease process that occupies volume in the thorax can reduce lung volume. Examples include tumors and pleural effusions.

Table 3-2 lists typical values for lung volumes for a healthy adult man, a patient with air trapping (as in emphysema), another with hyperinflation, and one with restriction (as in sarcoidosis). Restrictive processes usually cause lung volumes to be reduced equally. Proportional relationships between lung volume compartments, such as the RV/TLC ratio, may be relatively normal in restrictive diseases.

In obstruction, two different patterns may be observed. RV is almost always increased. This increase may be at the expense of a reduction in VC (Fig. 3-6), with TLC remaining close to normal. In other cases, RV may increase while VC is preserved, so TLC is greater than predicted. The term *air trapping* is sometimes used to describe an increase in FRC and RV, and the term *hyperinflation* is used to describe the absolute increase in TLC. TLC may be either normal or increased in obstructive processes such as asthma, chronic bronchitis, bronchiectasis, cystic

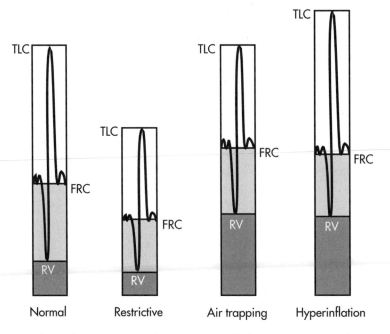

FIG. 3-6 *Lung volume changes in normal, restrictive, and obstructive patterns.* A comparison of the changes in lung volume compartments and VC (superimposed) shows the following: in restrictive patterns FRC, RV, and VC are all decreased proportionately, resulting in a decrease in the TLC, which defines restriction (see text). In obstruction (with air trapping) FRC and RV are both increased at the expense of the VC, and hence TLC remains relatively unchanged. Similar increases in RV and FRC may occur without reduction of VC, in which case the TLC increases (hyperinflation).

fibrosis, and emphysema. TLC does not change dynamically, even though FRC may increase acutely during exercise.

TLC may be decreased by processes that occupy space in the lungs such as edema, atelectasis, neoplasms, or fibrotic lesions. Other diseases that commonly result in decreased TLC include pulmonary congestion, pleural effusions, pneumothorax, or thoracic deformities. Pure restrictive defects show proportional decreases in most lung compartments as described for FRC and RV. When the TLC value is less than 80% of predicted or less than the 95% confidence limit, a restrictive process should be suspected. Reduced VC along with a normal or increased FEV_1/FVC ratio (see Chapter 2) is suggestive of restriction. If there is a contradiction between VC and TLC in defining restriction, the classification should be based on the TLC.

The RV/TLC ratio describes the percentage of total lung volume that must be ventilated by tidal breathing. In healthy adults the RV/TLC ratio may vary from 20% to 35%. Values greater than 35% may result from absolute increases of RV (as in emphysema) or from a decrease in TLC because of a loss of VC. A large RV/TLC in the presence of increased TLC is often indicative of hyperinflation. An increased RV/TLC with a normal TLC indicates that air trapping is present.

Thoracic Gas Volume

DESCRIPTION

The thoracic gas volume (VTG) is the gas contained in the thorax whether in communication with patent airways or trapped in any compartment of the thorax. VTG is usually measured at the end-expiratory level and is then equal to FRC. It may also be measured at other lung volumes and then corrected to relate to FRC. The VTG is reported in liters or milliliters, BTPS.

TECHNIQUE

VTG is measured using the body plethysmograph (Fig. 3-7). The technique is based on Boyle's law relating pressure to volume. A volume of gas varies in inverse proportion to the pres-

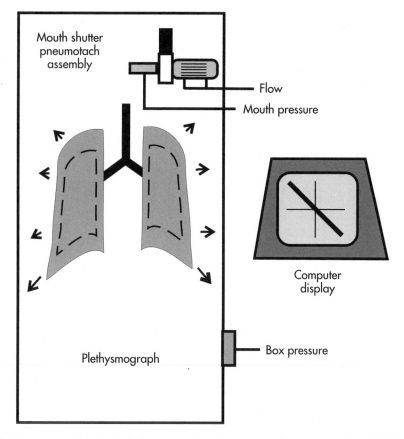

FIG. 3-7 *Components of the body plethysmograph used to measure thoracic gas volume (V$_{TG}$).* Boyle's law states that the volume varies inversely with the pressure if the temperature is held constant. A pressure-type plethysmograph, with pressure transducers for measurements of box pressure and mouth (alveolar) pressure is shown. The mouth shutter momentarily occludes the airway so that alveolar pressure can be estimated. The subject pants gently against the closed shutter. Gas in the lungs is alternately compressed and decompressed. Changes in lung volume are reflected by changes in box pressure. These changes are displayed as a sloping line on a computer display. When the original pressure (P), the new pressure (P'), and the new volume (V' or V + ΔV) are known, the original volume (V or V$_{TG}$) can be computed from Boyle's law (see text and Appendix E).

sure to which it is subjected if the temperature remains constant. The subject has an unknown volume of gas in the thorax (i.e., the FRC). The airway is momentarily occluded, allowing the subject to compress and decompress gas in the chest by breathing in and out against the occlusion. This causes a new volume and pressure to be generated. The changes in pressure are easily measured at the airway with a pressure transducer. Mouth pressure theoretically equals alveolar pressure when there is no airflow. Changes in pulmonary gas volume are measured by monitoring pressure changes in the plethysmograph (see Chapter 9). The pressure in the plethysmograph (sometimes called a body-box) is measured by a sensitive transducer. This transducer is calibrated by introducing a small, known volume of gas into the sealed box and expressing the pressure change as an index of volume. The calibration factor is then applied to measurements made on human subjects.

In the plethysmograph, the subject pants while the airway is momentarily occluded by an electrical shutter. Gas within the chest is alternately compressed and decompressed by the action of the ventilatory muscles. When flow is blocked by the shutter, mouth pressure theoretically equals alveolar pressure. Mouth pressure (P$_{MOUTH}$) is plotted on the vertical axis of a computer display. At the same time, box pressure (P$_{BOX}$) is plotted on the horizontal axis (see Fig. 3-7). Pressure changes on each axis are graphed continuously. The resulting figure appears as a sloping line, which is equal to ΔP/ΔV, where ΔP equals change in alveolar pressure and ΔV equals change in alveolar volume. Change in alveolar volume is measured indirectly by noting the reciprocal change in plethysmograph volume.

The V$_{TG}$ can then be obtained from the slope of the tracing by applying a derivation of Boyle's law:

$$V_{TG} = \frac{P_B}{\lambda V_{TG}} \times \frac{P_{BOX}cal}{P_{MOUTH}cal} \times K$$

where:

V$_{TG}$ = thoracic gas volume

P$_B$ = barometric pressure minus water vapor pressure

λV$_{TG}$ = slope of the displayed line equal to $\Delta P/\Delta V$

P$_{BOX}$cal = box pressure transducer calibration factor

P$_{MOUTH}$cal = mouth pressure transducer calibration factor

K = correction factor for volume displaced by the subject

For the complete derivation of the equation and sample calculations, see Appendixes E and F.

These measurements are usually made with the subject panting shallowly at a rate of 1 to 2 breaths/sec (i.e., 1 to 2 Hz) with an open **glottis**. Panting allows small pressure changes to be recorded near FRC. It also eliminates some artifact related to gas temperature and saturation. Some plethysmograph systems allow V$_{TG}$ measurements by occluding the airway during normal breathing without panting. If the mouth shutter is closed at precisely end-expiration, V$_{TG}$ equals FRC. Several panting efforts are recorded to obtain an average for the slope of $\Delta P/\Delta V$. The averaged slope is then used in the previous equation to derive the V$_{TG}$.

Computerized plethysmograph systems permit monitoring of tidal breathing in conjunction with the V$_{TG}$ maneuver. Instantaneous changes in lung volume can be monitored by continuously integrating the flow through the plethysmograph's pneumotachometer. The end-expiratory level can be determined from tidal breathing. The subject then pants with the shutter open. The computer records the change in lung volume above or below the resting level (i.e., FRC). When asked to pant, most subjects do so slightly above FRC. The mouth shutter then closes automatically, the subject continues panting, and V$_{TG}$ is measured as described. The computer then adds or subtracts the change in volume from the end-expiratory level (before panting began) to calculate the true FRC. This computerized technique allows the subject to pant at the correct frequency and depth before the shutter is closed. It also eliminates the necessity of closing the shutter precisely at end-expiration. Airway resistance (Raw) and conductance (SGaw) can also be measured simultaneously during the open-shutter panting (see Chapter 2).

A VC maneuver along with it subdivisions—ERV and IC—should be performed during the same testing session. Most plethysmograph systems allow these measurements using the built-in pneumotachometer. The same standards for accuracy should be applied to a slow VC measured in the plethysmograph as for any other spirometer. When FRC has been determined, the remaining lung volumes can be calculated as described for the open- or closed-circuit techniques.

Measurement of V$_{TG}$ is a complex procedure. Each patient must be carefully instructed in the required maneuvers. This is best done by allowing the subject to sit in the box with the door open. A few subjects may experience **claustrophobia** in the plethysmograph. The panting maneuver should be demonstrated by the technologist and then practiced by the subject. The subject should be instructed to place both hands against the cheeks. This prevents unwanted pressure changes in the mouth when the subject pants against the closed shutter. If practical, the shutter may be closed so that the patient knows what to expect during the test. The door of the plethysmograph can then be closed. The patient should understand that the plethysmograph can be opened if he or she becomes uncomfortable. Most systems allow the patient to open the door from within the box. If the plethysmograph is equipped with a communication device, it should be adjusted so the patient can hear instructions.

Depending on the construction of the plethysmograph, venting to the atmosphere is usually required to establish thermal equilibrium. Equilibrium can be presumed when the flow-volume recording stabilizes (i.e., does not **drift**). The subject is then instructed to pant at a frequency of approximately 1 Hz (i.e., once per second). When the correct panting frequency and depth have been established, the shutter may be closed. Some plethysmograph systems do this automatically. The subject should be allowed to pant against the closed shutter until a stable tracing is produced. If the subject pants too hard, the tracing may drift or appear as an "open" loop (Fig. 3-8). The

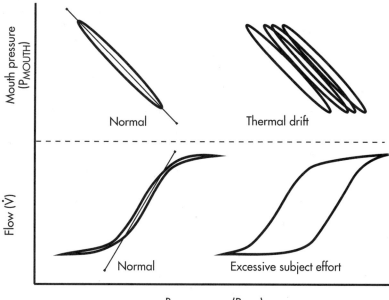

FIG. 3-8 *Normal and abnormal plethysmograph recordings. Top,* A normal closed-shutter maneuver in which mouth pressure is plotted against box pressure. The loop should be closed, or nearly so. If thermal equilibrium has not been reached the loop tends to be open and to drift across the screen. *Bottom,* A normal open-shutter measurement in which flow is plotted against box pressure. If the subject pants near FRC the loop takes on a nearly closed S-shaped appearance. If the subject pants too rapidly or too deeply, the tracing becomes open and flattened. Thermal drift can also cause the open-shutter tracing to resemble excessive patient effort.

BOX 3-4
CRITERIA FOR ACCEPTABILITY—VTG

1   The panting maneuver shows a closed loop without drift or other artifact.

2   Pressure changes are within calibration ranges; the tracing does not go off screen.

3   Panting frequency is approximately 1 Hz, preferably recorded.

4   Tangents or angles should agree within 10%; if shutter was closed at a volume other than FRC, calculated FRC values should be within 10%.

5   Reported VTG is averaged from 3 to 5 acceptable panting maneuvers.

---

recorded pressure changes should be within the range over which the transducers were calibrated. The entire tracing should be visible on the display. If the tracing goes off screen the pressure changes probably exceed the calibration ranges.

Three or more tangents (slopes) should be recorded (Box 3-4). These tangents should agree within 10% of the mean. Most computerized plethysmographs automatically measure the slope of the $\Delta P/\Delta V$ tracings. This is done by using least-squares **regression** to calculate "best-fit" line through the recorded data points. The technologist may need to correct computer-generated tangents, depending on data quality from the panting maneuvers. If the shutter is closed at volumes other than FRC, the tangents may vary by more than 10%. However, derived lung volumes (i.e., the FRC) should be within 10%.

It should be noted in the technologist's comments whether the subject cannot perform at least three acceptable maneuvers. VTG should be determined from three or more acceptable maneuvers. If the tangents or volumes vary by more than 10%, this too should be noted. It is often useful to compare lung volumes determined by two or more methods. The difference between lung volume (FRC) measured using the plethysmograph and either the open- or closed-circuit methods may be used as an index of gas trapping. In patients with airway obstruction, this difference can be significant. Plethysmographic lung volumes are usually larger in these subjects.

SIGNIFICANCE AND PATHOPHYSIOLOGY

See Box 3-5 for interpretive strategies. The V_{TG} is a quick and precise means of measuring lung volumes. It can be used in combination with simple spirometry to derive all lung volume compartments. The plethysmograph's primary advantage is that it measures all gas in the thorax, whether in ventilatory communication with the atmosphere or not. The plethysmographic measurement of FRC is often larger than that measured by He dilution or N_2 washout. This is the case in emphysema and other diseases characterized by air trapping, as well as in the presence of uneven distribution of ventilation. When open- or closed-circuit tests are continued for more than 7 minutes, the results for FRC determinations approach the V_{TG} value.

It is often useful to compare FRC values obtained by plethysmography with values obtained by gas dilution methods, particularly in subjects with obstructive disease. The ratio of FRC_{BOX}/FRC_{GAS} can be used as an index of gas trapping. This ratio is usually near 1.0 in subjects with normal lungs or even with restriction. Values greater than 1 indicate gas volumes detectable by the plethysmograph but hidden to the gas techniques. Care must be taken that lung volumes determined by the two separate methods are reliable before the values can be expressed as a ratio. This ratio has been used to evaluate candidates for **lung reduction** surgery. Lung reduction attempts to directly reduce gas trapping by removal of unperfused lung tissue. Patients with bullous emphysema may have 1 L or more difference in TLC when the methods are compared.

Some evidence suggests that in severe airways obstruction, FRC may actually be overestimated when plethysmographic technique is used. This occurs primarily because P_{MOUTH} (measured when the shutter is closed) may not equal alveolar pressure if the airways are severely obstructed. Rapid panting rates aggravate this inaccuracy. Care should be taken that patients with spirometric evidence of obstruction pant at a rate of 1 Hz.

Spirometry (e.g., FVC, FEV_1, VC) may be performed with the subject in the plethysmograph. The pneumotachometer must be capable of accurately measuring the entire range of gas flows required (i.e., up to 12 L/sec). For constant-volume plethysmographs, spirometry is done with the door open. Flow-based plethysmographs (see Chapter 9) have the advantage of allowing forced spirometry with the door closed. Flow boxes also allow a slightly different type of flow-volume curve to be recorded. Normal spirometry plots airflow at the mouth against volume at the mouth (as detected by the spirometer). With the subject in a flow box, flow at the mouth can be plotted against actual lung volume changes as detected by the box. This may be particularly useful in subjects with severe airways obstruction. It is possible to detect a significant compression volume during forced expiration and plot it against the flow generated. Spirometry, lung volumes, and airways resistance (see Chapter 2) can all be obtained in a single sitting using either type of plethysmograph.

BOX 3-5
INTERPRETIVE STRATEGIES—V_{TG}

1   Were the panting maneuvers performed acceptably? Was the panting frequency appropriate (1 Hz)? If not, interpret results cautiously.

2   Were at least three maneuvers averaged to obtain V_{TG} or FRC? Were individual values reproducible (within 10%)? If not, interpret cautiously.

3   Are reference values appropriate? Age, height, weight, race? Were they obtained plethysmographically?

4   Were other lung volumes (TLC) calculated appropriately? Were VC, ERV, and IC acceptable? If not, evaluate only FRC.

5   If the TLC is less than the lower limit of normal, suspect restriction.

6   If the TLC is greater than upper limit of normal, suspect hyperinflation.

7   Are lung volumes consistent with spirometric findings? If not, evaluate carefully for combined obstruction and restriction.

GAS DISTRIBUTION TESTS

Single-Breath Nitrogen Washout, Closing Volume, and Closing Capacity

DESCRIPTION

The single-breath nitrogen washout test (SBN_2), also called the SBO_2 or Fowler's test, measures the distribution of ventilation. Distribution is analyzed by measuring the change in N_2 concentration during expiration of the VC after a single breath of 100% O_2. Evenness of distribution is assessed by two parameters: the change in percentage of N_2 between the 750 to 1250 ml portion of the SBN_2 test ($\Delta\%N_2$ $_{750-1250}$) and the slope of Phase III. Each of these indices is recorded as percentage of change per unit of lung volume.

Closing volume (**CV**) is the portion of the VC that can be exhaled from the lungs after the on-set of airway closure. CV is usually expressed as a percentage of the VC. A related measurement, **closing capacity** (CC), is the sum of the CV and RV. CC is expressed as a percentage of the TLC.

TECHNIQUE

The test is performed with equipment similar to that used for the open-circuit FRC determination (see Fig. 3-1, *A*). The subject exhales to RV, then inspires a VC breath of 100% O_2 from a reservoir or demand valve. Without holding the breath, the subject exhales slowly and evenly at a flow of 0.3 to 0.5 L/sec. The N_2 analyzer monitors the N_2 concentration of the expired gas while the exhaled volume is measured by the spirometer. Volume expired is plotted against N_2 concentration on a graph (Fig. 3-9). This washout curve can be divided into four phases:

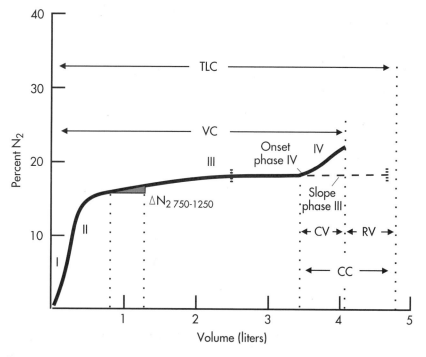

FIG. 3-9 *Single-breath nitrogen elimination (SBN$_2$).* A plot of the increasing N_2 concentration on expiration after a single vital capacity breath of 100% O_2. The curve is divided into four phases. *Phase I* is the extreme beginning of the expiration when only O_2 is being exhaled. *Phase II* shows an abrupt rise in N_2 concentration as mixed bronchial and alveolar air is expired. *Phase III* is the alveolar gas plateau, and N_2 concentration changes slowly as long as ventilation is uniformly distributed. *Phase IV* is an abrupt increase in N_2 concentration as basal airways close and a larger proportion of gas comes from the N_2-rich lung apices. Several useful parameters are derived from the SBN$_2$ tracing. The ΔN_2 $_{750-1250}$ and slope of Phase III are indices of the evenness of ventilation distribution. CV can be read directly from the onset of Phase IV until RV is reached; VC can also be read directly. RV, TLC, and CC can be calculated if the area under the curve is determined either by planimetry or electronic integration (see text).

Phase I: upper airway gas (from the **anatomic dead space** [VD]) consisting of 100% O_2

Phase II: mixed VD gas in which the relative concentrations of O_2 and N_2 change abruptly as the anatomic VD volume is expired

Phase III: a plateau caused by the exhalation of alveolar gas in which relative O_2 and N_2 concentrations change slowly and evenly

Phase IV: an abrupt increase in the concentration of N_2 that continues until RV is reached

The initial 750 ml of expired gas contains dead space gas from Phases I and II and is not used to assess distribution of ventilation. The difference in N_2 concentration between the 750 ml and 1250 ml points is called the delta N_2 ($\Delta\%N_{2\ 750-1250}$).

The slope of Phase III is the change in N_2 concentration from the point at which 30% of the VC remains up to the onset of Phase IV. It is recorded as $\Delta\%N_2$ per liter of lung volume.

The volume expired from the onset of Phase IV to the end of the breath is the CV. CV may be added to the RV, if the RV has been determined, and expressed as the CC. CV is reported as a percentage of the VC:

$$\frac{CV}{VC} \times 100$$

CC is recorded as a percentage of the TLC:

$$\frac{CC}{TLC} \times 100$$

TLC can be determined from the SBN$_2$ test by integrating the area of the washout curve. When the volume of N_2 is known, a dilution equation can be used to calculate RV. RV is then added to the measured VC to derive TLC. RV is calculated as follows:

$$RV = VC \times \frac{F\bar{E}N_2}{F_AN_2 - F\bar{E}N_2}$$

where:

$F\bar{E}N_2$ = mean expired N_2 concentration determined by **integration** of the area under the curve

F_AN_2 = N_2 concentration in the lungs at the beginning of inspiration, approximately 0.75 to 0.79

This method is accurate only in subjects who do not have significant obstructive or dead space–producing disease. CV and CC measurements may be in error if the subject does not perform an acceptable VC maneuver (Box 3-6). The inspired and expired VC should be within 5%. The VC during the SBN$_2$ should match the FVC or VC within 5% or 200 ml. Expiratory flow should be maintained between 0.3 and 0.5 L/sec.

SIGNIFICANCE AND PATHOPHYSIOLOGY

See Box 3-7 for interpretive strategies.

$\Delta N_{2\ 750-1250}$

The normal $\Delta\%N_{2\ 750-1250}$ is 1.5% or less for healthy young adults and slightly higher for healthy older adults (up to approximately 3%). Increased $\Delta\%N_{2\ 750-1250}$ is found in diseases characterized by uneven distribution of gas during inspiration or unequal emptying rates during expiration. In subjects with severe emphysema, $\Delta\%N_{2\ 750-1250}$ may exceed 10%.

BOX 3-6
CRITERIA FOR ACCEPTABILITY—SBN$_2$

1 Inspired and expired VC should be within 5% or 200 ml.

2 The VC during SBN$_2$ should be within 200 ml of a previously determined VC.

3 Expiratory flow should be maintained between 0.3 and 0.5 L/sec.

4 The N_2 tracing should show minimal cardiac oscillations.

Slope of Phase III

A best-fit line is drawn through the Phase III segment of the tracing from the point where 30% of the VC remains above RV to the onset of Phase IV. This slope of the line is used as an index of gas distribution, in a manner similar to the $\Delta\%N_2$ 750-1250. Values in healthy young adults range from 0.5% to 1.0% N_2/L of lung volume, with wide variability. Very slow expiratory flow rates may cause oscillations in the tracing of Phase III, making the accurate measurement of $\Delta\%N_2$ difficult. These oscillations are attributed to changes in alveolar N_2 concentrations as blood pulses through the pulmonary capillaries during cardiac systole. Increasing the expiratory flow rate slightly eliminates this artifact. Subjects who have small VC values may have difficulty exhaling enough gas to make the $\Delta\%N_2$ or slope of Phase III meaningful.

Closing Volume and Closing Capacity

After maximal expiration by an upright subject, more RV remains at the **apices** of the lungs than at the bases because of gravity. When the test gas (O_2) is inspired, the apices receive the gas occupying the subject's dead space, which consists largely of N_2. The O_2 then goes preferentially to the bases of the lungs. Gas concentrations in the lungs become widely different. The apices contain RV gas plus dead space gas rich in N_2. The bases of the lungs contain a higher concentration of the test gas O_2. Compression of the airways during the subsequent expiration causes airways to narrow and then close, as lung volume approaches RV. Airways at the bases close first because of gravity and the weight of the lung in subjects sitting upright. As airways at the bases close, proportionately more gas comes from the apices. This appears as an abrupt rise in the concentration of N_2 and is the onset of Phase IV.

The onset of Phase IV marks the lung volume at which airway closure begins. The point at which this occurs in the VC depends on the caliber of the small airways. In healthy young adults, airways begin closing after 80% to 90% of the VC has been expired. The CC in healthy young adults usually occurs at approximately 30% of the TLC, with wide variations. CV and CC may be increased, indicating earlier onset of airway closure in the following:

Elderly subjects

Restrictive disease patterns in which the FRC becomes less than the CV

Smokers and other subjects with early obstructive disease of small airways

Congestive heart failure when the caliber of the small airways is compromised by edema

---

Subjects with moderate or severe obstructive disease may have no sharp inflection separating Phases III and IV of the SBN₂. This lack of a clear point of airway closure is the result of grossly uneven distribution of gas in the lungs. Subjects who have airway obstruction typically show greater than normal $\Delta\%N_2$ 750-1250 values and slopes of Phase III.

In some subjects with no pulmonary disease, the onset of Phase IV cannot be accurately determined. Because of the variability in both the CV and CC, the mean of three tests is usually reported. Because of its poor reproducibility, the CV test is not widely used. Although it appears to be a sensitive indicator of abnormalities in the small airways, particularly in smokers, an increased CV/VC ratio is not highly predictive of which individuals will develop chronic airways obstruction. To calculate normal values for CV and CC according to age and sex, see Appendix B.

BOX 3-7
INTERPRETIVE STRATEGIES—SBN₂

1 Was the test performed acceptably? VC reproducible within 5% or 200 ml? Expiratory flow appropriate?

2 Are reference values appropriate? Age, height, sex, race?

3 Is $\Delta\%N_2$ 750-1250 greater than 1.5%? If so, suspect uneven distribution of ventilation.

4 Is slope of Phase III greater than 1.0% to 1.5%? If so, there is uneven distribution of ventilation.

5 Is CV/VC% greater than 20% (or age-related expected value)? If so, suspect small airways abnormalities. Correlate with clinical findings.

```
┌─────────────────────────────────────────────────────────────────────────┐
│ BOX 3-8                                                                    │
│ CRITERIA FOR ACCEPTABILITY—7 MINUTE N₂ WASHOUT                           │
├─────────────────────────────────────────────────────────────────────────┤
```

BOX 3-8
CRITERIA FOR ACCEPTABILITY—7 MINUTE N_2 WASHOUT

1 The rate and depth of breathing should be close to normal for the size of the subject (i.e., $\approx$500 ml and 10 to 12 breaths/min for an adult).

2 The washout curve should show a steady decrease in N_2 concentration without abrupt changes or increases.

3 The test should be continued for 7 minutes or until the N_2 concentration has fallen to 1.5% or less.

Nitrogen Washout Test (7 Minute)

DESCRIPTION

The N_2 washout test historically measured N_2 concentration in alveolar gas at the end of 7 minutes of breathing 100% O_2. Now, the pattern of N_2 washout and the time required to reduce the alveolar N_2 to 1.5% or less are used as indices of the evenness of ventilation. These measurements are usually made at the same time the FRC is determined.

TECHNIQUE

The simplest method of calculating the degree of N_2 washout from the lungs is by having the subject breathe 100% O_2 for 7 minutes or until the alveolar N_2 concentration has been reduced to less than 1.5%. If the alveolar N_2 concentration has not been reduced to 1.5% or less within 7 minutes, uneven distribution of ventilation exists. The length of time required to reduce the %N_2 to less than 1% with O_2 breathing is also used as an index of gas distribution (Box 3-8).

The washout of N_2 during O_2 breathing is usually graphed or displayed. Rapid analysis of expired gas allows the washout curve to be displayed breath-by-breath (see Fig. 3-2). The percent of N_2 or its **logarithm** is normally plotted against the expired volume or number of breaths. The washout of N_2 from a normal lung is nearly **exponential**. The end-expiratory points of a normal washout curve appear as a straight line when the log %N_2 is graphed on **semilog** paper. Because the same breathing circuit is used as for the open-circuit FRC determination, distribution of ventilation can be determined along with lung volumes.

The time to reach He equilibrium during the closed-circuit FRC determination can also be used as an index of distribution of ventilation. By simply recording the time to reach equilibrium and plotting the dilution curve, an estimate of the evenness of ventilation is obtained.

The multiple-breath N_2 test (as well as the He equilibration test) is independent of subject effort. The subject must maintain an adequate seal on the mouthpiece of the apparatus to prevent contamination of the O_2. Leaks in the breathing circuit or in the N_2 sampling device usually result in room air being mixed with the washed-out gas. A leak usually results in prolonged washout times or inability to reduce the alveolar N_2 to less than 2.5%, even in normal lungs. Leaks are usually identifiable by abrupt increases in the N_2 concentration during the maneuver (see Fig. 3-5, *B*).

SIGNIFICANCE AND PATHOPHYSIOLOGY

See Box 3-9 for interpretive strategies. The normal value for the concentration of N_2 in alveolar gas after 7 minutes of breathing O_2 is less than 2.5%. The results of the N_2 washout depend somewhat on the subject's tidal volume, dead space, and FRC. Increased tidal volume or breathing rate can lower the %N_2 in the alveoli to near normal levels despite marked unevenness of gas distribution. Subjects who do not have obstructive disease wash N_2 out of their lungs with 3 to 4 minutes of breathing O_2. Washout times longer than 3 to 4 minutes are usually consistent with poor distribution, increased FRC, reduced alveolar ventilation, or a combination of these.

The graphic method of displaying breath-by-breath washout provides a means of quantifying the evenness of ventilation. The slope of the washout curve is determined by the FRC, tidal volume, dead space volume, and frequency of breathing. If N_2 is washed out of the lungs evenly, the pattern appears as a straight line, regardless of the slope (see Fig. 3-5, *A*). Because the lung

---

BOX 3-9
INTERPRETIVE STRATEGIES—7 MINUTE N_2 WASHOUT

1   Was the test performed appropriately? Were the rate and depth of breathing regular?

2   Is the test free of leaks? If not, interpret results very cautiously.

3   Does the subject wash N_2 out to a concentration of 1.5% within 3 to 4 minutes? If so, distribution is normal.

4   Does the subject wash N_2 out to a concentration of 2.5% within 7 minutes? If so, distribution is probably normal. If not, correlate with other evidence of obstruction—spirometry, history, or physical examination.

5   Are additional tests indicated? Blood gases? Lung scan? Chest x-ray examination?

---

is not perfectly symmetric, the washout curve is usually slightly concave. The deviation from a straight line indicates the extent to which ventilation is uneven.

Uneven distribution of gas in the lungs is characteristic of all obstructive disease patterns. Emphysema, particularly in the advanced stages, shows the greatest degree of maldistribution. Patients who have bronchitis or asthma show similar unevenness of ventilation, particularly during acute exacerbations. The effect of uneven distribution of ventilation depends on ventilation-perfusion matching. Uneven ventilation often results in blood gas abnormalities, specifically hypoxemia (see Chapter 6). When ventilation is not matched to the same lung units that are receiving pulmonary capillary blood flow, the arterial saturation (Sa_{O_2}) falls. If the ventilation-perfusion mismatch is severe, the Pa_{CO_2} may rise. Some subjects who have marked maldistribution of ventilation (as in emphysema) may have relatively normal blood gases. If the disease process destroys pulmonary capillaries along with the other alveolar structures, ventilation distribution may be poor, but matches pulmonary capillary perfusion. As a result, blood gas values appear normal, with little or no hypoxemia.

Normal washout values are often produced by subjects who have a purely restrictive pattern. Tumors or other space-occupying lesions may block airways and cause regional differences in ventilation. Thoracic deformities, such as kyphoscoliosis and **pectus excavatum**, may also cause marked unevenness in the distribution of ventilation. The 7-minute washout test results may or may not appear abnormal in many of these types of restrictive disorders. Ventilation and perfusion lung scans offer the best means of assessing regional gas distribution and blood flow. Other imaging techniques, including MRI, positron emission tomography (**PET**), and ultrasonography, may be useful in identifying and localizing the causes of uneven gas distribution.

CASE STUDIES

CASE 3A

History

M.B. is a 27-year-old male high school teacher whose chief complaint is dyspnea on exertion. He states that his breathlessness has worsened over the past several months. He has smoked one pack of cigarettes a day for approximately 10 years (10 pack/years). He denies a cough or sputum production. No one in his family ever had emphysema, asthma, chronic bronchitis, carcinoma, or tuberculosis. There is no history of exposure to extraordinary environmental pollutants.

Pulmonary Function Testing

Personal data

Sex: Male
Age: 27 yr
Height: 65 in
Weight: 297 lb
BSA: 2.28 M^2

Spirometry and airway resistance

	Before drug	Predicted	%
FVC (L)	2.9	4.7	62
FEV_1 (L)	2.47	3.86	64
$FEV_{1\%}$ (%)	85	82	—
$FEF_{25\%-75\%}$ (L/sec)	4.62	4.35	106
$FEF_{50\%}$ (L/sec)	4.94	5.82	85
$FEF_{25\%}$ (L/sec)	2.49	3.22	77
MVV (L/min)	178	137	130
Raw (cm H_2O/L/sec)	2.33	0.6-2.4	—
SGaw (L/sec/cm H_2O/L)	0.23	0.12-0.50	—

Lung volumes (by plethysmograph)

	Before drug	Predicted	%
VC (L)	2.9	4.7	62
IC (L)	1.96	2.91	67
ERV (L)	0.94	1.8	59
FRC (L)	1.87	3.29	57
RV (L)	0.93	1.49	57
TLC (L)	3.83	6.2	62
RV/TLC (%)	25	24	—

Questions

1. What is the interpretation of:

   a. Spirometry?

   b. Lung volumes?

   c. Airway resistance?

2. What is the cause of the patient's symptoms?

3. What other tests might be indicated?

4. What treatment might be recommended based on these findings?

Discussion

1 **Interpretation**

All data from spirometry and lung volumes are acceptable. Spirometry shows a decreased FVC and FEV_1. The FEV_1 is normal. Flows are within normal limits, as is the maximal voluntary ventilation (MVV). Raw is near the upper limit of normal but SGaw is normal. Lung volumes are decreased, with the RV/TLC ratio preserved.

Impression: Moderate restrictive lung disease without evidence of obstruction. Restrictive pattern may be related to subject's weight. Recommend arterial blood gas testing to evaluate gas exchange abnormalities.

2 **Cause of symptoms**

This case is a good example of what might be considered a pure restrictive defect. Characteristic of a restrictive process is a proportional decrease in all lung volumes, including FVC and FEV_1. Flows such as $FEF_{25\%-75\%}$ or $FEF_{50\%}$ show little or no decrease (Fig. 3-10). Also characteristic of simple restriction is the well-preserved ratio of FEV_1 to FVC. The volume expired in the first second was in correct proportion to the VC, despite decreases in their absolute volumes. The MVV demonstrates the subject's ability to move a normal maximal volume. This may be accomplished despite moderately severe restriction by an increase in the rate rather than the tidal volume.

The explanation for the restrictive pattern lies in the subject's weight of 297 pounds. His actual weight is approximately 200% of his ideal weight. Obesity commonly causes restrictive patterns.

3 **Other tests**

The patient returned for analysis of arterial blood gases, which revealed resting hypoxemia and slightly elevated P_{CO_2}. The blood gas measurements confirmed the degree of impairment

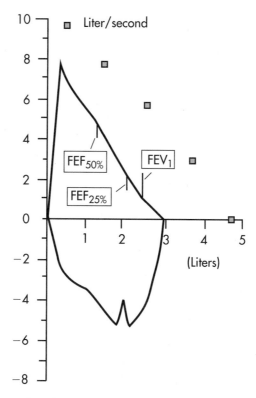

FIG. 3-10 *Case 3A.* Flow-volume loop from the subject. Upward tick mark superimposed on the loop denotes the FEV$_1$, whereas downward ticks show the FEF$_{50\%}$ and FEF$_{25\%}$, respectively. The small, shaded boxes represent the subject's reference values.

caused by the moderately severe restrictive pattern. Other tests that might be considered include ventilatory response tests for hypoxemia or hypercapnia (see Chapter 4). Studies to diagnose sleep **apnea** might be indicated if the subject had symptoms of disordered breathing during sleep. This subject's borderline Raw suggests upper airway involvement, which might predispose him to obstructive sleep apnea.

4   **Treatment**
    The subject was referred to a dietician for counseling in weight management.

CASE 3B

History

R.B. is a 37-year-old pipe fitter whose chief complaint is shortness of breath at rest and with exertion. His dyspnea has worsened in the past 6 months, so much so that he is no longer able to work. Additional symptoms include a dry cough. He admits some sputum production when he has a chest cold. He has smoked one pack of cigarettes a day since age 18 (19 pack/years). He quit smoking approximately 3 weeks before the tests. His father died of emphysema and his mother of lung cancer. His brother is in good health. His occupational exposure includes working for the past 13 years in the assembly room of a boiler plant. He admits to seldomly using the respirators provided at work despite the dusty environment.

Pulmonary Function Tests

Personal data

Sex: Male
Age: 37 yr
Height: 69 in
Weight: 143 lb

Spirometry

	Before drug	Predicted	%	After drug	%
FVC (L)	3.04	5.05	60	3.1	61
FEV_1 (L)	2.03	3.9	52	2.26	58
$FEV_{1\%}$(%)	67	77	—	73	—
$FEF_{25\%-75\%}$(L/sec)	1.3	4.09	32	1.6	39
$FEF_{50\%}$ (L/sec)	2.12	5.78	37	2.42	42
$FEF_{25\%}$ (L/sec)	0.78	2.95	26	1.2	41
MVV (L/min)	83	141	59	91	65
Raw (cm H_2O/L/sec)	2.51	0.6-2.4	—	2.47	—
SGaw (L/sec/cm H_2O/L)	0.14	0.11-0.44	—	0.15	—

Lung volumes (by N_2 washout)

	Before drug	Predicted	%
VC (L)	3.04	5.05	60
IC (L)	1.62	3.18	51
ERV (L)	1.42	1.87	76
FRC (L)	2.75	3.81	72
RV (L)	0.33	1.94	69
TLC (L)	4.37	6.99	63
RV/TLC (%)	30	28	—

Technologist's Comments

Spirometry results met all American Thoracic Society (ATS) recommendations, prebronchodilator and postbronchodilator.

Lung volumes by N_2 washout: all maneuvers were performed acceptably. Duplicate measurements were averaged.

Raw and SGaw efforts were performed appropriately.

Questions

1. What is the interpretation of:
    a. Prebronchodilator spirometry?
    b. Response to bronchodilator?
    c. Raw and SGaw?
    d. Lung volumes?
2. What is the cause of the patient's symptoms?
3. What other tests might be indicated?
4. What treatment might be recommended based on these findings?

Discussion

1   **Interpretation**

All data from spirometry and lung volumes are acceptable. Spirometry shows a reduced FVC and FEV_1. The $FEF_{25\%-75\%}$, $FEF_{50\%}$, and $FEF_{25\%}$ are all reduced. The MVV is low. Raw and SGaw are close to their respective limits of normal. Response to bronchodilators is borderline, with an increase in the FEV_1 of 230 ml (11%). The $FEF_{25\%}$ improved somewhat more than the other flows. The patient's lung volumes are all decreased. His RV/TLC ratio is normal.

Impression: There is moderate airway obstruction combined with a restrictive pattern. The response to inhaled bronchodilator medication is borderline. A trial of bronchodilators should be considered. Recommend arterial blood gas testing to evaluate possible hypoxemia.

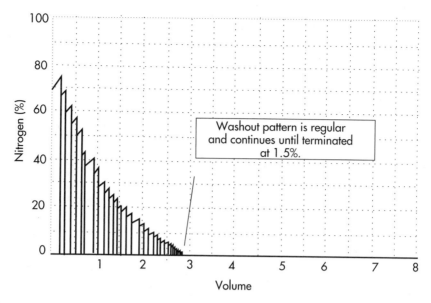

FIG. 3-11 *Case 3B.* Open-circuit N_2 washout from the subject. The tracing shows a normal pattern of washout with N_2 concentration plotted against lung volume (FRC). The test was terminated when the N_2 concentration fell to less than 1.5%.

2 Cause of symptoms

R.B. typifies the subject with combined obstructive and restrictive disease. His spirometry results indicate that a serious obstructive component is present, as revealed by the FEV_1 (52% of predicted) and the other flows. His $FEV_{1\%}$, however, is close to normal because his FVC is also reduced. Airway narrowing as a result of restriction is sometimes responsible for decreased flows. This is particularly evident when restriction is severe. R.B.'s symptoms of cough and sputum suggest a genuine obstructive process. His smoking and family history place him at risk. Because FVC can be reduced in either obstructive and restrictive processes, spirometry alone would not have adequately defined this subject's disease.

Lung volume measurements confirm the presence of a restrictive component (Fig. 3-11). All lung volumes are reduced in similar proportions. The reduction in VC matches decreases in FRC, RV, and TLC. The subject's history and symptoms suggest the possibility of restrictive or obstructive disease, or both. The obstructive component may be related to the subject's smoking history, but the etiology of the restrictive component is less clear. On further inquiry, it was learned that the subject's occupation involved exposure to asbestos, which can cause fibrosis or carcinoma. Chest x-ray studies revealed linear calcifications of the diaphragmatic pleura and pleural thickening, as well as fibrotic changes. These findings are all consistent with asbestos exposure.

3 Other tests

A sputum examination was performed and asbestos bodies were identified from the subject's sputum. Open-lung biopsy was deferred because both the obstructive and restrictive components were believed to be adequately identified. Measurement of pulmonary compliance (C_L) could have been used to document the severity of the fibrosis. Analysis of resting arterial blood gases is probably indicated because the patient has a significant degree of restriction. Diffusing capacity ($D_{L_{CO}}$) could also be used to identify possible gas exchange abnormalities.

Because of his dyspnea on exertion, the patient returned for an exercise evaluation. He walked on a treadmill with an arterial catheter in place. His Pa_{O_2} fell from 65 mm Hg (rest) to 55 mm Hg after only 2 minutes of walking at 2 miles per hour. The desaturation was corrected when the patient breathed O_2 by nasal cannula at 1 L/min.

4 Treatment

The patient was given a trial of bronchodilators and reported significant symptomatic improvement. He began using supplemental O_2 via a portable system and was able to return to work in a position modified to accommodate his abilities.

SELF-ASSESSMENT QUESTIONS

1 *Which of the following correctly describes the measurement of FRC by the closed-circuit method?*
  I.   The system volume of spirometer and circuitry must be calculated.
  II. The test is continued until the He changes by less than 2% in 30 seconds.
  III. A small amount of He is absorbed by blood and tissues.
  IV. A CO_2 absorber is required.
  a. I and II only
  b. III and IV only
  c. I, II, and III
  d. I, III, and IV

2 *A subject has the following lung volumes measured using a body plethysmograph:*

	Measured	Predicted
VC	4.91	5.20
FRC	4.66	3.90
RV	3.80	2.10
TLC	8.71	7.30

  These values are consistent with which of the following?
  a. An obstructive pattern such as emphysema
  b. A restrictive pattern such as sarcoidosis
  c. Normal lung volumes
  d. A calculation error involving the FRC

3 *The following data are obtained during a closed-circuit FRC determination:*

He added:	0.5 L
%He initial:	9.0%
%He final:	7.1%
Temperature:	24° C
He absorption correction:	0.1 L

  The FRC would be which of the following (see sample calculation in Appendix B)?
  a. 1.32 L BTPS
  b. 1.50 L BTPS
  c. 1.55 L ATPS
  d. 2.17 L ATPS

4 *A patient with pulmonary fibrosis has lung volumes measured using the open-circuit method and by plethysmography with the following results:*

FRC (N_2washout)	2.21 L
V_{TG}	2.34 L
FRC predicted	3.67 L

  Which of the following best explains these results?
  a. This is a normal pattern for the patient's diagnosis.
  b. The FRC by N_2 washout is erroneously low.
  c. The V_{TG} is erroneously low.
  d. The predicted FRC is incorrect.

5 *Which of the following combinations are characteristic of a restrictive pattern?*
  a. Reduced VC, reduced TLC, normal RV/TLC
  b. Reduced FRC, elevated TLC, normal RV/TLC
  c. Elevated RV, elevated TLC, elevated RV/TLC
  d. Reduced FRC, elevated V_{TG}

6 *To measure accurately the V_{TG} the patient should be instructed to do which of the following?*
  a. Breathe normally during closure of the shutter
  b. Pant rapidly and deeply
  c. Pant about one time per second
  d. Hold his or her breath as soon as the shutter closes

7 *The following data are obtained from spirometry and a He dilution FRC test (all values have been corrected to BTPS):*

VC	3.4 L
IC	2.1 L
ERV	1.3 L
FRC	3.9 L

  What is the patient's RV/TLC ratio?
  a. 22%
  b. 33%
  c. 38%
  d. 43%

8 *A subject has the following results from spirometry and N_2 washout FRC determination:*

	Measured	Predicted	% Predicted
VC	4.6	4.7	98
FRC	8.2	3.8	216
TLC	10.2	7.5	136
RV/TLC%	55	37	—

  Which of the following best explains these findings?
  a. The subject has normal lung volumes.
  b. The subject has severe air trapping.
  c. A leak occurred during the VC test.
  d. A leak occurred during the FRC test.

9 *The reported value for V_{TG} should be:*
  a. Averaged from three to five acceptable maneuvers
  b. The largest value from three acceptable maneuvers
  c. Reproducible within 1%
  d. Measured with the subject panting at 5 Hz

10 *A subject has the following measurements obtained during pulmonary function testing:*

FVC	3.90 L
FEV_1	1.10 L
FRC (He)	3.62 L
V_{TG}	4.77 L

These findings are consistent with:
a. Normal pulmonary function
b. Severe obstruction with air trapping
c. Mild restriction
d. A leak during the FRC determination

11 *An increased slope of Phase III during an SBN_2 test is:*
a. Consistent with severe restrictive disease
b. Indicative of uneven distribution of gas within the lungs
c. Usually caused by an accelerated heart rate
d. Diagnostic of increased anatomic dead space

12 *A subject with an FEV_1/FVC ratio of 37% performs a 7-minute N_2 washout test. After 7 minutes the alveolar N_2 concentration is 5.7%. This is consistent with which of the following?*
a. Chronic bronchitis
b. Idiopathic pulmonary fibrosis
c. Sarcoidosis
d. A right-to-left shunt

SELECTED BIBLIOGRAPHY

General References
Forster RE: *The lung: clinical physiology and pulmonary function tests,* ed 3, St Louis, 1988, Mosby.
Crapo RO, Morris AH, Clayton PD, et al: Lung volumes in healthy nonsmoking adults, *Bull Europ Physiopathol Respir* 18:419, 1982.
Goldman HI, Becklake MR: Respiratory function tests: normal values at median altitudes and the prediction of normal results, *Am Rev TB Pulm Dis* 79:457, 1959.
Hibbert ME, Lanigan A, Raven J, et al: Relation of armspan to height and the prediction of lung function, *Thorax* 43:657, 1988.

Thoracic Gas Volume
Begin P, Peslin R: Influence of panting frequency on thoracic gas volume measurements in chronic obstructive pulmonary disease, *Am Rev Respir Dis* 130:121, 1984.
Dubois AB, Bothelo SY, Bedell GH, et al: A rapid plethysmographic method for measuring thoracic gas volume: a comparison with a nitrogen washout method for measuring functional residual capacity, *J Clin Invest* 35:322, 1956.
Habib MP, Engel LA: Influence of the panting technique on the plethysmographic measurement of thoracic gas volume, *Am Rev Respir Dis* 117:265, 1978.
Leith DE, Mead J: Principles of body plethysmography, *DLD-NHLBI,* Nov, 1974.
Lourenco RV, Chung SYK: Calibration of a body plethysmograph for measurement of lung volume, *Am Rev Respir Dis* 95:687, 1967.
Rodenstein DO, Stanescu DC, Francis C: Demonstration of failure of body plethysmography in airway obstruction, *J Appl Physiol* 52:949, 1982.

Open- and Closed-Circuit Lung Volumes
Hathirat S, Renzetti AD, Mitchell M: Measurement of the total lung capacity by helium dilution in a constant volume system, *Am Rev Respir Dis* 102:760, 1970.
McMichael J: A rapid method of determining lung capacity, *Clin Sci* 4:167, 1939.

Meneely GR, Ball CO, Kory RC, et al: A simplified closed-circuit helium dilution method for the determination of the residual volume of the lungs, *Am J Med* 28:824, 1960.
Rodenstein DO, Stanescu DC: Reassessment of lung volume measurements by helium dilution and by body plethysmography in chronic airflow obstruction, *Am Rev Respir Dis* 126:1040, 1982.
Schaaning CG, Gulsvik A: Accuracy and precision of helium dilution technique and body plethysmography in measuring lung volume, *Scand J Clin Invest* 32:271, 1973.

Gas Distribution
Bouhuys A: Distribution of inspired gas in the lungs. In Fenn WO, Rahn H, eds: *Handbook of physiology—respiration I,* Washington, 1964, American Physiologic Society.
Darling RC, Cournand A, Richards DW: Studies of intrapulmonary mixture of gases: V. Forms of inadequate ventilation in normal and emphysematous lungs analyzed by means of breathing pure oxygen, *J Clin Invest* 23:55, 1944.
Fowler WS: Lung function studies: III. Uneven pulmonary ventilation in normal subjects and in patients with pulmonary disease, *J Appl Physiol* 2:283, 1949.
Hathirat S, Renzetti AD, Mitchell M: Intrapulmonary gas distribution: a comparison of the helium mixing time and nitrogen single-breath test in normal and diseased subjects, *Am Rev Respir Dis* 102:750, 1970.
Shinokazi T, Abajian JC Jr, Tabakin BS, et al: Theory of a digital nitrogen washout computer, *J Appl Physiol* 21:202, 1966.

Closing Volume
Abboud R, Morton J: Comparison of maximal midexpiratory flow, flow-volume curves, and nitrogen closing volumes in patients with mild airway obstruction, *Am Rev Respir Dis* 111:405, 1975.

Becklake MR, Permutt S: Evaluation of tests of lung function for "screening" for early detection of chronic obstructive lung disease. In Maclem PT, Permutt S, eds: *The lung in transition between health and disease,* New York, 1979, Marcel Dekker.

Berend N, Glanville AR, Grunstein MM: Determinants of the slope of phase III of the single-breath nitrogen test, *Bull Eur Physiopathol Respir* 20:521, 1984.

Cormier Y, Belanger J: The role of gas exchange in phase IV of the single-breath nitrogen test, *Am Rev Respir Dis* 125:396, 1982.

Martin R, Macklem PT: Suggested standardization procedures for closing volume determinations (nitrogen method), *DHD-NHLBI,* 1973.

Standards and Guidelines

American Association for Respiratory Care: Clinical practice guideline: static lung volumes, *Respir Care* 39:830-836, 1994.

American Association for Respiratory Care: Clinical practice guideline: body plethysmography, *Respir Care* 39:1184-1190, 1994.

American Thoracic Society: Lung function testing: selection of reference values and interpretive strategies, *Am Rev Respir Dis* 144:1202, 1991.

British Thoracic Society and Association of Respiratory Technicians and Physiologists: Guidelines for the measurement of respiratory function, *Respir Med* 88:165-194, 1994.

Quanjer PH, ed: Lung volumes and ventilatory flows. Report of the Working Party, Standardization of Lung Function Tests, European Community for Steel and Coal, *Bull Eur Physiopathol Respir* 16(suppl 6):5-40, 1993.

CHAPTER 4

Ventilation and Ventilatory Control Tests

OBJECTIVES

After studying this chapter and reviewing its tables and case studies, you should be able to do the following:

1 Calculate tidal volume and minute ventilation when given appropriate data

2 Describe two methods for measuring the breathing response to oxygen

3 Identify the normal ventilatory response to carbon dioxide

4 Calculate dead space and alveolar ventilation

THIS CHAPTER DISCUSSES THE measurement of ventilation and its components: tidal volume (V_T), respiratory frequency (f), and minute ventilation ($\dot{V}_E$). Wasted, or dead space, ventilation is also defined. Techniques for estimating dead space (V_D) and alveolar ventilation ($\dot{V}_A$) are described. Because a variety of diseases can affect V_D, its measurement is used to evaluate many disorders. Ventilation and V_D measurements are used in several different testing situations. These parameters may be measured in the critical care unit as well as in the pulmonary function laboratory.

Closely related to measurement of resting ventilation is assessment of ventilatory responses. The responses to two stimuli, carbon dioxide (CO_2) and oxygen (O_2), are commonly evaluated. Ventilatory response is usually assessed by measuring the change in ventilation that occurs with elevated CO_2 or decreased O_2. The output of the respiratory centers is also sometimes measured as the pressure developed during the first tenth of a second when the airway is blocked (P_{100}).

Tidal Volume, Respiratory Rate, and Minute Ventilation

DESCRIPTION

V_T is the volume of gas inspired or expired during each respiratory cycle (see Fig. 2-1). It is usually measured in milliliters and corrected to BTPS. Conventionally, the volume expired is expressed as the V_T. The respiratory rate is the number of breaths per unit of time, usually per minute. The total volume of gas expired per minute is the $\dot{V}_E$. It includes alveolar and dead space ventilation and is recorded in liters per minute, BTPS.

TECHNIQUE

V_T can be measured directly by simple spirometry (see Fig. 2-1). The subject breathes into a volume-displacement or flow-sensing spirometer. Volume change may be measured directly from the excursions of a volume spirometer. V_T may also be measured from an integrated flow signal (see Chapter 9). V_T can be recorded on either paper or a computer screen. Because no two breaths are the same, inhaled or exhaled tidal breaths should be measured for at least 1 minute and then divided by the rate to determine the average volume:

$$V_T = \frac{\dot{V}}{f}$$

BOX 4-1
CRITERIA FOR ACCEPTABILITY—TIDAL VOLUME, RATE, MINUTE VENTILATION

1   V_T averaged from at least 60 seconds of ventilatory data; either accumulated volume divided by respiratory rate or multiple breaths summed and averaged.

2   $\dot{V}_E$ measured for at least 60 seconds; one-way breathing circuit or appropriate rebreathing system used. Repeated measurements should be within 10%.

3   Respiratory rate measured for at least 15 seconds; longer intervals may be necessary for subjects with disordered breathing patterns.

where:

$$\dot{V} = \text{volume expired or inspired over a given interval, usually the } \dot{V}_E$$

$$f = \text{number of breaths for same interval (i.e., the respiratory rate)}$$

The inspired volume ($\dot{V}_I$) and V_T are normally slightly greater than the $\dot{V}_E$ because the body at rest produces a slightly lower volume of CO_2 than the volume of O_2 consumed. This exchange difference is termed the respiratory exchange ratio (**RER**). It is calculated as the $\dot{V}_{CO_2}/\dot{V}_{O_2}$, where $\dot{V}_{CO_2}$ is the volume of CO_2 produced and $\dot{V}_{O_2}$ is the volume of O_2 consumed per minute. RER is usually assumed to be approximately 0.8 in a resting subject. For most clinical purposes, expired volume is measured to calculate V_T.

V_T may also be estimated by means of the respiratory inductive plethysmography (RIP). The RIP uses coils of wire as transducers that respond to changes in the cross-sectional area of the rib cage and abdominal compartments. With appropriate calibration, RIP can be used to measure V_T without connections to the airway.

Respiratory frequency (f) may be determined by counting chest movements or the excursions of a spirometer (Box 4-1). Counting the rate for several minutes and taking an average produces a more accurate value than shorter measurements. Prolonged measurements of V_T and rate using a volume-displacement spirometer require a means of removing CO_2. This type of system is called a rebreathing system and uses a chemical CO_2 absorber (see Fig. 3-1, *B*). Sodium hydroxide crystals (Sodasorb) or barium hydroxide crystals (Baralyme) are commonly used to scrub CO_2 from rebreathing systems. Flow-sensing spirometers usually do not require a chemical absorber.

The $\dot{V}_E$ may be determined by allowing the subject to breathe into or out of a volume-displacement or flow-sensing spirometer for at least 1 minute. If a rebreathing system is used, a CO_2 absorber must be included, as well as means of replenishing O_2. Measuring expired gas volume for several minutes and dividing by the time gives an average $\dot{V}_E$. Because it is measured from expired gas, $\dot{V}_E$ is usually slightly smaller than the $\dot{V}_I$ because of the RER as described previously. For most clinical purposes this difference is negligible. BTPS corrections should be made.

SIGNIFICANCE AND PATHOPHYSIOLOGY

See Box 4-2 for interpretive strategies. Average V_T for healthy adults ranges between 400 and 700 ml, but there is considerable variation. Decreased V_T occurs in many types of pulmonary disorders, particularly those that cause severely restrictive patterns. Pulmonary fibrosis and neuromuscular diseases (e.g., myasthenia gravis) often cause reduced V_T. Decreased tidal breathing is usually caused by mechanical changes in the lungs or chest wall (i.e., compliance and resistance). These changes are almost always accompanied by increased respiratory rate required to maintain $\dot{V}_A$. Decreases in both V_T and respiratory rate are usually associated with respiratory center depression. Low V_T and rate usually result in alveolar hypoventilation. Rapid breathing rates and small V_T may suggest increased V_D or hypoventilation but must be correlated with arterial pH and P_{CO_2} values to be definitive.

Some subjects who have pulmonary disease may exhibit increased V_T, particularly at rest. The V_T alone is not an adequate indicator of $\dot{V}_A$. V_T should never be considered outside the context of respiratory rate and $\dot{V}_E$. Most healthy subjects display increased V_T simply as a result of breathing into the pulmonary function apparatus with the nose occluded. Estimates of resting ventilation may be artifactually increased when measured during pulmonary function testing.

> **BOX 4-2**
> **INTERPRETIVE STRATEGIES—TIDAL VOLUME, RATE, MINUTE VENTILATION**
>
> 1   Were V_T, respiratory rate, and $\dot{V}_E$ measured appropriately? Were adequate data collected? Did the ventilatory pattern change during the measurement? If so, suspect breathing circuit problems.
>
> 2   Were repeated measurements made? If so, were they reproducible within 10%?
>
> 3   Is the pattern of ventilation consistent with the subject's clinical status?
>
> 4   Is V_T, respiratory rate, or $\dot{V}_E$ excessive? If so, suspect hyperventilation. Arterial blood gas testing may be necessary.
>
> 5   Is V_T, respiratory rate, or $\dot{V}_E$ decreased? If so, suspect hypoventilation. Arterial blood gas testing is indicated.

Some subjects who have pulmonary disease may exhibit increased V_T, particularly at rest. The V_T alone is not an adequate indicator of $\dot{V}_A$. V_T should never be considered outside the context of respiratory rate and $\dot{V}_E$. Most healthy subjects display increased V_T simply as a result of breathing into the pulmonary function apparatus with the nose occluded. Estimates of resting ventilation may be artifactually increased when measured during pulmonary function testing.

The normal respiratory rate ranges from 10 to 20 breaths/min. Increased demand for ventilation, such as during exercise, usually results in increases in both the rate and depth of breathing. This is often a good indicator of the stimulus to breathe.

Increases or decreases in the respiratory rate are indications of a change in the ventilatory status. Breathing frequency, when evaluated with the V_T, may be used as an index of ventilation. **Hypoxia**, hypercapnia, **metabolic acidosis**, decreased lung compliance, and exercise all result in increased respiratory rate. Rapid breathing rates and small tidal volumes may suggest increased V_D or hypoventilation but must be correlated with arterial pH and P_{CO_2} values to be definitive if respiratory drive is normal. Decreased breathing frequency is common in central nervous system depression and in **CO_2 narcosis.** As with measurement of V_T, respiratory rate may be falsely elevated in subjects connected to unfamiliar breathing circuits, with or without a nose clip.

Normal $\dot{V}_E$ ranges from 5 to 10 L/min, with wide variations in normal subjects. The $\dot{V}_E$, when used in conjunction with blood gas values, indicates the adequacy of ventilation. $\dot{V}_E$ is the sum of both the V_D and $\dot{V}_A$. Because these components can change, absolute values for $\dot{V}_E$ do not necessarily indicate either hypoventilation or hyperventilation.

A large $\dot{V}_E$ at rest (i.e., greater than 20 L/min) may result from enlarged V_D because an increase in total ventilation is required to maintain adequate $\dot{V}_A$. $\dot{V}_E$ increases in response to hypoxia, hypercapnia, metabolic acidosis, anxiety, and exercise. Hyperventilation is ventilation in excess of that needed to maintain adequate CO_2 removal, with a resulting respiratory alkalosis.

Decreased ventilation may result from **hypocapnia, metabolic alkalosis,** respiratory center depression, or neuromuscular disorders which involve the ventilatory muscles. Hypoventilation is defined as inadequate ventilation to maintain a normal arterial P_{CO_2}, and the respiratory acidosis that results. The diagnosis of either hyperventilation or hypoventilation requires blood gas analysis (see Chapter 6).

Respiratory Dead Space and Alveolar Ventilation

DESCRIPTION

Respiratory dead space (V_D) is the lung volume that is ventilated but not perfused by pulmonary capillary blood flow. V_D can be divided into the conducting airways, or anatomic dead space, and the nonperfused alveoli, or alveolar dead space. The combination of alveolar and anatomic dead space is respiratory, or physiologic, dead space. V_D is recorded in milliliters or liters, BTPS.

$\dot{V}_A$ is the volume of gas that participates in gas exchange in the lungs. It equals $\dot{V}_E$ minus the V_D. For a single breath, the V_A equals the V_T minus the V_D. $\dot{V}_A$ is usually expressed in liters per minute, BTPS.

TECHNIQUE

Dead Space

Anatomic dead space is sometimes estimated from an individual's body size as 1 ml/lb of body weight. The actual respiratory dead space, however, is of greater clinical importance. V_D can be calculated in two ways. The first uses Bohr's equation defining V_D:

$$V_D = \frac{(F_{ACO_2} - F_{\bar{E}CO_2})}{F_{ACO_2}} V_T$$

where:

$$V_T = \text{tidal volume}$$

$$F_{ACO_2} = \text{fraction of } CO_2 \text{ in alveolar gas}$$

$$F_{\bar{E}CO_2} = \text{fraction of } CO_2 \text{ in } \textbf{mixed expired} \text{ gas}$$

Because the concentration of alveolar CO_2 is difficult to measure, partial pressure may be substituted and the equation written as follows:

$$V_D = \frac{(P_{ACO_2} - P_{\bar{E}CO_2})}{P_{ACO_2}} V_T$$

where:

$$P_{ACO_2} = \text{arterial } P_{CO_2}$$

$$P_{\bar{E}CO_2} = P_{CO_2} \text{ of mixed expired gas sample}$$

Note that the P_{ACO_2} is substituted for the alveolar P_{CO_2}. This substitution presumes perfect equilibration between alveoli and pulmonary capillaries. This may not be true in certain diseases. The test also assumes that little CO_2 is in the atmosphere. Therefore the P_{CO_2} in the expired gas is inversely proportional to the V_D. Gas is collected over a short interval, and arterial blood is obtained simultaneously to measure P_{ACO_2}. V_D is calculated by applying the previous equation. The estimate becomes more accurate as more expired gas is collected. Accuracy depends on measurement of $\dot{V}_E$, as well as the partial pressures of CO_2 in expired gas and arterial blood. The mixed expired gas sample is usually collected in a bag or balloon after filling and emptying it several times with expired gas to wash out room air from the valves, tubing, and bag itself. The volume of gas in the bag can be measured during collection by including a flow-sensing spirometer in the circuit. If $\dot{V}_E$ and respiratory rate are recorded, the volumes of V_D and V_T can be determined. If the volume expired is not measured, only the dilution ratio can be determined; this is called the V_D/V_T ratio.

The V_D/V_T ratio can also be estimated noninvasively. End-tidal P_{CO_2} can be used to estimate P_{ACO_2}. This technique is often used in systems that monitor expired CO_2 continuously. V_D/V_T is calculated as follows:

$$\frac{V_D}{V_T} = \frac{(P_{etCO_2} - P_{\bar{E}CO_2})}{P_{etCO_2}}$$

where:

$$P_{etCO_2} = \text{end-tidal } P_{CO_2}$$

$$P_{\bar{E}CO_2} = P_{CO_2} \text{ of mixed expired gas sample}$$

In some subjects, particularly those with severe obstruction, P_{etCO_2} does not accurately reflect P_{ACO_2}. As a result the V_D/V_T ratio may be incorrectly estimated. P_{ACO_2} should be used in the V_D calculation whenever possible.

Alveolar Ventilation

$\dot{V}_A$ can be calculated in two ways:

$$\dot{V}_A = f(V_T - V_D)$$

where:

$$V_T = \text{tidal volume}$$

$$V_D = \text{respiratory dead space}$$

$$f = \text{respiratory rate}$$

For the sake of convenience, V_D is often estimated as equal to anatomic dead space. This method is valid only when there is little or no alveolar dead space, as in individuals who do not have pulmonary disease.

Because atmospheric gas contains almost no CO_2, $\dot{V}_A$ can be calculated on the basis of CO_2 elimination from the lungs. A volume of expired gas is collected in a bag, balloon, or spirometer, and analyzed to determine the volume of CO_2 (see Chapter 7). The following equation can then be used:

$$\dot{V}_A = \frac{\dot{V}_{CO_2}}{F_{ACO_2}}$$

where:

$\dot{V}_{CO_2}$ = volume of CO_2 produced in liters per minute, **(STPD)**

F_{ACO_2} = fractional concentration of CO_2 in alveolar gas

If an end-tidal CO_2 monitor is used, a close approximation of the concentration of alveolar CO_2 is easily obtained and the equation simplified as follows:

$$\dot{V}_A = \frac{\dot{V}_{CO_2}}{\% alveolar CO_2} \times 100$$

End-tidal CO_2 may not equal alveolar CO_2 in subjects with grossly abnormal patterns of ventilation-perfusion (see Chapter 6).

The same equation can be used with a substitution of the Pa_{CO_2} for the alveolar P_{CO_2} (i.e., PA_{CO_2}), again presuming that arterial blood and alveolar gas are in equilibrium. The equation is then as follows:

$$\dot{V}_A = \frac{\dot{V}_{CO_2}}{Pa_{CO_2}} \times 0.863$$

where:

$\dot{V}_{CO_2}$ = CO_2 production in ml/min (STPD)

Pa_{CO_2} = partial pressure of arterial CO_2

0.863 = conversion factor from concentration to partial pressure and correcting $\dot{V}_{CO_2}$ to BTPS

SIGNIFICANCE AND PATHOPHYSIOLOGY

See Box 4-3 for interpretive strategies. Measurement of V_D yields important information regarding the ventilation-perfusion characteristics of the lungs. Anatomic dead space is larger in men than in women because of differences in body size; it increases along with the V_T during exercise, as well as in certain forms of pulmonary disease (e.g., bronchiectasis). It may be decreased in asthma or in diseases characterized by bronchial obstruction or mucous plugging. Because of the difficulty in measuring the anatomic dead space, estimates based on age, sex, functional residual capacity, or body size may be used. For clinical purposes the anatomic dead space in milliliters is sometimes considered equal to the subject's ideal body weight in pounds.

Of greater clinical significance is the measurement of respiratory dead space, which is accomplished reasonably well by applying Bohr's equation. The volume of ventilation wasted on the conducting airways and poorly perfused alveoli is usually expressed as the V_D/V_T ratio. The normal value is 0.2 to 0.4. Expressing dead space in this way eliminates the neccessity of measuring the volume of expired gas in the application of Bohr's equation. However, if V_T or $\dot{V}_E$ is known, the dead space volume can be easily calculated. Physiologic dead space measurements are a good index of ventilation-blood flow ratios because all CO_2 in expired gas comes from perfused alveoli (see Chapter 6). The V_D/V_T ratio decreases in normal subjects during exercise because of increases in the **cardiac output** and the increased perfusion of alveoli at the lung apices. This occurs despite absolute increases in the V_D itself.

Increased dead space, and V_D/V_T ratio, may be observed in **pulmonary embolism** and in pulmonary hypertension. In pulmonary embolism large numbers of arterioles may be blocked, resulting in little or no CO_2 removal in the associated alveoli. In pulmonary hypertension, increased

---

BOX 4-3
INTERPRETIVE STRATEGIES—VD AND V̇A

1 Was dead space determination based on Pa_{CO_2}? If not, interpret cautiously.

2 Was V̇E or VT measured? If not, then only VD/VT should be interpreted.

3 Is the VD/VT ratio greater than 0.40? If so, elevated dead space is likely. Consider clinical correlation, especially pulmonary embolism or pulmonary hypertension.

4 Is the VD/VT ratio less than 0.20 with subject at rest? Is there an elevated level of ventilation? Consider technical problems.

5 Is V̇A (if measured) consistent with the patient's clinical signs and symptoms?

---

pulmonary arterial pressure causes most alveoli to be perfused, so there is little or no recruitment of underperfused gas exchange units. This is most notable during exercise when the VD/VT ratio normally falls.

The V̇A at rest is approximately 4 to 5 L/min with wide variations in healthy individuals. The adequacy of the V̇A can be determined only by arterial blood gas studies. Low V̇A associated with acute respiratory acidosis (i.e., Pa_{CO_2} greater than 45 and pH less than 7.35) defines hypoventilation. Excessive V̇A (i.e., Pa_{CO_2} less than 35 and pH greater than 7.45) defines hyperventilation. Chronic hypoventilation and hyperventilation are associated with abnormal Pa_{CO_2} values but near normal pH values. Decreased V̇A can result from absolute increases in dead space as well as decreases in V̇E.

Ventilatory Response Tests for Carbon Dioxide and Oxygen

DESCRIPTION

Ventilatory response to CO_2 is the measurement of the increase or decrease in V̇E caused by breathing various concentrations of CO_2 under normoxic conditions ($Pa_{O_2} = 90$ to 100 mm Hg). It is recorded as L/min/mm Hg P_{CO_2}.

Ventilatory response to O_2 is the measurement of the increase or decrease in V̇E caused by breathing various concentrations of O_2 under isocapnic conditions ($Pa_{CO_2} = 40$ mm Hg). The change in ventilation (L/min) may be recorded in relation to changes in Pa_{O_2} or saturation as monitored by oximetry.

Occlusion pressure (P_{100}) is the pressure generated at the mouth during the first 100 msec of an inspiratory effort against an occluded airway. Changes in P_{100} are related to changes in the ventilatory stimulant (hypercapnia or hypoxemia). It is usually measured in centimeters of water (cm H_2O).

TECHNIQUE

CO_2 response can be measured in two ways:

---

1. *Open-circuit technique.* The subject breathes various concentrations (1% to 7%) of CO_2 in air or O_2 from a **demand valve** or reservoir until a steady state is reached. Measurements of Pet_{CO_2}, Pa_{CO_2}, P_{100}, and V̇E may be made at each concentration.

2. *Closed-circuit or rebreathing technique.* The subject rebreathes from a one-way circuit containing a reservoir of 7% CO_2 in O_2. Valves and pressure taps for monitoring P_{100}, and ports for extracting gas samples for Pet_{CO_2} determinations are included in the circuit. A pneumotachometer (see Chapter 9) is placed in line to record V̇E. Similarly, the gas reservoir bag may be placed in a rigid container or box, and volume change measured by connecting a spirometer to the container (i.e., "bag-in-box" setup). The subject rebreathes until the concentration of Pet_{CO_2} exceeds 9% or until 4 minutes have elapsed. The rebreathed gas may be analyzed to ascertain that the F_{IO_2} remains above 0.21. The subject's Sa_{O_2} may also be monitored by means of a pulse oximeter (see Chapter 9). Changes in V̇E are monitored and plotted against Pet_{CO_2} to obtain a response curve.

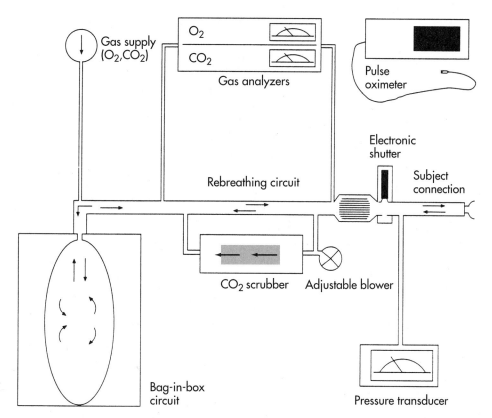

FIG. 4-1 *Closed-circuit system for the rebreathing O_2 response test.* The circuit allows the subject to rebreathe into a bag to which CO_2 or O_2 can be added. Gas analyzers allow continuous monitoring of gas concentrations in the circuit during testing. Ventilation is measured by integrating flow from the pneumotachometer or attaching a spirometer to the bag-in-box setup. A pressure transducer and mouth shutter allow the measurement of P_{100}, and a pulse oximeter provides data on the subject's saturation. A CO_2 scrubber with an adjustable blower allows the level of CO_2 in the system to be maintained at baseline levels (isocapnia). Increases in ventilation caused by the gradual consumption of the O_2 in the circuit can be measured by scrubbing just enough of the exhaled CO_2 to maintain a near normal alveolar P_{CO_2}. The same circuit can be used to measure response to CO_2 by rebreathing. The bag is this case is filled with 5% to 7% CO_2 in O_2 and the scrubber is removed from the circuit.

O_2 response can be measured by either open- or closed-circuit techniques:

1. *Open-circuit technique.* The subject breathes gas mixtures containing O_2 concentrations from 12% to 20%, to which CO_2 is added to maintain alveolar P_{CO_2} (P_{ACO_2}) at a constant level. When a steady state is reached, Pa_{O_2}, $\dot{V}_E$, and P_{100} can be measured. This procedure, often called a step test, is repeated with decreasing O_2 concentrations to produce the response curve. Continuous monitoring of Pet_{CO_2} is necessary to titrate the addition of CO_2 to the system to maintain **isocapnia** (Fig. 4-1). Pa_{O_2} should be monitored because it often varies from the alveolar P_{O_2} (P_{AO_2}). Pulse oximetry may be used to monitor changes in saturation. CO_2 response curves are sometimes measured at widely varying Pa_{O_2} levels, and the subsequent difference in ventilation or P_{100} at any particular P_{CO_2} is attributed to the response to hypoxemia.

2. *Closed-circuit technique (progressive hypoxemia).* The subject rebreathes from a system similar to that used for the closed-circuit CO_2 response but which contains a CO_2 **scrubber.** CO_2 can be added to the inspired gas to maintain isocapnia, or a variable blower may be used to direct a portion of the rebreathed gas through the scrubber to maintain isocapnia (see Fig 4-1). Response to decreasing inspired P_{O_2} is monitored by recording $\dot{V}_E$ or P_{100}, and the Pa_{O_2} or saturation is measured either directly by indwelling catheter or by pulse oximetry.

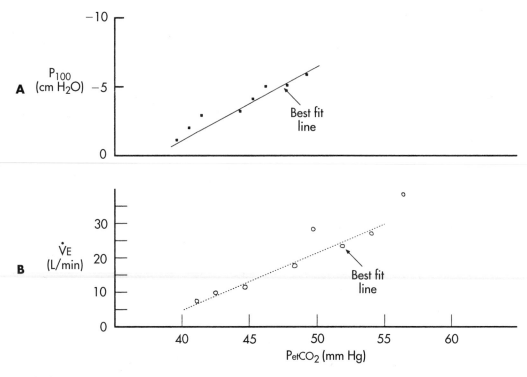

FIG. 4-2 A, P_{100} plotted against end-tidal CO_2 (Petco$_2$), as might be obtained during a CO_2 rebreathing study. **B,** Minute ventilation plotted against Petco$_2$ during the same study. Individual points may be plotted and a "best-fit" line constructed by statistical methods. The slope of the best-fit line is the rate at which ventilation or occlusion pressure increases with increasing stimulation from the rebreathed CO_2.

BOX 4-4
CRITERIA FOR ACCEPTABILITY—VENTILATORY RESPONSE TESTS

1 CO_2 response—Appropriate concentrations of CO_2 (i.e., 7% CO_2 in O_2 for rebreathing studies) must be used.

2 CO_2 response—**Normoxia** maintained; subject's Spo$_2$ should remain >95% during testing.

3 O_2 response—Fio$_2$ appropriate to induce hypoxic response; isocapnia demonstrated by monitoring Petco$_2$.

4 P_{100}—Pressure transducer and monitor capable of recording up to 50 cm H_2O at 50 to 100 mm/sec. Occlusion device should be hidden from subject.

5 Ventilatory responses (O_2, CO_2) should be reproducible within 10%; average of two trials should be reported if clinically practical.

6 Reported P_{100} should be the average of three or more occlusions at each level of challenge.

P_{100} is measured using a system similar to that in Fig. 4-1. A port at the mouth records pressure changes versus time on a storage **oscilloscope**, or by computer. A large-bore stopcock or electronic shutter mechanism is included in the inspiratory line so that inspiratory flow can be randomly occluded. The stopcock or shutter can be closed so that inspiration occurs against a complete occlusion near functional residual capacity. The entire apparatus is usually hidden from the subject so that he or she is unaware of the impending airway occlusion. A pressure-time curve is recorded. P_{100} is usually measured at varying Petco$_2$ values or levels of desaturation to assess the effect of changing stimuli to ventilation. P_{100} and $\dot{V}E$ are usually graphed against Petco$_2$ (Fig. 4-2) or versus O_2 saturation (O_2 response) (Box 4-4).

BOX 4-5

INTERPRETIVE STRATEGIES—VENTILATORY RESPONSE TESTS

1 CO_2 response—Were appropriate levels of elevated CO_2 attained? If rebreathing was used, was test terminated at 4 minutes or 9% CO_2?

2 CO_2 response—Was normoxia maintained? Did Sp_{O_2} demonstrate adequate saturation? If not, interpretation may be compromised.

3 O_2 response—Were appropriate low levels of FI_{O_2} attained? Was isocapnia maintained as demonstrated by Pet_{CO_2}? If not, interpretation may be compromised.

4 Were repeat tests reproducible? If not, interpret cautiously.

5 CO_2 response—Did ventilation increase by at least 1 L/mm Hg change in Pet_{CO_2}? If not, decreased ventilatory response to CO_2 is likely.

6 O_2 response—Did ventilation increase exponentially at Sp_{O_2} levels less than 90%? If not, suspect decreased ventilatory response to hypoxia.

7 P_{100}—Was the occlusion pressure appropriate for the baseline Pa_{CO_2} (1.5-5.0 cm H_2O at a Pa_{CO_2} of 40 mm Hg)? Did P_{100} increase by at least 0.5 cm H_2O/mm Hg change in Pet_{CO_2}? If not, there is likely a decreased central ventilatory drive.

SIGNIFICANCE AND PATHOPHYSIOLOGY

See Box 4-5 for interpretive strategies. The response to an increase in Pa_{CO_2} in a normal individual is a linear increase in $\dot{V}E$ of approximately 3 L/min/mm Hg (P_{CO_2}). The normal range of response varies from 1 to 6 L/min/mm Hg P_{CO_2}, and some variation is present in repeated testing of the same individual. The response to CO_2 in subjects who have obstructive disease may be reduced; this is partially attributable to increased airway resistance, which has been shown to reduce ventilatory drive in healthy individuals. It is unclear why some subjects who have obstructive disease increase ventilation to maintain a normal Pa_{CO_2}, whereas others tolerate an increased Pa_{CO_2}. A plot of $\dot{V}E$ versus Pet_{CO_2} may be used to determine a slope or response curve.

The normal response to a decrease in Pa_{O_2} appears to be exponential once the Pa_{O_2} has fallen to the range of 40 to 60 mm Hg. Again, responses vary widely among individuals. The hypoxic response is increased in the presence of hypercapnia and decreased in hypocapnia. Subjects who have severe chronic obstructive pulmonary disease (COPD) with CO_2 retention receive their primary respiratory stimulus from the hypoxemic response. This group of subjects may experience severe or even fatal respiratory depression if that response is obliterated by uncontrolled O_2 therapy.

Some subjects with minimal intrinsic lung disease show markedly decreased response to hypoxemia or hypercapnia. These include subjects with **myxedema,** obesity-hypoventilation syndrome, obstructive sleep apnea, and idiopathic hypoventilation. CO_2 and O_2 response measurements, along with tests of pulmonary mechanics, may be particularly valuable in the evaluation and treatment of these types of subjects.

The P_{100} ($P_{0.1}$) has been suggested as a measurement of ventilatory drive independent of the mechanical properties of the lungs. Because no airflow occurs during occlusion of the airway, significant interference from mechanical abnormalities (e.g., increased resistance or decreased compliance) is omitted. Reflexes from the airways and chest wall are also of little influence during the first 100 msec of the occluded breath. Therefore, the pressure generated can be viewed as proportional to the neural output of the **medullary centers** that drive the rate and depth of breathing. This proportionality may be influenced by other factors, however, such as body position and the contractile properties of the respiratory muscles.

Subjects whose Pa_{CO_2} values are normal have P_{100} values in the range of 1.5 to 5 cm H_2O. P_{100} has been shown to increase in hypercapnia and hypoxia and appears to correlate well with the observed ventilatory responses. Increasing P_{CO_2}, and thereby inducing hypercapnia, in healthy subjects typically results in an increase in the occlusion pressure of 0.5 to 0.6 cm H_2O/mm Hg P_{CO_2}, with as much as 20% variability. Some subjects who have chronic airway obstruction demonstrate no increase in P_{100} in response to an increase in their P_{CO_2}, even with increased airway resistance. Normal subjects increase their P_{100} when breathing through artificial resistance on challenge with high P_{CO_2} or low P_{O_2}. This failure to respond to increased resistance in the airways may predispose individuals with COPD to respiratory failure when lung infections occur. Similarly, subjects being maintained on mechanical ventilation may experience difficulty in weaning if their ventilatory drive is compromised, as demonstrated by failure to increase the P_{100} when challenged with increased Pco_2. Determination of the P_{100} may prove helpful in determining the effects of treatment in subjects who have abnormal ventilatory responses.

CASE STUDIES

CASE 4A

History

T.J. is a 45-year-old man admitted to the hospital for acute shortness of breath. He has never smoked but has a family history of heart disease. His lungs are clear during auscultation. He becomes breathless just moving around his hospital room. He denies any recent respiratory infections. Because of his rapid respiratory rate, his attending physician requested an arterial blood gas test using room air and a VD/VT ratio determination.

Pulmonary Function Studies

Personal data

Age: 45
Height: 67 in
Weight: 175 lb
Race: Caucasian

Blood gas analysis

pH	7.49
Pco_2 (mm Hg)	29
Po_2 (mm Hg)	102
HCO_3^- (mEq/L)	21
Hb (g/dl)	14.2
Sao_2 (%)	98

Exhaled gas analysis

$\dot{V}E$ (L/min)	24.20
f (breaths/min)	20
$Peco_2$ (mm Hg)	14

Questions

1. Determine the following for this patient.
    a. VT
    b. VD/VT
    c. $\dot{V}A$
2. What is the interpretation of the patient's ventilation?
3. What other tests might be indicated?
4. What treatment might be recommended?

Discussion

1   Calculations
    a.

$$V_T = \frac{\dot{V}_E}{f}$$

$$= \frac{24.2}{20}$$

$$V_T = 1.21 \text{ L}$$

b.

$$V_D/V_T = \frac{(Pa_{CO_2} - Pe_{CO_2})}{Pa_{CO_2}}$$

$$= \frac{(29 - 14)}{29}$$

$$V_D/V_T = 0.517$$

c.

$$\dot{V}_A = f (V_T - V_D)$$

where:

$$V_D = V_D/V_T(V_T)$$

or:

0.517 (1.21) which equals 0.626

Substituting this value in the alveolar ventilation equation:

$$\dot{V}_A = 20 (1.21 - 0.626)$$

$$= 20 (0.584)$$

$$\dot{V}_A = 11.68$$

2   **Ventilation**

This patient has a rapid respiratory rate and a large V_T. The result of this is a large $\dot{V}_E$ (i.e., 24.2 L/min). The blood gas analysis shows hyperventilation (respiratory alkalosis, see Chapter 6) consistent with excessive ventilation. The V_D/V_T ratio is increased at 52% (0.517 as a fraction). Healthy subjects have V_D/V_T ratios of 30% to 40% at rest. In effect, this patient is wasting more than half of each breath. Calculation of the $\dot{V}_A$ similarly reveals that less than half of his $\dot{V}_E$ is actually available for gas exchange. To maintain a normal Pa_{CO_2} (or in this case, to hyperventilate), patients who have increased dead space must increase their total ventilation. Large increases in dead space can occur as a result of obstruction of pulmonary arterial vessels by blood clots or similar lesions. Congestion of pulmonary vessels (resulting from pulmonary hypertension) can also cause imbalances in ventilation-perfusion ratios, especially during exercise.

3   **Other tests**

Other diagnostic procedures that might be indicated include perfusion or ventilation-perfusion scanning of the lungs. Perfusion scans can identify areas of the lung in which there is little or no blood flow. $\dot{V}/\dot{Q}$ scans can detect which areas of the lungs have decreased blood flow in relation to their ventilation. These imaging tests are often used when pulmonary **emboli** are suspected. Ventilation-perfusion scans of T.J. indicated multiple areas of decreased perfusion in both lower lobes, consistent with multiple pulmonary emboli.

4   **Treatment**

The patient had been given O_2 therapy after the blood gas test results were obtained. Because there was adequate oxygenation on room air, the O_2 therapy was inappropriate and discontinued. After the lung scans, the patient was started on anticoagulant therapy (**heparin**). During the next week, the pattern of pulmonary embolization gradually resolved. His ventilation and V_D/V_T ratio returned to normal.

CASE 4B

History

T.B. is a 37-year-old Caucasian man who weighs 245 lb. He was referred to the pulmonary function laboratory after an evaluation in the sleep laboratory revealed obstructive sleep apnea. He admits to daytime somnolence. Baseline pulmonary function studies revealed the following:

	Actual	% Predicted
FVC (L)	3.2	72%
FEV$_1$ (L)	2.7	81%
TLC (L)	4.1	71%
RV/TLC	22%	

Baseline blood gas results were as follows:

pH	7.36
Pco$_2$ (mm Hg)	47
Po$_2$ (mm Hg)	77
HCO$_3^-$ (mEq/L)	28
Sao$_2$ (%)	93

A CO_2 response test was performed to assess T.B.'s respiratory drive. The rebreathing method was used. T.B. rebreathed a mixture of 7% CO_2 in O_2 for 4 minutes. Triplicate measurements of P_{100} were made at intervals throughout the test using a pneumatically operated occlusion valve. The following data were obtained:

Petco$_2$ (mm Hg)	V̇E (L/min)	P_{100} (cm H$_2$O)
43	4.5	2.2
46	4.4	—
50	5.9	—
54	7.9	7.8
57	15.1	—
59	17.1	12.0

Questions

1. What is the interpretation of:
   a. Ventilatory response to CO_2 stimulation?
   b. Respiratory drive response to CO_2 stimulation?
2. What is the cause of the patient's daytime somnolence?
3. What treatment might be recommended based on these findings?

Discussion

1 **Interpretation**

All data obtained during the CO_2 rebreathing test were acceptable. The Petco$_2$ increased appropriately, and the test was terminated after 4 minutes of rebreathing. P_{100} was obtained at baseline, after 2 minutes, and near the end of the test. All pressures were reproducible and the average values were reported. Ventilatory response was diminished at 0.8 L/mm Hg Pco$_2$. P_{100} appeared to increase appropriately.

Impression: Markedly reduced ventilatory response to CO_2, with a normal occlusion pressure.

2 **Cause of symptoms**

This subject, who has documented sleep apnea, also displays a reduced sensitivity to increasing levels of CO_2. Spirometry and total lung capacity suggest a restrictive pattern. His baseline blood gases indicate mild CO_2 retention. His slightly elevated HCO$_3^-$ suggests that this is a chronic condition. The Po$_2$ is mildly reduced as a result of hypoventilation.

The rebreathing test documents that the subject does not increase his ventilation appropriately in response to an increasing load of CO_2 (Fig. 4-3). At the same time, the subject's P_{100} shows a relatively normal response to hypercapnia. This pattern suggests that the subject does not increase ventilation even though his respiratory center is signaling otherwise. These findings are consistent with his obstructive sleep apnea. Subjects who retain CO_2 because of large- or small-airway obstruction often have reduced sensitivity to elevated CO_2.

3 **Treatment**

This patient was given nasal continuous positive airway pressure (CPAP) at night. Nasal CPAP alleviates much of the obstruction occurring in the upper airway. The patient reported a marked decrease in daytime hypersomnolence.

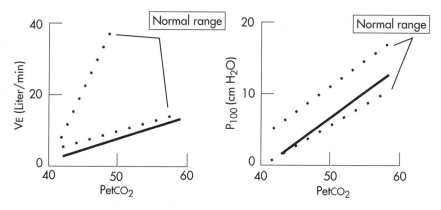

FIG. 4-3 *Plot of data from Case 4A.*

SUMMARY

T HIS CHAPTER HAS DISCUSSED measurement of $\dot{V}_E$, V_T, and respiratory rate. Resting ventilatory measurements can be used in conjunction with blood gases to evaluate respiratory status. One of the most important parameters is the respiratory or physiologic dead space. An estimate of wasted ventilation can be made by comparing expired CO_2 with the arterial P_{CO_2}. Dead space and reduced $\dot{V}_A$ are common to a wide range of pulmonary disorders. When dead space increases, ventilation must increase to maintain a normal acid-base status.

Disorders of ventilatory control are also common to many diseases. Evaluation of responses to hypoxemia and hypercapnia are often useful in characterizing types of ventilatory response disorders. Different techniques of assessing responses have been described. The rebreathing techniques for O_2 and CO_2 are used most often. Measurement of P_{100} can discriminate central ventilatory drive problems from other causes of abnormal responses.

SELF-ASSESSMENT QUESTIONS

1 *A circuit is set up to perform a CO_2 rebreathing response test; the reservoir bag in the circuit should contain which of the following?*
a. Room air
b. 3% CO_2 in air
c. 7% CO_2 in O_2
d. 100% O_2

2 *A subject has the following results after 4.0 minutes of a CO_2 rebreathing test:*

	Time 0	4 Minutes
P_{ETCO_2}	37	57
$\dot{V}_E$ (L/min)	5.0	12.5

These findings are consistent with which of the following?
a. Normal lung function
b. Obesity-hypoventilation syndrome
c. Chronic asthma
d. Interstitial pulmonary fibrosis

3 *Exhaled gas is collected for 5 minutes; the mixed expired P_{CO_2} is measured. Blood gases are drawn during the last minute of gas collection and the following data are recorded:*

P_{ECO_2}:	24 mm Hg
pH:	7.38
Pa_{CO_2}:	32
Pa_{O_2}:	71

What is this subject's V_D/V_T ratio?
a. 0.75
b. 0.33
c. 0.25
d. 0.11

4 *A patient has her respiratory dead space measured as 0.3 L (BTPS). If she is breathing at a rate of 22/min with a V_T of 0.7 L (BTPS), what is her $\dot{V}_A$?*
   a. 22.0 L (BTPS)
   b. 15.4 L (BTPS)
   c. 8.8 L (BTPS)
   d. 6.6 L (BTPS)

5 *A patient with COPD has the following data recorded:*

$\dot{V}_E$:	7.6 L/min (BTPS)
Respiratory rate:	18/min

What is this subject's V_T?
   a. 0.42 L (BTPS)
   b. 0.33 L (BTPS)
   c. 0.23 L (BTPS)
   d. 0.14 L (BTPS)

6 *The V_D/V_T ratio may be estimated noninvasively by measuring which of the following?*
   a. V_T and mixed expired P_{CO_2}
   b. Mixed expired P_{CO_2} and end-tidal P_{CO_2}
   c. End-tidal P_{CO_2} and V_T
   d. Arterial P_{CO_2} and mixed expired P_{CO_2}

7 *Which of the following measurements confirm the diagnosis of hypoventilation?*
   I.   Respiratory rate of 7/min
   II. Ventilation of 4.0 L/min (BTPS)
   III. Pa_{CO_2} of 49 mm Hg
   IV. pH of 7.29
   a. II only
   b. III only
   c. I and II
   d. III and IV

8 *P_{100} is the:*
   a. Ventilation in liters per minute when the patient is breathing 100% O_2
   b. Pet_{CO_2} when the subject is breathing 100 L/min
   c. Pressure developed during the first 100 msec of an occluded breath
   d. Mean alveolar pressure extrapolated to a respiratory rate of 100/min

9 *A rebreathing CO_2 response test should be terminated in which of the following situations?*
   I.   When the Pet_{CO_2} exceeds 9% in the circuit
   II. If the $F_{I_{O_2}}$ drops below 0.21
   III. When the subject has rebreathed for 4 minutes
   IV. As soon as the P_{100} has been measured
   a. I only
   b. II and III only
   c. I, II, and III
   d. I, II, III, and IV

10 *A subject has the following data recorded during a rebreathing O_2 (hypoxic) response test:*

Time (min)	0	1	2	3	4
Pet_{CO_2} (mm Hg)	38	39	39	38	37
Sp_{O_2} (%)	95	94	92	88	85
$\dot{V}_E$ (L/min)	4.1	5.2	9.5	20.4	44.5

These findings are consistent with which of the following?
   a. A normal ventilatory response to hypoxemia
   b. A blunted ventilatory response to hypoxemia
   c. An improperly calibrated pneumotachometer
   d. A malfunctioning end-tidal CO_2 analyzer

SELECTED BIBLIOGRAPHY

General References
Forster RE: *The lung, clinical physiology and pulmonary function tests,* ed 3, St Louis, 1986, Mosby.
West JB: *Pulmonary pathophysiology: the essentials,* ed 4, Baltimore, 1992, Williams & Wilkins.
West JB: *Respiratory physiology: the essentials,* ed 5, Baltimore, 1994, Williams & Wilkins.

Ventilation
Clark AL, Coats AJ: Relationship between ventilation and carbon dioxide production in normal subjects with induced changes in anatomical dead space, *Eur J Clin Invest* 23:428-432, 1993.
Riley RL, Cournand A: "Ideal" alveolar air and the analysis of ventilation-perfusion relationships in the lungs, *J Appl Physiol* 1:825, 1949.
Severinghaus JW, Stipfel M: Alveolar dead space as an index of distribution of blood flow in pulmonary capillaries, *J Appl Physiol* 10:335, 1957.

Zimmerman MI, Miller A, Brown LK, et al: Estimated vs actual values for dead space/tidal volume ratios during incremental exercise in patients evaluated for dyspnea, *Chest* 106:131-136, 1994.

Control of Ventilation
Benlloch E, Cordero P, Morales P, et al: Ventilatory pattern at rest and response to hypercapnic stimulation in patients with obstructive sleep apnea, *Respiration* 62:4-9, 1995.
Cherniack NS, Lederer DH, Altose MD, et al: Occlusion pressure as technique in evaluating respiratory control, *Chest* 70(suppl):137, 1976.
Howard LS, Robbins PA: Problems with determining the hypoxic response in humans using stepwise changes in end-tidal P_{O_2}, *Respir Physiol* 98:241-249, 1994.
Johnson DC, Kazemi H: Central control of ventilation in neuromuscular disease, *Clin Chest Med* 15:607-617, 1994.

McGurk SP, Blanksby BA, Anderson MJ: The relationship of hypercapnic ventilatory responses to age, gender, and athleticism, *Sports Med* 19:173-183, 1995.

Read DJC: A clinical method for assessing the ventilatory response to carbon dioxide, *Australas Ann Med* 16:20, 1967.

Rebuck AS, Campbell EJM: A clinical method for assessing the ventilatory response to hypoxia, *Am Rev Respir Dis* 109:345, 1974.

Scano G, Spinelli A, Duranti R, et al: Carbon dioxide responsiveness in COPD patients with and without chronic hypercapnia, *Eur Respir J* 8:78-85, 1995.

Shaw RA, Schonfeld SA, Whitcomb ME: Progressive and transient hypoxic ventilatory drive tests in healthy subjects, *Am Rev Respir Dis* 126:37, 1982.

Smith JM, Bogard JM, Goorden G, et al: A quasi steady state ramp method for the estimation of the ventilatory response to CO_2, *Respiration* 59:9-15, 1992.

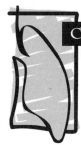

CHAPTER 5

Diffusing Capacity Tests

OBJECTIVES

After studying this chapter and reviewing its tables and case studies, you should be able to do the following:

1 Compare and contrast diffusing capacity measurements made using the single-breath and steady-state methods

2 Determine whether a single-breath diffusing capacity test is acceptable according to recognized standards

3 Apply corrections to the measured diffusing capacity for hemoglobin, carboxyhemoglobin, and altitude

4 Differentiate between obstructive lung disease and restrictive lung disease as causes of decreased diffusing capacity

THIS CHAPTER DESCRIBES MEASUREMENT of diffusion in the lungs. Diffusing capacity is measured using small volumes of carbon monoxide (CO) and is referred to as DL_{CO} or D_{CO}. DL_{CO} is used to assess the gas exchange ability of the lungs, specifically oxygenation of mixed venous blood. A number of different methods have evolved, all of which use CO. The most common method is the single-breath, or breath-hold, technique.

The technique section of the chapter describes the various methods. A major portion of the discussion is dedicated to the single-breath technique. Its wide use has been accompanied by efforts at standardization, which are discussed in detail. Many of the concepts involved in the single-breath method are applicable to the other methods as well.

DL_{CO} measurements are used in the diagnosis and management of both obstructive and restrictive pulmonary disorders. The importance of standards and guidelines in the overall interpretation of DL_{CO} are highlighted. Interpretive strategies are presented in a format similar to those of previous chapters.

Carbon Monoxide Diffusing Capacity

DESCRIPTION

DL_{CO} measures the transfer of a diffusion-limited gas (CO) across the **alveolocapillary** membrane. The DL_{CO} is reported in milliliters of CO per minute per millimeter of mercury at 0° C, 760 mm Hg, dry (i.e., STPD).

TECHNIQUE

CO combines with hemoglobin (Hb) approximately 210 times more readily than oxygen (O_2). In the presence of normal amounts of Hb and normal ventilatory function, the primary limiting factor to diffusion of CO is the status of the alveolocapillary membrane. A small amount of CO in inspired gas produces measurable changes in the concentration of inspired versus expired gas. Because there is normally little or no CO in pulmonary capillary blood, the pressure **gradient** causing diffusion is basically the alveolar pressure (P_{ACO}). If the partial pressure of CO in the alveoli and the rate of uptake of the gas can be measured, the DL_{CO} of the lung can be determined. There are several methods for determining the DL_{CO} (Table 5-1). All of these methods are based on the following equation:

TABLE 5-1 Advantages and Disadvantages of $D_{L_{CO}}$ Testing Methods

Method	Technique	Advantages	Disadvantages	Applications
$D_{L_{CO}}SB$ (breath hold)	He and CO analysis relatively simple; 10 seconds breath hold	Easy calculations, simple; fast; no COHb back pressure; can be automated	Sensitive to distribution of ventilation and $\dot{V}/\dot{Q}$; "nonphysiologic"; not practical for exercise	Screening and clinical application; good standardization
$D_{L_{CO}}SS_1$ (Filey technique)	CO, CO_2, O_2 analysis; arterial blood sample; relatively simple	Most accurate steady-state method; good for exercise testing	Arterial puncture and blood gas analysis; sensitive to uneven $\dot{V}/\dot{Q}$	Clinical application; exercise studies
$D_{L_{CO}}SS_2$ (end-tidal CO)	End-tidal sample, F_{ECO} simultaneously; CO analysis only	No arterial puncture or breath hold; easy calculation	COHb back pressure; V_T must be maintained high; very sensitive to $\dot{V}/\dot{Q}$	Fast, easy screening and clinical method; not used for exercise studies
$D_{L_{CO}}SS_3$ (assumed V_D)	CO analysis (slow or fast); large V_T improves accuracy	Relatively simple calculations; good for exercise studies	Large error if V_T is too small; sensitive to COHb	Screenings and clinical applications; exercise studies
$D_{L_{CO}}SS_4$ (mixed venous P_{CO_2})	CO, CO_2 analysis (rapid); rebreathing required	No arterial puncture; easy calculations; slow CO analysis acceptable	Sensitive to COHb; rebreathing must be controlled closely	Not widely used clinically
$D_{L_{CO}}RB$ (rebreathing)	He and CO analysis (rapid); rebreathing required	Less sensitive to V_A than $D_{L_{CO}}SB$; less sensitive to $\dot{V}/\dot{Q}$ abnormalities	Complex calculations; rapid CO and He analyzers required; sensitive to COHb	Clinically applicable; provides most accurate $D_{L_{CO}}$
$D_{L_{CO}}SS_{He}$ (washout equilibration)	CO, He analysis (rapid): sequencing required	Eliminates V_A, $\dot{V}/\dot{Q}$, and distribution problems	Complex calculations (computerized)	Research applications
$D_{L_{CO}}IB$ (intra-breath)	Rapid responding CO, CH_4 analyzers required	Breath holding not required	Complex calculations (computerized); flow must be controlled; sensitive to uneven $\dot{V}/\dot{Q}$	Screening; may be useful in subjects who cannot hold their breath
F_{CO} (fractional CO uptake)	CO analysis; may be done with $D_{L_{CO}}SS_2$	Simple; CO analysis of inspired and expired gas only	Sensitive to $\dot{V}_E$, $\dot{V}/\dot{Q}$, and V_D/V_T	Screening or correlation to $D_{L_{CO}}SS_2$
$1/D_m + 1/\Theta V_c$ (membrane and red blood cell resistance)	$D_{L_{CO}}SB$ repeated before and after O_2 breathing	Differentiates membrane from red cell components; calculates V_c	Complex calculations; estimates of alveolar P_{O_2} critical	Research with limited clinical applications

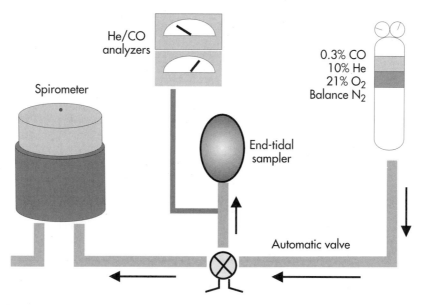

FIG. 5-1 $D_{L_{CO}}$ *apparatus.* The basic equipment for performing the $D_{L_{CO}}$ test (specifically the $D_{L_{CO}}SB$) is illustrated. The test gas used contains 0.3% CO, 10% He, 21% O_2, and balance N_2. Gas is delivered to the automated valve from a large volume bag (not shown), from the spirometer, or by a demand valve (not shown). The automatic valve allows the subject to inhale the test gas rapidly. The valve then closes, assisting the breath-hold maneuver. After 10 seconds the valve opens, allowing exhalation to the spirometer to measure dead space (washout). It then directs exhaled gas to the alveolar sampling device. Gas analyzers for CO and the tracer gas (usually He) then measure the concentrations of gas from the alveolar sample. Some systems measure exhaled gas continuously with rapid responding analyzers (see text). In these systems gas is sampled directly at the mouth without an alveolar sample bag. Not shown is the computer display, which records a volume-time display of the entire maneuver (see Fig. 5-2). Timing of the maneuver may be accomplished automatically by the computer or from a recording device such as a kymograph.

$$D_{L_{CO}} = \frac{\dot{V}_{CO}}{P_{ACO} - P_{CCO}}$$

where:

$\dot{V}_{CO}$ = milliliters of CO transferred per minute (STPD)

P_{ACO} = mean alveolar partial pressure of CO

P_{CCO} = mean capillary partial pressure of CO, assumed to be 0

$D_{L_{CO}}$ is essentially a measure of transfer of CO across the alveolocapillary membranes. $D_{L_{CO}}$ is expressed as milliliters of gas per minute per unit of driving pressure. An additional method of quantifying $D_{L_{CO}}$, fractional uptake of CO (F_{UCO}), simply relates the inspired and expired CO concentrations during normal breathing.

Modified Krogh Technique—Single Breath

The subject inspires a vital capacity breath from a system as described in Fig. 5-1. A spirometer or reservoir contains a gas mixture of 0.3% CO, 10% helium (He), 21% O_2, and the balance nitrogen (N_2). The subject holds the breath at total lung capacity (TLC) for approximately 10 seconds. The subject then exhales. A sample of alveolar gas is collected in a small volume bag (approximately 500 ml), after a suitable washout volume (750 to 1000 ml) has been discarded (Fig. 5-2). The sample is analyzed to obtain the fractional CO and He concentrations in alveolar gas, F_{ACO_T} (where T is the time of the breath hold) and $F_A He$, respectively. The concentration of CO in the alveoli at the beginning of the breath hold (F_{ACO_0}) must be determined as well. It is computed with the following equation:

$$F_{ACO_0} = F_{ICO} \times \frac{F_A He}{F_I He}$$

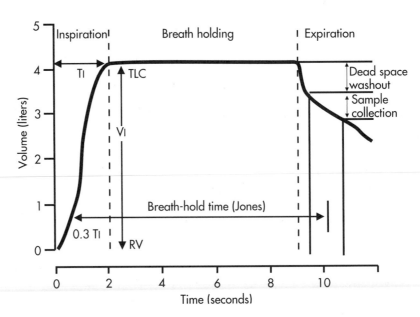

FIG. 5-2 *$DL_{co}SB$ maneuver tracing.* A tracing of the single-breath DL_{co} maneuver proceeding from left to right (*heavy line*). Inspiration is up. After exhaling to RV, the subject rapidly inspires a vital capacity breath (VI) of the test gas, then holds the breath at TLC for approximately 10 seconds. At the end of the breath hold, the subject exhales the dead space washout volume (usually 0.750 to 1.0 L). Then a sample of alveolar gas is collected (usually 0.5 to 1.0 L). Any remaining volume is exhaled. The recommended timing method is illustrated. The Jones method measures from 0.3 of the inspiratory time (TI) to the midpoint of the alveolar sample.

where:

$$FACO_0 = \text{fraction at the beginning of the breath hold (time = 0)}$$

$$FICO = \text{fraction of CO in the reservoir (usually 0.003)}$$

$$FAHe = \text{fraction of He in alveolar gas in the end-tidal sample}$$

$$FIHe = \text{fraction of He in inspired gas (usually 0.10)}$$

The change in He concentration reflects dilution by the gas remaining in the lungs (residual volume [RV]). This change is used to determine what the initial CO concentration must have been, before any gas diffused from the alveoli into the pulmonary capillaries. The $DL_{co}SB$ is then calculated as follows:

$$DL_{co}SB = \frac{VA \times 60}{(PB - 47) \times (T)} \times Ln \frac{FACO_0}{FACO_T}$$

where:

$$VA = \text{alveolar volume, ml (STPD)}$$

$$60 = \text{correction from seconds to minutes}$$

$$PB = \text{barometric pressure, mmHg}$$

$$47 = \text{water vapor pressure } (PH_2O) \text{ at } 37° \text{ C, mm Hg}$$

$$T = \text{breath-hold interval, seconds}$$

Ln = natural logarithm

$$FACO_0 = \text{fraction of CO in alveolar gas at the beginning of the breath hold}$$

$$FACO_T = \text{fraction of CO in alveolar gas at the end of breath hold}$$

VA may be calculated from the single-breath dilution of He:

$$VA = (VI - VD) \times \frac{FIHe}{FAHe} \times STPD \text{ correction factor}$$

where:

V_I = volume of test gas inspired, ml (see Fig. 5-2)

V_D = dead space volume (anatomic and instrumental), ml

$F_A He$ = fraction of He in alveolar gas

$F_I He$ = fraction of He in inspired gas (usually 0.10 or 10%)

The dilution of He is used again, in this case to determine the lung volume at which the breath hold occurred.

A simplification of the above single-breath method is widely used. The He and CO analyzers may be calibrated to read full scale (100% or 1.000) when sampling the diffusion mixture and to read zero when sampling air (no He or CO). If the analyzers have a linear response to each other, the $F_A He$ obtained from the end-tidal sample equals the $F_A CO_0$. This technique assumes that both He and CO are diluted equally during inspiration. Because no He leaves the lung during the breath hold, its concentration in the alveolar sample must equal that of the CO before any diffusion occurred. The exponential rate of CO diffusion from the alveoli can then be expressed as follows:

$$Ln\left(\frac{F_A He}{F_A CO_T}\right)$$

where:

$F_A He$ = fraction of He in the alveolar sample, equal to $F_A CO_0$

$F_A CO_T$ = fraction of CO in the alveolar sample after the breath hold

Ln = natural logarithm of the ratio

This technique avoids the necessity of analyzing the absolute concentrations of the two gases. However, it requires that the analyzers be linear with respect to each other. Analysis of CO is often done using infrared analyzers (see Chapter 9), and their output is nonlinear. Care must be taken to ensure that corrected CO readings are used in the computation. This correction is easily accomplished either electronically or via software in computerized systems. The **linearity** of the system should be within 1% of full scale. This means that any drift or nonlinearity should cause no more than a 1% error when analyzing a known gas concentration.

Other approaches to $D_{L_{CO}}$ gas analysis include rapidly responding multigas analyzers and gas chromatography. Multigas analyzers are specialized infrared analyzers capable of detecting several gases simultaneously. These systems use methane (CH_4) as a tracer gas in place of He. An advantage of multigas analysis is that CO and CH_4 are measured rapidly and continuously (Fig. 5-3). Gas chromatography (see Chapter 9) can also be used for $D_{L_{CO}}$ gas analysis. Neon (Ne) is used as the tracer gas in place of He (Fig. 5-4). He is used as a "carrier" gas for the chromatograph. Although gas analysis using chromatography is slow (60 to 90 seconds), it is extremely accurate.

The resistance of the breathing circuit should be less than 1.5 cm $H_2O/L/sec$, a flow of 6 L/sec. This is important in allowing the subject to inspire rapidly from RV to TLC. A demand valve may be used instead of a reservoir for the test gas. In a demand-flow system, the maximal inspiratory pressure to maintain a flow of 6 L/sec should be less than 10 cm H_2O. The timing device for the maneuver should be accurate to within 100 msec over a 10-second interval (1%). Most computerized systems time the maneuver automatically. However, a means of verifying the accuracy of the breath-hold time should be available. The Jones method of timing the breath hold should be used (see Fig. 5-2).

Corrections must be made for the subject's anatomic dead space (V_D) as well as dead space in the valve and sample bag. Anatomic V_D should be calculated as 2.2 ml/kg of ideal body weight. Instrument V_D should be specified by the equipment manufacturer. Instrument V_D should not exceed 100 ml, including any filters that might be used. Anatomic and instrument V_D are subtracted from inspired volume (V_I) before the alveolar volume (V_A) is calculated.

All gas volumes must be corrected from ATPS to STPD for the $D_{L_{CO}}$ calculations. The V_A, however, when used to calculate the ratio of $D_{L_{CO}}$ to lung volume (D_L/V_A) is normally expressed in BTPS units. Accurate measurement of lung volumes requires that the spirometer has an accuracy of 3% over a range of 8 L. The system must also be free from leaks.

Gas analyzers that are affected by carbon dioxide (CO_2) or water vapor require appropriate absorbers. Absorption of CO_2 is usually accomplished with a chemical absorber using $Ba(OH)_2$ or NaOH. Each of these reactions produce water vapor. Therefore CO_2 absorbers should be

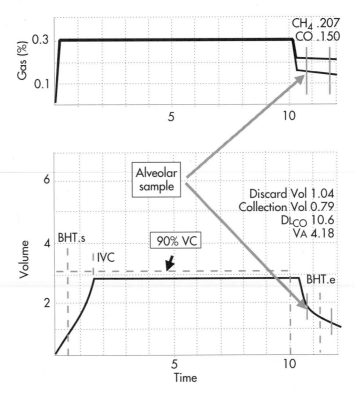

FIG. 5-3 $DL_{co}SB$ *maneuver using continuous gas analysis.* The *top graph* shows changes in gas concentrations. The test gases (CO and CH_4) rise rapidly to their initial values of 0.3% during the breath hold. During exhalation both gas concentrations fall with dead space washout. CH_4 shows a plateau as alveolar gas is exhaled. CO shows a similar pattern but with a lower concentration because of diffusion during the breath hold. Gas concentration measurements are made from an alveolar "window" (*gray lines*) which can be adjusted. The *lower graph* shows changes in lung volumes. *IVC* indicates the inspiratory volume. In this test the subject failed to inspire at least 90% of vital capacity (*VC*) (*dashed gray line*). *BHTs* indicates the start of breath-hold timing; *BHTe* denotes the end of the breath hold at the midpoint of the alveolar sample "window." The calculated DL_{co} and related measurements are displayed (on the computer screen), allowing inspection of changes as the alveolar sample "window" is adjusted. (Courtesy Sensormedics, Inc., Yorba Linda, CA.)

placed upstream of an H_2O absorber. Anhydrous $CaSO_4$ is commonly used to remove water vapor. Selectively permeable tubing (PERMAPURE) can also be used to remove or establish a known water vapor content. Gas conditioning devices must be routinely checked to ensure accurate gas analysis.

$DL_{co}SB$ maneuvers should be performed after the subject has been seated for at least 5 minutes. Because exercise increases DL_{co}, the subject should refrain from exertion immediately before the test. The subject should be instructed about the requirements of the maneuver. After expiration to RV, inspiration should be rapid but not forced. Healthy subjects should be able to inspire at least 90% of their VC within 2.5 seconds (Box 5-1). Patients with moderate or severe airway obstruction should inspire the same volume within 4.0 seconds. The breath hold should be relaxed, either against the closed glottis or a closed valve. The subject should avoid excessive positive intrathoracic pressure (Valsalva maneuver) or excessive negative intrathoracic pressure (**Müller's maneuver**). Expiration after the breath hold should be smooth and uninterrupted. A sample volume of 0.5 to 1.0 L should be collected within 4 seconds. In $DL_{co}SB$ systems that analyze expired gas continuously (see Fig. 5-3), inspection of the washout of the tracer gas is used to select an appropriate alveolar sample.

Two or more acceptable $DL_{co}SB$ maneuvers are usually averaged (see Box 5-1). Duplicate determinations should be within 10% or 3 ml CO/min/mm Hg, whichever is greater. The difference between two tests may be calculated:

$$\frac{\text{Test 1} - \text{Test 2}}{\text{Average}} \times 100$$

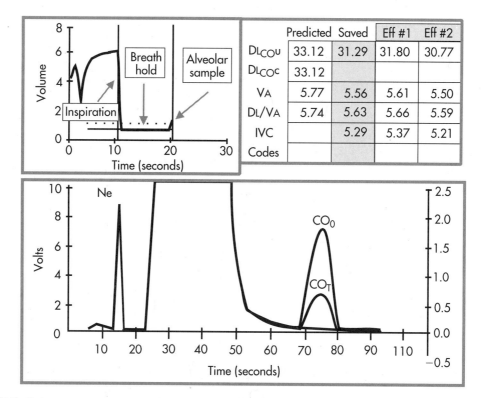

	Predicted	Saved	Eff #1	Eff #2
$D_{L_{CO}}u$	33.12	31.29	31.80	30.77
$D_{L_{CO}}c$	33.12			
V_A	5.77	5.56	5.61	5.50
D_L/V_A	5.74	5.63	5.66	5.59
IVC		5.29	5.37	5.21
Codes				

FIG. 5-4 *$D_{L_{CO}}SB$ test using gas chromatography.* The *upper left panel* depicts the volume-time tracing with inspiration, breath hold, and alveolar sampling. In this scheme, inspiration causes a downward deflection. The *lower graph* shows the output of the gas chromatograph. Neon (*Ne*) (the tracer gas) and CO show distinct peaks. The CO concentrations from the beginning (CO_o) and end (CO_T) of the breath hold are superimposed. The *upper right panel* shows the calculated $D_{L_{CO}}$ and related values for multiple efforts. (Courtesy Medical Graphics, Inc., St. Paul, MN.)

BOX 5-1
CRITERIA FOR ACCEPTABILITY—$D_{L_{CO}}SB$

1 Volume-time tracing should show a smooth, rapid inspiration from RV to TLC.

2 Inspiration should be rapid but not forced; less than 2.5 seconds in healthy subjects and less than 4 seconds in patients with obstruction.

3 Dead space washout should be 0.75 to 1.00 L (0.5 L if the VC is less than 2.0 L). If continuous analysis of expired gas is used, visual inspection of dead space washout should be made.

4 Alveolar sample volume should be 0.5 to 1.0 L, unless continuous analysis is used.

5 The V_I should be at least 90% of the previously recorded best VC.

6 Breath hold time should be within 9 to 11 seconds, using the Jones method.

7 The average of two or more acceptable tests should be reported. Duplicate determinations should be within 10% of 3 ml CO/min/mm Hg.

There should be a 4-minute delay between repeated maneuvers to allow for washout of the test gas from the lungs. Corrections for abnormal Hb concentrations should be applied using a current Hb value. The measured $D_{L_{CO}}$ should be corrected so that the value reported is standardized to an Hb of 14.6 g% for adult men and adolescent boys, and to 13.4 g% for women and children of either sex under 15 years of age. The correction factor for men may be calculated as follows:

$$\text{Hb correction} = \frac{(10.22 + \text{Hb})}{1.7 \times \text{Hb}}$$

Similarly, the equation for women and children under 15 years of age is as follows:

$$\text{Hb correction} = \frac{(9.38 + \text{Hb})}{1.7 + \text{Hb}}$$

The DL_{CO} may then be corrected:

$$\text{Hb adjusted } DL_{CO} = \text{Hb correction} \times \text{observed } DL_{CO}$$

Both uncorrected and corrected DL_{CO} values should be reported, along with the Hb value itself. Correction for the presence of carboxyhemoglobin (COHb) in the subject's blood is also recommended. The DL_{CO} may be adjusted as follows:

$$\text{COHb-adjusted } DL_{CO} = \text{Measured } DL_{CO} \times \left(1.00 + \frac{\%\text{COHb}}{100} \right)$$

CO **back pressure** corrections can also be made by estimating the partial pressure of CO in the pulmonary capillaries and subtracting this value from the $FACO_0$ and the $FACO_T$. Subjects should be asked to refrain from smoking for 24 hours before the test to reduce the CO back pressure in the blood.

DL_{CO} varies inversely with changes in alveolar oxygen pressure (PAO_2). PAO_2 changes as a function of altitude, as well as with the oxygen pressure of the test gas. DL_{CO} increases approximately 0.35% for each mm Hg decrease in the PAO_2. When test gas mixtures that produce an inspired O_2 pressure of 150 mm Hg (i.e., 21% at sea level) are used, DL_{CO} values will be equivalent to those measured at sea level. Alternatively, standard test gas ($FIO_2 = 0.21$) can be used and DL_{CO} corrected by adjusting either PAO_2 or PIO_2.

For a PAO_2 of 120 mm Hg, the equation is as follows:

$$\text{Altitude-adjusted } DL_{CO} = \text{Measured } DL_{CO} \times (1.0 + 0.0035[PAO_2 - 120])$$

For a PIO_2 of 150 mm Hg (sea level), the equation is as follows:

$$\text{Altitude-adjusted } DL_{CO} = \text{Measured } DL_{CO} \times (1.0 + 0.0031[PIO_2 - 150])$$

Filey Technique—Steady State

The subject breathes a gas mixture of 0.1% to 0.2% CO in air for 5 to 6 minutes. During the final 2 minutes, expired gas is collected in a bag or balloon, and an arterial blood sample is drawn. Exhaled volume is measured. Expired gas is analyzed for CO, CO_2, and O_2. The arterial blood is analyzed for PCO_2. Steady-state diffusing capacity is calculated by using the following equation:

$$DL_{CO}SS_1 = \frac{\dot{V}CO}{PACO}$$

where:

$$\dot{V}CO = \text{volume of CO transferred in milliliters per minute (STPD)}$$

$$PACO = \text{mean alveolar partial pressure of CO}$$

$\dot{V}CO$ is determined by analyzing inspired and expired CO ($FICO$ and $FECO$ respectively), $\dot{V}E$, inspired N_2 (FIN_2), and expired N_2 (FEN_2), determined indirectly from the fractions of O_2, CO_2, and H_2O vapor in the exhaled gas as follows:

$$\dot{V}CO = \dot{V}E \left(FICO \, \frac{FEN_2}{FIN_2} - FECO \right)$$

The $PACO$ is determined by using a form of Bohr's equation, as follows:

$$PACO = PB - 47 \left(\frac{FECO - rFICO}{1 - r} \right)$$

where:

$$r = \frac{PACO_2 - PECO_2}{PECO_2}$$

where:

$$Paco_2 = \text{partial pressure of arterial } CO_2$$

$$Peco_2 = \text{partial pressure of mixed expired } CO_2$$

Estimating Paco in this way avoids the necessity of obtaining a direct alveolar sample.

End-Tidal CO Determination

The end-tidal CO determination ($DL_{co}SS_2$) method resembles the $DL_{co}SS_1$ in $\dot{V}co$ and is derived similarly. Paco, however, is determined by taking the average end-tidal CO tension (Petco) from instantaneous analysis of multiple breaths. The end-tidal value is assumed to be equal to the mean Paco.

Assumed VD Technique

The assumed VD technique ($DL_{co}SS_3$) is also similar to the $DL_{co}SS_1$. $\dot{V}co$ is determined as in $DL_{co}SS_1$, but the Paco is measured differently. The fraction of CO in alveolar gas (Faco), which can be used to derive Paco when PB is known, is computed as follows:

$$Faco = \frac{V_T(Feco) - V_D(Fico)}{V_T - V_D}$$

where:

$$V_T = \text{tidal volume}$$

$$V_D = \text{dead space volume}$$

$$Feco = \text{fraction of expired CO}$$

$$Fico = \text{fraction of inspired CO}$$

V_T is measured by averaging multiple breaths. V_D is often assumed to be equal to 2.2 ml/kg of ideal body weight. The mechanical V_D of the breathing circuit is subtracted.

Mixed Venous Pco$_2$ Technique

$\dot{V}co$ is obtained as in $DL_{co}SS_1$. The Paco is calculated by estimating the mixed venous Pco$_2$ from an equilibration technique. The Paco$_2$ is then determined from the $P\bar{v}co_2$ and the normal gradient. When the Paco$_2$ is derived, an equation similar to that used to determine Paco in the $DL_{co}SS_1$ technique can be used. Using mixed venous Pco$_2$ avoids the necessity of arterial puncture.

Rebreathing Technique

The subject rebreathes from a reservoir containing a mixture of 0.3% CO, 10% He, and the remaining air for 30 to 60 seconds at a rate of approximately 30 breaths/min. After this interval, measurements of the final CO, He, and O$_2$ concentrations in the reservoir are made. An equation similar to that used for the single-breath technique is used (see $DL_{co}SB$):

$$DL_{co}RB = \frac{V_S \times 60}{(P_B - 47)(T2 - T1)} \times Ln\left(\frac{Faco_{T1}}{Faco_{T2}}\right)$$

where:

$$V_S = \text{volume of the lung reservoir system (initial volume} \times FiHe/FA_{He})$$

$$60 = \text{correction from seconds to minutes}$$

$$P_B = \text{barometric pressure, mm Hg}$$

$$47 = \text{water vapor pressure (P}H_2O), \text{ mm Hg}$$

$$T2 - T1 = \text{rebreathing interval, seconds}$$

$$Ln = \text{natural logarithm}$$

$$Faco_{T1} = \text{fraction of CO in alveolar gas before diffusion}$$

$$Faco_{T2} = \text{fraction of CO in alveolar gas at the end of diffusion}$$

Equilibration—Washout Method

The subject rebreathes from a reservoir containing 0.3% CO, 10% He, and the remaining air until equilibrium is reached. Then the subject again breathes room air, and the washouts of both CO and He are recorded by a rapid gas analyzer. During the washout, CO is removed at a rapid rate by diffusion as well as by ventilation, while He is removed more slowly by ventilation alone. The difference in washout rates is caused by the rate of CO diffusion. An equation similar to the $DL_{co}SB$ equation is used to calculate $DL_{co}SS_{He}$. A logarithmic expression of the ratio of final He concentration to initial He concentration is included as a factor with the CO concentration ratio. Representation of these washout curves requires computerization.

Slow Exhalation Single Breath—Intrabreath Method

In this technique the subject inspires a vital capacity (VC) breath of test gas containing 0.3% CO, 0.3% CH_4, 21% O_2, and balance N_2. The subject then exhales slowly and evenly at approximately 0.5 L/sec from TLC to RV. Gas concentrations are monitored by a rapidly responding infrared analyzer. The rate of disappearance of CO can be calculated in a manner similar to the washout method. Change in VA is calculated from the change in concentration of the CH_4 tracer gas. CH_4 is used in place of He because it can be rapidly measured using an infrared analyzer. Multiple estimates of DL_{co} can be made during a single exhalation, recording DL_{co} as a function of lung volume. This is done using an equation similar to that used for the single-breath method. Instead of one estimate of VA (equal to the lung volume at breath hold) multiple increments of VA are made, and DL_{co} is plotted against lung volume. A single estimate of the overall DL_{co} can also be obtained.

Fractional CO Uptake

The subject first inspires a mixture of 0.1% CO in air from a reservoir to establish a steady-state breathing pattern, then exhales into a spirometer or reservoir, from which an average expired CO sample is analyzed. The F_{UCO} is expressed as follows:

$$F_{UCO} = \frac{F_{ICO} - F_{ECO}}{F_{ICO}}$$

where:

$$F_{ICO} = \text{fraction of inspired CO}$$
$$F_{ECO} = \text{fraction of expired CO}$$

The resulting fraction may be multiplied by 100 and expressed as a percentage. The level of $\dot{V}_E$ is critical for a valid determination of F_{UCO} and should be monitored closely.

Membrane Diffusion Coefficient and Capillary Blood Volume

The subject performs two $DL_{co}SB$ tests, each at a different level of alveolar Po_2. The first $DL_{co}SB$ is performed as described previously. The subject then breathes an elevated concentration of O_2 (balance N_2) for approximately 5 minutes, exhales to RV, and performs the second $DL_{co}SB$ maneuver. The DL_{co} values are calculated for both the air- and oxygen-breathing maneuvers. The total resistance caused by the alveolocapillary membrane (Dm) and the resistance caused by the rate of chemical combination with Hb and transfer into the red blood cell (ΘQc) is calculated according to the following equation:

$$1/DL_{co} = 1/Dm + 1/\Theta Qc$$

where:

$1/DL_{co}$ = reciprocal of diffusing capacity, or resistance

$1/Dm$ = alveolocapillary membrane resistance

$1/\Theta Qc$ = resistance caused by the red blood cell membrane and rate of reaction with Hb

Θ = transfer rate of CO per milliliter of capillary blood

Qc = capillary blood volume

Because CO and O_2 compete for binding sites on Hb, measurement of diffusion of CO at different levels of alveolar Po_2 can be used to distinguish resistance caused by the alveolocapillary membrane from resistance caused by the red blood cell membrane and Hb reaction rate. **Qc** is presumed to remain the same for both tests, but Θ varies in response to changes in Po_2. Resistance caused by the alveolocapillary membrane can be calculated by plotting Θ at two points against $1/DL_{co}$ and extrapolating back to zero (as if no O_2 were present).

SIGNIFICANCE AND PATHOPHYSIOLOGY

See Box 5-2 for interpretive strategies. The average DL_{CO} value for resting adult subjects by the single-breath method is 25 ml CO/min/mm Hg (STPD). The expected DL_{CO} value in a healthy subject varies directly with the subject's lung volume. Values derived using one of the steady-state methods are usually slightly less than the single-breath method in healthy subjects, but they may vary by as much as 30%. Women have slightly lower normal values, presumably in correlation with smaller normal lung volumes. DL_{CO} values can increase two to three times in healthy individuals during exercise.

Most **reference equations** use height, sex, and age to predict DL_{CO}. Some equations use VA or body surface area (**BSA**) to calculate expected values. If the subject's weight is used (i.e., to calculate BSA), the ideal body weight is recommended. Using the actual body weight in obese subjects can result in erroneous predicted values. Significant differences exist among reference equations. These discrepancies result from different methods used to measure DL_{CO} in various laboratories. Laboratories should check the appropriateness of their reference equations by comparing the results obtained from normal subjects. Fifteen to 20 healthy subjects of each sex should have their DL_{CO} measured. If the reference equations used are appropriate, the differences between the measured and expected values for the healthy subjects should be minimal. Regression equations for calculation of expected DL_{CO} values are included in Appendix B.

DL_{CO} is often decreased in restrictive lung diseases. Many restrictive disorders result from pulmonary fibrosis. Fibrotic changes in the lung **parenchyma** are associated with asbestosis, **berylliosis**, and silicosis. Many other diseases with causes related to inhalation of dusts also cause fibrotic changes in lung tissue. Idiopathic pulmonary fibrosis, sarcoidosis, systemic lupus erythematosus, and scleroderma are also commonly associated with reduction in DL_{CO}. Inhalation of toxic gases or organic agents may cause inflammation of the alveoli (**alveolitis**) and decrease DL_{CO}. These disease states are sometimes categorized as *diffusion defects*. The decrease in DL_{CO} is probably more closely related to the loss of lung volume, alveolar surface area, or capillary bed than to thickening of the alveolocapillary membranes.

DL_{CO} also falls when there is loss of lung tissue or replacement of normal parenchyma by space-occupying lesions such as tumors. DL_{CO} may also be reduced in the presence of pulmonary edema. The reduction in DL_{CO} in edema is caused by not only congestion of the alveoli but also disruption of alveolar ventilation and reduction of lung volume. In the early stages of congestive heart failure (CHF), DL_{CO} may actually be increased. As the left ventricle decompensates, pulmonary vessels become engorged. The increased blood volume causes the DL_{CO} to increase, until the congestion becomes advanced.

DL_{CO} may be reduced as a result of medical or surgical intervention for cardiopulmonary disease. Lung resection for cancer or other reasons typically results in decreased DL_{CO}. The extent of reduction is usually directly proportional to volume of lung removed. An exception to this pattern occurs in lung volume reduction surgery or **bullectomy.** These surgical procedures resect areas of the lung that have little or no blood flow. Lack of perfusion is documented by a lung scan. Excision of tissue in such areas reduces lung volume without necessarily reducing the surface area available for diffusion. Improved ventilation-perfusion matching in the remaining lung often results in increased DL_{CO}.

Radiation therapy that involves the lungs almost always causes a loss of DL_{CO}. Radiation causes **pneumonitis** that commonly results in fibrotic changes. Drugs used in chemotherapy (e.g., bleomycin) and those used to suppress rejection in organ transplantation may cause reductions in DL_{CO}. These drugs appear to directly affect the alveolocapillary membranes. Some drugs used in the treatment of cardiac arrhythmias (e.g., amiodarone) have been shown to reduce DL_{CO}. DL_{CO} is commonly used to monitor drug toxicity.

DL_{CO} may also be decreased in both acute and chronic obstructive lung disease. DL_{CO} is reduced in emphysema for several reasons. Emphysematous lungs have a reduced surface area, with the loss of both alveolar walls and their associated capillary beds. As a result of the decreased surface area, less gas can be transferred per minute even if the remaining gas exchange units are structurally normal. In addition to loss of surface area for gas exchange, the distance from the terminal bronchiole to the alveolocapillary membrane increases in emphysema. As alveoli break down, terminal lung units become larger. Gas must diffuse farther just to reach the alveolocapillary surface. There is also mismatching of ventilation and pulmonary capillary blood flow in emphysema. Disruption of alveolar structures causes loss of support for terminal airways. Airways collapse and gas trapping result in ventilation-perfusion (V/Q) abnormalities.

BOX 5-2
INTERPRETIVE STRATEGIES—DL_{CO}

1   Were the test maneuvers performed acceptably? Were the tests reproducible within 10% or 3 ml CO/min/mm Hg of the mean?

2   Were all appropriate corrections made? Hb? COHb? Altitude?

3   Are reference values appropriate? Age? Height? Sex? Weight?

4   Is DL_{CO} less than the lower limit of normal? If not explained by abnormal Hb or COHb, check DL/VA.

5   Is the DL/VA ratio within normal limits? If so, suspect reduced diffusing capacity related to decreased lung volumes or parenchymal changes. Consider clinical correlation.

6   Is the DL/VA ratio reduced? If so, suspect reduced diffusing capacity related to obstruction or increased dead space. Look for clinical correlation.

7   Is DL_{CO} increased? If not explained by abnormal Hb, consider increased pulmonary blood volume or **hemorrhage.** Look for clinical correlation.

8   Is the DL_{CO} less than 50% of predicted? If so, consider additional tests (blood gases, exercise desaturation study).

Other obstructive diseases (e.g., chronic bronchitis, asthma) may not reduce the DL_{CO} unless they result in markedly abnormal $\dot{V}/\dot{Q}$ patterns. DL_{CO} is sometimes used to differentiate among these obstructive patterns. Low DL_{CO} in the presence of obstruction is sometimes assumed to be evidence of emphysema. However, $\dot{V}/\dot{Q}$ mismatching can cause DL_{CO} to appear to be reduced in asthma, chronic bronchitis, or emphysema. Some asthmatic patients may have elevated DL_{CO}, but the cause is not completely understood.

DL_{CO} measurements at rest have been suggested to estimate the probability of O_2 desaturation during exercise. Not all clinicians agree that a reduction in DL_{CO} can predict desaturation. However, there does appear to be a correlation between resting DL_{CO} and gas exchange during exercise. In some subjects who have chronic obstructive pulmonary disease (COPD), DL_{CO} less than 50% of predicted is accompanied by O_2 desaturation during exercise. Low DL_{CO} (i.e., less than 50% of predicted) may indicate the need for assessment of oxygenation during exertion.

DL_{CO} is directly related to lung volume (VA). Analysis of this relationship can be useful to differentiate whether decreased DL_{CO} resulted from loss of lung volume (restriction) or from uneven $\dot{V}/\dot{Q}$ (obstruction). DL_{CO} may be divided by the lung volume at which the measurement was obtained to express DL_{CO} per unit of VA. This ratio is reported as DL/VL or DL/VA. This calculation is simple because VA must be measured to derive DL_{CO} (see Fig. 5-4). In healthy subjects, DL/VA is approximately 4 to 5 ml of CO transferred per minute, per liter of lung volume. In obstruction, low DL_{CO} without reduction in VA results in a low ratio. In a purely restrictive process, loss of DL_{CO} reflects loss of VA and the ratio is preserved. For example, a subject who has a DL_{CO} of 12 ml CO/min/mm Hg (50% of predicted) and a VA of 3.0 L would have a DL/VA ratio of 4. This reduction in DL_{CO} is caused by a loss of lung volume.

The $DL_{CO}SB$ is the most widely used method because of its relative simplicity and noninvasive nature. The rapidity with which repeated maneuvers can be performed also lends to its popularity. Many automated systems use the $DL_{CO}SB$, thus contributing a certain degree of standardization to the methodology. Large differences in reported DL_{CO} values exist between laboratories. This variability has been attributed to different testing techniques, problems in the gas analysis involved in the test, and differences in computations. Breath holding at TLC is not a physiologic maneuver. This and the fact that DL_{CO} varies with lung volume cause some concerns about $DL_{CO}SB$ as an accurate description of diffusing capacity. $DL_{CO}SB$ is not practical for use during exercise. Some subjects have difficulty expiring fully, inspiring fully, or holding their breath. The American Thoracic Society (ATS) has provided guidelines to improve standardization of the single-breath maneuver (Table 5-2).

The steady-state methods ($DL_{CO}SS_{1-4}$) all use various methods of estimating the mean alveolar PCO. $DL_{CO}SS_1$ has the broadest application of the steady-state methods. Availability of arterial blood gas analysis is a primary requirement for $DL_{CO}SS_1$. $DL_{CO}SS_2$ has gained popularity because of the

TABLE 5-2 Dl$_{co}$SB Recommendations

A. Equipment
  1. Volume accuracy same as for spirometry (±3% over 8 L range, all gases)
  2. Documented analyzer linearity from 0 to full span ± 1%
  3. Circuit resistance less than 1.5 cm H_2O at 6 L/sec
  4. Demand valve sensitivity less than 10 cm H_2O to generate 6 L/sec flow
  5. Timing mechanism accurate to ±1% over 10 sec; checked quarterly
  6. Documented instrument dead space (inspiratory/expiratory) less than 0.1 L
  7. Check for leaks and volume accuracy (3 L calibration) daily
  8. Validate system by testing healthy, nonsmokers (biologic controls) quarterly
B. Technique
  1. Subject should refrain from smoking for 24 hours before test
  2. Subject should be instructed carefully before procedure
  3. Subject should inspire rapidly; 2.5 seconds or less for healthy subjects, 4 seconds or less in obstruction
  4. Subject should achieve an inspired volume greater than 90% of VC
  5. Subject should perform breath hold for 9-11 sec, relaxing against closed glottis or closed valve (no Valsalva or Müller maneuver)
  6. V$_D$ washout should be 0.75-1.0 L, (0.5 L if VC less than 2.0 L)
  7. Alveolar sample volume should be 0.5-1.0 L collected in less than 4 sec.
  8. Visual inspection of V$_D$ washout and alveolar sampling should be used for system that continuously analyzes expired gas
  9. Test gas should contain 21% O_2 at sea level; supplemental O_2 should be discontinued 5 min before testing if possible
  10. Four minutes should elapse between repeat tests
C. Calculations
  1. Average at least two acceptable tests; duplicate determinations should be within 10% or 3 ml CO/min/mm Hg
  2. Use Jones method of timing breath hold
  3. Alveolar volume should be determined by the single-breath dilution of tracer gas
  4. Adjust for V$_D$ volumes (instrument and subject)
  5. Determine inspired gas conditions (ATPS or ATPD)
  6. Correct for CO_2 and H_2O absorption
  7. Report Dl/V$_A$ in ml CO (STPD)/min/mmHg per L (BTPS)
  8. Correct for Hb concentration (see text)
  9. Adjust for COHb (recommended)
  10. Adjust for altitude (recommended)
  11. Use reference equations appropriate to the laboratory method and patient population

Summarized from Single-breath carbon monoxide diffusing capacity (transfer factor): recommendations for a standard technique—1995 update, *Am J Respir Crit Care Med* 152:2185-2198, 1995.

availability of fast-response CO analyzers (see Chapter 9). Dl$_{co}$SS$_3$ may be used to measure Dl$_{co}$ during exercise because small differences in the assumed V$_D$ become less significant as V$_T$ increases. All of the steady-state methods can be applied to exercise testing, but Dl$_{co}$SS$_1$ and Dl$_{co}$SS$_4$ are most commonly used.

The rebreathing method (Dl$_{co}$RB) requires somewhat complicated calculations but offers the advantages of a normal breathing pattern without arterial puncture. Dl$_{co}$RB is less sensitive to $\dot{V}/\dot{Q}$ abnormalities and uneven ventilation distribution than either the Dl$_{co}$SB or the steady-state methods. The rebreathing method and the steady-state methods may have some inaccuracy from accumulation of COHb in the capillary blood and the resultant back pressure. Capillary Pco is routinely assumed to be zero. The actual alveolocapillary CO gradient at the time of testing can be estimated, although with some difficulty.

Dl$_{co}$SS$_{He}$ is the most sophisticated technique. It is relatively insensitive to $\dot{V}/\dot{Q}$ and ventilation abnormalities. However, it is probably limited to research applications.

The measurement of Dl$_{co}$ by the intrabreath method (Dl$_{co}$IB) offers the advantage of not requiring a breath hold at TLC. However, the subject must inspire a large enough volume of test gas so that the subsequent exhalation will clear the instrument and anatomic V_D. In addition, the single-breath exhalation must be slow and even. In some systems a flow restrictor may be necessary to limit expiratory flow. The single-breath slow exhalation technique produces values similar to those obtained by the breath-hold method in healthy subjects when flow is maintained at 0.5 L/sec. Uneven distribution of ventilation may produce intrabreath DL_{CO} values that are artificially elevated. Because the evenness of distribution of ventilation can be assessed from the washout of CH_4, unacceptable DL_{CO} values can be detected. Table 5-1 compares some of the advantages and disadvantages of the different DL_{CO} testing methods.

Measurement of membrane and red blood cell components of diffusion resistance in healthy subjects reveals that each factor accounts for approximately half of the total resistance. Difficulty in quantifying the partial pressure of O_2 in the lungs (pulmonary capillaries) restricts the use of the membrane diffusing capacity determination.

Numerous other factors can influence the observed DL_{CO}:

1. *Hemoglobin and* **hematocrit** *(Hct).* Decreased Hb or Hct reduces the DL_{CO}, whereas increased Hb and Hct elevate the DL_{CO}. DL_{CO} may be corrected if the subject's Hb is known. CO uptake varies approximately 7% for each gram of Hb. The measured DL_{CO} may be corrected so that the value reported is standardized to an Hb level of approximately 14.6 g% for men and 13.4% for women and children younger than 15 years of age, as discussed earlier. When this correction is applied, DL_{CO} will be reduced if the subject's Hb is greater than standardized value (14.6 or 13.4 g%, respectively). Conversely, DL_{CO} increases if the Hb is less than the standard value. Both the corrected and uncorrected values should be reported. Care should be taken to use an Hb value that is representative of the subject's true Hb level at the time of the DL_{CO} test.

2. *COHb.* Elevated COHb levels, as found in smokers, reduce DL_{CO}. Smokers may have COHb levels of 10% or even greater, causing significant CO back pressure. The diffusion gradient for CO across alveolocapillary membranes is assumed to equal the alveolar pressure of CO. In healthy, nonsmoking subjects, very little CO is present in pulmonary capillary blood. When there is carboxyhemoglobinemia, diffusion of CO is reduced because the gradient across the membrane is reduced. COHb also shifts the oxyhemoglobin dissociation curve, further altering gas transfer. Each 1% increase in COHb causes an approximate 1% decrease in the measured DL_{CO}. CO back pressure corrections can also be made by estimating the partial pressure of CO in the pulmonary capillaries. This pressure can be subtracted from the $FACO_0$ and the $FACO_T$.

3. *Alveolar* PCO_2. Increased PCO_2 raises DL_{CO} because the alveolar PO_2 is necessarily decreased. Significant increases in the alveolar PCO_2 lower the alveolar PO_2 (i.e., hypoventilation).

4. *Pulmonary capillary blood volume.* Increased blood volume in the lungs (Qc) causes increased DL_{CO}. Increases in pulmonary capillary blood volume may result from increased cardiac output as occurs during exercise. Pulmonary hemorrhage may also cause an increase in the blood volume in the lungs. In each of these cases the increase in DL_{CO} is related to the increased volume of Hb available for gas transfer. Excessive negative intrathoracic pressure during breath holding can increase pulmonary capillary volume and raise the DL_{CO}. Conversely, excessive positive intrathoracic pressure (Valsalva maneuver) can reduce pulmonary blood flow and decrease DL_{CO}.

5. *Body position.* The supine position increases DL_{CO}. Changes in body position affect the distribution of capillary blood flow.

6. *Altitude above sea level.* DL_{CO} varies inversely with changes in alveolar oxygen pressure (PAO_2). At altitude the DL_{CO} increases unless corrections are made (see "Technique," p. 118).

Several additional technical considerations may affect the measurement of DL_{CO} (particularly the $DL_{CO}SB$). VA is calculated from He dilution during the single-breath maneuver. This technique underestimates lung volume in subjects who have moderate or severe obstruction. Low estimated VA results in low DL_{CO} values. Some clinicians prefer to use a separately determined lung volume to estimate VA. RV, as measured by one of the gas techniques or by plethysmography, can be added to the inspired volume (VI) to derive VA. VA calculated this way may be larger in airway-obstructed patients than VA calculated from the single-breath dilution method. The resulting estimate of DL_{CO}

is larger. This approach may be questionable because the single-breath He dilution value (FAHe) is also used in the exponential ratio that describes transfer of CO from the alveoli. Some laboratories report DL_{CO} calculated by both methods.

The method of measuring the time of breath hold also influences the calculation of DL_{CO} (see Fig. 5-2). Most systems measure breath-hold time by one of three methods:

1. *Ogilvie method:* from the beginning of inspiration (VI) to the beginning of alveolar sampling
2. *Epidemiology Standardization Project (ESP) method:* from the midpoint of inspiration (half of the VI) to the beginning of alveolar sampling
3. *Jones method:* includes 0.7 of the inspiratory time to the midpoint of the alveolar sample

Theoretically, breath-hold time is considered the time during which diffusion occurs. However, because some gas transfer may take place early in inspiration, DL_{CO} may be greater if timing starts at the midpoint of VI, as when the ESP method is used. Similarly, some diffusion occurs during washout and alveolar sampling. If the timing period is extended into the alveolar sampling phase, as is done in the Jones method, the actual time of breath holding is increased and the additional diffusion accounted for. The timing method may become significant if the reference values used for comparison were generated by one of the other methods. The Jones method is the recommended method (see Table 5-2). Rapid inspiration and rapid expiration to the alveolar sampling phase reduces differences resulting from the timing methods.

The volume of gas discarded before collecting the alveolar sample may affect the measured DL_{CO}. Most automated systems allow variable washout volumes, with 0.75 to 1.0 L most commonly used. Washout volume may need to be reduced to 0.5 L if the subject's VC is less than 2.0 L. In subjects who have obstructive disease, reducing the washout volume may result in increased VD gas being added to the alveolar sample. Because dead-space gas resembles the diffusion mixture, DL_{CO} tends to be underestimated.

Alveolar sampling technique also affects the measurement of DL_{CO}. Alveolar samples should be collected within 4 seconds, including washout and alveolar sampling. A sample volume of 0.5 to 1.0 L is recommended. Subjects with a small VC (i.e., less than 2.0 L) may require a smaller volume, just as with the washout. When only a small sample is obtained, the gas may not accurately reflect alveolar concentrations of CO and He, particularly in the presence of $\dot{V}/\dot{Q}$ abnormalities. Continuous analysis of the expirate using a rapidly responding analyzer allows identification of alveolar gas. Infrared analyzers that can simultaneously analyze the tracer gas and CO allow the entire breath to be analyzed. These instruments permit adjustment of the alveolar sampling window so that a representative gas sample can be obtained (see Fig. 5-3).

CASE STUDIES

CASE 5A

History

P.M. is a 55-year-old woman referred to the pulmonary function laboratory because of shortness of breath on exertion. She has a 38 pack/year smoking history, but stopped smoking 6 months ago. She still coughs each morning, but her sputum volume has decreased since she stopped smoking. She has no significant environmental or family history of pulmonary disease. She had been using an inhaled β-agonist but withheld it for 12 hours before the test.

Pulmonary Function Testing

Personal data

Age: 55
Height: 65 in
Weight: 137 lb
Race: African-American

Spirometry

			Before drug			After drug		
		Predicted	Actual	% Predicted	Actual	% Predicted	% Change
FVC	(L)	2.81	2.77	99%	2.82	100%	2%
FEV$_1$	(L)	2.11	1.91	91%	2.01	95%	5%
FEV$_{1\%}$	(%)	75	69		71		
FEF$_{25\%-75\%}$	(L/sec)	2.80	1.44	51%	1.51	54%	5%
PEF	(L/min)	5.99	4.01	67%	5.13	86%	28%
FEF$_{25\%}$	(L/sec)	5.59	3.31	59%	3.60	64%	9%
FEF$_{50\%}$	(L/sec)	4.19	2.27	54%	2.60	62%	15%
FEF$_{75\%}$	(L/sec)	1.79	0.69	39%	1.01	56%	46%

Lung volumes

		Predicted	Actual	% Predicted
TLC	(L)	4.39	4.97	113%
FRC	(L)	2.45	3.10	127%
RV	(L)	1.58	2.20	139%
VC	(L)	2.81	2.77	99%
IC	(L)	1.94	1.87	96%
ERV	(L)	0.87	0.90	103%
RV/TLC	(%)	36	44	

Diffusing capacity

	Predicted	Actual	% Predicted
DL$_{co}$SB (ml CO/ min/mm Hg)	19.7	10.0	51%
DL$_{co}$SB adjusted (ml CO/min/mm Hg)	19.7	10.3	52%
VA (L)	4.39	4.81	109%
DL/VA	4.49	2.08	46%

Technologist's Comments

All spirometry maneuvers meet ATS criteria. Lung volumes by body plethysmography were performed acceptably. All DL$_{co}$ maneuvers exceeded 11 seconds for breath hold, otherwise acceptable (two tests were averaged). DL$_{co}$ was corrected for Hb.

Questions

1. Interpret the following:
   a. Spirometry, prebronchodilator and postbronchodilator
   b. Lung volumes
   c. DL$_{co}$
2. What is the cause of the patient's symptoms?
3. What other tests might be indicated?
4. What treatment should be considered?

Discussion

1 **Interpretation**

All maneuvers were performed acceptably except for the breath-hold time during the DL$_{co}$SB. Spirometry is normal but there is a mild reduction in the FEV$_{1\%}$. The FEF$_{50\%}$ and FEF$_{75\%}$ are also reduced. After bronchodilator therapy there is only a 100 ml improvement (5%) in FEV$_1$. Lung volumes reveal a slightly increased functional residual capacity and moderately increased RV. The RV/TLC ratio is increased, consistent with air trapping. DL$_{co}$ markedly decreased, even after correction for Hb. DL/VA is reduced, consistent with an obstructive process.

Impression: Mild obstruction with minimal response to bronchodilator; this should not preclude a therapeutic trial if clinically indicated. Lung volumes suggest air trapping. DL_{CO} is severely reduced even when corrected for Hb.

2 **Cause of symptoms**

This patient has symptoms characteristic of airway obstruction that has progressed to the point where dyspnea on exertion prompted a visit to the physician. Her obstruction appears mild. Instantaneous flows, particularly $FEF_{50\%}$ and $FEF_{75\%}$, suggest peripheral airway involvement. Her response to bronchodilator therapy seems to indicate obstruction caused by inflammation rather than reversible bronchospasm. Lung volumes testing confirms that enough obstruction is present to cause some air trapping. This pattern is not unusual for patients with chronic bronchitis and emphysema.

Her gas exchange, as measured by DL_{CO}, is markedly impaired. Emphysema reduces DL_{CO} by reducing the alveolar-capillary surface area available for diffusion. Chronic bronchitis can reduce DL_{CO} by causing a ventilation-perfusion mismatch. This subject appears to have both of these diseases disrupting gas transfer. Subjects who have reduced DL_{CO} values seldom have normal blood gases. Exertion or exercise often aggravates the gas exchange impairment. Many patients with markedly reduced DL_{CO} (less than 50% of predicted) display exercise desaturation. That is, their Pao_2 falls to levels of 55 mm Hg or less with exercise. The reduction in DL_{CO} cannot, however, accurately predict the degree of desaturation that will occur.

3 **Other tests**

An obvious additional test for this patient would be measuring resting arterial blood gases while the patient breathes room air. Resting hypoxemia would explain dyspnea on exertion. P.M. had blood gas samples drawn. Her Pao_2 while breathing air was 63 mm Hg, with a saturation of 91%. Because this value did not qualify her for supplemental O_2, an exercise test was performed with an arterial catheter in place (see Chapter 7). At a low workload her Pao_2 fell to 51 mm Hg. She was then retested while breathing O_2 via nasal cannula at 1 L/min. She then tolerated more exercise, and her Pao_2 never fell below 68 mm Hg.

4 **Treatment**

Based on the results of the exercise evaluation, supplemental O_2 was prescribed for the patient to use during exertion. She was given a portable liquid O_2 system. Because she showed little response to bronchodilators, she was told to stop taking the inhaled β-agonist. However, a trial of inhaled steroids (beclamethasone) resulted in noticeable improvement in symptoms.

CASE 5B

History

B.C. is a 63-year-old woman with a history of cardiomyopathy, hypertension, and pernicious **anemia.** She has had episodes of ventricular tachycardia that have been managed by means of an automatic implantable cardiac **defibrillator** (AICD). She has never smoked and denies cough or sputum production. She does get short of breath with exertion. Her family history includes a sister who had asthma and chronic bronchitis. She has no history of environmental toxin exposure. To manage her arrhythmias her physician prescribed the drug amiodarone. To monitor the effects of this medication, she was referred for tests before starting the drug and again after 3 months of therapy.

Pulmonary Function Testing

Personal data

Sex: Female
Age: 63
Height: 62 in
Weight: 131 lb
Race: Caucasian

Spirometry

	Pretreatment			3 months	
	Predicted	*Actual*	*% Predicted*	*Actual*	*% Predicted*
FVC (L)	2.77	2.5	90	1.97	70
FEV_1 (L)	2.01	2.09	104	1.81	90
$FEV_{1\%}$ (%)	72	84		92	
$FEF_{25\%-75\%}$ (L/sec)	2.38	2.82	118	2.77	116

Lung volumes (He dilution)

	Pretreatment			3 months	
	Predicted	Actual	% Predicted	Actual	% Predicted
TLC (L)	4.88	3.92	87	3.50	78
FRC (L)	2.54	2.26	89	2.23	88
RV (L)	1.71	1.50	87	1.52	89
VC (L)	2.77	2.42	87	1.97	71
IC (L)	1.94	1.66	85	1.26	65
ERV (L)	0.83	0.76	91	0.71	85
RV/TLC (%)	38	38		44	

Diffusing capacity ($D_{L_{CO}}$SB)

	Pretreatment			3 months	
	Predicted	Actual	% Predicted	Actual	% Predicted
$D_{L_{CO}}$ (ml/min/mm Hg)	18.0	12.6	69	9.7	54
$D_{L_{CO}}$ adj (ml/min/mm Hg)	18.0	15.5	86	10.9	60
V_ASB (L)	4.48	3.26	72	3.25	72
D_L/V_A	4.0	3.9	96	3.0	74

Technologist's Comments

Pretreatment

Spirometry: All ATS criteria are met.

Lung voumes: Maneuver was performed acceptably.

$D_{L_{CO}}$: Inspired volume was less than 90% of best VC (83%, 83%); $D_{L_{CO}}$ was corrected for Hb of 10.7 g%.

3 months

Spirometry: All ATS criteria are met.

Lung volumes: Maneuver was performed acceptably.

$D_{L_{CO}}$: Inspired volume was less than 90% of best VC (81%, 76%); $D_{L_{CO}}$ was corrected for Hb of 11.3 g%.

Questions

1. Interpret the following:

    a. Pretreatment spirometry, lung volumes

    b. $D_{L_{CO}}$ before treatment

    c. $D_{L_{CO}}$ after 3 months of treatment

2. What caused the change in the patient's $D_{L_{CO}}$?

3. What technical problems might have affected the interpretation of the $D_{L_{CO}}$ both before and after treatment?

Discussion

1   **Interpretation**

Pretreatment, FVC is normal, as are FEV_1 and $FEV_{1\%}$. Lung volumes by He dilution are normal. The diffusing capacity was substandard in performance because the patient could not inspire fully. The best efforts show mildly reduced $D_{L_{CO}}$ that is normal when corrected for the patient's Hb of 10.7.

After 3 months, FVC is reduced, but FEV_1 is normal. This makes the $FEV_{1\%}$ appear greater than expected. Lung volumes by He dilution show a TLC that is mildly reduced but a normal FRC and RV. The $D_{L_{CO}}$ maneuver is substandard because of poor inspiratory volume. The $D_{L_{CO}}$ is moderately reduced, even when corrected for an Hb of 11.3 g%. Since the previous test, the patient's VC has decreased slightly, and the $D_{L_{CO}}$ has decreased significantly.

2   **Cause of changes in diffusing capacity**

This case presents a good example of one application of $D_{L_{CO}}$: monitoring drug therapy. B.C. had basically normal lung function. Initially, her $D_{L_{CO}}$ was slightly reduced. However, because she had a history of anemia, her Hb level was checked. The Hb-adjusted $D_{L_{CO}}$ was within normal limits. Because the drug amiodarone has been shown to cause changes to the lung parenchyma, her physician ordered pulmonary function studies, including DL_{CO}.

On her return visit after 3 months of the antiarrhythmic therapy, some significant changes had occurred. As pointed out in the interpretation of the 3-month follow-up, her FVC and FEV_1 had decreased slightly. TLC also decreased by a similar volume (400 to 500 ml). Her other lung volumes (FRC, RV) remained largely unchanged. These changes suggest that something happened that primarily affected the VC.

Her DL_{CO} showed the greatest decrement during the 3-month period. The Hb-adjusted DL_{CO} decreased by approximately 30%. This marked decrease occurred even though the measured VA did not change. As a result, DL/VA was reduced. The DL/VA ratio is usually preserved when DL_{CO} decreases simply because of loss of lung volume. When the DL/VA ratio falls in conjunction with a low DL_{CO}, factors other than loss of lung volume are assumed responsible for the change. In this patient it appears that drug therapy did affect the DL_{CO}. However, a pattern of pneumonitis and fibrosis causing reduced lung volumes is not clearly evident. Because of the changes in DL_{CO}, amiodarone therapy was discontinued.

3   **Technical factors influencing DL_{CO}**

Two noteworthy technical factors are illustrated by this case. Correction of the DL_{CO} for the effects of abnormal levels of Hb is very important. In this mildly anemic patient, correction for Hb resulted in a significant difference in DL_{CO} in both tests. Her pretreatment DL_{CO} looks mildly reduced until corrected for Hb. After 3 months of amiodarone therapy, both the uncorrected and corrected DL_{CO} values are below normal. Comparison of serial DL_{CO} measurements can be compromised if one test is Hb-adjusted and the other is not.

A second factor is that none of the patient's DL_{CO} tests met established criteria for acceptability. In all efforts she was unable to inspire at least 90% of her VC for the breath-hold maneuver. This information is documented in the technologist's comments for each test. When the patient fails to inspire maximally, the breath hold does not occur at TLC. As a result, the DL_{CO} may appear low compared with predicted values. This technical difficulty may have influenced these test results. However, because a similar pattern was seen on both the initial and follow-up tests, the data can be cautiously interpreted.

SUMMARY

T HIS CHAPTER HAS ADDRESSED the measurement of DL_{CO}. DL_{CO} can be measured by various techniques. These techniques include the single-breath method and steady-state methods, as well as others. The single-breath method, or $DL_{CO}SB$, is the most commonly used. $DL_{CO}SB$ is noninvasive and can be repeated easily to obtain multiple tests. Many automated $DL_{CO}SB$ systems are available. The ATS and others have published standardization guidelines for $DL_{CO}SB$. Careful attention to standards and clinical practice guidelines can reduce the variance in $DL_{CO}SB$ measurements in different laboratories. The steady-state and other methods, although not used as widely, have advantages for measuring DL_{CO} in special situations (e.g., exercise).

DL_{CO} measurements are used diagnostically for a variety of diseases. Because DL_{CO} assesses gas exchange, it is useful in both obstructive and restrictive disease patterns. DL_{CO} and DL/VA are commonly used to assess the course of diseases such as idiopathic pulmonary fibrosis and sarcoidosis. DL_{CO} is often measured in subjects with obstructive breathing patterns to characterize the physiology of the obstructive process. DL_{CO} is also used to assess gas exchange abnormality in patients with obstruction. In both obstructive and restrictive disorders, DL_{CO} is used to measure response to surgical or medical interventions.

SELF-ASSESSMENT QUESTIONS

1   *Why is CO an ideal gas for measuring diffusing capacity of the lungs?*
   a. It is taken up by Hb in a manner similar to O_2.
   b. It is always present in capillary blood at 0.3%.
   c. It is quickly converted into CO_2 in the lungs.
   d. It does not react with He or other tracer gases.

2   *The fractional concentration of CO after 10 seconds of breath-holding ($FACO_t$) is determined by which of the following?*
   a. $(FAHe/FIHe) \times FICO$
   b. Volume inspired divided by $FAHe/FIHe$
   c. Estimation of the ratio $FICO/FAHe$
   d. Measurement of CO from an alveolar sample

3 *The Jones method of timing the breath hold for* $D_{L_{CO}}SB$ *measures from:*
   a. Beginning of inspiration to beginning of alveolar sampling
   b. 0.3 of inspiratory time to the middle of alveolar sampling
   c. 0.5 of inspiratory time to the middle of alveolar sampling
   d. Beginning of breath-hold to the end of alveolar sampling

4 *A Valsalva maneuver during the* $D_{L_{CO}}SB$:
   a. is required to properly perform the breath hold
   b. may cause the D_L/V_A to appear artificially elevated
   c. may cause the $D_{L_{CO}}SB$ to appear artificially reduced
   d. helps keep breath-hold time between 9 and 11 seconds

5 *Which of the following* $D_{L_{CO}}$ *methods requires an arterial blood sample to be drawn during the test?*
   a. $D_{L_{CO}}SS_1$
   b. $D_{L_{CO}}SS_2$
   c. $D_{L_{CO}}SB$
   d. $D_{L_{CO}}IB$

6 *A nonsmoking subject performs two* $D_{L_{CO}}SB$ *maneuvers and the following results are obtained:*

   Test 1:   24.3 ml CO/min/mm Hg
   Test 2:   18.7 ml CO/min/mm Hg

   Which of the following is appropriate?
   a. Report the largest value as the $D_{L_{CO}}$.
   b. Report the average of the two values.
   c. Perform an additional maneuver.
   d. Correct the value from Test 2 for COHb.

7 *In which of the following disorders would a reduction in* $D_{L_{CO}}$ *be expected?*
   I.   Sarcoidosis
   II. Scleroderma
   III. Polycythemia
   IV. Interstitial pulmonary fibrosis
   a. I and III only
   b. II and IV only
   c. I, II, and IV
   d. II, III, and IV

8 *Diffusing capacity is reduced in emphysema because of which of the following?*
   a. Loss of alveolar surface area
   b. Engorgement of pulmonary capillaries
   c. Dynamic airway compression
   d. Elevated pulmonary arterial pressure

9 *A subject has a* $D_{L_{CO}}SB$ *of 10.2 ml CO/min/mm Hg (STPD), which is 51% of her predicted value. Her* D_L/V_A *ratio is 4.1. Which of the following is most consistent with these values?*
   a. Pulmonary emphysema
   b. Pulmonary resection
   c. Cystic fibrosis
   d. Carboxyhemoglobin of 5.5%

10 *Which of the following is an advantage of continuous analysis of expired gas during a* $D_{L_{CO}}SB$ *test?*
   a. Instrument dead space is eliminated.
   b. Exhaled gas concentrations can be visually inspected.
   c. CO back pressure is reduced.
   d. Breath-hold times longer than 11 seconds are acceptable.

SELECTED BIBLIOGRAPHY

General References

Crapo RO, Forster RE: Carbon monoxide diffusing capacity, *Clin Chest Med* 10:187, 1989.

Epler GR, Saber FA, Gaensler EA: Determination of severe impairment (disability) in interstitial lung disease, *Am Rev Respir Dis* 121:647-659, 1980.

Ferris BG, ed: Epidemiology standardization project: recommended standardized procedure for pulmonary function testing, *Am Rev Respir Dis* 118(suppl 2:55):1, 1978.

Forster RE: Diffusion of gases across the alveolar membrane. In Farhi LE, Tenney SM, eds: *Handbook of physiology,* vol 4, Bethesda, Md, 1987, Physicologic Society.

Morris AH, Kanner RE, Crapo RO, et al: *Clinical pulmonary function testing,* ed 2, Salt Lake City, 1984, Intermountain Thoracic Society.

Owens GR, Rogers RM, Pennock BE, et al: The diffusing capacity as a predictor of arterial oxygen desaturation during exercise in patients with chronic obstructive pulmonary disease, *N Engl J Med* 310:1218-1221, 1984.

Symonds G, Renzetti AD Jr, Mitchell MM: The diffusing capacity in pulmonary emphysema, *Am Rev Respir Dis* 109:391, 1974.

West JB: *Pulmonary pathophysiology: the essentials,* ed 4, Baltimore, 1992, Williams & Wilkins.

$D_{L_{CO}}SB$

Crapo RO, Morris AH: Standardized single breath normal values for carbon monoxide diffusing capacity, *Am Rev Respir Dis* 123:185, 1981.

Cotes JE, Dabbs JM, Elwood PC, et al: Iron-deficiency anaemia: its effects on transfer factor for the lung (diffusing capacity) and ventilation and cardiac frequency during submaximal exercise, *Clin Sci* 42:325, 1972.

Dinakara P, Blumenthal WS, Johnston RF, et al: The effect of anemia on pulmonary diffusing capacity with derivation of a correction equation, *Am Rev Respir Dis* 102:965, 1970.

Forster RE: The single-breath carbon monoxide transfer test 25 years on: a reappraisal: physiologic considerations (editorial), *Thorax* 38:1, 1983.

Gaensler EA, Smith AA: Attachment for automated single breath diffusing capacity measurement, *Chest* 63:136, 1973.

Graham BL, Mink JT, Cotton DJ: Overestimation of the single breath carbon monoxide diffusing capacity in patients with air-flow obstruction, *Am Rev Respir Dis* 129:403, 1984.

Graham BL, Mink JT, Cotton DJ: Effect of breath hold time on $D_{L_{CO}}SB$ in patients with airway obstruction, *J Appl Physiol* 58:1319-1325, 1985.

Huang Y-C, MacIntyre NR: Real-time gas analysis improves the measurement of single-breath diffusing capacity, *Am Rev Respir Dis* 146:946-950, 1992.

Leech JA, Martz L, Liben A, et al: Diffusing capacity for carbon monoxide: the effects of different durations of breath hold time and alveolar volume and of carbon monoxide back pressure on calculated results, *Am Rev Respir Dis* 132:1127, 1985.

Kanner RE, Crapo RO: The relationship between alveolar oxygen tension and the single breath carbon monoxide diffusing capacity, *Am Rev Respir Dis* 133:676, 1986.

Mohsenifar Z, Tashkin DP: Effect of carboxyhemoglobin on the single breath diffusing capacity: derivation of an empirical correction factor, *Respiration* 37:185, 1979.

Ogilvie CM, Forster RE, Blakemore WS, et al: A standardized breath holding technique for the clinical measurement of the diffusing capacity of the lung for carbon monoxide, *J Clin Invest* 36:1, 1957.

$D_{L_{CO}}SS$

Filey GF, Macintosh DJ, Wright GW: Carbon monoxide uptake and pulmonary diffusing capacity in normal subjects at rest and during exercise, *J Clin Invest* 33:530, 1954.

Davies NJH: Does the lung work? 4. What does the transfer of carbon monoxide mean? *Br J Dis Chest* 76:105, 1982.

$D_{L_{CO}}IB$

Newth CJL, Cotton DJ, Nadel JA: Pulmonary diffusing capacity measured at multiple intervals during a single exhalation in man, *J Appl Physiol Respirat Environ Physiol* 43:617, 1977.

Wilson AF, Hearne J, Brennan M, et al: Measurement of transfer factor during constant exhalation, *Thorax* 49:1121-1126, 1994.

Standards and Guidelines

American Association for Respiratory Care: Single-breath carbon monoxide diffusing capacity, *Respir Care* 38:511-515, 1993.

American Thoracic Society: Single-breath carbon monoxide diffusing capacity (transfer factor): recommendations for a standard technique—1995 update, *Am J Respir Crit Care Med* 152:2185-2198, 1995.

British Thoracic Society and the Association of Respiratory Technicians and Physiologists: Guidelines for the measurement of respiratory function, *Respir Med* 88:165-194, 1994.

European Respiratory Society: Standardization of transfer factor (diffusing capacity), *Eur Respir J* 6(suppl 16):41-52, 1993.

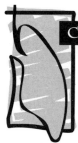

CHAPTER 6

Blood Gases and Related Tests

OBJECTIVES

After studying this chapter and reviewing its tables and case studies, you should be able to do the following:

1 Describe the measurement of pH and P_{CO_2} and how they are used to assess acid-base status

2 Interpret P_{O_2} and oxygen saturation to assess oxygenation

3 List situations in which pulse oximetry can be used to evaluate a patient's oxygenation

4 Describe the use of capnography to assess changes in the ventilation-perfusion patterns of the lung

5 Calculate the shunt fraction using appropriate laboratory data

BLOOD GAS ANALYSIS IS THE MOST basic pulmonary function test. Evaluation of the acid-base and oxygenation status of the body provides information about the function of the lungs themselves. Other measures of gas exchange (e.g., pulse oximetry and capnography) have the advantage of monitoring patients noninvasively. Noninvasive techniques have drawbacks. Understanding of their limitations allows them to be used to provide appropriate patient care. Calculating the shunt fraction uses blood gas measurements to assess gas exchange as it applies to oxygenation.

This chapter addresses how blood gas measurements are used in the pulmonary function laboratory. A complete description of blood gas electrodes is included in Chapter 9. The use of pulse oximetry and capnography as adjuncts to traditional invasive measures are discussed. Two methods of calculating shunt fraction are detailed so that the most appropriate method may be used.

BLOOD GAS ANALYSIS

pH

pH is the negative logarithm of the hydrogen ion (H^+) concentration in the blood, used as a positive number. The pH scale is unitless. The pH of water (7.00) represents the center of the pH scale. The physiologic range of pH in blood in clinical practice is from approximately 6.90 to 7.80.

Carbon Dioxide Tension

P_{CO_2} is a measurement of the partial pressure exerted by CO_2 in solution in the blood. The measurement is expressed in millimeters of mercury (mm Hg or torr) or in **kilopascals** (kPa) used in the International System of Units (1 mm Hg = 0.133 kPa). The normal range for P_{CO_2} in arterial blood is 35 to 45 mm Hg. In mixed venous blood, P_{CO_2} varies from 40 to 46 mm Hg.

Oxygen Tension

Po_2 measures the partial pressure exerted by oxygen (O_2) dissolved in the blood. Like Pco_2, it is recorded in millimeters of mercury or in kilopascals. The normal range for arterial Po_2 is 80 to 100 mm Hg for healthy young adults. Mixed venous Po_2 averages 40 mm Hg in healthy subjects.

TECHNIQUE

pH

Blood pH is measured by exposing the specimen to a glass electrode (see Fig. 9-21) under **anaerobic** conditions. pH measurements are made at 37° C. The pH of arterial blood is related to the $Paco_2$ by the Henderson-Hasselbalch equation:

$$pH = pk + \log\frac{[HCO_3^-]}{[CO_2]}$$

where:

$$pK = \text{negative log of dissociation constant for carbonic acid (6.1)}$$

$$[HCO_3^-] = \textbf{molar} \text{ concentration of serum bicarbonate}$$

$$[CO_2] = \text{molar concentration of } CO_2$$

$Paco_2$, measured directly by the CO_2 electrode, may be multiplied by 0.03 (the **solubility coefficient** for CO_2) to express the $Paco_2$ in mEq/L. The equation then may be written as follows:

$$pH = 6.1 + \log\frac{[HCO_3^-]}{[0.03\,(Paco_2)]}$$

Carbon Dioxide Tension

Pco_2 is measured by submitting blood to a modified pH electrode (i.e., a Severinghaus electrode) that is contained in a jacket with a Teflon membrane at its tip (see Chapter 9). Inside the jacket is a bicarbonate buffer. As CO_2 diffuses through the membrane, it combines with water to form **carbonic acid** (H_2CO_3). The H_2CO_3 dissociates into H^+ and HCO_3^- thereby changing the pH of the bicarbonate buffer. The change in pH is measured by the electrode and is proportional to the Pco_2. The blood must be **anticoagulated** and kept in an anaerobic state in an ice-water bath until analysis. The Pco_2 may also be estimated using a **transcutaneous** electrode. Measurement of end-tidal CO_2 ($Petco_2$) is sometimes used to track Pco_2 (see "Capnography," p. 146).

pH and Pco_2 are usually measured from the same sample, so bicarbonate can be easily calculated. Automated blood gas analyzers perform this calculation along with others to derive values such as total CO_2 (dissolved CO_2 plus HCO_3^-) and standard bicarbonate (i.e., HCO_3^- corrected to a $Paco_2$ of 40 mm Hg). If the hemoglobin (Hb) is measured or estimated, the base excess (BE) can be calculated. BE is the difference between the actual buffering capacity of the blood and the normal buffer base at a pH of 7.40, approximately 48 mEq/L. The main buffers which affect the BE are HCO_3^- and Hb.

Oxygen Tension

The Po_2 (either arterial or mixed venous) is measured by exposing whole blood, obtained anaerobically, to a platinum electrode covered with a thin polypropylene membrane. This type of electrode is called a **polarographic** electrode or Clark electrode. Oxygen molecules are reduced at the platinum cathode after diffusing through the membrane (see Chapter 9). Po_2 may also be measured using a transcutaneous electrode (see Chapter 9).

pH may change depending on the body temperature of the subject. Alteration of body temperature affects the partial pressure of dissolved CO_2, which influences pH as described in the previous equations (Table 6-1). Although pH measurements are made at 37° C, the value reported is often corrected to the patient's temperature.

Technical problems with blood gas electrodes include contamination by protein or blood products. Depletion of the potassium chloride (KCl) bridge between the pH measuring and reference electrodes (see Chapter 9) is also a common problem. Depletion of the bicarbonate buffer in the Pco_2 electrode may reduce accuracy and cause unacceptable drift. **Oxidation-reduction** reactions in the Po_2 electrode cause metal ions to deposit on the platinum cathode. After a period of use, the tip of the O_2 electrode must be abraded to expose the platinum wire. This is usually accomplished by brushing the tip with a mild abrasive. Tears or ruptures of the membranes used to cover the Pco_2 and Po_2 electrodes are also common malfunctions.

TABLE 6-1 Effects of Body Temperature on Blood Gas Values*

Temperature (°C)	34°	37°	40°
pH	7.44	7.40	7.36
P_{CO_2}	35	40	46
P_{O_2}	79	95	114

*Temperature corrections based on algorithms from *NCCLS: definitions of quantities and conventions related to blood pH and gas analysis,* ed 2, (Tentative Standard), vol 12, No. 11, 1991.

TABLE 6-2 Complications of Arterial Puncture for Blood Gases Testing

Pain and discomfort
Hematoma
Air or blood emboli
Infection or contamination
Inadvertent needle stick
Vascular trauma or occlusion
Vasovagal response
Arterial spasm

Specimen Collection for Blood Gases

Arterial samples are usually obtained from either the radial or **brachial** artery. Arterial specimens may also be drawn from the femoral or dorsalis pedis arteries. The radial artery is the preferred site. Before a radial artery puncture, the adequacy of collateral circulation to the hand via the ulnar artery should be established using the modified **Allen's test.** The technologist occludes both the radial and ulnar arteries by pressing down over the wrist. The subject is instructed to make a fist, then open the hand and relax the fingers. The palm of the hand is pale and bloodless because both arteries are occluded. The ulnar artery is released while the radial remains occluded. The hand should be reperfused rapidly (5 to 10 seconds) if the ulnar supply is adequate. If perfusion is inadequate, an alternate site should be used.

Arterial puncture should not be performed through any type of lesion. Similarly, puncture distal to a surgical shunt (i.e., as used for dialysis) should be avoided. Infection or evidence of peripheral vascular disease should prompt selection of an alternative site. Many patients may be using anticoagulant drugs such as heparin, coumadin, or streptokinase. High dosages of these drugs or a history of prolonged clotting times may be relative contraindications to arterial puncture. Table 6-2 lists some of the potential hazards associated with arterial puncture.

Mixed venous samples are drawn from a pulmonary artery **(Swan-Ganz) catheter.** Contamination of the mixed venous specimen with flush solution is a common problem. Withdrawing a small volume of blood into a "waste" syringe ensures that the sample is not diluted by flush solution in the catheter. Care should be taken to limit the volume of blood removed in this process. Significant blood loss can occur with repetitive measurements. Another common problem with mixed venous specimen collection is displacement of the catheter tip. If the catheter is advanced too far, it may "wedge" into a pulmonary arteriole. Specimens drawn from this position often reflect arterialized pulmonary capillary blood. Similarly, if the catheter tip is withdrawn or "loops back," it may be in the right ventricle or atrium rather than the pulmonary artery. Specimens obtained from this location may not represent true mixed venous blood.

Venous samples from peripheral veins are not useful for assessing oxygenation. Venous blood only reflects the metabolism of the area drained by that particular vein. Venous samples may be used for measurement of pH or blood **lactate** during exercise.

Blood is usually collected in a heparinized syringe and sealed from the atmosphere immediately (Box 6-1). Care must be taken that heparin solution (if used) does not dilute the sample. Heparin solution (sodium heparin) has a P_{O_2} of approximately 150 mm Hg and a P_{CO_2} near 0. If the volume of heparin solution is large in relation to the blood sample, P_{O_2} and P_{CO_2} will be altered. The P_{O_2} will increase, if it is less than 150 mm Hg, and the P_{CO_2} will decrease. Although liquid heparin is slightly acidic compared with blood, pH is usually not directly affected. The large buffering capacity of whole blood prevents large changes in pH. To prevent dilution effects when a heparin solution is used, the following guidelines are helpful:

1.   Draw up a small volume of sterile heparin in the syringe. Typically, 0.25 ml of 1000 μ/ml is sufficient for a 3-ml syringe.

2.   Hold the syringe with the needle pointed up. Pull back the plunger so that the heparin solution coats the interior walls of the syringe.

3.   Expel all of the heparin solution through the needle, leaving liquid only in the hub and lumen of the needle.

4.   Obtain a blood sample volume of 2 to 4 ml, if possible.

Blood gas kits that feature dry (lyophilyzed) heparin are available. Dry heparin is applied to the lumen of the needle and the interior of the syringe. A small heparin pellet is often placed in the syringe to provide additional anticoagulation. After the syringe has been capped (see "Infection Control and Safety," Chapter 10), the sample should be thoroughly mixed by rolling or gently shaking. Mixing helps prevent the sample from clotting, whether dry or liquid heparin is used. Lithium heparin or a similar preparation should be used for specimens that will also be used for electrolyte analysis.

Air contamination of arterial or mixed venous blood specimens can seriously alter blood gas values. Room air at sea level has a P_{O_2} of approximately 150 mm Hg, and a P_{CO_2} near 0. If air bubbles are present in a blood gas specimen, equilibration of gases between sample and air begins to occur (Table 6-3). Contamination commonly happens during sampling when air is left in the syringe after the sample is collected. Small bubbles may also be introduced if the needle does not connect tightly to the syringe. Other sources of air contamination include poorly fitting plungers and failure to properly cap the syringe.

TABLE 6-3   Air Contamination of Blood Gas Samples

	In vivo values	Air contamination*
pH	7.40	7.45
P_{CO_2}	40	30
P_{O_2}	95	110

*Typical values that might occur when a blood gas specimen is exposed to air, either directly or by mixing with a solution that has been exposed to air (i.e., heparinized flush solution). The change in pH occurs because of the change in P_{CO_2}.

BOX 6-1
CRITERIA FOR ACCEPTABILITY—BLOOD GASES

1   Blood should be collected anaerobically. Syringe body and plunger should be tight fitting. Commercially available blood gas kits should be used according to manufacturers' specifications. Air bubbles should be expelled immediately.

2   The specimen must be adequately anticoagulated; sodium or lithium heparin is preferred. If liquid heparin is used, all excess should be expelled. Choice of anticoagulant should be determined by analyses to be performed (e.g., electrolytes).

3   A sample volume of 2 to 4 ml is recommended.

4   The specimen should be analyzed as soon as possible. If immediate analysis is not available, the specimen should be stored in an ice-water slurry at 0° C and analyzed within 1 hour.

5   The specimen should be adequately identified, including patient name and/or number, date/time, ordering physician, and accession number. Information provided with the specimen should be the site from which it was obtained, F_{IO_2} (if applicable) and ventilator settings (if applicable).

6   Analysis should be performed on an instrument that has been recently calibrated and whose function is documented by appropriate **controls.**

The sample should be stored in an ice-water slush if analysis is not done within a few minutes. Ice water reduces the metabolism of red and white blood cells in the sample. Specimens with O_2 tensions in the normal physiologic range (i.e., 50 to 150 mm Hg) show minimal changes over 1 to 2 hours if kept in ice water. Changes in specimens held at room temperature are related to cellular metabolism in the blood, particularly in white blood cells and platelets. Specimens with PO_2 values above 150 mm Hg are most susceptible to alterations resulting from gas leakage or cell metabolism. When the PO_2 is 150 mm Hg or more, Hb is almost completely bound with O_2. In such cases a small change in O_2 content results in a large change in PO_2.

Capillary samples are useful in infants when arterial puncture is impractical. The area for collection (the heel is commonly chosen) should be heated by a warm compress and lanced. Blood is then allowed to fill the required volume of heparinized glass capillary tubes. Squeezing the tissue should be avoided because predominately venous blood will be obtained. The capillary tubes should be carefully sealed to avoid air bubbles. Guidelines for quality control of blood gas analyzers and for the safe handling of blood specimens are included in Chapter 10.

SIGNIFICANCE AND PATHOPHYSIOLOGY

See Box 6-2 for interpretive strategies.

pH

The pH of arterial blood in healthy adults averages 7.40 with a range of 7.35 to 7.45. Arterial pH below 7.35 constitutes **acidemia.** A pH above 7.45 constitutes **alkalemia.** A change of 0.3 pH units represents a twofold change in H^+ concentration. When the pH falls from 7.40 to 7.10 with no change in PCO_2, the concentration of hydrogen ions has doubled. Conversely, if the concentration of H^+ is halved, the pH rises from 7.40 to 7.70, assuming the PCO_2 remains at 40 mm Hg. Changes of this magnitude represent marked abnormalities in the acid-base status of the blood and are almost always accompanied by clinical symptoms such as cardiac arrhythmias.

BOX 6-2
INTERPRETIVE STRATEGIES—BLOOD GASES

1   Was the blood gas specimen obtained acceptably? Free of air bubbles and clots? Analyzed promptly and/or iced appropriately?

2   Did the blood gas analyzer function properly? Was there a recent acceptable calibration of all electrodes? Was analyzer function validated by appropriate quality controls?

3   Is pH within normal limits (7.35 to 7.45)? If so, go to Step 4. If below 7.35, **acidosis** is present; if above 7.45, **alkalosis** is present. Otherwise, look for compensatory changes or combined disorders.

4   Is the PCO_2 within normal limits (35 to 45 mm Hg)? If so, go to Step 5.
    If PCO_2 >45 and pH <7.35, then respiratory acidosis.
    If PCO_2 >45 and pH >7.35, then compensated respiratory acidosis.
    If PCO_2 <35 and pH >7.45, then respiratory alkalosis.
    If PCO_2 <35 and pH <7.45, then compensated respiratory alkalosis.

5   Is calculated HCO_3^- within normal limits (22 to 27 mEq/L)? If so, acid-base status is probably normal; go to Step 6.
    If HCO_3^- <22 and pH <7.35, then metabolic* acidosis.
    If HCO_3^- <22 and pH >7.35, then compensated metabolic* acidosis.
    If HCO_3^- >27 and pH >7.45, then metabolic* alkalosis.
    If HCO_3^- >27 and pH <7.45, then compensated metabolic* alkalosis.

6   Is PO_2 within normal limits (80 to 100 mm Hg)? If so, oxygenation status is probably normal; check O_2Hb saturation via co-oximetry. Is PO_2 appropriate for FIO_2? Is **A-a gradient** increased? If PO_2 <55, significant hypoxemia is present.

7   Are blood gas results consistent with patient's clinical history and status? Are additional tests indicated (co-oximetry, shunt study)?

---

*Metabolic = nonrespiratory.

Acid-base disorders arising from lung disease are often related to P_{CO_2} and its transport as carbonic acid. If the pH is outside of its normal range and P_{CO_2} is inconsistent with the observed disorder (i.e., acidemia or alkalemia), the condition is termed nonrespiratory or metabolic (Table 6-4). The calculated HCO_3^- is a useful indicator of the relationship between pH and P_{CO_2}. In the presence of acidemia (i.e., pH less than 7.35) and normal CO_2 (i.e., P_{CO_2} of 35 to 45 mm Hg), HCO_3^- will be low and a nonrespiratory acidosis is present. If P_{CO_2} is less than 35 mm Hg in the presence of acidosis, ventilatory compensation for acidemia is likely occurring. The acid-base status would be considered partially compensated nonrespiratory (i.e., metabolic) acidosis. Complete compensation occurs if pH returns to the normal range. This happens when ventilation reduces P_{CO_2} to match the HCO_3^-.

In the presence of alkalemia (i.e., pH more than 7.45) and a normal P_{CO_2} (i.e., 35 to 45 mm Hg), calculated bicarbonate will be increased and nonrespiratory (i.e., metabolic) alkalosis is present. If ventilatory compensation occurs, the P_{CO_2} will be slightly elevated. However, decreased ventilation is required so that the CO_2 can increase. Reduced ventilation may interfere with oxygenation. For this reason, Pa_{CO_2} seldom rises above 50 to 55 mm Hg to compensate for nonrespiratory (i.e., metabolic) alkalosis. Compensation may be incomplete if the alkalosis is severe.

Combined respiratory and nonrespiratory acid-base disorders are characterized by abnormal P_{CO_2} and HCO_3^-. In combined acidosis, P_{CO_2} is elevated (i.e., more than 45 mm Hg) and HCO_3^- lowered (i.e., less than 22 mEq/L). In combined alkalosis, the HCO_3^- is high (i.e., more than 26 mEq/L) and P_{CO_2} is low (i.e., less than 35 mm Hg).

Carbon Dioxide Tension

The arterial carbon dioxide tension (Pa_{CO_2}) of a healthy adult is approximately 40 mm Hg; it may range from 35 to 45 mm Hg. The P_{CO_2} of venous or mixed venous blood is seldom used clinically. Body temperature affects the Pa_{CO_2} as described in Table 6-1.

Pa_{CO_2} is inversely proportional to alveolar ventilation ($\dot{V}A$) (see Chapter 4). When $\dot{V}A$ decreases, CO_2 is not removed by the lungs as fast as it is produced. This causes the Pa_{CO_2} to rise. The pH falls as CO_2 is hydrated to form carbonic acid:

$$CO_2 + H_2O \leftrightarrows H_2CO_3 \leftrightarrows H^+ + HCO_3^-$$

Increasing levels of CO_2 in the blood drive the reaction to the right. The subject develops respiratory acidosis resulting from hypoventilation. Conversely, when alveolar ventilation removes CO_2 more rapidly than it is produced, Pa_{CO_2} falls. The pH rises as the subject becomes alkalotic. This condition is called hyperventilation, or respiratory alkalosis.

TABLE 6-4 Acid-Base Disorders

Status	pH	P_{CO_2}	HCO_3^-
Simple disorders			
Metabolic acidosis	Low	Normal	Low
Metabolic alkalosis	High	Normal	High
Respiratory acidosis	Low	High	Normal
Respiratory alkalosis	High	Low	Normal
Compensated disorders			
Compensated respiratory acidosis, or metabolic alkalosis	Normal*	High	High
Compensated metabolic acidosis, or respiratory alkalosis	Normal*	Low	Low
Combined disorders			
Metabolic/respiratory acidosis	Low	High	Low
Metabolic/respiratory alkalosis	High	Low	High

*Compensation cannot return values to within normal limits in severe acid-base disturbances. In addition, a normal pH may result in instances of respiratory and metabolic disturbances that occur together but are not compensatory.

If dead space increases, high minute ventilation ($\dot{V}E$) may be required to adequately ventilate alveoli and keep $Paco_2$ within normal limits. Respiratory dead space occurs because some lung units are ventilated but not perfused by pulmonary capillary blood. Pulmonary embolization is an example of dead space–producing disease. Emboli may block pulmonary arterioles causing ventilation of the affected lung units to be "wasted." To maintain normal $Paco_2$, total ventilation must be increased to compensate for wasted ventilation.

The $Paco_2$ may be normal, or even reduced, when significant pulmonary disease is present. Subjects who have disorders such as lobar pneumonia may increase their $\dot{V}E$ to produce more alveolar ventilation of functioning lung units. This mechanism compensates for lung units that do not participate in gas exchange. Hypoxemia is a common cause of hyperventilation (i.e., respiratory alkalosis). Hyperventilation may be seen in subjects with asthma, emphysema, bronchitis, or foreign body obstruction. Anxiety or central nervous system disorders may also cause hyperventilation.

Increased $Paco_2$ (i.e., hypercapnia) is commonly found in subjects who have advanced obstructive or restrictive disease. These individuals are characterized by markedly abnormal ventilation-perfusion ($\dot{V}/\dot{Q}$) patterns. They are unable to maintain adequate alveolar ventilation. Not all subjects with advanced pulmonary disease retain CO_2. Those who become hypercapnic often have a low ventilatory response to CO_2 (see Chapter 4). Their response to the increased work of breathing caused by obstruction or restriction is to allow CO_2 to rise rather than increase ventilation. The respiratory acidosis that results from the increased Pco_2 is managed by renal compensation (see Table 6-4).

Elevated $Paco_2$ may also be seen in subjects who hypoventilate as a result of central nervous system or neuromuscular disorders. Whether CO_2 retention is the result of lung disease, central nervous system dysfunction, or neuromuscular disease, pH is maintained close to normal. The kidneys retain and produce bicarbonate (HCO_3^-) to match the increased $Paco_2$. This response may completely compensate for a mildly elevated $Paco_2$. However, it can seldom produce normal pH when the $Paco_2$ is greater than 65 mm Hg. If the disorder causing the increased $Paco_2$ is acute (e.g., foreign body aspiration), little or no renal compensation may be observed.

Hypoxemia is always present in subjects who retain CO_2 while breathing air. As alveolar CO_2 increases, alveolar O_2 decreases. If the cause of hypercapnia is either obstructive or restrictive lung disease, hypoxemia may be severe because of $\dot{V}/\dot{Q}$ abnormalities. Because O_2 therapy is commonly used in these subjects, changes in Pco_2 while breathing supplementary O_2 must be carefully monitored. Some subjects with chronic hypoxemia have a decreased ventilatory response to CO_2. O_2 administered to these patients may reduce their hypoxic stimulus to ventilation. As a result, $Paco_2$ may increase further. O_2 therapy must be titrated to maintain $Paco_2$ values less than 60 mm Hg without hypercapnia and acidosis.

Oxygen Tension

The Pao_2 of a healthy young adult at sea level varies from 85 to 100 mm Hg and decreases slightly with age. Hyperventilation may increase Pao_2 as high as 120 mm Hg in a subject with normal lung function. Healthy persons breathing 100% O_2 may exhibit Pao_2 values higher than 600 mm Hg. The alveolar Po_2 (Pao_2) for a particular inspired O_2 fraction can be calculated as described in the shunt calculation section. Decreased Pao_2 can result from hypoventilation, diffusion defects, $\dot{V}/\dot{Q}$ imbalances, and inadequate atmospheric O_2 (high altitude).

Table 6-1 lists the changes that occur in Pao_2 as a result of body temperatures above and below normal (37° C). The changes in Po_2 and Pco_2 reflect solubility of the gas. Partial pressure of each gas is a measure of its activity. Hypothermia (low body temperature) is accompanied by decreased partial pressure. Hyperthermia (elevated body temperature) causes elevated gas tensions. All blood gas analyzers perform analyses at 37° C and allow temperature corrections to be made. Although blood gas tensions vary with temperature, the clinical significance of correcting measurements is unclear. Blood gas values should be reported at 37° C. Care must be taken to ensure that blood gas analyzers are maintained at 37° C. Measurements made at other temperatures can significantly alter results.

Po_2 is the pressure of O_2 dissolved in blood. It is not influenced by the amount of Hb present or whether the Hb is capable of binding O_2. Hypoxemia (decreased O_2 content of the blood) may occur even though Pao_2 is normal or elevated by breathing O_2. Hypoxemia commonly results from inadequate or abnormal Hb. Many automated blood gas analyzers calculate oxygen saturation

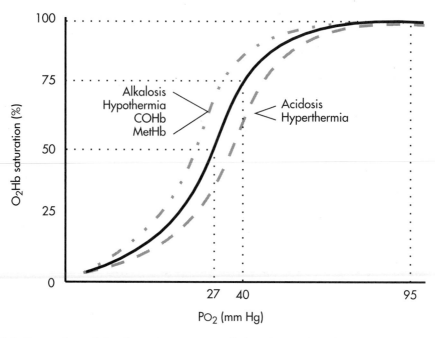

FIG. 6-1 *Oxygen-hemoglobin dissociation curve.* An S-shaped curve describes the relationship between partial pressure of O_2 in blood (X axis) and Hb saturation (Y axis). The solid curve represents the reaction occurring when the Hb is normal, pH is 7.40, and temperature is 37° C. When Po_2 is 95 mm Hg, Hb is approximately 97% saturated; at a Po_2 of 60 mm Hg, saturation falls to approximately 90%. At a Po_2 of 40 mm Hg (normal level for mixed venous blood), the saturation of Hb is 75%. The P_{50} identifies the O_2 tension at which Hb is 50% saturated. For normal Hb, this is approximately 27 mm Hg. Conditions such as alkalosis, hypothermia, or elevated COHb or MetHb shift the dissociation curve to the left. This causes Hb to bind O_2 more tightly with less oxygen being unloaded as partial pressure falls. Similarly, acidosis and hyperthermia shift the curve to the right, enhancing the delivery of O_2 as pressure falls.

(Sao_2). Saturation is calculated from the Pao_2 and pH, assuming a normal oxygen-hemoglobin reaction occurs (Fig. 6-1). Calculated Sao_2 may be quite different from the true saturation measured by a **spectrophotometer** (see "Oxygen Saturation," p. 141). A common example is the subject with elevated carboxyhemoglobin (COHb) resulting from smoking or smoke inhalation. The subject's Pao_2 may be normal while O_2 saturation is markedly decreased. Calculating saturation from Po_2 in this case overestimates the O_2 content of the blood. Measured Sao_2 is preferred to a calculated value.

The ability of Hb to bind O_2 is measured by the P_{50}. P_{50} specifies the partial pressure at which Hb is 50% saturated (see Fig. 6-1). The P_{50} of normal Hb is approximately 26.7 mm Hg. The P_{50} may be determined by **tonometering** (i.e., equilibrating) blood with several gases at low oxygen tensions. An Hb-O_2 dissociation curve is then constructed to estimate the partial pressure at which Hb is 50% saturated.

A second method estimates P_{50} by comparing measured Sao_2 using a spectrophotometer to the expected saturation. Calculated saturations presume a P_{50} of 26 to 27 mm Hg, but it may differ significantly depending on the types of Hb and interfering substances present.

Severity of impaired oxygenation is indicated by the Pao_2 at rest. Pao_2 is a good index of the lungs' ability to match pulmonary capillary blood flow with adequate ventilation. If ventilation matches perfusion, pulmonary capillary blood leaves the lungs with a Po_2 close to that of the alveoli. If ventilation is adequate, pulmonary capillary blood is almost completely saturated. When either of these conditions is not met (i.e., poor ventilation or $\dot{V}/\dot{Q}$ mismatching), pulmonary capillary blood has reduced O_2 content. Pao_2 is reduced in proportion to the number of lung units contributing blood with low O_2 content. Lung units with good $\dot{V}/\dot{Q}$ cannot compensate for their poorly functioning counterparts because pulmonary capillary blood leaving them is already almost fully oxygenated. O_2 binding to Hb is almost complete when the Pao_2 is greater than 60 mm Hg (i.e., 90% saturation). As the Pao_2 falls from 60 to 40 mm Hg, saturation decreases from 90% to 75%, with increasing symptoms of hypoxia (i.e., mental confusion, shortness of breath).

Delivery of O_2 to the tissues, however, depends on Hb concentration and cardiac output. Arterial oxygen content (CaO_2, ml/dl) is defined as follows:

$$CaO_2 = (1.34 \times Hb \times SaO_2) + (PaO_2 \times 0.0031)$$

where:

$$1.34 = O_2 \text{ binding capacity of Hb (ml/gm)}$$
$$Hb = \text{hemoglobin concentration (ml/dl)}$$
$$SaO_2 = \text{arterial oxygen saturation as a fraction}$$
$$PaO_2 = \text{arterial oxygen tension (mm Hg)}$$
$$0.0031 = \text{solubility coefficient for } O_2$$

Because most O_2 transported is bound to Hb, there must be an adequate supply (12 to 15 g/dl) of functional Hb. Adequate cardiac output (4 to 5 L/min) is necessary to deliver the oxygenated arterial blood to the tissues. Signs and symptoms of hypoxia may be present despite adequate PaO_2 because of severe anemia and/or reduced cardiac function.

The mixed venous oxygen tension ($P\bar{v}O_2$) in healthy subjects at rest ranges from 37 to 43, with an average of 40 mm Hg (see Fig. 6-1). In healthy persons the CaO_2 averages 20 ml/dl; mixed venous O_2 content averages 15 ml/dl, resulting in a content difference of 5 ml/dl (or vol%). Although PaO_2 varies with the inspired O_2 fraction and matching of V/Q, $P\bar{v}O_2$ changes in response to alterations in cardiac output and O_2 consumption. If cardiac output increases while oxygen consumption ($\dot{V}O_2$) remains constant, the a-$\bar{v}$ content difference ($C(a-\bar{v})O_2$) decreases. Conversely, if cardiac output falls without a change in O_2 consumption, the $C(a-\bar{v})O_2$ increases. Increased cardiac output sometimes occurs in response to pulmonary shunting. This allows mixed venous oxygen content to rise, reducing the deleterious effect of the shunt. Critically ill subjects often have low $P\bar{v}O_2$ values and increased $C(a-\bar{v})O_2$ as a result of poor cardiovascular performance. Alterations in the $P\bar{v}O_2$ often occur even though the PaO_2 may be within normal limits. $P\bar{v}O_2$ values less than 28 mm Hg in critically ill patients, accompanied by $C(a-\bar{v})O_2$ greater than 6 vol%, suggest marked cardiovascular decompensation.

Resting subjects who have severe obstructive or restrictive diseases may have decreased PaO_2, occasionally as low as 40 mm Hg. Mild pulmonary disease may show little decrease in PaO_2 if hyperventilation is present. PaO_2 may be normal if the disease process affects ventilation and perfusion similarly. In subjects with emphysema, destruction of alveolar septa may eliminate pulmonary capillaries as well, resulting in poor ventilation and equally poor blood flow. These subjects may have severe airways obstruction but little or no decrease in PaO_2. Subjects with chronic bronchitis or asthma, particularly during acute exacerbations, may have moderate or severe resting hypoxemia because of V/Q abnormalities.

Analysis of PaO_2 during exercise in subjects with obstructive disease often shows a decrease in PaO_2 commensurate with the extent of the disease. PaO_2 during exercise is correlated with the subject's diffusing capacity (DL_{CO}) and FEV_1, but wide variability exists. Subjects with markedly decreased DL_{CO} (i.e., less than approximately 50% of predicted) typically show low PaO_2 values at rest that fall during exercise. The degree of arterial desaturation cannot be predicted from static pulmonary function measurements.

PaO_2 may be decreased for nonpulmonary reasons such as anatomic shunts (intracardiac) or neuromuscular hypoventilation. Tissue hypoxia can occur because of inadequate or nonfunctional Hb or because of poor cardiac output. PaO_2 should be correlated with spirometry (i.e., FEV_1), DL_{CO}, ventilation (i.e., $\dot{V}E$, tidal volume, dead space), and lung volumes (i.e., vital capacity, residual volume, total lung capacity) to distinguish pulmonary from nonpulmonary causes of inadequate oxygenation.

Oxygen Saturation

DESCRIPTION

Oxygen saturation is the ratio of oxygenated Hb (O_2Hb) to either total available Hb or functional Hb. Functional Hb is that portion of the total Hb that is capable of binding oxygen. This ratio of content to capacity is normally expressed as a percentage but is sometimes recorded as a simple fraction. The values may differ significantly depending on the method of calculation:

1. Oxyhemoglobin fraction of total Hb:

$$\frac{O_2Hb}{O_2Hb + RHb + COHb + MetHb}$$

2. Oxygen saturation of available Hb:

$$\frac{O_2Hb}{O_2Hb + RHb}$$

where:

$$RHb = \text{reduced hemoglobin concentration}$$

$$COHb = \text{carboxyhemoglobin concentration}$$

$$MetHb = \text{methemoglobin concentration}$$

Measurement of O_2 saturation using multiple wavelength spectrophotometers (i.e., **co-oximeters**) uses the first equation, and pulse oximeters normally uses the second.

TECHNIQUE

O_2 saturation of Hb may be measured in one of several ways. In the first technique O_2 content of arterial blood is measured volumetrically. Then the blood is exposed to the atmosphere so that the Hb may combine with O_2 under ambient conditions. The content is measured again and represents the oxygen binding capacity. Saturation is the original content divided by the capacity, determined after corrections for dissolved O_2 are made.

In the second technique, O_2 saturation is measured using a spectrophotometer (see Chapter 9). The spectrophotometer, or co-oximeter as it is sometimes described, uses Equation 1 just described. The total Hb, O_2Hb, COHb, and MetHb are usually reported.

In a third method, saturation is estimated noninvasively using a pulse oximeter (see Chapter 9). Pulse oximeters may use either the ear, finger, or other capillary bed for attachment of the probe. Pulse oximeters typically use only two wavelengths of light and use Equation 2 just described.

A fourth technique measures mixed venous oxygen saturation. $S\bar{v}O_2$ may be measured by a reflective spectrophotometer in a pulmonary artery catheter (i.e., Swan-Ganz catheter). A special catheter that includes fiberoptic bundles is used to perform **in vivo** measurements. Descriptions of both the spectrophotometers and pulse oximeters are included in Chapter 9.

Blood specimens for co-oximetry should be prepared as described for arterial blood gas specimens (see "Blood Gases," p. 136). Guidelines for quality control of blood gas analysis are included in Chapter 10.

Measurement of percent saturation allows calculation of the O_2 content of either arterial or mixed venous blood (CaO_2 and $C\bar{v}O_2$, respectively) (see "Significance and Pathophysiology, Oxygen Tension," p. 139).

SIGNIFICANCE AND PATHOPHYSIOLOGY

See Box 6-3 for interpretive strategies. SaO_2 for a healthy young adult with a PaO_2 of 95 mm Hg is approximately 97%. The O_2Hb dissociation curve is relatively flat when the PaO_2 is above 60 mm Hg (i.e., SaO_2 is 90% or greater). Saturation changes only slightly even when there is a marked change in PaO_2 at partial pressures above 60 mm Hg (see Fig. 6-1). Therefore, PaO_2 is a more sensitive indicator of oxygenation in lungs that do not have gross abnormalities. At PaO_2 values of approximately 150 mm Hg, Hb becomes completely saturated (i.e., SaO_2 is 100%). At PaO_2 values above 150 mm Hg, further increases in O_2 content are caused by increased dissolved oxygen. Alterations in $\dot{V}/\dot{Q}$ patterns in the lungs can be monitored by allowing the subject to breath 100% O_2, and measuring the changes in dissolved oxygen. In practice this is accomplished by using the clinical shunt equation (see "Shunt Calculation," p. 148).

When PaO_2 falls below 60 mm Hg, SaO_2 decreases rapidly. Small changes in PaO_2 result in large changes in saturation. As the SaO_2 falls below 90%, O_2 content decreases proportionately. At saturations less than 85% (i.e., PaO_2 less than 55 mm Hg) symptoms of hypoxemia increase and supplementary O_2 may be indicated.

Healthy persons have small amounts of Hb that cannot carry O_2. COHb is present in blood from metabolism and from environmental exposure to carbon monoxide (CO) gas. Normal COHb, expressed as a percentage, ranges from 0.5% to 2% of the total Hb. CO comes from smoking (cigarettes, cigars, and pipes), smoke inhalation, improperly vented furnaces, automobile emis-

---

BOX 6-3
INTERPRETIVE STRATEGIES—OXYGEN SATURATION

1   How was the estimate of saturation obtained? Co-oximeter? Calculated saturation? Pulse oximeter?

2   For co-oximetry or calculated saturation: was the specimen obtained anaerobically and handled properly?

3   Is the Hb within normal limits? If low, oxygenation may be compromised; if elevated, look for clinical correlation.

4   Is the O_2Hb >90%? If so, oxygenation is probably adequate; if not hypoxemia is likely.

5   Is O_2Hb <85%? If so, supplementary oxygen may be indicated. Correlate to Pao_2 and clinical history.

6   Is COHb >3%? If so, check for smoking history and/or environmental exposure.

7   Is MetHb >1.5%? If so, check for environmental exposure to oxidizers.

---

sions, and other sources of air pollution. In smokers, levels may increase from 3% to 15%, depending on recent smoking history. Smoke inhalation or CO poisoning from other sources also results in elevated COHb levels, sometimes as high as 50%. CO combines rapidly with Hb. Exposures of short duration can cause a high level of COHb if high concentrations of CO are present. Because O_2Hb saturation falls as COHb rises, COHb levels greater than 15% almost always result in hypoxemia. High levels of COHb can be rapidly fatal because of the profound hypoxemia that occurs.

COHb absorbs light at wavelengths similar to O_2Hb. When COHb is elevated arterial blood appears bright red. Cyanosis, which appears when there is an increased concentration of reduced Hb, is absent. In addition, Pao_2 may be close to normal limits. Blood gas analysis that includes calculated saturation may give erroneously high O_2 saturations. For this reason O_2Hb and COHb should be measured by co-oximetry whenever possible.

COHb interferes with O_2 transport in two ways. It binds competitively to Hb and it shifts the O_2Hb curve to the left (see Fig. 6-1). Increased COHb causes reduced O_2Hb with a decrease in O_2 content. The left shift of the dissociation curve causes O_2 to be bound more tightly to Hb. The combination of these two effects can seriously alter O_2 delivery to the tissues. COHb concentrations in blood begin to decrease once the source of CO has been removed. Removal of CO from the blood depends on the minute ventilation. Breathing air may require several hours to reduce even moderate levels to normal. Breathing 100% O_2 speeds the washout of CO. High concentrations of O_2 are indicated whenever dangerously high levels of COHb are encountered.

Methemoglobin (MetHb) forms when iron atoms of the Hb molecule are oxidized from Fe^{++} to Fe^{+++}. The normal MetHb level is less than 1.5% of the total Hb. High levels of MetHb can result from ingestion of or exposure to strong oxidizing agents. Like COHb, MetHb reduces O_2 carrying capacity of the blood by reducing the available Hb and shifting the O_2Hb dissociation curve to the left (see Fig. 6-1).

The saturation of mixed venous blood ($S\bar{v}o_2$) in healthy subjects averages 75% at a $P\bar{v}o_2$ of 40 mm Hg. Healthy subjects have a content difference, $C(a-\bar{v})o_2$, of 5 vol%. Arterial blood typically carries approximately 20 vol% O_2, and mixed venous blood carries 15 vol% O_2. Pulmonary diseases that cause arterial hypoxemia may reduce $S\bar{v}o_2$ if **oxygen uptake** and cardiac output remain constant. Cardiac output often increases to combat arterial hypoxemia caused by intrapulmonary shunting. Increased cardiac output increases O_2 delivery to the tissues. This results in a reduced extraction of O_2 from the blood. Mixed venous blood then returns to the lungs with normal or even increased O_2 saturation. When this blood is shunted it has a higher O_2 content, thereby reducing the shunt effect. With or without arterial hypoxemia, $S\bar{v}o_2$ falls if the cardiac output is compromised.

$S\bar{v}o_2$ is useful in assessing cardiac function in the critical care setting and during exercise. Patients who have good cardiovascular reserves maintain a mixed venous saturation of 70% to 75%. Patients whose $S\bar{v}o_2$ values are in the 60% to 70% range have a limited ability to deliver more O_2 to the tissues. $S\bar{v}o_2$ values less than 60% usually indicate cardiovascular decompensation and tissue hypoxemia. The indwelling reflective spectrophotometer (see Chapter 9) allows continuous monitoring of this important parameter. $S\bar{v}o_2$ also decreases during exercise. Despite increased cardiac output, O_2 extraction by the exercising muscles reduces the content of blood returning to the lungs.

Estimation of Sa_{O_2} by most pulse oximeters (Sp_{O_2}) is based on absorption of light at two wavelengths. When only two wavelengths are analyzed, only two species of Hb can be detected. Absorption in the red and near-infrared portions of the visible spectrum allows measurement of the oxyhemoglobin and reduced Hb, providing an estimate of the oxygen saturation of available Hb (see "Pulse Oximetry," below).

Pulse Oximetry

DESCRIPTION

Sp_{O_2} estimates Sa_{O_2} by analyzing absorption of light passing through a capillary bed. Pulse oximetry is noninvasive. Sp_{O_2} is reported as percent saturation.

TECHNIQUE

Pulse oximeters (see Chapter 9) measure the light absorption of a mixture of two forms of Hb: O_2Hb and reduced Hb (RHb). The relative absorptions at 660 nm (red) and 940 nm of light (near infrared) can be used to calculate the combination of the two Hb forms. Absorption at two wavelengths provides an estimate of the saturation of available Hb (see "Oxygen Saturation," p. 141). Most pulse oximeters use a stored calibration curve to estimate the oxygen saturation.

Pulse oximetry may be used in any setting in which a noninvasive measure of oxygenation status is sufficient. This includes monitoring of O_2 therapy and ventilator management. Pulse oximetry is commonly used during diagnostic procedures such as bronchoscopy, sleep studies, or stress testing. It is also used for monitoring during patient transport or rehabilitation. Pulse oximetry may be used for continuous monitoring with inclusion of appropriate alarms to detect desaturation. Many pulse oximeter systems use memory (RAM) to record Sp_{O_2} and heart rate for extended periods. Alternatively, pulse oximetry can be used for discrete measurements or "spot checks."

Most pulse oximeters use a sensor that attaches to the finger (nail bed) or ear lobe. The choice of attachment site should be dictated by the type of measurement being made. The ear site may be preferred in patients undergoing exercise testing or in whom arm movement precludes use of the finger site. Both finger and ear lobe sites presume pulsatile blood flow. Most oximeters adjust light

---

BOX 6-4
CRITERIA FOR ACCEPTABILITY—PULSE OXIMETRY

1 Documentation of adequate correlation with measured Sa_{O_2} should be available. Sp_{O_2} and Sa_{O_2} should be within 2% from 85% to 100% saturation. Elevated COHb (>3%) or MetHb (>5%) may invalidate Sp_{O_2}.

2 Adequate perfusion of the sensor site should be documented by agreement between oximeter and patient's heart rate (ECG or palpation) and reproducible pulse waveforms (if available).

3 Known interfering substances or agents should be eliminated or accounted for.

4 Pulse oximeter readings should be stable long enough to answer the clinical question being investigated. Readings should be consistent with the patient's clinical history and presentation.

TABLE 6-5   Pulse Oximeter Limitations

Interfering substances	Interfering factors
Carboxyhemoglobin (COHb)	Motion artifact, shivering
Methemoglobin (MetHb)	Bright ambient lighting
Intravascular dyes (indocyanine green)	Hypotension, low perfusion (sensor site)
Nail polish or coverings (finger sensor)	Hypothermia
	Vasoconstrictor drugs
	Dark skin pigmentation

output to compensate for tissue density or pigmentation. In some subjects, impaired perfusion to one site determines which site is preferred. Low perfusion or poor vascularity can cause the oximeter to be unable to detect pulsatile blood flow. Rubbing or warming of the site often improves local blood flow and may be indicated to obtain reliable data.

Some pulse oximeters display a representation of the pulse waveform derived from the absorption measurements (see Chapter 9). Such waveforms may be helpful in selecting an appropriate site or trouble-shooting questionable SpO_2 values. Most pulse oximeters report heart rate (HR), also detected from pulsatile blood flow at the sensor site. Comparison of oximeter HR with palpated pulse or with an electrocardiograph (ECG) signal can assist with selection of an appropriate site. Inability to obtain a valid HR reading or acceptable pulse waveform suggests that SpO_2 values should be interpreted cautiously (Box 6-4).

A number of factors limit the validity of SpO_2 measurements (Table 6-5). To validate pulse oximetry readings, direct measurement of arterial saturation is required. Simultaneous measurement of SpO_2 and SaO_2 can be used initially to validate pulse oximetry. Pulse oximetry used during exercise testing has been shown to produce variable results. Co-oximetry may be necessary to validate pulse oximetry readings at peak exercise.

COHb absorbs light at wavelengths similar to oxyhemoglobin. The pulse oximeter senses COHb as O_2Hb and overestimates the O_2 saturation. MetHb increases absorption at both wavelengths used by pulse oximeters. This causes the ratio of the two Hb forms to approach 1.0, which is usually represented as a saturation of 85% (see "Pulse Oximeters," Chapter 9). Other interfering substances may cause the pulse oximeter to underestimate saturation.

SIGNIFICANCE AND PATHOPHYSIOLOGY

See Box 6-5 for interpretive strategies. Arterial oxygen saturation estimated by pulse oximetry should equal that measured by blood oximetry in healthy nonsmoking adults. Most pulse oximeters are capable of accuracy of ±2% of the actual saturation when SaO_2 is above 90%. For SaO_2 values of 85% to 90%, accuracy may be slightly less. For very low saturations (i.e., less than 80%), pulse oximeter accuracy is less of an issue because the clinical implications are the same.

Pulse oximetry is most useful when it has been shown to correlate with blood oximetry in an individual patient in a known circumstance. When this is the case, pulse oximetry can be used for noninvasive monitoring, either continuously or by taking discrete measurements. Uses include monitoring of O_2 therapy, ventilatory support, pulmonary or cardiac rehabilitation, bronchoscopy, surgical procedures, sleep studies, and cardiopulmonary exercise testing. In each of these applications, careful attention must be paid to minimizing known interfering agents or substances (see Table 6-5).

Because of its limitations, pulse oximetry should be used cautiously when assessing oxygen need. This is particularly true when using pulse oximetry to detect exercise desaturation. Pulse oximetry may not accurately reflect SaO_2 during exertion. For this reason, SpO_2, even if demonstrated to correlate with SaO_2 at rest, may yield **false-positive** or **false-negative** results during

---

BOX 6-5
INTERPRETIVE STRATEGIES—PULSE OXIMETRY

1 Is the SpO_2 reading supported by blood oximetry? If not, interpret very cautiously.

2 Is there evidence of adequate perfusion at the sensor site? Consistent pulse waveform (if available)? Good correlation with palpated pulse or ECG heart rate? If not, consider alternate site or blood oximetry.

3 Is the patient a current smoker or smoke inhalation victim? If so, blood oximetry is indicated.

4 Is the indicated SpO_2 >90%? If so, Hb saturation is probably adequate; correlate with clinical presentation.

5 Is indicated SpO_2 between 85% to 90%? If so, oxygen supplementation may be indicated; correlate with clinical presentation.

6 If indicated SpO_2 <85%, supplementary O_2 is indicated unless there is reason to suspect invalid SpO_2 data.

7 Does supplementary O_2 improve SpO_2 reading? If not, suspect shunt or invalid SpO_2 data.

exercise. Blood gas analysis with blood oximetry should be used to resolve discrepancies between the SpO_2 reading and the patient's clinical presentation.

Pulse oximetry may not be appropriate in all situations. To evaluate hyperoxemia (i.e., PaO_2 greater than 100 to 150 mm Hg) or acid-base status in an individual patient, blood gas analysis is required. Measurement of O_2 delivery, which depends on Hb concentration, cannot be adequately assessed by pulse oximetry alone.

Capnography

DESCRIPTION

Capnography includes continuous, noninvasive monitoring of expired CO_2 and analysis of the single-breath CO_2 waveform. Continuous monitoring of expired CO_2 allows trending of changes in alveolar and dead space ventilation. Analysis of a single breath of expired CO_2 measures the uniformity of both ventilation and pulmonary blood flow. End-tidal PCO_2 ($PetCO_2$) is reported in mm Hg.

TECHNIQUE

Continuous monitoring of expired CO_2 is performed by sampling gas from the proximal airway. This gas may be pumped to an infrared analyzer (see Chapter 9) or to a mass spectrometer. An alternative method inserts a "mainstream" sample window directly into the expired gas stream. The analyzer signal is then passed to either a recorder or computer. CO_2 waveforms may be displayed either individually (Fig. 6-2) or as a series of peaks to form a trend plot. $PetCO_2$ may be read from the peaks of the waveforms. It can also be obtained by a simple peak detector and displayed digitally. Continuous CO_2 monitoring is commonly used in subjects with artificial airways in the critical care setting. $PaCO_2$ can be measured at intervals to establish a gradient with $PetCO_2$. Respiratory rate may be determined from the frequency of the CO_2 waveforms. The change in CO_2 concentration during a single expiration may be analyzed to detect ventilation-perfusion abnormalities (see Fig. 6-2).

Technical problems involved in capnography include the necessity of accurate calibration and management of the gas sampling system (Box 6-6). Calibration using known gases (preferably two

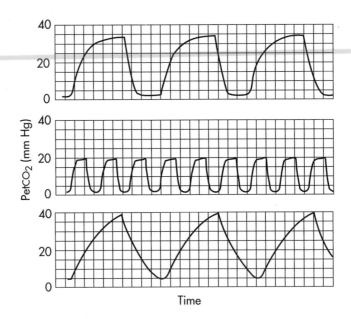

FIG. 6-2 *Capnography tracings.* Expired CO_2 is plotted versus time in three subjects; in each example expiration is marked by the rapid increase in carbon dioxide to a peak ($PetCO_2$) followed by a return to baseline during inspiration. *Top,* A normal respiratory pattern with $PetCO_2$ near 40 mm Hg and a relatively flat alveolar phase. *Middle,* A rapid respiratory rate and low $PetCO_2$ (20 mm Hg) such as might be found in a subject who is hyperventilating; the expiratory waveform has a normal configuration. *Bottom,* An abnormal expired CO_2 waveform consistent with $\dot{V}/\dot{Q}$ abnormalities; no alveolar plateau is present and the baseline does not return to zero.

gas concentrations) is required if the system will be used to monitor $Paco_2$. Many systems use room air, containing minimal CO_2, and a 5% CO_2 mixture for calibration (see Chapter 10). Condensation of water in sample tubing, connectors, or in the sample chamber itself can affect accuracy. Some infrared analyzers (see Chapter 9) may be affected if flow changes after calibration. Saturation of a **dessicator** column, if used, can also lead to inaccurate readings. Long sample lines or low sample flows can cause **damping** of the CO_2 waveform, invalidating any analysis of the shape of the expired gas curve.

SIGNIFICANCE AND PATHOPHYSIOLOGY

See Box 6-7 for interpretive strategies. In healthy subjects, CO_2 rises to a plateau as alveolar gas is expired (see Fig. 6-2). If all lung units empty CO_2 evenly, this plateau appears flat. However, even healthy lungs have ventilation and blood flow imbalances. Healthy lung units empty CO_2 at varying rates. Alveolar CO_2 concentration rises slightly as the breath continues. $Petco_2$ theoretically should not exceed $Paco_2$. In healthy subjects the $Petco_2$ is usually close to the arterial value. When ventilation and perfusion become grossly mismatched (e.g., in severe obstruction), CO_2 concentration at the end of the alveolar plateau may exceed the $Paco_2$. $Paco_2$ reflects gas exchange characteristics of the entire lung. Hence, $Petco_2$ may differ significantly if some lung units are poorly ventilated.

Continuous CO_2 analysis provides useful data for monitoring critically ill patients, particularly those requiring ventilatory support. $Petco_2$ measurements allow trending of changes in $Paco_2$ provided there is little or no change in the shape of the CO_2 waveform (i.e., indicating $\dot{V}/\dot{Q}$ abnormalities). When a reference blood gas sample is obtained, $Petco_2$ can be used as a continuous, noninvasive monitor. Respiratory rate can be measured from the frequency of expired CO_2 waveforms. Marked changes (e.g., **hyperpnea** or apnea) can be detected quickly. Analysis of the individual CO_2 waveforms, along with $Paco_2$, may help identify abrupt changes in dead space. This can be useful in detecting pulmonary embolization or reduced cardiac output.

Problems related to ventilatory support devices can also be detected. Disconnection or leaks in breathing circuits can be quickly recognized by the loss of the CO_2 signal. Increased mechanical

---

BOX 6-6
CRITERIA FOR ACCEPTABILITY—CAPNOGRAPHY

1   The CO_2 analyzer should be calibrated on a frequency consistent with the types of measurements being made. Calibration with air and 5% CO_2 is suitable for most purposes.

2   Sample flow (except in mainstream analyzers) should be high enough to prevent damping of CO_2 waveforms. Sample flow should not be changed after calibration. The sample chamber and tubing should be free of secretions or condensation that might affect the accuracy of the results.

3   $Paco_2$ should be obtained to establish the gradient with $Petco_2$.

4   CO_2 waveforms (if displayed) should be consistent with the subject's clinical condition.

5   CO_2 waveforms (if displayed) should return to baseline during inspiration, indicating appropriate washout of dead space.

BOX 6-7
INTERPRETIVE STRATEGIES—CAPNOGRAPHY

1   Was there an appropriate calibration of the CO_2 analyzer? If not, arterial to end-tidal CO_2 gradients may be inaccurate.

2   Are CO_2 waveforms (if available) consistent with the patient's clinical condition? Do waveforms show an obvious alveolar plateau?

3   Was $Paco_2$ measured? If so, what is the $Paco_2$-$Petco_2$ gradient? If greater than 5 mm Hg, consider marked ventilation-perfusion abnormalities.

4   Has $Petco_2$ changed (serial measurements)? Consider acute changes in dead space or cardiac output.

dead space (i.e., gas rebreathed in the ventilator circuit) can be identified by a baseline CO_2 concentration greater than zero. Irregularities in the CO_2 waveform often signal that the patient is "out of phase" with the ventilator.

The shape of the expired CO_2 curve is determined by ventilation-perfusion matching. Only lung units that are both ventilated *and* perfused contribute CO_2 to expired gas. The CO_2 waveform in subjects without lung disease shows a flat initial segment of anatomic dead space gas containing little or no CO_2. This phase is followed by a rapid increase in CO_2 concentration reflecting a mixture of dead space and alveolar gas. Finally, an "alveolar" plateau occurs in which gas composition changes only slightly. This slight change is caused by different emptying rates of various lung units. The absolute concentration of CO_2 at the alveolar plateau depends on factors such as minute ventilation and CO_2 production. Dead space–producing disease (e.g., pulmonary embolization or marked decrease in cardiac output) may show a profound decrease in the expired CO_2 concentration. Subjects who have pulmonary disease, especially obstruction, show poorly delineated phases of the CO_2 washout curve. The alveolar plateau may actually be a continuous slope throughout expiration, making measurement of Pet_{CO_2} misleading.

Shunt Calculation

DESCRIPTION

A shunt is that portion of the cardiac output that traverses the pulmonary capillaries without participating in gas exchange. The shunt calculation determines the ratio of shunted blood ($\dot{Q}s$) to total perfusion ($\dot{Q}t$). Shunt is reported as a percent of total cardiac output, or sometimes as a simple fraction.

TECHNIQUE

Two techniques for measuring the shunt fraction are commonly used. The first uses O_2 content differences between arterial and mixed venous blood. This method is called the physiologic shunt equation:

1.
$$\frac{\dot{Q}s}{\dot{Q}t} = \frac{Cc_{O_2} - Ca_{O_2}}{Cc_{O_2} - C\bar{v}_{O_2}}$$

where:

$Cc_{O_2} = O_2$ content of end-capillary blood, estimated from saturation associated with calculated Pa_{O_2}

$Ca_{O_2} =$ arterial O_2 content, measured from an arterial sample (see "Oxygen Saturation")

$C\bar{v}_{O_2} =$ mixed venous O_2 content, measured from a sample obtained from a pulmonary artery catheter

The term in the denominator of this equation reflects potential arterialization of mixed venous blood. The term in the numerator reflects the actual arterialization.

In the second technique, the subject breathes 100% O_2 until the Hb is completely saturated (Fig. 6-3). Twenty minutes of O_2 breathing is usually sufficient. Percent shunt is then calculated from differences in dissolved O_2. This method is called the clinical shunt equation:

2.
$$\frac{\dot{Q}s}{\dot{Q}t} = \frac{(P_{AO_2} - Pa_{O_2}) \times 0.0031}{C(a-\bar{v})_{O_2} + [(P_{AO_2} - Pa_{O_2}) \times 0.0031]}$$

where:

$P_{AO_2} =$ alveolar O_2 tension

$Pa_{O_2} =$ arterial O_2 tension

$C(a-\bar{v})_{O_2} =$ arteriovenous O_2 content difference

$0.0031 =$ conversion factor to volume percent for O_2

When the subject is breathing 100% O_2, P_{AO_2} can be estimated as follows:

$$P_{AO_2} = P_B - P_{H_2O} - \left(\frac{P_{ACO_2}}{0.8}\right)$$

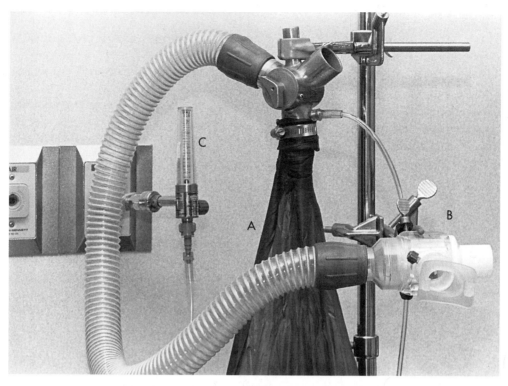

FIG. 6-3 *Equipment used for clinical shunt measurement.* **A,** A large bag or balloon is used as a reservoir for 100% oxygen. **B,** A two-way nonrebreathing valve allows the subject to breathe gas from the balloon. **C,** An oxygen source allows the balloon to be refilled as necessary so the subject can breathe O_2 for at least 20 minutes. A blood gas syringe (not shown) is set up to obtain an arterial specimen at the end of the oxygen breathing. A pulse oximeter may be used to monitor the subject's saturation during the test. An oxygen analyzer (or appropriate blood gas analyzer) can be used to measure the actual FIO_2.

where:

$$P_B = \text{barometric pressure}$$

$$P_{H_2O} = \text{partial pressure of water vapor at body temperature (47 mm Hg)}$$

$$P_{ACO_2} = \text{alveolar } CO_2 \text{ tension (estimated from arterial } P_{CO_2})$$

$$0.8 = \text{normal respiratory exchange ratio}$$

This calculation of alveolar P_{O_2} assumes that the inspired gas is 100% O_2. If the FIO_2 is measured and found to be less than 1.00, the standard alveolar air equation can be used (see Appendix E).

The clinical shunt calculation is accurate only when Hb is completely saturated. This normally requires a PaO_2 of greater than 150 mm Hg. A saturation of 100% is usually easily accomplished if O_2 is breathed long enough. If breathing 100% O_2 does not raise the PaO_2 high enough to completely saturate Hb, the content difference method (physiologic method) should be used. With either method, shunt fraction may be multiplied by 100 and reported as a percentage (i.e., 0.20 ratio × 100 equals a 20% shunt).

Several technical considerations should be noted regarding shunt measurement (Box 6-8). Using O_2 content differences (Equation 1) requires a pulmonary artery catheter to obtain mixed venous O_2 content. Using dissolved O_2 differences (Equation 2) also relies on measured $C(a-\bar{v})O_2$. If placement of a pulmonary artery catheter is not practical, the clinical shunt equation may be used with an assumed a-$\bar{v}$ content difference (see "Significance and Pathophysiology," p. 150).

The physiologic shunt equation may be used for patients on any known FIO_2. The clinical shunt measurement requires O_2 breathing for 20 minutes or longer. Prolonged O_2 breathing may be contraindicated in subjects whose respiration is driven by hypoxemia. Breathing 100% O_2 washes nitrogen (N_2) out of the lungs. Washout of N_2 combined with O_2 uptake by perfusing blood flow can reduce the size of alveoli to their critical limit. In poorly ventilated lung units, this may

---

BOX 6-8
CRITERIA FOR ACCEPTABILITY—SHUNT CALCULATION

1 For physiologic shunt, patient must have simultaneous arterial and mixed venous blood specimens drawn over a 30-second interval.

2 For clinical shunt, patient should breathe 100% O_2 for at least 20 minutes, or until Hb is completely saturated (PaO_2 >150 mm Hg). If PaO_2 >150 mm Hg cannot be achieved, clinical shunt calculation may underestimate true shunt.

3 CaO_2 and $C\bar{v}O_2$ must be measured for physiologic shunt. Measured contents should be used for clinical shunt if available; otherwise estimated a-$\bar{v}$ content difference should be based on clinical status.

4 FIO_2 should be accurately determined; this is required to calculate capillary content for physiologic shunt. FIO_2 of 1.00 can be assumed for clinical shunt calculation, but measured value improves accuracy.

---

cause alveolar collapse. The effect of this "nitrogen shunting" may be shunt values that are falsely high because some shunting was induced by the test itself.

SIGNIFICANCE AND PATHOPHYSIOLOGY

See Box 6-9 for interpretive strategies. In healthy subjects, approximately 5% of the cardiac output is shunted through the pulmonary system. An increased shunt fraction indicates that some lung units have little ventilation in relation to their blood flow. These patterns may be found in both obstructive and restrictive diseases. However, even in severe obstruction or restriction, blood flow to areas of poor ventilation may be reduced by the lesions themselves. In emphysema, destruction of the alveolar septa obliterate pulmonary capillaries. As the terminal airways loose their support, they also have reduced blood flow. In poorly ventilated lung units, **vasoconstriction** of pulmonary arterioles redirects blood flow away from the affected area. In these cases there may be minimal shunting, even though severe ventilatory impairment exists.

Increased shunting is commonly caused by acute disease patterns such as atelectasis or foreign body aspiration. Diseases such as pneumonia or adult respiratory distress syndrome (ARDS) often result in a shunt-like effect. This is caused by reduced ventilation in relation to blood flow in many lung units. Foreign body aspiration may cause shunting by blocking an airway and depriving all distal lung units of ventilation. Blood flow to the affected units cannot participate in gas exchange. The degree of shunting is directly related to the number of lung units with V/Q ratios close to 0.

Very large shunt values (greater than 30%) suggest that a significant volume of blood is moving from the right to left ventricle without participating in gas exchange. Further testing may be required to determine whether the shunt occurs in the lungs or in the heart. **Echocardiography** with contrast media or cardiac catheterization may be necessary to identify intracardiac shunts.

The accuracy of the clinical shunt measurement (i.e., dissolved O_2 differences) depends on the accuracy of PO_2 determinations. In small shunts Hb becomes 100% saturated. The difference between alveolar and arterial PO_2 values results simply from the amount of O_2 dissolved. The difference between the actual content of dissolved oxygen and that which could potentially dissolve is the basis for the calculation. Measurements of PO_2 used for shunt calculations (200 to 600 mm Hg) are much higher than the normal physiologic range. Additional calibration and quality control of the PO_2 electrode may be necessary.

The calculated shunt fraction also depends on the O_2 content difference between arterial and mixed venous blood. $C(a-\bar{v})O_2$ is a component of the denominator in the clinical shunt equation. The a-$\bar{v}$ content difference is determined not only by the lungs but by cardiac output and perfusion status of the tissues. Ideally, the value used in the equation should be measured rather than estimated. Arterial content can be determined easily from a sample taken from a peripheral artery. However, mixed venous content can only be measured accurately from a pulmonary artery sample. In subjects who do not have a pulmonary artery catheter in place, an estimated value must be used. $C(a-\bar{v})O_2$ values from 4.5 to 5.0 vol% are reasonable a-$\bar{v}$ content differences in subjects who have good cardiac output and perfusion status. Values of 3.5 vol% are more realistic in patients who are critically ill.

In some instances, a-$\bar{v}$ content difference cannot be reliably estimated, or Hb cannot be maximally saturated by breathing 100% oxygen. In such cases, the alveolar-arterial oxygen gradient (A-aD_{O_2}) may be useful as an index for matching of ventilation to blood flow. The $\dot{Q}s/\dot{Q}t$

BOX 6-9
INTERPRETIVE STRATEGIES—SHUNT CALCULATION

1 For physiologic shunt: Were arterial and mixed venous samples obtained correctly? Analyzed properly? FIO_2 accurately determined?

2 For clinical shunt: Did patient breathe O_2 long enough to maximally saturate Hb? Was estimated or measured content difference used?

3 Was calculated shunt ≤5%? If so, no significant shunting exists.

4 Was calculated shunt >5% but <10%? If so, some shunting is likely. Consider technical causes (assumed content differences, assumed FIO_2).

5 Was calculated shunt >10% but <30%? If so, significant shunting is present. Consider clinical correlation.

6 Was calculated shunt >30%? If so, severe shunting is present. Further testing is indicated to determine the site and physiologic basis for the shunt.

---

does not directly provide absolute values for $\dot{Q}s$, but if the cardiac output ($\dot{Q}t$) is known, $\dot{Q}s$ can be determined simply.

Measurement of the shunt fraction is often performed in conjunction with the determination of the VD/VT ratio (see Chapter 4) to assess both types of gas exchange abnormalities together.

CASE STUDIES

CASE 6A

History

C.O. was a 57-year-old man referred to the pulmonary function laboratory for increasing shortness of breath. He admitted to having a chronic cough with production of thick white sputum, mainly upon waking in the morning. He reported that he was a former smoker and averaged approximately two packs of cigarettes per day before quitting 3 months ago. His referring physician performed pulse oximetry in an outpatient clinic and obtained readings of 90% to 91%. Complete pulmonary function studies with arterial blood gases were requested.

Personal data

Sex: Male
Age: 57 yr
Height: 66 in
Weight: 197 lb

Spirometry

	Before drug	Predicted	%	After drug	%	% Chg
FVC (L)	3.97	4.10	97	4.04	99	2
FEV_1 (L)	2.31	2.99	77	2.50	84	8
$FEV_{1\%}$ (%)	58	73	—	62	—	7
$FEF_{25\%-75\%}$ (L/sec)	1.01	3.05	33	1.32	43	31
MVV (L/min)	83	116	72	92	79	11

Lung volumes

	Before drug	Predicted	%
VC (L)	3.97	4.10	97
IC (L)	2.66	2.76	96
ERV (L)	1.31	1.35	97
FRC (L)	3.65	3.42	107
RV (L)	2.34	2.07	113
TLC (L)	6.31	6.18	102
RV/TLC (%)	37	34	—

DL$_{CO}$

	Before drug	*Predicted*	*%*
DL$_{CO}$ (ml/min/mm Hg)	16.7	26.3	63
DL$_{CO}$(adj)	17.0	26.3	65
DL/VA (ml/min/mm Hg/L)	76	4.38	86

Blood gases

pH	7.37
PCO$_2$ (mm Hg)	44
PO$_2$ (mm Hg)	57
HCO$_3^-$ (mEq/L)	26.4
BE (mEq/L)	−1.7
Hb (gm/dl)	16.2
O$_2$Hb (%)	80.1
COHb (%)	5.9
MetHb (%)	0.2

Technologist's Comments

All spirometry maneuvers were performed acceptably. Lung volumes by helium (He) dilution were also performed acceptably. DL$_{CO}$ was performed acceptably; DL$_{CO}$ was corrected for an Hb of 16.2 and COHb of 5.9.

Questions

1. What is the interpretation of:
   a. Spirometry, prebronchodilator and postbronchodilator?
   b. Lung volumes?
   c. DL$_{CO}$?
   d. Blood gases?
2. What is the cause of the patient's symptoms?
3. What treatment or additional tests might be indicated?

Discussion

1   **Interpretation**
All spirometry, lung volumes, and diffusing capacity maneuvers were performed acceptably. Spirometry reveals moderate airway obstruction with minimal response to inhaled bronchodilators. Lung volumes by He dilution show a normal TLC, but with increased FRC, RV, and RV/TLC ratio. These changes are consistent with air trapping. DL$_{CO}$ is moderately decreased even after correction for increased Hb and elevated COHb. Arterial blood gas results reveal normal acid-base status with a PCO$_2$ of 44. There is moderate to severe hypoxemia as indicated by PO$_2$ of 57 and oxyhemoglobin saturation of 80%. The hypoxemia is further aggravated by an increased COHb consistent with cigarette smoking or environmental exposure.

   Impression: Moderate obstructive airways disease with no significant improvement after inhaled bronchodilator. There appears to be mild air trapping and a moderate loss of diffusing capacity. There is significant hypoxemia on room air, which is further increased by an elevation of COHb. Recommend further investigation of source of CO and clinical evaluation of O$_2$ supplementation.

2   **Cause of symptoms**
This case demonstrates the importance of arterial blood gas analysis in the diagnosis of pulmonary disorders. The subject's complaint of increased shortness of breath was not explained by the borderline value of SpO$_2$. The referring physician correctly suspected a pulmonary problem resulting from the patient's previous smoking history.

   The spirometric measurement shows moderate obstruction as evidenced by the FEV$_{1\%}$ of 58%. The response of FEV$_1$ to inhaled bronchodilator is less than 200 ml and represents only an 8% improvement over prebronchodilator values. Lung volumes are also consistent with an obstructive pattern showing a mild degree of air trapping.

Diffusing capacity is also reduced in a pattern consistent with mild to moderate airway obstruction. This abnormality persists even after the DL_{CO} is corrected for the elevated COHb. Correction for elevated CO in the blood increases the measured diffusing capacity. In this patient, the correction was offset by the elevated Hb level. When adjusted for the higher than normal Hb, his DL_{CO} decreased.

Of the variables measured, the arterial blood gas values are most abnormal. Although pH and Pco_2 are within normal limits, Po_2 is markedly reduced. As a result, oxygen saturation is low. Further complicating oxygenation is elevated CO. This level is characteristic of individuals who currently smoke or who are chronically exposed to low levels of CO in their environment. The patient's spouse reported that he was still smoking 5 to 10 cigarettes per day.

3   **Treatment and other tests**

The patient was advised to refrain from smoking, which he did within a few days. Blood gases analysis 2 weeks later confirmed his smoking cessation (i.e., COHb was 1.7%). However, his Po_2 improved only slightly to 61 mm Hg (Sao_2 was 87%). He was referred for evaluation of possible exercise desaturation. His arterial oxygenation was shown to actually increase with exercise, so O_2 supplementation was unnecessary. His lung function continued to improve over several months, presumably as a result of his smoking cessation.

CASE 6B

History

Y.M. is a 31-year-old woman referred to the pulmonary function laboratory for a shunt study. Her chief complaint is shortness of breath with exertion as well as at other times. Her referring physician suspected a shunt and requested a shunt study. Y.M. was in no apparent distress on arrival at the laboratory. She had never smoked and had no significant environmental exposure to respiratory irritants. Her mother had died of a stroke at age 50, but there was no heart or lung disease in her immediate family.

Shunt Study

Personal data

Age: 31 yr
Height: 69 in
Weight: 200 lb
Race: Caucasian

Blood gases (drawn after 20 minutes of O_2 breathing)

FIO_2	1.00
P_B	752
pH	7.43
Pco_2	38
Po_2	557
HCO_3^-	24.1
BE	0.1
Hb	7.4
O_2Hb	99.6
COHb	0.3
MetHb	0.1

Questions

1. What is the subject's calculated shunt?
2. What is the interpretation of:
   a. Blood gases?   b. Shunt?
3. What is the cause of the patient's symptoms?
4. What other tests or treatments might be indicated?

Discussion

1   Calculations

The P_{AO_2} is calculated as follows:

$$P_{AO_2} = P_B - P_{H_2O} - \left(\frac{P_{ACO_2}}{0.8}\right)$$

$$= 752 - 47 - \left(\frac{38}{0.8}\right)$$

$$= 705 - 48$$

$$P_{AO_2} = 657$$

Substituting this value in the clinical shunt equation and assuming an a-$\bar{v}$ content difference of 4.5:

$$\frac{\dot{Q}s}{\dot{Q}t} = \frac{(P_{AO_2} - P_{aO_2}) \times 0.0031}{C(a-\bar{v})_{O_2} + [(P_{AO_2} - P_{aO_2}) \times 0.0031]}$$

$$= \frac{(657 - 557) \times 0.0031}{4.5 + [(657 - 557) \times 0.0031]}$$

$$= \frac{0.31}{4.5 + (0.31)}$$

$$\frac{\dot{Q}S}{\dot{Q}t} = 0.06$$

2   Interpretation

This subject's blood gas results show a normal acid-base status. The P_{aO_2} reflects an appropriate increase after breathing 100% O_2 for 20 minutes. The Hb as measured by co-oximetry is markedly reduced. The patient's shunt is 6% (0.06 as a fraction). This is very close to the normal range.

Impression: Normal arterial blood gas results and normal shunt with markedly reduced Hb. Recommend clinical correlation.

3   Cause of symptoms

This patient's primary symptom of dyspnea does not appear to be caused by any significant shunting. In a shunt, blood passes from the right side of the heart to the left side without coming into contact with alveolar gas. The shunt may be in the heart or in the lungs themselves. Breathing high concentrations of oxygen will not relieve this problem. This patient increased her P_{aO_2} appropriately, which rules out a large shunt.

A more likely cause of the symptoms described is the patient's low Hb level. Severe anemia reduces the arterial oxygen content dramatically. Oxygen delivery to the tissues is reduced. Dyspnea can result during exertion or times of increased metabolic demand. This patient's arterial content (ml/dl) can be calculated as follows:

$$C_{aO_2} = (1.34 \times Hb \times O_2Hb) + (P_{aO_2} \times 0.0031)$$

$$= (1.34 \times 7.4 \times 0.996) + (557 \times 0.0031)$$

$$= (9.9) + (1.7)$$

$$C_{aO_2} = 11.6$$

This value is much lower than the normal content of 20 ml/dl. It should be noted that the term in the second parentheses represents dissolved O_2, and would be much lower when the patient breathes room air.

4   Other tests and treatment

This subject's anemia could have been diagnosed by any test that measures total Hb. Co-oximetry, in addition to providing accurate saturation data, also provides an estimate of total Hb. The shunt study could have been performed using calculated Hb saturation, but the low arterial content would have been missed.

No treatment is indicated for this patient until the cause of the anemia can be identified. Y.M. was referred to a hematologist for further evaluation. Additional testing revealed a hemolytic form of anemia, which was successfully treated.

SUMMARY

THIS CHAPTER HAS DESCRIBED THE measurement of pH, P_{CO_2}, P_{O_2}, and blood oximetry used as part of pulmonary function testing. The technical aspects of obtaining samples was covered in some detail because accurate interpretation makes numerous assumptions regarding proper specimen handling. The design and function of blood gas electrodes and blood oximeters is more fully described in Chapter 9. Calibration and quality control issues as they apply to blood gas analyzers are discussed in Chapter 10.

Two noninvasive methods of assessing gas exchange are commonly used: pulse oximetry and capnography. Pulse oximetry offers a simple means of assessing oxyhemoglobin saturation. Attention to interfering factors and correlation with blood gases is necessary to make optimal use of pulse oximetry. Capnography is useful to monitor changes in Pet_{CO_2}, particularly for patients in critical care settings.

Shunt measurements allow estimates of severe ventilation-perfusion imbalances in the lungs. Two methods were described: the clinical and physiologic equations. The advantages and disadvantages of each were discussed.

SELF-ASSESSMENT QUESTIONS

1 *If a patient has a fever of 40° C, the pH as measured by an automated blood gas analyzer will be which of the following?*
   a. Higher than measured at 37° C
   b. Lower than measured at 37° C
   c. Unchanged with temperature correction
   d. Dependent on the corrected P_{O_2}

2 *Before drawing a specimen for blood gas analysis from the radial artery, the modified Allen's test should be performed. Collateral circulation is adequate if the hand is reperfused within:*
   a. 1 to 2 seconds
   b. 10 seconds
   c. 30 to 40 seconds
   d. Less than 60 seconds

3 *A blood gas syringe is prepared using liquid heparin. A volume of 0.5 ml of heparin solution is left in the syringe and a 1.5 ml specimen is obtained. Which of the following problems will occur with this specimen?*
   a. The pH will be more acidotic than expected.
   b. The P_{CO_2} will be lower because of dilution.
   c. The P_{O_2} will be altered because of dilution.
   d. Calculated HCO_3^- will be higher because of changes in P_{CO_2}.

4 *A patient complaining of shortness of breath has the following blood gases obtained on an F_{IO_2} of 0.21:*

pH	7.28	HCO_3^-	25.8 mEq/L
P_{CO_2}	51 mm Hg	BE	−2.1 mEq/L
P_{O_2}	55 mm Hg	O_2Hb	82%

Which of the following best describes the acid-base status of this patient?
   a. Metabolic acidosis
   b. Respiratory acidosis
   c. Compensated metabolic alkalosis
   d. Partially compensated respiratory alkalosis

5 *A patient has the following blood gas results reported:*

pH	7.41
P_{CO_2}	38 mm Hg
P_{O_2}	77 mm Hg
Hb	10 g/dl
O_2Hb	94%

What is this patient's calculated oxygen content (Ca_{O_2})?
   a. 12.5 ml/dl
   b. 12.8 ml/dl
   c. 13.4 ml/dl
   d. 13.7 ml/dl

6 *A patient is referred for arterial blood gas testing. She has an SpO_2 of 84% by pulse oximetry, but blood oximetry reveals an SaO_2 of 94%. Which of the following best explains the difference between results?*
   a. The patient may be severely anemic (Hb less than 8 g/dl).
   b. The patient may have respiratory alkalosis (hyperventilation).
   c. The patient may have an elevated COHb level.
   d. The pulse oximeter reading may have been in error.

7 *A subject referred for shortness of breath has the following arterial blood gas test results:*

pH	7.46
$PaCO_2$	34
PaO_2	57
HCO_3^-	22

   Which of the following best describes these?
   a. Normal acid-base and oxygenation status
   b. Respiratory alkalosis with moderate hypoxemia
   c. Uncompensated respiratory acidosis with mild hypoxemia
   d. Partially compensated metabolic alkalosis with moderate hypoxemia

8 *How should an infrared analyzer used for capnography be calibrated?*
   a. Using 5% CO_2 and room air
   b. Using 5% CO_2 and 15% CO_2
   c. Using 10% CO_2 and 16% O_2
   d. With 100% CO_2

9 *A patient is connected to a 12-lead ECG monitor and pulse oximeter before an exercise test. The HR displayed by the ECG monitor is 97; the pulse oximeter reads an HR of 121 with an SpO_2 of 85%. Which of the following would be the most appropriate action?*
   a. Move the pulse oximeter sensor to an alternate site.
   b. Check all ECG lead wires for good connection.
   c. Obtain an arterial blood gas sample as quickly as possible.
   d. Document the readings and proceed with the test.

10 *An outpatient is referred for a shunt study. After 25 minutes of breathing 100% O_2 the following arterial blood gas values are obtained:*

PO_2 (mm Hg)	290
PCO_2 (mm Hg)	40
Saturation (%)	100
Hb (vol%)	10.2

   If the barometric pressure is 750 and a content difference of 4.5 vol% is assumed, what is this subject's shunt?
   a. 20%
   b. 22%
   c. 24%
   d. 25%

SELECTED BIBLIOGRAPHY

General References
Morris AH, Kanner RE, Crapo RO, et al: *Clinical pulmonary function testing*, ed 2, Salt Lake City, 1984, Intermountain Thoracic Society.
Shapiro BA, Kozlowski-Templin R, Peruzzi WT: *Clinical application of blood gases*, ed 5, St Louis, 1994, Mosby.
Shapiro BA, Cane RD: Blood gas monitoring: yesterday, today, and tomorrow, *Crit Care Med* 17:573, 1989.
West JB: *Pulmonary pathophysiology: the essentials*, ed 4, Baltimore, 1992, Williams & Wilkins.
West JB: *Respiratory physiology: the essentials*, ed 5, Baltimore, 1995, Williams & Wilkins.

Blood Gases
Bageant RA: Variations in arterial blood gas measurements due to sampling techniques, *Respir Care* 20:565, 1975.
Hansen JE: Arterial blood gases, *Clin Chest Med* 10:277, 1989.
Raffin TA: Indications for arterial blood gas analysis, *Ann Intern Med* 105:390, 1986.
Severinghaus JW: Blood gas calculator, *J Appl Physiol* 21:1108, 1966.

Siggard-Anderson O: Acid-base and blood gas parameters: arterial or capillary blood, *Scand J Clin Lab Invest* 21:28 9, 1968.

Pulse Oximetry
Barker SJ, Tremper KK, eds: Pulse oximetry: applications and limitations, *Int Anesthesiol Clin* 25:155-175, 1987.
Hannhart B, Habberer J-P, Saunier C, et al: Accuracy and precision of fourteen pulse oximeters, *Eur Respir J* 4:115-119, 1991.
Raener DB, Elliott WR, Topulos GP, et al: The theoretical effect of carboxyhemoglobin on the pulse oximeter, *J Clin Monit* 5:246-249, 1989.
Ries AL, Prewitt LM, Johnson JJ: Skin color and ear oximetry, *Chest* 96:287-290, 1989.
Severinghaus JW, Kelleher JF: Recent developments in pulse oximetry, *Anesthesiology* 76:1018-1038, 1992.

Capnography
Carlon GC, Ray C, Miodownik S, et al: Capnography in mechanically ventilated patients, *Crit Care Med* 16:550-556, 1988.

Graybeal JM, Russel GB: Capnometry in the surgical ICU: an analysis of the arterial-to-end-tidal carbon dioxide difference, *Respir Care* 38:923-928, 1993.

Hess DR, Branson RD: Noninvasive respiratory monitoring equipment. In Branson RD, Hess DR, Chatburn RL, eds: *Respiratory care equipment,* Philadelphia, 1994, JB Lippincott.

Hess D: Capnometry and capnography: technical aspects, physiologic aspects, and clinical applications, *Respir Care* 35:557-573, 1990.

Wiedemann HP, McCarthy K: Noninvasive monitoring of oxygen and carbon dioxide, *Clin Chest Med* 10:239, 1989.

Shunt Calculation

Cane RD, Shapiro BA, Harrison RA, et al: Minimizing errors in intrapulmonary shunt calculations, *Crit Care Med* 8:294, 1980.

Harrison RA, Davison R, Shapiro BA, et al: Reassessment of the assumed a-v oxygen content difference in the shunt calculation, *Anesth Analg* 54:198, 1975.

Standards and Guidelines

Definitions of quantities and conventions related to blood pH and gas analysis, ed 3, (tentative standard), National Committee for Clinical Laboratory Standards, Publication C12-T2, 1991.

Blood gas preanalytical considerations: specimen collection, calibration, and controls (tentative guideline), National Committee for Clinical Laboratory Standards, Publication C27-T, 1989.

Oxygen content, hemoglobin oxygen "saturation," and related quantities in blood: terminology, measurements, and reporting, National Committee for Clinical Laboratory Standards, Publication C25-P; 10:1-49.

American Association for Respiratory Care: Capnography/capnometry during mechanical ventilation, *Respir Care* 40:1321-1324, 1995.

American Association for Respiratory Care: In-vitro pH and blood gas analysis and hemoximetry, *Respir Care* 38:505-510, 1993.

American Association for Respiratory Care: Sampling for arterial blood gas analysis, *Respir Care* 37:913-917, 1992.

American Association for Respiratory Care: Pulse oximetry, *Respir Care* 36:1406-1409, 1991.

Task Force on Guidelines, Society of Critical Care Medicine: Guidelines for standards of care for patients with acute respiratory failure on mechanical ventilatory support, *Crit Care Med* 19:275-278, 1991.

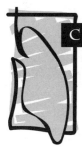

CHAPTER 7

Cardiopulmonary Exercise Testing

OBJECTIVES

After studying this chapter, you should be able to do the following:

1 Select an appropriate exercise protocol based on the reason for performing the test

2 Describe the normal changes that occur in ventilation when workload is increased

3 Classify exercise limitation as caused by cardiovascular, ventilatory, gas exchange, or blood gas abnormalities

4 Describe two methods for measuring ventilation, oxygen consumption, and carbon dioxide production during exercise

5 Identify indications for terminating a cardiopulmonary stress test

THE EFFICIENCY OF THE CARDIOPULMONARY system may be different during increased metabolic demand than at rest. Tests designed to assess ventilation, gas exchange, and cardiovascular function during exercise can provide information not obtainable with the subject at rest. Cardiopulmonary exercise testing allows evaluation of the heart and lungs under conditions of increased metabolic demand. Limitations to work are not entirely predictable from any single resting measurement of pulmonary function. To define work limitations, a cardiopulmonary exercise test is necessary. In most exercise tests, cardiopulmonary variables are assessed in relation to the workload (i.e., the level of exercise). The patterns of change in any particular variable (e.g., heart rate) are then compared with the expected normal response.

The primary indications for performing exercise tests are dyspnea on exertion, pain (especially angina), and fatigue. Other indications include exercise-induced bronchospasm and arterial desaturation. Exercise testing can detect the following:

1. The presence and nature of ventilatory limitations to work
2. The presence and nature of cardiovascular limitations to work
3. The extent of conditioning or **deconditioning**
4. The maximum tolerable workload and safe levels of daily exercise
5. The extent of disability for rehabilitation purposes
6. O_2 desaturation and appropriate levels of supplemental O_2 therapy

Exercise testing may be indicated in apparently healthy individuals, particularly in adults over 40 years of age. Cardiopulmonary exercise testing is indicated to assess fitness before engaging in vigorous physical activities (e.g., running). Cardiopulmonary exercise testing may be useful in assessing risk of postoperative complications, particularly in subjects undergoing **thoracotomy.**

This chapter deals primarily with cardiopulmonary measurements during exercise. This does not include simple cardiac stress testing during which only the electrocardiogram (ECG) and blood pressure (BP) are monitored, or more sophisticated tests involving injection of radioisotopes.

Exercise Protocols

Cardiopulmonary exercise tests can be divided into two general categories depending on the protocols used to perform the test: (1) progressive multistage tests and (2) **steady-state tests.**

Progressive multistage exercise tests examine the effects of increasing workloads on various cardiopulmonary variables, without necessarily allowing a steady state to be achieved. These protocols are often used to determine the workload at which the subject reaches a maximum oxygen uptake ($\dot{V}O_{2max}$). Multistage protocols can determine maximal ventilation, maximal heart

TABLE 7-1   Exercise Protocols

Treadmill	Speed (mph)/grade (%)	Interval (min)	Comment
Bruce	1.7/10 2.5/12 3.4/14 4.2/16 5.0/18 5.5/20 6.0/22	3	Large workload increments; 1.7/0 and 1.7/5 may be used as preliminary stages for deconditioned subjects
Balke	3.3-3.4/0 increasing grade by 2.5% to exhaustion	1	Small workload increments; may use 3 mph and 2-minute intervals for deconditioned subjects, or reduce slope changes to 1%
Jones	1.0/0 2.0/0 2-3.5/2.5 increasing grade by 2.5% to exhaustion	1	Small workload increments and low starting workload

Cycle ergometer	Workload	Interval (min)	Comment
Astrand	50 W (300 kpm) to exhaustion	4	Large workload increments and long intervals; 33 W (200 kpm) may be used for women
"RAMP"	10 W/min to exhaustion	Continuous	Requires electronically braked ergometer; different work rates may be used to alter ramp slope
Jones	16 W/min (100 kpm) to exhuastion	1	Smaller increments (50 kpm) may be used for deconditioned subjects

Other	Description	Interval (min)	Comment
Master step test	Either constant or variable step height combined with increasing step rates	Variable	Simple to perform; workload may be difficult to qualify
6-Minute walk	Distance covered in 6 minutes of free walking	6	Simple; useful in subjects with limited reserves or for evaluation of rehabilitation; can also be done for 12 minutes

rate, or a symptom limitation (i.e., chest pain) to exercise. Progressive multistage protocols (also called **incremental** tests) allow cardiopulmonary variables to be compared with expected patterns as workload increases.

In a typical incremental test, the subject's workload increases at predetermined intervals (Table 7-1). The workload may be increased at intervals of 1 to 6 minutes. Measurements (e.g., BP or obtaining blood gas levels) are usually made during the last 30 to 60 seconds of each interval. Complex measurements (e.g., cardiac output) may require longer intervals. Computerized systems that measure ventilation, gas exchange, and cardiopulmonary variables continuously permit shorter intervals to be used. The combination of intervals and work increments should allow the subject to reach exhaustion or symptom limitation within a reasonable period. An incremental test lasting 8 to 10 minutes after a warm-up is usually appropriate. If a computerized **cycle ergometer** is used, a "ramp" test may be performed. In a ramp protocol the ergometer's resistance is increased continuously at a predetermined rate (**watts** per minute).

During incremental tests with short intervals (1 to 3 minutes or a ramp protocol), a steady state of gas exchange, ventilation, and cardiovascular response may not be attained. Healthy subjects may reach a steady state in 2 to 3 minutes at low and moderate workloads. Attainment of a steady state, however, is unnecessary if the primary objective of the evaluation is to determine the maximum values (oxygen uptake, heart rate [HR], or ventilation). Short exercise intervals also lessen muscle fatigue that may occur with prolonged tests. Short interval or ramp protocols may allow better delineation of gas exchange ($\dot{V}O_2$, $\dot{V}CO_2$) **kinetics.** Progressive multistage tests using intervals of 4 to 6 minutes may result in a steady state.

STEADY-STATE TESTS

Steady-state tests are designed to assess cardiopulmonary function under conditions of constant metabolic demand. Steady-state conditions are usually defined in terms of HR, oxygen consumption ($\dot{V}O_2$), or ventilation ($\dot{V}E$). If the HR remains unchanged for 1 minute at a given workload, a steady state may be assumed. Steady-state tests are useful for assessing responses to a known workload. Steady-state protocols may be used to evaluate the effectiveness of various therapies or pharmacologic agents on exercise ability. For example, an incremental test may be performed initially to determine a subject's maximum tolerable workload. Then a steady-state test may be used to evaluate specific variables at a submaximal level, such as 50% and 75% of the highest $\dot{V}O_2$ achieved. The subject exercises for 5 to 8 minutes at a predetermined level to allow a steady state to develop. Measurements are performed during the last 1 or 2 minutes of the period. Successive steady-state determinations at higher power outputs may be made continuously or spaced with short periods of light exercise or rest. A similar protocol may be used for evaluation of exercise-induced bronchospasm (see Chapter 8).

Two methods of varying exercise workload are commonly used: the treadmill and the cycle ergometer (Figs. 7-1 and 7-2). Each device has advantages and disadvantages. Other methods sometimes used include arm ergometers, steps, and free running or walking.

Workload on a treadmill is adjusted by changing the speed and/or slope of the walking surface. The speed of the treadmill may be calibrated in either miles per hour or in kilometers per hour. Treadmill slope is registered as **"percent grade."** Percent grade refers to the relationship between the length of the walking surface and the elevation of one end above level. A treadmill with a 6-foot surface and one end elevated 1 foot above level would have an elevation of $\frac{1}{6} \times 100$, or approximately 17%. The primary advantage of a treadmill is that it elicits walking, jogging, or running, which are familiar forms of exercise. An additional advantage is that maximal levels of exercise can be easily attained, even in conditioned healthy subjects. However, the actual work performed during treadmill walking is a function of the weight of the subject. Subjects of different weights walking at the same speed and slope perform different workloads. Different walking patterns, or stride length, may also affect the actual amount of work being done. Subjects who grip the handrails of the treadmill may use their arms to reduce the amount of work being performed. For these reasons, estimating $\dot{V}O_2$ from a subject's weight and the speed and slope of the treadmill may produce erroneous results. $\dot{V}O_{2max}$ has been shown to be measured slightly higher (approximately 7% to 10%) on a treadmill compared to a cycle ergometer.

The cycle ergometer allows workload to be varied by adjustment of the resistance to pedaling and by the pedaling frequency, usually specified in revolutions per minute. The flywheel of a mechanical ergometer turns against a belt or strap, both ends of which are connected to a weighted

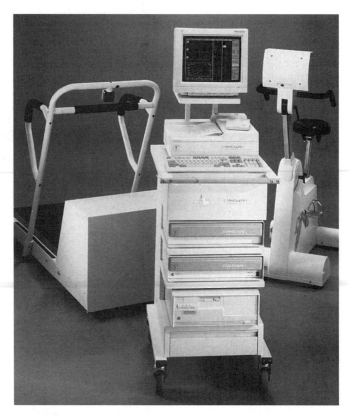

FIG. 7-1 *Treadmill with computerized electrocardiogram (ECG) and controller.* The treadmill is controlled by a programmable interface so that different protocols (i.e., speeds and percent grade) can be selected. Manual control is also provided. Cardiac monitoring and exhaled gas analysis are integrated in a single computer system. The 12-lead ECG recordings or rhythm strips can be taken automatically at each exercise level. Most automated systems provide storage of data regarding significant arrhythmia during the test for later review. The same system can be interfaced to a cycle ergometer (see Fig. 7-2). (Courtesy Medical Graphics Inc., St. Paul, MN.)

physical balance. The diameter of the wheel is known and the resistance can be easily measured. When pedaling speed (usually 50 to 90 rpm) is determined, the amount of work performed can be accurately calculated. One of the chief advantages of the cycle ergometer is that the workload is independent of the weight of the subject. Unlike the treadmill, $\dot{V}o_2$ can be reasonably estimated if the pedaling speed and resistance are carefully measured. In addition, workload can be changed rapidly by adjusting the tension on the flywheel. Another advantage of ergometers is better stability of the subject for gas collection, blood sampling, and blood pressure monitoring. Electronically braked cycle ergometers (see Fig. 7-2) provide a smooth, rapid, and more reproducible means of changing exercise workload than mechanical ergometers. Electronically braked ergometers allow continuous adjustment of workload independent of pedaling speed. This feature permits the exercise level to be ramped (i.e., the workload increases continuously rather than in increments). The **ramp test** allows the subject to advance from low to high workloads quickly and provides all the information normally sought during a progressive maximal exercise test. A ramp protocol typically requires computerization for adjustment of the workload and rapid collection of physiologic data.

Some differences in the maximal performance exist between the treadmill and the cycle ergometer. These differences primarily result from the muscle groups used. In most subjects, cycling does not produce as high a maximum O_2 consumption as walking on the treadmill (approximately 7% to 10% less). Ventilation and lactate production may be slightly greater on the cycle ergometer because of the different muscle groups used. Differences between the treadmill and cycle ergometer are not significant in most clinical situations. The choice of device may be dictated by the subject's clinical condition (i.e., orthopedic impairments) or the types of measurements to be made.

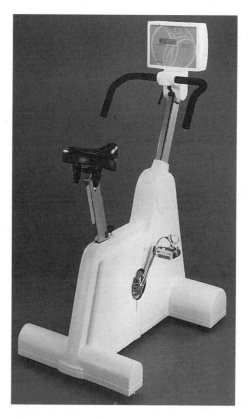

FIG. 7-2 *Electronically braked cycle ergometer.* A typical cycle ergometer with continuous adjustable electronic braking. Workload (i.e., resistance) is usually managed by interfacing the ergometer to a computer. The computer allows selection of various cycle ergometer protocols. Changes in pedaling rate by the subject causes resistance to be altered to maintain a constant workload. (Courtesy Medical Graphics Inc., St. Paul, MN.)

Workload may be expressed quantitatively in several ways:

Work is normally expressed in kilopond-meters **(kpm).** One kpm equals the work of moving a 1 kg mass a vertical distance of 1 m against the force of gravity.

Power is expressed in kilopond-meters per minute (i.e., work per unit of time) or in watts. One watt equals 6.12 kpm/min (100 watts ≈ 600 kpm/min).

Energy is expressed by oxygen consumption ($\dot{V}_{O_2}$), in liters or milliliters per minute (STPD), or in terms of multiples of the resting O_2 uptake **(METS).** Resting or baseline $\dot{V}_{O_2}$ can be measured as described in the following paragraphs or estimated. For purposes of standardization, 1 MET is often considered to be 3.5 ml O_2/min/kg.

For cardiopulmonary exercise evaluation, it is particularly useful to relate the ventilatory, blood gas, and hemodynamic measurements to the $\dot{V}_{O_2}$ as the independent variable. This requires measurement of ventilation and analysis of expired gas during exercise.

A number of cardiopulmonary exercise variables may be used depending on the clinical questions to be answered. Schemes for measuring these variables are described in Table 7-2. Graded exercise with monitoring of only BP and ECG may be limited to evaluation of subjects with suspected or known coronary artery disease. Addition of pulse oximetry may add little to this noninvasive protocol because pulse oximetry accuracy can be affected by changes in perfusion during exercise.

Measurement of ventilation, oxygen consumption, carbon dioxide production, and related variables permits a comprehensive evaluation of the cardiovascular system. Addition of these measurements to ECG, BP, and pulse oximetry makes it possible to grade the adequacy of cardiopulmonary function. In addition, analysis of exhaled gas allows the relative contributions of

TABLE 7-2   Cardiopulmonary Exercise Variables

Variables measured	Uses
ECG, blood pressure, Sp_{O_2}	Limited to suspected or known coronary artery disease; pulse oximetry may be misleading if used without blood gases
All of the above plus ventilation, $\dot{V}_{O_2}$, $\dot{V}_{CO_2}$, and derived measurements	Noninvasive estimate of ventilatory threshold (AT), quantify workload, discriminate between cardiovascular and pulmonary limitation to work
All of the above plus arterial blood gases	Detailed assessment of gas exchange abnormalities; calculation of V_D/V_T; titration of O_2 in exercise desaturation; measurement of pH and lactate possible
All of the above plus mixed venous blood gases	Cardiac output by Fick method, calculation of shunt, thermodilution cardiac output, pulmonary artery pressures, calculation of pulmonary and systemic vascular resistances

cardiovascular, pulmonary, or conditioning limitations to work to be determined. All of these variables can be measured noninvasively.

Addition of blood gases to the exercise protocol enables detailed analysis of the pulmonary limitations to exercise. Placement of an arterial catheter is preferrable to a single sample obtained at peak exercise. Multiple specimens permit comparison of blood gases at each workload. A single sample at peak exercise may be difficult to obtain and may not adequately describe the pattern of gas exchange abnormality. In some patients, a pulmonary artery (Swan-Ganz) catheter may be indicated. The addition of mixed venous blood gases allows cardiac output to be determined via the **Fick method,** along with many derived variables. Thermal dilution cardiac output is also practical with most pulmonary artery catheters.

Cardiovascular Monitors During Exercise

Continuous monitoring of HR and ECG during exercise is essential to safe performance of the test. Intermittent or continuous monitoring of BP is equally important to assure that exercise testing is safe. Recording of HR, ECG, and BP allows work limitations caused by cardiac or vascular disease to be identified and quantified. The level of fitness or conditioning can be gauged from the HR response in relation to the maximal work rate achieved during exercise.

HEART RATE AND ELECTROCARDIOGRAM

HR and rhythm should be monitored continuously using one or more modified chest leads. Standard **precordial** chest lead configurations (V_1 to V_6) allow comparison with resting 12-lead tracings (Box 7-1). Twelve-lead monitoring during exercise is practical with electrocardiographs designed for exercise testing. These instruments incorporate filters (digital or analog) that eliminate movement artifact and provide **ST segment** monitoring. Limb leads normally must be moved to the torso for ergometer or treadmill testing (modified leads). A resting ECG should be performed to record both the standard and modified leads. Single-lead monitoring allows only for gross arrhythmia detection and HR determination. It may not be adequate for testing subjects with known or suspected cardiac disease.

The ECG monitor should allow assessment of intervals and segments up to the subject's maximum heart rate (HR_{max}). Computerized arrhythmia recording, or manual "freeze-frame" storage, allows later evaluation of conduction abnormalities while the testing protocol continues (Fig. 7-3). Some digital ECG systems generate computerized "median" complexes averaged from a series of beats. These may be helpful in analyzing ST-segment depression. The "raw," or nondigitized, ECG should also be available. Significant ST-segment changes should be easily identifiable from the tracing up to the predicted HR_{max}.

HR should be analyzed by visual inspection of the ECG, with manual measurement of the rate rather than by an automatic sensor. Most HR meters average **RR intervals** over multiple beats. Inaccurate HR measurements may occur with **nodal** or ventricular arrhythmias or because of

---

BOX 7-1
CRITERIA FOR ACCEPTABILITY—CARDIOVASCULAR
MONITORS DURING EXERCISE

1 Heart rate and rhythm (ECG) should be monitored continuously. At least one precordial lead is required; full 12-lead monitoring using modified limb leads is recommended.

2 A resting 12-lead ECG should be available for comparison with exercise tracings.

3 All exercise tracings should be free from artifact caused by motion or electrical interference.

4 ECG monitoring devices should allow manual or automated storage of arrhythmia events for later review.

5 "Raw" ECG tracings should be available for comparison to computer averaged complexes.

6 Heart rates should be checked by visual inspection of the ECG tracing.

7 Systemic blood pressure (BP) should be monitored at appropriate intervals (i.e., at least once per exercise stage).

8 BP may be monitored using an appropriate sized cuff or by automated noninvasive blood pressure (NIBP) monitor. A cuff/stethoscope should be available as back-up for NIBP.

9 If BP is monitored by indwelling arterial catheter, the pressure transducer must be zeroed and calibrated appropriately. The catheter should be secured to minimize movement artifact.

---

motion artifact. Tall P or T waves may be falsely identified as R waves causing automatic calculation of HR to be incorrect. Accurate measurement of HR is necessary to determine the subject's maximum in comparison with their age-related predicted value.

Motion artifact is the most common cause of unacceptable ECG recordings during exercise. Allowing the subject to practice pedaling on the ergometer or walking on the treadmill permits adequacy of the ECG signal to be checked. Carefully applied electrodes, proper skin preparation, and secured lead wires greatly minimize movement artifact (see Box 7-1). Electrodes specifically designed for exercise testing are helpful. Most of these use extra adhesive to ensure electrical contact even when the subject begins perspiring. The skin sites should be carefully prepared. Removal of surface skin cells by gentle abrasion is recommended. Subjects with excessive body hair may require shaving of the electrode site to ensure good electrical contact. Lead wires must be securely attached to the electrodes. Devices that limit the movement of the lead wires can greatly reduce motion artifact. Spare electrodes and lead wires should be available to avoid test interruption in the event of an electrode failure.

HR increases linearly with increasing workload, up to an age-related maximum. Several formulas are available for predicting HR_{max}. For most predicted HR_{max} values a variability of ± 10 to 15 beats/min exists in healthy adult subjects. Two commonly used equations for predicting HR_{max} are as follows:

$$1.\ HR_{max} = 220 - Age_{years}$$
$$2.\ HR_{max} = 210 - (0.65 \times Age_{years})$$

Equation 1 yields slightly higher predicted values in young adults. Equation 2 produces higher values in older adults. Other methods of predicting HR_{max} vary depending on the type of exercise protocol used in deriving the regression data. Specific criteria for terminating an exercise test should include factors based on symptom limitation as well as HR and BP changes (see "Safety," p. 170).

HR increases almost linearly with increasing $\dot{V}O_2$. The increase in cardiac output (CO) depends on both HR and stroke volume (**SV**) according to the following equation:

$$CO = HR \times SV$$

Increases in stroke volume account for a smaller portion of the increase in CO, primarily at low and moderate workloads (Fig. 7-4). While HR increases from 70 beats/min up to 200 beats/min in healthy upright subjects, SV increases from 80 ml to approximately 110 ml. At low workloads, increase in CO depends on the subject's ability to increase both HR and SV. At high workloads, further increases in CO result almost entirely from the increase in HR.

Deconditioned subjects usually have a limited SV. High HR values occur with moderate

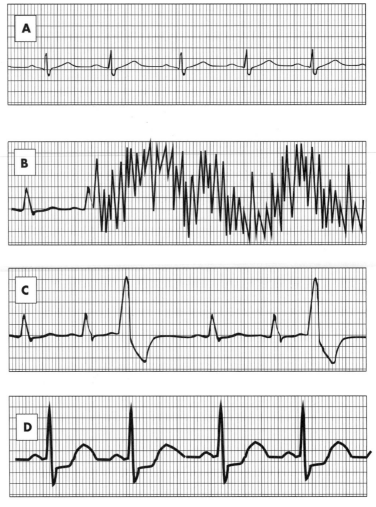

FIG. 7-3 *Electrocardiographic (ECG) monitoring during exercise.* **A,** A standard rhythm lead showing normal sinus rhythm. Although testing can be done with 1 to 3 leads, 12-lead monitoring during exercise allows comparison with resting ECG tracings and better detection of ischemic changes. **B,** Motion artifact. The most common monitoring problem during exercise is poor ECG signals because of motion. These problems can be minimized by careful skin preparation and electrode application. Lead wires and cables should be supported so that movement and traction on electrodes is kept to a minimum. **C,** Premature ventricular contractions (PVCs). PVCs are a common occurrence during exercise in patients with underlying cardiac disease. Increased rate of PVCs, couplets (two in a row), or triplets (three in a row) may be indications for limiting the exercise test. **D,** ST segment changes. Depression (and sometimes elevation) of the ST segment of the ECG is usually considered evidence of cardiac ischemia. Depression (or elevation) of the ST segment greater than 1 to 2 mm for 0.08 seconds or longer is consistent with significant ischemia. ST segments should be checked in multiple leads before, during, and after exercise.

workloads in deconditioned individuals because that is the primary mechanism for increasing CO. Training (i.e., endurance or **aerobic**) typically improves SV. This allows the same cardiac output to be achieved at a lower HR. Training usually results in a lower resting HR as well as a higher tolerable maximum workload. Except in highly trained subjects, maximal exercise in healthy individuals is limited by the inability to further increase the CO. Reductions in SV are usually related to the **preload** or afterload of the left ventricle. Increased HR response, in relation to the workload, implies that the SV is compromised.

Reduced HR response may occur in subjects who have **ischemic** heart disease or complete heart block (Box 7-2). Low HR is also common in subjects who have been treated with drugs that block the effects of the sympathetic nervous system (β-blockers). HR response may also be reduced if the autonomic nervous system is impaired or the heart is **denervated,** as occurs in cardiac transplantation.

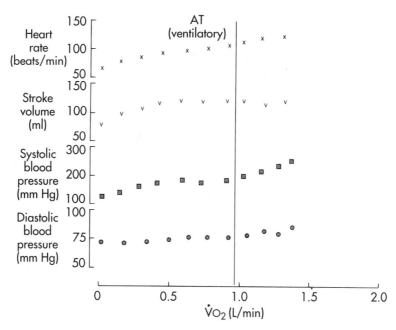

FIG. 7-4 *Normal cardiovascular responses during exercise.* Four cardiovascular parameters are plotted against $\dot{V}o_2$ as a measure of work rate, as they might appear in a normal healthy adult. Heart rate (HR) increases linearly with work. The maximum HR is predicted by the age of the subject. Stroke volume (SV) increases initially at low to moderate work loads, but then becomes relatively constant. Cardiac output, which equals HR × SV, increases at low and moderate work loads because of increases in both HR and SV (see text). At higher levels of work, increases in HR are responsible for increasing cardiac output. Systolic BP increases by approximately 100 mm Hg in a linear fashion, whereas diastolic pressure increases only slightly.

BOX 7-2
INTERPRETIVE STRATEGIES—CARDIOVASCULAR MONITORS DURING EXERCISE

1   Is the ECG recording acceptable? Free from motion and other artifact?

2   Is the resting tracing consistent with previous 12-lead ECGs? If not, are differences caused by lead placement?

3   What is the rate and rhythm at rest? Is there evidence of heart block at rest? Is there evidence of ischemia (ST-segment changes) at rest?

4   Was maximal heart rate greater than 85% of predicted? If so, patient probably exerted maximal effort. If not, what factors limited exercise? Ventilation? Pain? Fatigue? Other?

5   Did the rhythm change with exercise? Increased or decreased PVCs? Was there evidence of ischemia (ST- or T-wave changes)?

6   Were symptoms (chest pain, dizziness) consistent with ECG findings?

7   Was BP normal at rest? If not, consider clinical correlation.

8   Did systolic BP increase appropriately? Did it exceed 250 mm Hg at maximal exercise?

9   Did diastolic BP remain constant or increase slightly? If not, consider clinical correlation.

In subjects who have heart disease (e.g., coronary artery disease, cardiomyopathy), increased HR is typically accompanied by ECG changes such as arrhythmias or ST-segment depression. Deconditioned subjects without heart disease show a high HR at lower than maximal workloads but usually without ECG abnormalities. Depression of the ST segment greater than 1 mm (from the resting baseline) for a duration of 0.08 seconds is usually considered evidence of ischemia. ST depression at low workloads that increases with HR and continues into the postexercise period is usually indicative of multivessel coronary artery disease. ST depression accompanied by exertional **hypotension** or marked increase in **diastolic** pressure is usually associated with significant

TABLE 7-3   Exercise Variables and Dyspnea*

	Cardiac	Ventilatory	Deconditioned	Poor effort
$\dot{V}O_{2max}$	Less than 80% of predicted	Less than 80% of predicted	Less than 80% of predicted	Less than 80% of predicted
$\dot{V}E_{max}$	Less than 50% of MVV	Greather than 70% of MVV	Less than 50% of MVV	Variable
Anaerobic threshold	Achieved at low $\dot{V}O_2$	Usually not achieved	Achieved at low $\dot{V}O_2$	Not achieved
HR	Greater than 85% of predicted	Less than 85% of predicted	Greater than 85% of predicted	Less than 85% of predicted
ECG/signs of ischemia	ST changes, arrhythmias, chest pain	Usually normal	Normal	Normal
Sao_2	Greater than 90%	Often less than 90%, hypoxemia	Greater than 90%	Greater than 90%

*This table compares the usual findings for the exercise variables listed in subjects with dyspnea caused by cardiac disease, pulmonary disease, or deconditioning. Some subjects may have dyspnea because of a combination of causes. Poor effort during exercise may result from improper instruction, lack of understanding by the subject, or lack of motivation by the subject.

MVV, Maximal voluntary ventilation; *Sao_2* arterial oxygen saturation.

coronary disease. The predictive value of ST-segment changes during exercise must be related to the subject's clinical history and risk factors for heart disease.

The most common arrhythmia that occurs during exercise testing is the premature ventricular contraction (**PVC**) (see Fig. 7-3). PVCs are associated with an increased incidence of myocardial ischemia and are considered dangerous because they may precede more serious, lethal arrhythmias. Exercise-induced PVCs occurring at a rate of more than 10 per minute are often found in ischemic heart disease. Increased PVCs during exercise may also be seen in mitral valve prolapse. Coupled PVCs (**couplets**) often precede ventricular tachycardia or ventricular **fibrillation.** Occurrence of couplets or frequent PVCs may be indications for terminating the exercise evaluation. Some subjects with PVCs at rest or at low workloads may have these **ectopic** beats suppressed as exercise intensity increases. The most serious ventricular dysrhythmias are sometimes seen in the immediate postexercise phase.

Shortness of breath brought on by exertion is perhaps the most widespread indication for cardiopulmonary exercise evaluation. The combination of cardiovascular parameters (i.e., HR, SV) with data obtained from analysis of exhaled gas (i.e., $\dot{V}O_2$, AT) permits assessment of dyspnea on exertion. Table 7-3 generalizes some of the basic relationships between cardiovascular and pulmonary exercise responses. These relationships help delineate whether exertional dyspnea is a result of cardiac or pulmonary disease or whether the subject is simply deconditioned. In some instances, poor effort may mimic exertional dyspnea. Comparison of data from cardiovascular and exhaled gas variables can confirm inadequate subject effort.

BLOOD PRESSURE

Systemic BP may be monitored intermittently using the standard cuff method. Automated noninvasive cuff devices for monitoring BP are also available. Although these methods work well at rest and at low workloads, they may be difficult to implement during high levels of exercise. BP sounds may be difficult to detect because of treadmill noise or subject movement. It is important to monitor the pattern of BP response at low and moderate workloads to establish that both **systolic** and diastolic pressure are responding as anticipated.

Continuous monitoring of BP may be accomplished by connection of a pressure transducer to an indwelling arterial catheter (Fig. 7-5). An indwelling line allows continuous display and recording of systolic, diastolic, and mean arterial pressures. In addition, the catheter provides ready access for arterial blood sampling. Arterial catheterization may be easily accomplished using either the radial or brachial site. The catheter must be adequately secured to prevent loss of patency during vigorous exercise. Insertion of arterial catheters presents some risk of blood splashing or spills. Adequate protection for the individual inserting the catheter, as well as for those withdrawing

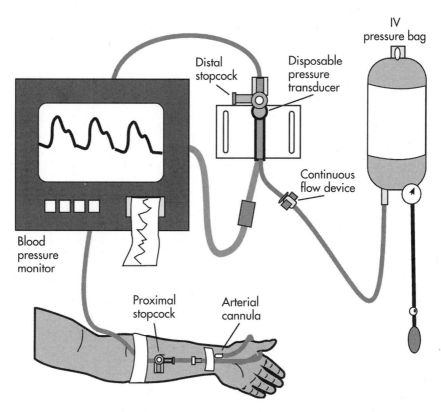

FIG. 7-5 *Pressure transducer setup for continuous arterial monitoring.* A catheter is normally inserted into the radial or brachial artery. Pressure tubing connects the catheter to a continuous flow device that maintains a constant pressure (and a small flow of solution) against the arterial line to prevent backflow of blood into the system. The continuous flow device also allows flushing of the system. Connected in line with the tubing is a pressure transducer assembly. Pressure changes in the system are transmitted via a thin membrane to the transducer. Blood samples may be drawn by inserting a heparinized syringe at a stopcock located near the indwelling catheter (the blood pressure signal is temporarily lost during sampling). A similar assembly can be used for connection to a Swan-Ganz catheter for pulmonary artery monitoring during exercise.

specimens, is essential. See Chapter 10 for specific recommendations regarding arterial sampling via catheters.

Systolic BP increases in healthy subjects during exercise from 120 mm Hg up to approximately 200 to 250 mm Hg. Diastolic pressure normally rises only slightly (10 to 15 mm Hg) or not at all. The mean arterial pressure rises from approximately 90 mm Hg to approximately 110 mm Hg, depending on the changes in systolic and diastolic pressures. The increase in systolic pressure is caused almost completely by increased CO, particularly the SV. Even though the CO may increase fivefold, (i.e., from 5 to 25 L/min), the systolic pressure only increases twofold. Systolic pressure only doubles because of the tremendous decrease in peripheral vascular resistance. Most of this decrease in resistance results from vasodilatation in exercising muscles. Increases in the systolic pressure to greater than 250 to 300 mm Hg should be considered an indication for terminating the exercise evaluation. Similarly, if the systolic pressure fails to rise with increasing workload, the CO is not increasing appropriately. The exercise test should be terminated and the subject's condition stabilized. Variations in BP during exercise are often caused by the subject's respiratory effort. Phasic changes with respiration are particularly common in subjects who develop large transpulmonary pressures because of lung disease. Differences of as much as 30 mm Hg between inspiration and expiration may be seen during continuous monitoring of arterial pressure.

In maximal tests (i.e., the subject reaches HR_{max}), it may be impossible to obtain a reliable BP at peak exercise. Even with an arterial catheter, motion artifact may prevent recording of a usable tracing. Systolic pressure may transiently drop and diastolic pressure may fall to zero at the termination of exercise. To minimize the degree of hypotension resulting from abrupt cessation of heavy exercise, the subject should "cool down." This is accomplished easily by having the subject continue exercising at a low work rate until BP and HR have stabilized at or slightly above baseline levels.

SAFETY

Safe and effective exercise testing for cardiopulmonary disorders requires careful pretest evaluation to identify contraindications to the test procedure (Box 7-3). A preliminary workup should include a complete history and physical examination by either the referring physician or the physician performing the stress test. Preliminary laboratory tests should include a 12-lead ECG, chest x-ray study, baseline pulmonary function studies before and after bronchodilator therapy, and routine laboratory examinations such as complete blood count and serum electrolytes. Subjects who take

---

BOX 7-3
CONTRAINDICATIONS TO EXERCISE TESTING*

Pa_{O_2} less than 40 mm Hg on room air
Pa_{CO_2} greater than 70 mm Hg
FEV_1 less than 30% of predicted
Recent (within 4 weeks) myocardial infarction
Unstable angina pectoris
Second- or third-degree heart block
Rapid ventricular/atrial arrhythmias
Orthopedic impairment
Severe **aortic stenosis**
Congestive heart failure
Uncontrolled hypertension
Limiting neurologic disorders
Dissecting/ventricular **aneurysms**
Severe pulmonary hypertension
Thrombophlebitis or intracardiac **thrombi**
Recent systemic or pulmonary embolus
Acute **pericarditis**

*These conditions represent *relative* contraindications to exercise testing; the risk to the patient must be evaluated on a case-by-case basis.

BOX 7-4
INDICATIONS FOR TERMINATING EXERCISE TESTS

Monitoring system failure
2-mm horizontal or down-sloping ST depression or elevation
T-wave inversion or Q waves
Sustained supraventricular tachycardia
Ventricular tachycardia
Multifocal premature ventricular beats
Development of second- or third-degree heart block
Exercise-induced left or right **bundle branch block**
Progressive chest pain (angina)
Sweating and **pallor**
Systolic pressure greater than 250 mm Hg
Diastolic pressure greater than 120 mm Hg
Failure of systolic pressure to increase or a drop of 10 mm Hg with increasing workload
Light-headedness, mental confusion, or headache
Cyanosis
Nausea or vomiting
Muscle cramping

methylxanthine bronchodilators should have a recent theophylline level measurement, particularly if the primary indication for exercise testing is ventilatory limitation.

The risks and benefits of the entire exercise procedure should be explained to the subject. Appropriate informed consent should be obtained. A physician experienced in exercise testing should supervise the test. Submaximal tests on subjects younger than 40 years of age with no known risk factors may be performed by qualified technologists or nurses, provided a physician is immediately available. Criteria for terminating the exercise evaluation before the specified end point or symptom limitation occurs are listed in Box 7-4.

After termination of the exercise evaluation for whatever reason, the subject should be monitored until HR, BP, and ECG return to pretest levels. Electrocardiographic monitoring should continue for at least 15 minutes, and tracings should be made at frequent intervals immediately after exercise.

Personnel conducting exercise tests should be trained in handling cardiovascular emergencies and should be certified in cardiopulmonary resuscitation. The laboratory should have available resuscitation equipment, including the following:

1. Standard intravenous (IV) medications (epinephrine, atropine, lidocaine, isoproterenol, propanolol, procainamide, sodium bicarbonate, and calcium gluconate)
2. Syringes, needles, IV infusion apparatus
3. Portable O_2 and suction equipment
4. Airway equipment, endotracheal tubes, and **laryngoscope**
5. DC defibrillator and appropriate monitor

All emergency equipment should be checked daily or immediately before any cardiopulmonary exercise evaluation. Equipment such as defibrillators, laryngoscopes, and suction apparatus should be routinely evaluated for proper function according to institutional policies.

Ventilation During Exercise

Collection and analysis of expired gas during cardiopulmonary exercise testing provides a noninvasive means of obtaining the following variables:

- Minute ventilation ($\dot{V}E$)
- Tidal volume (VT)
- Frequency of breathing; respiratory rate (f_b)
- Oxygen consumption; oxygen uptake ($\dot{V}O_2$)
- Carbon dioxide production ($\dot{V}CO_2$)
- Respiratory exchange ratio (RER)
- Ventilatory equivalent for oxygen ($\dot{V}E/\dot{V}O_2$)
- Ventilatory equivalent for CO_2 ($\dot{V}E/\dot{V}CO_2$)

EQUIPMENT SELECTION AND CALIBRATION

The traditional method of measuring ventilation collected exhaled gas using a one-way breathing circuit and a collection system, usually a bag or balloon (Fig. 7-6). The collected gas was then measured using a spirometer. Exhaled gas was analyzed by submitting a sample to an analyzer. A similar method included a flow transducer (Fig. 7-7) to measure ventilation and a **mixing chamber** for sampling gas. Many modern systems use computerized breath-by-breath measurements (Fig. 7-8).

Whatever volume measuring device is used should be calibrated before each procedure (see Chapter 10). Pneumotachometers are used in both mixing chamber and breath-by-breath systems and should be calibrated using a known volume or flow signal (Box 7-5). They may also be calibrated by being connected in series with a volume-based spirometer of known accuracy. Gas analyzers should also be calibrated and checked before each test procedure. Some laboratories perform calibration before and after testing to detect instrument drift. Two-point calibration using gases that approximate the physiologic range to be tested provide the most appropriate means of

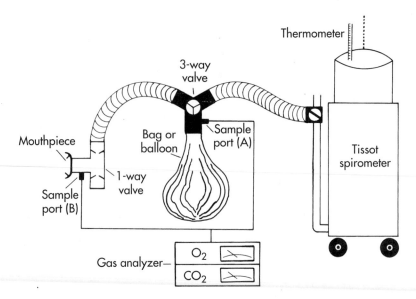

FIG. 7-6 *System for collection and analysis of expired gas.* The subject inspires from a one-way valve and expires through large-bore tubing into a Douglas bag, a meteorologic balloon, or directly into an appropriate spirometer. A three-way valve can be used to direct expired gas to the bag or spirometer. A sample of expired gas may be collected over a timed interval into the bag. F_{EO_2} and F_{ECO_2} are determined by extracting a sample from *port A.* The volume in the bag/balloon may then be emptied into the spirometer to determine volume. Temperature of the gas in the spirometer is measured for conversion of gas volumes to BTPS and STPD. Gas may also be sampled at *port B,* allowing determination of end-tidal CO_2 and respiratory rate. Although this type of manual system is no longer widely used for exercise testing, it can be used to validate computerized systems, or for collecting/analyzing expired gas for specific purposes (e.g., V_D/V_T).

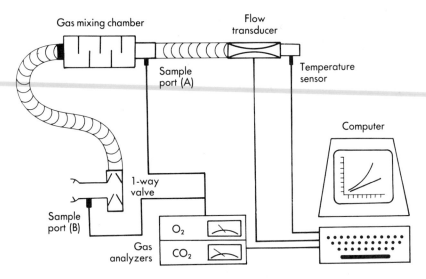

FIG. 7-7 *Mixing chamber type system for analysis of expired gas.* The subject inspires room air through a one-way valve and expires through large-bore tubing into a mixing chamber that has a volume of approximately 5 L. Baffles in the chamber cause the gas to be thoroughly mixed so that it is representative of mixed expired gas. A small volume is extracted at *sample port A* and directed to the O_2 and CO_2 analyzers for determination of the F_{EO_2} and F_{ECO_2}. The expired gas then passes through a flow-sensing (i.e., pneumo-tachometer) device from which volume can be obtained by integration. A temperature probe at the flow transducer provides data for conversion of the gas volume from ambient temperature to BTPS and STPD. Signals from the gas analyzers, flow transducer, and temperature sensor may be recorded directly on an analog recorder or converted to digital signals for processing by computer. Analysis of individual breaths of expired gas can be obtained by sampling at *port B.* This technique allows end-tidal CO_2 and O_2 concentrations, as well as respiratory rate, to be determined. The mixing chamber type of system can be used for exercise protocols as well as for resting metabolic measurements.

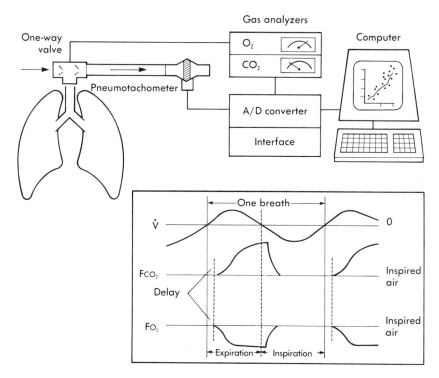

FIG. 7-8 *Breath-by-breath system for determination of $\dot{V}O_2$, $\dot{V}CO_2$, and ventilation.* The subject inspires room air through a one-way valve and expires through a *pneumotachometer* or similar flow-sensing device. Gas is continuously sampled at the subject's mouth to determine fractional concentrations of O_2 and CO_2. The flow signal and signals from the gas analyzers are integrated to measure volume, F_{EO_2}, and F_{ECO_2}, and to calculate $\dot{V}E$, $\dot{V}O_2$, $\dot{V}CO_2$, rate, and VT. To perform the necessary calculations and corrections, computerization is required. The insert shows the simultaneous recording of flow ($\dot{V}$) and fractional concentrations of O_2 and CO_2. During expiration F_{CO_2} rises and F_{O_2} falls. Gas concentrations and flow are out of phase because of the time required to transport gas from the mouthpiece to the analyzers and because of the response time of the analyzers themselves. The signals can be aligned by storing appropriate phase delay corrections (determined during calibration) in the computer. Ventilatory and gas exchange parameters can be monitored and displayed on a breath-by-breath basis. For exercise tests or metabolic measurements, breath-by-breath data are averaged over a short interval (10 to 60 seconds) or specific number of breaths.

BOX 7-5
CRITERIA FOR ACCEPTABILITY—VENTILATORY MEASUREMENTS DURING EXERCISE

1. Volume transducer calibration before exercise measurements should be documented.

2. Temperature and other environmental factors should be recorded.

3. Breathing valve resistance and dead space should be appropriate for the patient tested.

4. Ventilatory variables should be measured over intervals appropriate for the type of exercise (incremental versus steady-state).

5. Recent FEV_1 and MVV maneuvers should be available for interpretive purposes.

---

ensuring accuracy. Three-point calibration is necessary to check the linearity of the analyzers. Table 7-4 lists some recommended gas concentrations for calibration of analyzers to be used for exercise tests.

The gas collection valve (see Chapter 9) used in the breathing circuit should have a low resistance (1 to 2 cm H_2O at 100 L/min) and a small dead space. In healthy adult subjects, a valve dead space of 100 ml is acceptable. In children or subjects who have dead space-producing disease or very small tidal volumes, a valve with reduced dead space (i.e., 25 to 50 ml) may be more appropriate. Some breath-by-breath systems can be programmed to reject small breaths (less than

TABLE 7-4 Recommended Calibration Gases for Exercise Systems

Type of exercise test	Suggested calibration gases
Maximal or submaximal with subject breathing room air	20.9% O_2, 0% CO_2; and 15% O_2, 5% CO_2
Maximal or submaximal with subject breathing supplementary O_2 (may also be used to check linearity)	20.9% O_2, 0% CO_2; and 15% O_2, 5% CO_2; and 26% O_2, 0% CO_2

100 ml). If this feature is used, the volume of the rejected breath should be matched to valve dead space. Breaths that do not clear valve dead space should be discarded. If valve dead space is too large for the subject, significant rebreathing may occur. In breath-by-breath exercise systems, this may show up as a CO_2 level that does not fall to zero during inspiration.

If a gas collection system (either a bag or balloon or mixing chamber) is being used, the subject should be allowed to breathe through the circuit with a nose clip in place long enough to wash out room air with expired gas. The exact washout volume, or time, depends on the volume of the collection system. A bag or balloon should be filled and emptied at least once before collecting gas. Circuits using a mixing chamber and pneumotachometer can usually be washed out quickly. Breath-by-breath systems (see Fig. 7-8) normally require minimal washout because fractional gas concentrations are sampled directly at the mouthpiece. If supplemental O_2 is breathed, the inspiratory portion of the breathing circuit as well as the subject's lungs should be in equilibrium before gas sampling starts.

Depending on the protocol and equipment used, gas collection and analysis are performed over a specified interval during each exercise level. For steady-state protocols, gas collection is usually performed after 4 to 6 minutes at a constant workload. For incremental protocols, sampling may be performed during the last minute of each stage. In breath-by-breath systems, sampling is done continuously, with data being displayed for each breath. Breath-by-breath data may also be averaged over several breaths.

In gas collection or mixing chamber systems, raw data collected includes the following:

1. *Volume* expired, in liters
2. *Temperature* of the gas at the measuring device (°C)
3. *Time* of the collection, in seconds or minutes
4. *Respiratory rate* during the collection interval
5. Fraction of mixed expired O_2 (F_{EO_2})
6. Fraction of mixed expired CO_2 (F_{ECO_2})

These data can be recorded manually or by a multichannel recorder with appropriate analog signals. Similarly, the data may be entered into a computer either manually, or *on-line,* by means of an analog-to-digital (A/D) converter (see Chapter 9). On-line data reduction offers the advantage of immediate feedback for all measurements. Automated data collection also offers greater flexibility for using different exercise protocols (see Table 7-1). Breath-by-breath gas analysis requires that signals from the volume transducer be integrated with the gas analyzer signals for F_{EO_2} and F_{ECO_2}. The **phase delay** between volume and gas concentration signals must be considered (see Fig. 7-8). This is done by measuring phase delay time (for each gas analyzer) during calibration. The phase delay is then stored, and subsequent measurements use this factor to align the volume and gas signals. Sampling flow or sample lines should not be altered after calibration because phase delay values may change.

MINUTE VENTILATION

$\dot{V}_E$ is the volume of gas expired per minute by the exercising subject, expressed in liters, BTPS. $\dot{V}_E$ may be calculated as follows:

$$\dot{V}_E = \frac{\text{Volume expired} \times 60}{\text{Collection time (sec)}} \times \text{BTPS factor}$$

Sample calculations and BTPS factors are contained in Appendix F.

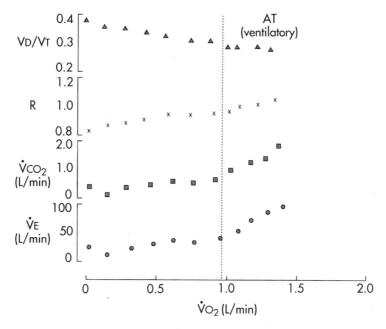

FIG. 7-9 *Normal ventilation/gas exchange responses during exercise.* Four variables as they might appear in a healthy young adult are plotted against $\dot{V}o_2$. The *dotted vertical line* represents the anaerobic threshold *(AT)*. $\dot{V}e$ increases linearly with work rate at low and moderate work loads up to the AT, as does $\dot{V}co_2$. At higher levels, both $\dot{V}e$ and $\dot{V}co_2$ increase at a faster rate, as lactic acid is buffered by HCO_3^- and CO_2 is produced. The ratio of $\dot{V}co_2$ to $\dot{V}o_2$ (RER) follows a similar pattern as RER approaches, then exceeds 1.00. V_D/V_T initially decreases rapidly as the V_T increases; it then continues to fall but at a slower rate (see text).

Healthy adults at rest breathe 5 to 10 L/min. During exercise this value may increase to more than 200 L/min in trained subjects. It commonly exceeds 100 L/min in healthy adults (Figs. 7-9 and 7-10). The increase in ventilation removes CO_2, the primary product of exercising muscles, as the workload increases. Ventilation increases linearly with an increasing workload (i.e., $\dot{V}o_2$) at low and moderate levels of exercise. In healthy subjects this increase in ventilation during exercise follows the rise in $\dot{V}co_2$. As higher levels of work are achieved (i.e., greater than approximately 60% of the $\dot{V}o_{2max}$), metabolic demand exceeds the capacity for energy production solely by aerobic pathways. To meet the increasing energy demands, anaerobic glycolysis assumes an increasing role. The main product of these reactions is lactate. As blood lactate rises, buffering occurs via the carbonic acid (H_2CO_3) pathway. The result is an increase in the total $\dot{V}co_2$. In healthy subjects, ventilation increases further to remove CO_2 produced by the buffering of **lactic acid.**

Relating the $\dot{V}e_{max}$ to resting ventilatory function provides an index of ventilatory limitations to exercise. The **dyspnea index** compares ventilation during exercise with a routine pulmonary function measurement, the maximal voluntary ventilation (MVV) (see Chapter 2). This index relates the $\dot{V}e$ achieved during a submaximal exercise level, usually 6 minutes at 0% grade and 2 mph, to the MVV, and is calculated as follows:

$$\text{Dyspnea index} = \frac{\dot{V}e \text{ during the last minute}}{\text{MVV}} \times 100$$

Values greater than 50% for this calculation are consistent with severe dyspnea. A valid MVV maneuver is essential or the dyspnea index may be overestimated.

MVV can be similarly related to the $\dot{V}e$ achieved at the highest workload attained, ($\dot{V}e_{max}$). $\dot{V}e_{max}$ may approach the MVV if there is a primary ventilatory limitation to exercise because MVV is often reduced by lung disease. $\dot{V}e_{max}$ may also be compared with the FEV_1 multiplied by a factor of 35 (some clinicians prefer a factor of 40). The $FEV_1 \times 35$ provides a satisfactory estimate of ventilation that can be maintained for 1 to 4 minutes, both in healthy subjects and in those with moderate ventilatory impairment. In healthy subjects, maximal exercise will produce a $\dot{V}e$ that may range from 20% to 50% of the MVV. The difference between $\dot{V}e_{max}$ and MVV is often called the ventilatory reserve. Ventilatory reserve is calculated as follows:

$$\text{Ventilatory reserve} = \left[1 - \left(\frac{\dot{V}e_{max}}{\text{MVV}} \right) \right] \times 100$$

where:

$$\dot{V}_{E_{max}} = \text{ventilation at the highest exercise level reached}$$

$$MVV = \text{maximal voluntary ventilation in liters per minute}$$

The ventilatory reserve is usually expressed as a percentage. The $FEV_1 \times 35$ is often used in place of the MVV.

In healthy subjects the ventilatory reserve seldom exceeds 50%. In subjects with pulmonary disease, it typically exceeds 70% (see Table 7-3). Patients who have airways obstruction may actually achieve a $\dot{V}_E$ during exercise that equals the MVV. Exercise is limited by their inability to further increase ventilation.

In patients with chronic airflow limitation, inability to increase ventilation may be related to **dynamic compression** of the airways and **dynamic hyperinflation** (i.e., increased lung volume) that can occur during exertion. These subjects have large resting lung volumes. During exercise, the end-expiratory lung volume (EELV) tends to increase even more as the subject attempts to optimize expiratory flow to meet ventilatory demands. The dynamic shift in lung volume places the respiratory muscles at an even greater disadvantage. The sensation of dyspnea increases tremendously, and the patient is unable to continue exercise.

At high levels of ventilation in healthy subjects (greater than 120 L/min), increases in O_2 uptake gained by increased ventilation serve mainly to supply O_2 to the respiratory muscles. The same phenomenon may occur at much lower levels of ventilation in subjects with severe lung disease because of the increased work of breathing. Because of the enormous ventilatory reserve in

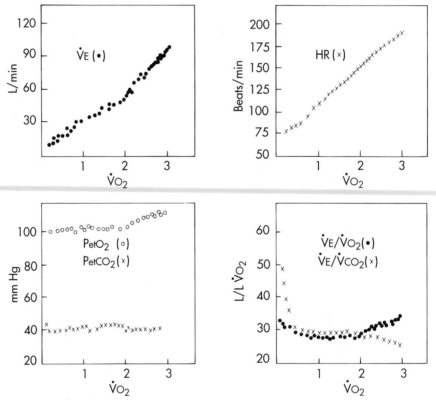

FIG. 7-10 *Breath-by-breath exercise data.* Four plots of data obtained using a breath-by-breath technique, as in Fig. 7-8. Although data are recorded for each breath the plots represent 30 second averages. All parameters are plotted against $\dot{V}_{O_2}$ as the measure of work being performed. $\dot{V}_E$ increases linearly up to approximately 2 L/min $\dot{V}_{O_2}$; HR increases linearly throughout the test. Pet_{O_2} and Pet_{CO_2} (end-tidal partial pressures of O_2 and CO_2, respectively) remain relatively constant up to approximately 2 L/min $\dot{V}_{O_2}$. At this point end-tidal O_2 begins to increase and end-tidal CO_2 begins to fall. A similar pattern is seen on the plot of ventilatory equivalents for oxygen and carbon dioxide ($\dot{V}_E/\dot{V}_{O_2}$ and $\dot{V}_E/\dot{V}_{CO_2}$, respectively). A primary advantage of breath-by-breath analysis is that these plots may be viewed in "real time" as they occur, thus allowing modification of the testing protocol as required. The data in this example indicates the occurrence of the ventilatory threshold (AT) at approximately 2 L/min of $\dot{V}_{O_2}$.

healthy subjects, exercise is seldomly limited by ventilation. Maximal exercise is normally limited by inability to further increase cardiac output, or inability to extract more O_2 at the tissue level in exercising muscles. Some highly trained athletes may achieve ventilatory limitation. Aerobic training can improve cardiovascular function so that ventilation, not cardiac output, limits maximal work.

TIDAL VOLUME AND RESPIRATORY RATE

V_T during exercise may be calculated by dividing the $\dot{V}_E$ by the f_b. Breath-by-breath systems record individual breaths and then report an average V_T over a short interval, or after a fixed number of breaths have been analyzed. In healthy subjects, V_T increases with low and moderate workloads. Increased V_T accounts for most of the rise in ventilation at these workloads; only a small amount results from increased f_b. This pattern continues until the V_T approaches approximately 60% of vital capacity (VC). Further increases in total ventilation are accomplished by increasing the f_b.

Subjects who have airway obstruction may be able to increase their $\dot{V}_E$ but cannot attain predicted values (Box 7-6). If VC is markedly reduced by the obstructive process, there may be little reserve to accommodate an increased V_T. Obstructed subjects, who have a normal VC but increased resistance to flow, may increase their V_T at a low f_b during exercise in an effort to minimize the work of breathing. This pattern continues until the V_T reaches a plateau, as described previously. Then the f_b must be augmented to further increase $\dot{V}_E$. Because of flow limitations, particularly during the expiratory phase, increases in f_b must be accomplished by shortening the inspiratory portion of each breath. Reduction of the inspiratory time in relation to the total breath time (i.e., T_I/T_{tot}) requires the inspiratory muscles to generate increasingly greater flows. The increased load placed on the muscles of inspiration typically results in dyspnea.

Unlike the pattern in obstruction, in restrictive disease V_T may remain relatively fixed. Increases in $\dot{V}_E$ during exercise are accomplished primarily by rapid respiratory rates. It is usually more efficient for subjects who have "stiff" lungs to move small tidal volumes at fast rates to increase ventilation. Flow limitation may be close to normal, whereas the work of distending the lung is increased in restrictive patterns. The mechanism of increasing ventilation primarily by increasing flow places a load on the respiratory muscles. In combination with hypoxemia, this increased load often results in extreme shortness of breath.

Oxygen Consumption, Carbon Dioxide Production, and Respiratory Exchange Ratio in Exercise

OXYGEN CONSUMPTION

$\dot{V}_{O_2}$ is the volume of O_2 taken up by the exercising (or resting) subject in liters, or milliliters per minute, STPD. Oxygen consumption is also commonly reported in milliliters per kilogram of body weight (ml/kg). $\dot{V}_{O_2}$ is the product of ventilation per minute and the rate of extraction from the gas

---

BOX 7-6
INTERPRETIVE STRATEGIES—VENTILATORY MEASUREMENTS DURING EXERCISE

1   Were data collected over an interval appropriate to the type of exercise test?

2   Was resting ventilation within normal limits ($\approx$5 to 10 L/min)? If not, why?

3   Did minute ventilation increase appropriately with workload?

4   Was $\dot{V}_{E_{max}}$ less than 70% of MVV or $FEV_1 \times 35$? If so, some ventilatory reserve is present. If not, ventilatory limitation to exercise is present.

5   Did V_T increase to approximately 60% of VC? If not, why? Was increased respiratory rate primarily responsible for increased $\dot{V}_E$? If so, suspect a restrictive ventilatory pattern.

6   What reason did the patient offer for stopping exercise (if applicable)? Was this finding consistent with the pattern of ventilation observed?

breathed (i.e., the difference between the F_{IO_2} and the F_{EO_2}, see the following paragraph). Healthy subjects at rest have a $\dot{V}_{O_2}$ of approximately 0.25 L/min (STPD), or approximately 3.5 ml O_2/min/kg. During exercise, $\dot{V}_{O_2}$ may increase to over 4.0 L/min (STPD) in trained subjects. $\dot{V}_{O_2}$ is the best single measure of external work being performed. Exercise limitation caused by gas exchange abnormalities or inappropriate cardiovascular responses may be quantified by relating specific variables to the $\dot{V}_{O_2}$. Figs. 7-4 and 7-9 provide examples of ventilatory and cardiovascular variables related to $\dot{V}_{O_2}$ in healthy subjects. The causes of work limitation may be defined by comparing these patterns in the exercising subject. Exercise limitation may be a result of pulmonary disease, cardiovascular disease, muscular abnormalities, deconditioning, poor effort, or a combination of these factors.

To calculate $\dot{V}_{O_2}$ and $\dot{V}_{CO_2}$, the fractional concentrations of O_2 and CO_2 in expired gas must be analyzed (Box 7-7). Exhaled gas is sampled from a collection device (see Fig. 7-6), a mixing chamber (see Fig. 7-7), or a breath-by-breath system (see Fig. 7-8). In systems that accumulate gas (i.e., a bag, balloon, spirometer, or mixing chamber), a pump is used to draw the sample through the O_2 and CO_2 analyzers. Water vapor is removed from the mixed expired sample by passing the gas through a drying tube (usually containing calcium chloride). If the sample is removed before volume is measured, $\dot{V}_E$ should be corrected for the volume withdrawn. If exhaled gas is sampled continuously, gas from the pump may be returned to the volume measuring device. In breath-by-breath systems, fractional gas concentrations are sampled at the mouth using rapid gas analyzers. Gas concentration signals from the analyzers are integrated with the expiratory flow signal to provide the volumes of O_2 and CO_2 exchanged for each breath (see Fig. 7-8).

$\dot{V}_{O_2}$ is calculated from an accumulated gas volume using the following equation:

$$\dot{V}_{O_2} = \left(\left[\left(\frac{1 - F_{EO_2} - F_{ECO_2}}{1 - F_{IO_2}} \right) \times F_{IO_2} \right] - F_{EO_2} \right) \times \dot{V}_E(STPD)$$

where:

F_{EO_2} = fraction of O_2 in the expired sample

F_{ECO_2} = fraction of CO_2 in the expired sample

F_{IO_2} = fraction of O_2 in inspired gas (room air = 0.2093)

The term

$$\left(\frac{1 - F_{EO_2} - F_{ECO_2}}{1 - F_{IO_2}} \right)$$

is a factor to correct for the small differences between inspired and expired volumes when only expired volumes are measured. Ventilation is corrected to STPD as follows:

$$\dot{V}_E(STPD) = \dot{V}_E(BTPS) \times \left(\frac{P_B - 47}{760} \right) \times 0.881$$

BOX 7-7
CRITERIA FOR ACCEPTABILITY—$\dot{V}_{O_2}$, $\dot{V}_{CO_2}$

1 There should be documentation of appropriate gas analyzer calibrations; 2-point calibration recommended for room air exercise, 3-point for exercise with supplemental oxygen.

2 Phase delay calibration (breath-by-breath systems) should be documented within manufacturer's specifications.

3 Volume transducer should be calibrated before testing.

4 Breathing valve (if used) should have appropriate resistance and dead space volume for patient tested.

5 There should be evidence of appropriate washout of collection device or mixing chamber (if used).

6 RER at rest should be within the physiologic range of 0.70 to 1.10; RER values greater than 1.0 may be present because of hyperventilation.

7 $\dot{V}_{O_2}$ and $\dot{V}_{CO_2}$ should be within normal limits with the subject at rest; each should increase with increasing workloads.

O_2 consumption at the highest level of work attainable by normal subjects is termed the $\dot{V}O_{2max}$. $\dot{V}O_{2max}$ is characterized by a plateau of the oxygen uptake despite increasing external work loads. $\dot{V}O_{2max}$ is useful for comparing exercise capacity between subjects. $\dot{V}O_{2max}$ may also be used to compare a subject with his or her age-related predicted value of $\dot{V}O_{2max}$. Equations for deriving predicted $\dot{V}O_{2max}$ are included in Appendix B.

One measure of impairment is the percentage of expected $\dot{V}O_{2max}$ attained by the exercising subject. Height, gender, age, and fitness level all affect the "normal" maximal oxygen consumption. Because of these factors, most reference equations show a large variability ($\pm20\%$). Subjects who have reductions in their $\dot{V}O_{2max}$ of 20% to 40% have mild to moderate impairment. Those who have $\dot{V}O_{2max}$ values less than 60% of their predicted values have severe exercise impairment.

Some studies have attempted to estimate $\dot{V}O_2$ based on the height and weight of the subject and the speed and slope of a treadmill. O_2 consumption estimated from treadmill walking is sufficiently variable so that its use is limited. Power output from a calibrated cycle ergometer may be used to estimate $\dot{V}O_2$ more accurately than from treadmill exercise. Values obtained during cycle ergometry are not influenced by weight or stride. Actual $\dot{V}O_2$ may differ significantly from the estimated value even using an ergometer. Cycle ergometry usually produces slightly lower maximal $\dot{V}O_2$ values than treadmill walking in healthy subjects (see "Exercise Protocols," p. 160).

CARBON DIOXIDE PRODUCTION

$\dot{V}CO_2$ is a direct reflection of metabolism. It is expressed in liters or milliliters per minute, STPD. $\dot{V}CO_2$ may be calculated using the following equation:

$$\dot{V}CO_2 = (FECO_2 - 0.0003) \times \dot{V}E$$

where:

$$FECO_2 = \text{fraction of } CO_2 \text{ in expired gas}$$

$$0.0003 = \text{fraction of } CO_2 \text{ in room air (may vary)}$$

$$\dot{V}E \text{ (STPD)} = \text{calculated as in the equation for } \dot{V}O_2$$

Pulmonary ventilation, consisting of alveolar ventilation ($\dot{V}A$) and dead space ventilation ($\dot{V}D$), may be related in terms of the $\dot{V}CO_2$. The fraction of alveolar carbon dioxide ($FACO_2$) is directly proportional to $\dot{V}CO_2$ and inversely proportional to the $\dot{V}A$. The concentration of CO_2 in the lung is determined by CO_2 production and the rate of removal from the lung by ventilation. This relationship may be expressed as follows:

$$FACO_2 = \frac{\dot{V}CO_2}{\dot{V}A}$$

$\dot{V}CO_2$ in a healthy person at rest is approximately 0.20 L/min (STPD). It may increase to more than 4 L/min (STPD) during maximal exercise in trained individuals. The adequacy of $\dot{V}A$ in response to the increase in $\dot{V}CO_2$ is indicated by how well $PaCO_2$ is maintained near normal levels. Alveolar ventilation keeps $PaCO_2$ in equilibrium with alveolar gas at low and moderate workloads. At high workloads $\dot{V}A$ increases dramatically to reduce $PaCO_2$ when buffering of lactic acid takes place. At maximal workloads, even high levels of ventilation cannot keep pace with CO_2 production. As a result, acidosis develops.

RESPIRATORY EXCHANGE RATIO

RER is defined as the ratio of $\dot{V}CO_2$ to $\dot{V}O_2$ at the mouth. RER is calculated by dividing the $\dot{V}CO_2$ by the $\dot{V}O_2$; it is expressed as a fraction. In some circumstances RER is assumed to be equal to 0.8. For exercise evaluation or metabolic studies, however, the actual value is calculated. RER normally varies between 0.70 and 1.00 in resting subjects, depending on the nutritional substrate being metabolized (see "Metabolic Measurements," Chapter 8). RER reflects the respiratory quotient (**RQ**) at the cellular level only when the subject is in a true steady state. RER may differ significantly from RQ depending on the subject's ventilation.

RER typically increases from a resting level of between 0.75 and 0.85 as work increases. When anaerobic metabolism (see the next paragraph) begins to produce CO_2 from the buffering of lactate, the $\dot{V}CO_2$ approaches the $\dot{V}O_2$. As exercise continues, the $\dot{V}CO_2$ exceeds $\dot{V}O_2$ and the RER becomes greater than 1.00. RER is commonly elevated at rest because many subjects hyperventilate while breathing into the gas collection apparatus (see Box 7-7). In steady-state exercise tests (i.e., 4 to 6 minutes at a constant workload), RER may equal the RQ, and then reflects the ratio of $\dot{V}_{CO_2}/\dot{V}_{O_2}$ at the cellular level. Under steady-state conditions, the $\dot{V}_{CO_2}$ reflects the CO_2 produced metabolically at the cellular level.

ANAEROBIC THRESHOLD

Measurement of $\dot{V}_E$ and analysis of exhaled gases during exercise allows a noninvasive estimate of the AT. The AT occurs when the energy demands of the exercising muscles exceed the body's ability to produce energy by aerobic metabolism. The workload at which AT occurs is considered an index of fitness in healthy subjects. The AT is also used to assess cardiac performance in subjects with heart disease.

Historically, anaerobic metabolism was detected by noting an increase in the blood lactate level of an exercising subject. Analysis of $\dot{V}_E$ and $\dot{V}_{CO_2}$ in relation to workload ($\dot{V}_{O_2}$) can be used to detect the onset of anaerobic metabolism without drawing blood. This threshold is commonly referred to as the **ventilatory threshold.**

At low and moderate workloads $\dot{V}_E$ increases linearly with increases in $\dot{V}_{CO_2}$. When the body's energy demands exceed the capacity of aerobic pathways, further increases in energy are produced anaerobically. The primary product of anaerobic metabolism is lactate. The increased lactic acid (from lactate) is buffered by HCO_3^- resulting in an increase in CO_2 in the blood. $\dot{V}_{CO_2}$ measured from exhaled gas increases because CO_2 is being produced by both the exercising muscles and by the buffering of lactate. To maintain the pH near normal, $\dot{V}_E$ increases to match the increased $\dot{V}_{CO_2}$. This pattern of increasing ventilation and CO_2 production can be detected when these parameters are plotted against $\dot{V}_{O_2}$ (see Fig. 7-9). Determination of the ventilatory AT may be accomplished by visual inspection of an appropriate plot. Statistical analysis can also be used to determine the inflection point as displayed by the graph in Fig. 7-11. Several different algorithms have been used to determine the ventilatory AT. One of the most common techniques uses regression analysis to determine the "breakpoint" at which $\dot{V}_E$ and $\dot{V}_{CO_2}$ change abruptly (Beaver method).

Noninvasive AT determination may be useful in assessing cardiovascular or pulmonary diseases (Box 7-8). In healthy subjects, AT occurs at 60% to 70% of the $\dot{V}_{O_2max}$. Patients who have cardiac disease reach their AT at a lower workload ($\dot{V}_{O_2}$). Early onset of anaerobic metabolism occurs when the demands of exercising muscles exceed the capacity of the heart to supply O_2. Occurrence of the anaerobic threshold at less than 40% of the $\dot{V}_{O_2max}$ is considered abnormally low. Patients who have a ventilatory limitation to exercise (i.e., pulmonary disease) may be unable to exercise at a high enough workload to reach their anaerobic threshold. In these subjects, O_2 delivery is limited by the lungs, rather than by cardiac output or extraction by the exercising muscle.

Aerobic training improves cardiac performance, specifically the stroke volume (SV). This delivers more O_2 to the tissues, resulting in a delay in the AT until higher workloads are reached.

BOX 7-8
INTERPRETIVE STRATEGIES—$\dot{V}_{O_2}$, $\dot{V}_{CO_2}$

1   Were the data obtained acceptably? Were all calibrations appropriate? Gas analyzers? Volume transducer? Phase delay?

2   Were appropriate reference values selected? Age? Sex? Height? Weight?

3   Was $\dot{V}_{O_2max}$ (ml/kg) achieved? If so, there is no aerobic impairment.

4   Was $\dot{V}_{O_2max}$ (ml/kg) less than 80% of predicted? If so, some aerobic impairment is present. Was $\dot{V}_{O_2max}$ (ml/kg) less than 60% of predicted? If so, there is moderate to severe exercise limitation.

5   Was ventilatory AT reached? If so, at what % $\dot{V}_{O_2max}$? If less than 50% to 60%, early onset of anaerobic metabolism is likely. Consider clinical correlation.

6   What factors contributed to the reduced $\dot{V}_{O_2max}$?
    Cardiac (arrhythmias, ischemic changes)?
    Vascular (BP response)?
    Pulmonary (ventilation, hypoxemia, V_D/V_T)?
    Other (poor effort, deconditioning, pain, orthopedic problems)?

7   What reason did the patient cite for stopping exercise (incremental tests)? Is it consistent with physiologic patterns observed?

Measurement of the AT is often used to select a training level. Maximum training effects seem to occur when the subject exercises at a workload slightly below the AT. In sedentary subjects, deconditioning may occur. Deconditioning is characterized by reduced SV and poor O_2 extraction by the muscles from lack of use. Deconditioning may be present when the AT occurs at a lower than expected workload and there is no evidence of cardiovascular disease.

The AT may also be determined by inspecting graphs of the ventilatory equivalents for O_2 and CO_2 (see the next section) plotted against $\dot{V}O_2$. When the $\dot{V}E/\dot{V}O_2$ increases without an increase in $\dot{V}E/\dot{V}CO_2$, the AT has been reached. A similar pattern can be seen when the end-tidal O_2 and CO_2 gas tensions are plotted (see Fig. 7-10).

Sample calculations of $\dot{V}E$, $\dot{V}O_2$, $\dot{V}CO_2$, and RER, as used with one of the gas collection methods, are included in Appendix F.

VENTILATORY EQUIVALENT FOR OXYGEN

Minute ventilation during exercise may be related to the work being performed (expressed as the $\dot{V}O_2$). This ratio is termed the ventilatory equivalent for O_2, or $\dot{V}E/\dot{V}O_2$. It is calculated by dividing the $\dot{V}E$ (BTPS) by the $\dot{V}O_2$ (STPD) and expressing the ratio in liters of ventilation per liter of O_2 consumed per minute. The $\dot{V}E/\dot{V}O_2$ is a measure of the efficiency of the ventilatory pump at various workloads.

Ventilation at low and moderate workloads increases linearly with increasing $\dot{V}O_2$ and $\dot{V}CO_2$. The absolute level of ventilation depends on the response to CO_2, on the adequacy of $\dot{V}A$, and on the VD/VT ratio. In healthy subjects the ratio remains in the range of 20 to 30 L/L $\dot{V}O_2$ until higher levels of work are reached. At workloads above 60% to 75% of the $\dot{V}O_{2max}$, $\dot{V}E$ is more closely related to $\dot{V}CO_2$. As ventilation increases to match the $\dot{V}O_2$ above the AT, the ventilatory equivalent for O_2 also increases.

Ventilation helps determine how much O_2 can be transported per minute. Therefore, it is often useful to evaluate the level of total ventilation required for a particular workload to assess the role of the lungs in exercise limitations. In some pulmonary disease patterns, the $\dot{V}E/\dot{V}O_2$ may be close to normal at rest, but increases with exercise out of proportion to increases in either $\dot{V}O_2$ or $\dot{V}CO_2$. This usually occurs in individuals who have $\dot{V}/\dot{Q}$ abnormalities that worsen as cardiac output

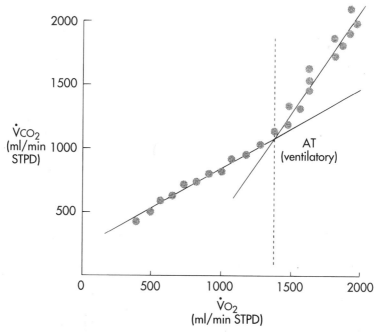

FIG. 7-11 *V-slope determination of the ventilatory threshold (AT).* By plotting $\dot{V}CO_2$ against $\dot{V}O_2$ an infection point can typically be identified, indicating an abrupt increase in CO_2 production. A more precise method fits two regression lines to the data gathered. One line is a best-fit line through the low and moderate workload portion of the data; the second is fit through the high workload points. These lines are recalculated repeatedly until the best statistical "fit" is obtained. The point at which the two lines intersect is representative of the onset of lactate production, the anaerobic threshold.

increases during exercise. Some subjects who have pulmonary disease may have an elevated $\dot{V}E/\dot{V}O_2$ at rest (i.e., greater than 40 L/L $\dot{V}O_2$) that falls during exercise but does not return to the normal range. Many subjects hyperventilate during the resting phase at the beginning of an exercise evaluation. The result is an increased $\dot{V}E/\dot{V}O_2$ that usually returns to the normal range during exercise. This pretest hyperventilation is also usually denoted by an RER of greater than 1.0 that returns to a normal level when the subject begins exercise.

VENTILATORY EQUIVALENT FOR CARBON DIOXIDE

The ventilatory equivalent for CO_2 ($\dot{V}E/\dot{V}CO_2$) is calculated in a manner similar to that used for the $\dot{V}E/\dot{V}O_2$. Minute ventilation (BTPS) is divided by CO_2 production (STPD). The normal level is in the range of 25 to 35 L/L $\dot{V}CO_2$. The $\dot{V}E$ tends to match $\dot{V}CO_2$ from low up to high workloads. Hence the $\dot{V}E/\dot{V}CO_2$ remains constant in healthy subjects until the highest workloads are reached. The $\dot{V}E/\dot{V}CO_2$ may be useful for estimating the maximum tolerable workload in subjects who have moderate or severe ventilatory limitations. The ventilatory equivalents for O_2 and CO_2, measured using a breath-by-breath technique, may be useful in identifying the onset of the AT. Anaerobic metabolism is usually accompanied by a steady increase in the $\dot{V}E/\dot{V}O_2$ while the $\dot{V}E/\dot{V}CO_2$ remains constant, or falls slightly. This same pattern may also be seen on a breath-by-breath display of $PetO_2$ and $PetCO_2$ (see Fig. 7-10). A markedly elevated $\dot{V}E/\dot{V}CO_2$ (greater than 50 L/L $\dot{V}CO_2$) may also be observed in pulmonary hypertensive disease.

OXYGEN PULSE

The efficiency of the circulatory pump may be related to the workload (i.e., $\dot{V}O_2$) during exercise by the **O_2 pulse.** O_2 pulse is defined as the volume of O_2 consumed per heartbeat. The HR may be read manually from a standard ECG or from a computerized display. The $\dot{V}O_2$ in milliliters per minute (STPD) is divided by the HR per minute. The quotient is expressed as milliliters of O_2 per heartbeat. In healthy subjects, O_2 pulse varies between 2.5 and 4.0 ml O_2/beats at rest. It increases to 10 to 15 ml O_2/beat during strenuous exercise.

In patients with cardiac disease, the O_2 pulse may be normal or even low at rest but does not rise to expected levels during exercise. This pattern is consistent with an inappropriately high HR for a particular level of work. The CO is the product of the HR and SV. Cardiac output normally increases linearly with increasing exercise (see Fig. 7-4). A low O_2 pulse is consistent with an inability to increase the SV. O_2 pulse may even fall in subjects with poor left ventricular function. The pattern of low O_2 pulse with increasing work rate may be seen in subjects with coronary artery disease or **valvular insufficiency,** but it is most pronounced in cardiomyopathy. Tachycardia, or tachyarrythmias, tend to lower the O_2 pulse because of the abnormally elevated heart rate. Conversely, β-blocking agents, which tend to reduce HR, may falsely elevate the O_2 pulse.

O_2 pulse is often used as an index of fitness. At similar power outputs, a fit subject will have a higher O_2 pulse than one who is deconditioned. Fitness is generally accompanied by a lower HR, both at rest and at maximal workloads. Lower HR occurs because conditioning exercises (e.g., aerobic training) tend to increase SV. As a result, the heart beats less frequently but produces the same CO. Trained subjects can thus achieve higher work rates before reaching their limiting cardiac frequency (i.e., attain a higher O_2 pulse).

Exercise Blood Gases

ARTERIAL CATHETERIZATION

Although invasive, blood gas sampling during exercise testing is often indicated in subjects with primary pulmonary disorders. An indwelling arterial catheter permits analysis of blood gas tensions (i.e., PaO_2, $PaCO_2$), saturation (SaO_2), O_2 content (CaO_2), pH, and lactate levels at various workloads. Table 7-5 lists some of the indications for arterial catheterization for exercise testing.

Arterial catheterization, at either the radial or brachial sites, has been demonstrated to be relatively safe. The modified Allen's test is performed to ascertain adequate collateral circulation (see Chapter 6). The site is cleaned with povidone-iodine or similar disinfectant. Local anesthetic (2% xylocaine) is injected subcutaneously. An appropriate-size catheter is inserted **percutaneously.** The catheter may be secured with one or two sutures, depending on the type of exercise to be performed. The catheter is then connected to a high-pressure flush system to maintain patency. Care must be taken when drawing blood samples from the catheter not to contaminate the specimen with flush solution (Box 7-9). If flush solution mixes with the specimen, dilution occurs and can affect pH, PCO_2, PO_2, and hemoglobin (Hb) values.

TABLE 7-5 Indications for Arterial Catheterization with Exercise Testing

Moderate or severe pulmonary disease
Low diffusion capacity for carbon monoxide (less than 50% predicted)
Low or borderline Pao_2 at rest (55 to 60 mm Hg)
Multiple blood specimens required (blood gases, lactate)
Titration of supplemental O_2

BOX 7-9
CRITERIA FOR ACCEPTABILITY—EXERCISE BLOOD GASES

1   Blood gases should be drawn from either a radial or brachial catheter. Care should be taken that specimens are not contaminated with flush solution.

2   Exercise blood gas specimens should be handled like any other sample for blood gas analysis. They should be obtained aerobically and kept in an ice-water slush if not analyzed within a few minutes.

3   Specimens from multiple exercise levels should be labeled to indicate the exercise workload and related conditions.

4   Blood obtained by a single arterial puncture at peak exercise should be obtained within 15 seconds of the observed maximal workload.

5   If pulse oximetry is used to evaluate exercise desaturation, it should be validated by correlation to co-oximetry, preferrably at rest and peak exercise.

6   If pulse oximetry is used to titrate supplemental O_2 administration and the Spo_2 does not increase, an arterial blood specimen may be required.

The catheter may also be connected to a suitable pressure transducer (see Fig. 7-5) for continuous monitoring of systemic BP. The BP transducer should be balanced ("zeroed") at the level of the left ventricle during exercise. See Chapter 10 for precautions concerning insertion of arterial catheters.

ARTERIAL PUNCTURE

An alternate technique is to obtain a specimen by a simple arterial puncture at peak exercise. Use of a cycle ergometer for testing allows better stabilization of the radial or brachial artery sites. The site should be identified and the modified Allen's test performed before beginning exercise. The sample should be obtained within 15 seconds of peak exercise. Blood gas tensions, particularly Pao_2, may change rapidly as blood recirculates. A serious disadvantage of the single puncture is that if the specimen cannot be obtained within 15 seconds, the procedure must be repeated. If any of the conditions listed in Table 7-5 are present, arterial catheterization should be considered.

PULSE OXIMETRY

Oxygen saturation during exercise may be monitored using a pulse oximeter (Spo_2) using either the ear or finger sites (see Chapter 9). Whether the pulse oximeter is attached to the finger or ear, the probe should be adequately secured. Motion artifact is a common problem, particularly with treadmill exercise.

An advantage of pulse oximetry is that it provides continuous measurements of saturation, compared with discrete measurements of arterial sampling. Continuous measurements can be very helpful in evaluating subjects who have pulmonary disease. These patients often display rapid changes in Pao_2 and Sao_2 during exercise. A decrease of 4% to 5% in Sao_2 is indicative of exercise desaturation, even if some other factor (e.g., ventilation, arrythmias) limits exercise.

Pulse oximetry may overestimate the true saturation if a significant concentration of COHb is present (see Box 7-9). A low total Hb level (i.e., anemia) sometimes contributes to exercise limitation. This condition may not be detected by pulse oximetry alone. Inadequate perfusion of the ear or finger may also cause erroneous readings during exercise testing. Motion artifact, light scattering within the tissue at the probe site, and dark skin pigmentation may all cause discrepancies between the Spo_2 and the actual Sao_2 (see Chapter 6). A single arterial sample, preferably at peak exercise, may be used to correlate the SpO_2 reading with true saturation if the specimen is analyzed with a multiwavelength blood oximeter (see Chapter 9). If adequate correlation between SaO_2 and SpO_2 during exercise is established, further blood sampling may be unnecessary.

PaO_2 DURING EXERCISE

In healthy subjects, PaO_2 remains relatively constant even at high workloads (Box 7-10). Alveolar PO_2 increases at maximal exercise from the increased ventilation accompanying the rise in $\dot{V}CO_2$. The alveolar-arterial (A-a) gradient (normally approximately 10 mm Hg) widens as a result of the increase in alveolar oxygen tension. The A-a gradient also increases somewhat because of a lower mixed venous O_2 content during exercise. The A-a gradient may increase to 20 to 30 mm Hg in healthy subjects during heavy exercise because of these mechanisms.

A fall in the PaO_2 with increasing exercise can result from increased right-to-left shunting. Similarly, inequality of $\dot{V}A$ in relation to pulmonary capillary perfusion may result in reduced PaO_2. Diffusion limitation at the alveolocapillary interface can also affect PaO_2. Because exercise reduces the mixed venous oxygen tension ($P\bar{v}O_2$), a shunt or $\dot{V}/\dot{Q}$ inequality may result in a decrease in the PaO_2 or widening of the A-a gradient. This change in PaO_2 may occur without an absolute change in the magnitude of the shunt. Mixed venous blood with a lowered O_2 content (from extraction by the exercising muscles) passes through abnormal lung units and then mixes with normally arterialized blood.

In some subjects who have decreased PaO_2 and increased $P(A-a)O_2$ at rest, oxygenation may improve with exercise. Increased cardiac output or redistribution of ventilation during exercise may actually cause an increase in the PaO_2. Some improvement of PaO_2 may occur as a result of an increased PAO_2 caused by a reduction of $PaCO_2$ at moderate to high work rates. Improved $\dot{V}/\dot{Q}$ relationships resulting directly from the changes in ventilation or cardiac output may also improve the PaO_2. Because PaO_2 may either increase or decrease during exercise, measuring PaO_2 during exercise may be particularly valuable in subjects with pulmonary disorders.

When PaO_2 falls to less than 55 mm Hg or SaO_2 decreases to less than 85%, the exercise evaluation should be terminated. Subjects with hypoxemia at rest or who desaturate at very low work rates should be tested with supplemental O_2 (e.g., a nasal cannula) to determine an appropriate exercise O_2 prescription. Different flows of supplemental O_2 may be required at rest and for various levels of exertion. Correlation of PaO_2 while breathing supplemental O_2 at different exercise workloads allows precise titration of therapy to the patient's needs. Measurement of $\dot{V}O_2$ while the patient breathes supplemental O_2 presents special problems. A closed system in which the subject breathes from a reservoir containing blended gas is usually required.

$PaCO_2$ DURING EXERCISE

In healthy subjects, $PaCO_2$ remains relatively constant at low and moderate work rates (see Box 7-10). $\dot{V}A$ increases to match the increase in $\dot{V}CO_2$. End-tidal CO_2 increases at submaximal workloads, indicating that less ventilation is "wasted" (VD/VT decreases). At workloads in excess of 50% to 60% of the $\dot{V}O_{2max}$ metabolic acidosis from anaerobic metabolism stimulates an increase in $\dot{V}E$. This occurs in response to the augmented $\dot{V}CO_2$ from the buffering of lactic acid. Ventilation thus increases in excess of that required to keep the $PaCO_2$ constant. A progressive decrease in $PaCO_2$ results, causing respiratory compensation for the acidosis associated with anaerobic metabolism (see Figs. 7-9 and 7-10). The $PetCO_2$ decreases along with the $PaCO_2$ at high work rates.

Some individuals who have airways obstruction can increase their $\dot{V}A$ to maintain a normal $PaCO_2$ at low workloads. At higher workloads, however, they may be unable to reduce the $PaCO_2$ to compensate for the metabolic acidosis. In many subjects with airway obstruction, maximal exercise is limited by lack of ventilatory reserve. These individuals typically do not reach the AT. Ventilatory limitation prevents them from attaining a workload high enough to induce anaerobic metabolism. In subjects with severe airflow obstruction, $\dot{V}A$ may be unable to match any increment in $\dot{V}CO_2$, resulting in hypercapnia and respiratory acidosis. Increased work of breathing and reduced sensitivity to CO_2, combined with the increased $\dot{V}CO_2$ of exercise, allow the $PaCO_2$ to rise.

ACID-BASE STATUS DURING EXERCISE

The pH, like $PaCO_2$, is regulated by the $\dot{V}A$ at low work rates. $\dot{V}A$ increases in proportion to the $\dot{V}CO_2$ up to the AT. At work rates above AT, proportional increases in ventilation maintain the pH at near-normal levels. Most of the buffering of lactic acid is provided by HCO_3^- and a decrease in the

---

BOX 7-10
INTERPRETIVE STRATEGIES—EXERCISE BLOOD GASES

1   Were blood gas samples obtained acceptably? No dilution or contamination with flush solution or air?

2   Were blood gas samples obtained at each exercise level or just at peak exercise? If drawn by arterial puncture at peak exercise only, were they obtained within 15 seconds?

3   Did Pa_{O_2} fall with increasing workloads? Did the A-a gradient increase to greater than 30 mm Hg? If so, exercise desaturation is probably occurring.

4   Did Pa_{O_2} fall to less than 55 mm Hg or Sa_{O_2} to less than 85%? If so, supplemental O_2 is indicated. Retesting on O_2 may be indicated.

5   Did Pa_{CO_2} remain constant or fall slightly with increasing workloads? If not, respiratory acidosis may be contributing to work limitation.

6   Did pH fall to the range of 7.20 to 7.35 (or lower) at the highest workload? If so, metabolic acidosis occurred; the patient made a good effort. If not, did ventilation limit work below the anaerobic threshold?

7   Was the V_D/V_T normal at rest? Did it fall with increasing workloads? If not, suspect pulmonary hypertension or similar condition.

8   Are the blood gas test results consistent with observed changes in ventilatory and cardiovascular variables during exercise?

Pa_{CO_2}. At the highest work rates (above 80% of the Vo_{2max}), pH decreases despite hyperventilation because compensation for lactic acidosis becomes incomplete. In the presence of airways obstruction, ventilatory limitations may prevent compensation above the anaerobic threshold, with the development of significant respiratory acidosis. However, subjects who have moderate or severe obstruction generally cannot exercise up to a level that elicits anaerobic metabolism. Acidosis in these subjects may be primarily caused by increased Pa_{CO_2} (respiratory acidosis).

EXERCISE VARIABLES CALCULATED FROM BLOOD GASES

Arterial blood gases drawn during exercise allow several other parameters of gas exchange to be determined (see Box 7-10). These include physiologic dead space, alveolar ventilation, and the V_D/V_T ratio.

Calculation of V_D, $\dot{V}_A$, and V_D/V_T requires measurement of the Pa_{CO_2}. V_D may be calculated using the following equation:

$$V_D = \left(V_T \times \left[1 - \frac{F_{ECO_2} \times (P_B - 47)}{Pa_{CO_2}} \right] \right) - V_{D_{sys}}$$

where:

V_T = tidal volume, in liters (BTPS)

F_{ECO_2} = fraction of expired CO_2

$P_B - 47$ = dry barometric pressure

Pa_{CO_2} = arterial CO_2 tension

$V_{D_{sys}}$ = dead space of the one-way breathing valve, in liters

When V_D has been determined, $\dot{V}_A$ can be calculated using the following equation:

$$\dot{V}_A = \dot{V}_E - (f_b \times V_D)$$

where:

$\dot{V}_E$ = minute ventilation (BTPS)

f_b = respiratory rate

V_D = respiratory dead space (BTPS)

The V_D/V_T ratio may be calculated as the quotient of the V_D (as just determined) and the V_T, averaged from the $\dot{V}_E$ and f_b. Alternately, the V_D/V_T may be derived simply from the difference between arterial and mixed expired CO_2 at each exercise level:

$$V_D/V_T = \frac{(Pa_{CO_2} - P\bar{E}_{CO_2})}{Pa_{CO_2}}$$

where:

$$P\bar{E}_{CO_2} = \text{partial pressure of } CO_2 \text{ in expired gas}$$

Most breath-by-breath systems calculate V_D/V_T ratio noninvasively by substituting end-tidal CO_2 for Pa_{CO_2}. This method assumes that Pet_{CO_2} and Pa_{CO_2} are equal. This may not be the case in patients who have pulmonary disease.

V_D, comprised of anatomic and alveolar dead space (see Chapter 2), is that part of the $\dot{V}_E$ that does not participate in gas exchange. V_D/V_T ratio expresses the relationship between "wasted" and tidal ventilation for the average breath. The healthy adult subject at rest has a $\dot{V}_A$ of 4 to 7 L/min (BTPS), and a V_D/V_T ratio of approximately 0.25 to 0.35. The absolute volume of dead space increases during exercise in conjunction with increased $\dot{V}_E$. Because of increases in V_T and increased perfusion of well-ventilated lung units (e.g., at the apices), the V_D/V_T ratio falls. This pattern is expected in healthy subjects (see Fig. 7-9). The V_D/V_T may fall in mild or moderate pulmonary disease states as well. In severe airway obstruction or in pulmonary vascular disease, V_D/V_T remains fixed or may even increase. An increase in V_D/V_T with exertion indicates ventilation increasing in excess of perfusion. This pattern is often associated with pulmonary hypertension. The vascular "space" is fixed in pulmonary hypertension; additional lung units cannot be recruited to handle the increased CO during exercise.

$\dot{V}_A$ during exercise in healthy subjects increases more than $\dot{V}_E$ as V_D/V_T falls. In subjects whose V_D/V_T ratio remains fixed or rises, adequacy of $\dot{V}_A$ must be assessed in terms of the Pa_{CO_2} and not simply by the magnitude of the $\dot{V}_E$.

Cardiac Output During Exercise

CO is commonly measured by the direct Fick method or by thermal dilution. Both methods can be used to measure CO during exercise. Both methods require placement of a pulmonary artery catheter (Swan-Ganz) (Box 7-11).

DIRECT FICK METHOD

The direct Fick method is based on measurement of O_2 consumption and arterial-venous content difference for O_2:

$$\dot{Q}_T = \frac{\dot{V}_{O_2}}{C(a - \bar{v})_{O_2}} \times 100$$

where:

$$\dot{Q}_T = \text{cardiac output, in liters per minute}$$

$$\dot{V}_{O_2} = \text{oxygen consumption, in liters per minute}$$

$$C(a-\bar{v})_{O_2} = \text{arterial–mixed venous } O_2 \text{ content difference, in vol\%}$$

$$100 = \text{factor to correct } C(a-\bar{v})_{O_2} \text{ to liters (content differences are normally reported in vol\% or milliliters per deciliter)}$$

$\dot{V}_{O_2}$ is measured using one of the methods described previously. $C(a-\bar{v})_{O_2}$ is obtained by measuring or calculating oxygen content in both the arterial and mixed venous blood (see Chapter 6). Arterial and mixed venous blood specimens should be drawn simultaneously during the last 15 to 30 seconds of each exercise level. Oxygen consumption averaged over the same interval should be used for the calculation.

THERMODILUTION METHOD

Most pulmonary artery (Swan-Ganz) catheters use circuitry for measurement of CO by **thermodilution**. A sensitive **thermistor** is placed near the tip of the catheter. This thermistor is connected to a small, dedicated computer. A cool saline solution (usually 10° to 20° C) is injected through a

---

BOX 7-11
CRITERIA FOR ACCEPTABILITY—CARDIAC OUTPUT
DURING EXERCISE

1   For Fick cardiac output method, the pulmonary artery catheter must be properly placed. The distal port should be located in a pulmonary arteriole and must not be in the "wedge" position. For thermodilution the catheter must also be properly placed; the proximal (injection) port must be in the right atrium with the thermistor in a pulmonary arteriole.

2   For Fick measurements, arterial and mixed venous blood should be drawn simultaneously over 15 to 30 seconds (or longer). Care should be taken to avoid dilution with flush solution; dilution can markedly alter content calculations and hence cardiac output.

3   Oxygen consumption should be measured over the same time period as blood sampling for the Fick method.

4   Thermodilution measurements should be performed according to the manufacturers' recommendations, particularly in regard to temperature of injectate and rate of injection.

5   With either method, two or more acceptable measurements should be averaged; multiple measurements may not be practical with the Fick method if short exercise intervals are used.

---

port in the right atrium. The thermistor senses the change in temperature as the solution is pumped through the right ventricle and into the pulmonary artery. The computer then integrates the change in temperature and the time required for the change to occur. From these inputs, flow per unit of time or CO can be calculated.

The thermodilution method is commonly used in critical care settings. It is also practical for exercise testing. Multiple measurements (2 to 4) should be made at each exercise level and the results averaged. Some automated systems allow other cardiopulmonary variables (e.g., **ejection fraction**) to be calculated as well.

CARDIAC OUTPUT DURING EXERCISE

CO in healthy adult subjects is approximately 4 to 6 L/min at rest. During exercise, it may rise to 25 to 35 L/min (Box 7-12). CO is the product of HR and SV:

$$\dot{Q}_T = HR \times SV$$

where:

$$\dot{Q}_T = \text{cardiac output}$$

$$HR = \text{heart rate in beats per minute}$$

$$SV = \text{stroke volume in liters or milliliters}$$

In healthy upright adults SV is approximately 70 to 100 ml at rest. SV may be slightly higher if the subject is supine or semirecumbent because of increased venous return from the lower extremities. SV increases to 100 to 140 ml with low or moderate exercise. HR increases almost linearly with increasing work rate as described earlier, so that at low work loads an increase in CO is caused by a combination of HR and SV. At moderate and high workloads, further increases in CO result mainly from increased HR. Derivation of the SV (dividing $\dot{Q}_T$ by HR) is useful in quantifying poor cardiac performance in subjects with coronary artery disease, cardiomyopathy, or other diseases which affect myocardial contractility.

Subjects who reach their predicted $\dot{V}_{O_{2max}}$ and their predicted HR_{max} typically have normal CO and SV. A subject who has a reduced $\dot{V}_{O_{2max}}$ but achieves maximal predicted HR often has low CO because of low SV. Limited CO during increasing workload is often accompanied by an early onset of anaerobic metabolism. Reduced CO may be seen in both atrial and ventricular arrhythmias, in valvular insufficiency, and in cardiomyopathies.

In subjects who are fit, SV is increased both at rest and during exercise. Endurance (aerobic) training normally results in increased SV. Other benefits of aerobic training include reductions in systolic BP and ventilation. Fit subjects typically have a lower resting HR than their sedentary counterparts. Because HR (i.e., cardiac output) is the limiting factor to exercise in most individuals, fit subjects reach a higher $\dot{V}_{O_{2max}}$. Depending on the frequency, intensity, and duration of train-

---

BOX 7-12
INTERPRETIVE STRATEGIES—CARDIAC OUTPUT DURING EXERCISE

1 Were acceptable cardiac output measurements obtained? Were the measurements reproducible within 10% (if applicable)? If not, interpret cautiously.

2 Did cardiac output increase appropriately with increasing workloads? If not, consider cardiomyopathy, valvular insufficiency.

3 Was stroke volume normal at rest? Did it increase at low and medium workloads?

4 Was there evidence of ischemic changes or arrhythmias (on ECG) that might explain reduced cardiac output?

5 Was cardiac output compromised by increased systemic or pulmonary vascular resistance?

---

ing, fit individuals are able to maintain a higher level or work for longer periods because of improved CO.

The main disadvantage of the Fick method is that placement of a pulmonary artery catheter is required to obtain mixed venous samples. An indirect Fick method using CO_2 rebreathing is sometimes used. However, this technique is somewhat complicated and may not be accurate in all subjects. In patients who have obstructive pulmonary disease, this may be a serious limitation.

The thermodilution method also requires placement of a pulmonary artery catheter, which is a highly invasive procedure. Thermodilution CO measurements may be in error if the subject has significant valvular disease, particularly if regurgitation of blood through the tricuspid valve occurs.

CASE STUDIES

CASE 7A

History

T.S. is a 65-year-old man with a history of chronic obstructive pulmonary disease. He was referred for exercise evaluation as part of pulmonary rehabilitation. He experiences shortness of breath on exertion. He claims these episodes have grown worse in the last year. He has a smoking history of 72 pack/years but has recently quit smoking. A chest x-ray examination showed emphysematous changes and flattening of the diaphragms. Family history and occupational exposure were not significant.

Pulmonary Function Tests

Personal data

Sex: Male
Age: 65 yr
Height: 69 in
Weight: 125 lb

Spirometry

	Before drug	Predicted	%	After drug	% Chg
FVC (L)	2.42	4.35	56	2.51	4
FEV_1 (L)	1.2	3.01	40	1.3	8
$FEV_{1\%}$ (%)	50	69	—	52	—
$FEF_{25\%-75\%}$ (L/sec)	0.77	2.83	27	0.85	10
$\dot{V}max_{50}$ (L/sec)	1.37	4.94	28	1.51	10
$\dot{V}max_{25}$ (L/sec)	0.59	1.8	33	0.57	−3
MVV (L/min)	45	118	38	48	7
Raw (cm H_2O/L/sec)	2.8	0.6-2.4	—	2.71	−3
SGaw (L/sec/cm H_2O/L)	0.07	0.11-0.44	—	0.07	0

Lung volumes (by plethysmograph)

	Before drug	Predicted	%
VC (L)	2.42	4.35	56
IC (L)	1.74	2.96	59
ERV (L)	0.68	1.39	49
FRC (L)	5.11	3.81	134
RV (L)	4.43	2.42	183
TLC (L)	6.85	6.77	101
RV/TLC (%)	65	36	—

Diffusing capacity (single-breath)

	Before drug	Predicted	%
DL_{CO} (ml CO/min/mm Hg)	11.8	25.7	46
$\dot{V}A$ (L)	6.7	—	—
DL/VA	1.76	3.79	—

Technologist's Comments

Spirometry testing was performed acceptably, but best efforts were not within 200 ml after seven attempts. Lung volumes testing by plethysmography was performed acceptably. DL_{CO} maneuvers all had breath-hold times of 12 seconds or more. DL_{CO} was not corrected for Hb or carboxyhemoglobin (COHb).

Questions

1. What is the interpretation of:

   a. Spirometry, prebronchodilator and postbronchodilator?

   b. Lung volumes and diffusing capacity?

2. What is the interpretation of:

   a. Ventilation during exercise?

   b. Gas exchange during exercise?

   c. Blood gas levels during exercise?

3. What is the cause of the patient's exercise limitation?

4. What treatment might be recommended based on these findings?

Discussion

1 **Interpretation (pulmonary function)**

Seven acceptable FVC maneuvers were obtained but the two best FVC values were not within 200 ml. Lung volumes were acceptable. Diffusing capacity tests were substandard because breath-hold times exceeded 11 seconds.

   Spirometry is consistent with severe obstructive lung disease without significant response to bronchodilator therapy. Lung volumes show marked air trapping with residual volume replacement of the vital capacity. The diffusing capacity is severely reduced.

2 **Interpretation (exercise)**

The exercise test (Table 7-6) was terminated because the subject exceeded 85% of his age-related predicted maximum HR. He was also very short of breath. His maximum $\dot{V}E$ exceeded his MVV. VT increased with exercise, as did VD, and the VD/VT fell slightly. His gas exchange shows a $\dot{V}O_2$ of 1.2 L/min, which is approximately 57% of expected. $\dot{V}CO_2$ rose so that a respiratory exchange ratio (RER) slightly greater than one occurred at the highest workload. The ventilatory equivalent for oxygen ($\dot{V}E/\dot{V}O_2$) is elevated, and the O_2 pulse is slightly reduced.

   Blood gas testing during exercise reveal a mild hypoxemia that worsened slightly with exercise. Saturation remained adequate. No hypercapnia or acidosis occurred.

   No arrhythmias or ischemic changes were observed. The highest HR achieved was 88% of his predicted maximum. Mild systolic hypertension was present.

   Impression: (1) Marked aerobic impairment, (2) ventilatory limitation with hypoxemia, and (3) inappropriate cardiovascular response for the workload achieved.

TABLE 7-6   Exercise Test—Case 7A

Exercise level	1	2	3	4	5	6
Workload						
mph	0	1.5	2	2	2.5	3
Grade (%)	0	0	4	8	8	8
Duration (min)	10	3	3	3	3	3
METS	1	3.1	3.4	4.0	4.5	5.1
Ventilation						
f (breaths/min)	30	24	26	30	36	39
$\dot{V}_E$ (L/BTPS)	13.52	24.83	27.57	33.30	48.08	51.98
$\dot{V}_A$ (L/BTPS)	5.99	14.37	17.34	21.57	31.64	34.31
V_T (L/BTPS)	0.451	1.035	1.055	1.110	1.335	1.340
V_D (L/BTPS)	0.251	0.436	0.391	0.392	0.457	0.456
V_D/V_T	0.556	0.421	0.371	0.352	0.342	0.340
Gas exchange						
$\dot{V}_{O_2}$ (L/STPD)	0.237	0.745	0.797	0.954	1.056	1.204
$\dot{V}_{CO_2}$ (L/STPD)	0.244	0.655	0.733	0.896	1.044	1.298
RER	1.030	0.880	0.920	0.940	0.989	1.078
$\dot{V}_E/\dot{V}_{O_2}$ (L/L)	57	33	35	35	46	43
$\dot{V}_{O_2}$/HR (ml/beat)	2.7	7.8	8.4	9.1	8.5	8.9
Blood gases						
pH	7.47	7.43	7.42	7.39	7.39	7.38
Pa_{CO_2} (mm Hg)	33	35	34	36	33	35
Pa_{O_2} (mm Hg)	74	72	72	70	73	68
Sa_{O_2} (%)	95.5	95	95	94	94	93
$A-a_{O_2}$ (mm Hg)	36	31	38	38	41	46
Hemodynamics						
HR (beats/min)	85	95	95	105	124	135
Systolic BP (mm Hg)	124	162	178	194	200	210
Diastolic BP (mm Hg)	90	86	90	100	104	108

3   **Cause of exercise limitation**

T.S. walked a total of 15 minutes on the treadmill, reaching a rate of 3 mph at 8% grade. This equaled an energy production of 5 METS.

His ventilatory pattern is characteristic of moderate airway obstruction. His respiratory rate is elevated at the beginning of the procedure, falls slightly and then increases, particularly at the last two levels of work. The minute ventilation increases dramatically from rest to the beginning of exercise. It then increases slowly until the last two levels. The $\dot{V}_A$ increases in approximately the same pattern. His V_T increases to approximately 1 L and stays near that level throughout the test. This is a normal response. Healthy subjects generally accomplish increases in ventilation by increasing their V_T until they are using approximately 60% of their VC. Further increases are obtained by increasing the rate of breathing. In this case the subject immediately increased his V_T to 50% to 60% of his VC. He then increased $\dot{V}_E$ by raising his rate, particularly at the end of the test. His MVV was measured as 45 L/min and the $FEV_1 \times 35$ was 42 L/min. Compared with these values, the subject exceeded the maximal level of total ventilation that might have been expected. The V_D rose during exercise and fluctuated. The V_D/V_T ratio decreased slightly, as might be expected even with moderate obstruction. The ratio fell because the V_T increased more rapidly than the V_D.

At rest the subject has an RER slightly greater than 1.0. $\dot{V}_{CO_2}$ is elevated in relation to $\dot{V}_{O_2}$. The subject also has respiratory alkalosis, indicating hyperventilation. This pattern is not uncommon in resting subjects before beginning exercise. When he begins walking on the treadmill, his gas exchange parameters return to a normal pattern. There is a steady increase in both $\dot{V}O_2$ and $\dot{V}CO_2$, with an RER exceeding 1.0 at the final level. The subject may have reached his anaerobic threshold at this point, although the arterial pH is well within normal limits. The marked increase in $\dot{V}E$ during the last two levels may have resulted from the increased $\dot{V}CO_2$ of anaerobic metabolism.

The ventilatory equivalent for oxygen is inappropriately high at rest (level 1). This finding might be expected with moderate airway obstruction. The $\dot{V}E/\dot{V}O_2$ falls during the first few stages of exercise but rises again at the higher workloads. At all levels, the subject is performing an abnormally high level of ventilation compared with the work being performed. This finding is also consistent with airway obstruction.

The O_2 pulse ($\dot{V}O_2/HR$) rose with exercise, but not to 10-15 ml/beat, as might be expected. This suggests an inappropriate cardiovascular response. O_2 pulse is a function of the SV and the $C(a-\bar{v})O_2$. It is unclear which factor was responsible for the low ratio of $\dot{V}O_2$ to HR in this case. Cardiac pathology usually results in decreased SV. Deconditioning can also be accompanied by reduced SV. Deconditioning results in a low $C(a-\bar{v})O_2$ caused by poor extraction of O_2 by the muscles. Because the subject's HR and BP rose to near maximal levels without arrhythmias or ST-segment changes on the ECG, some element of deconditioning may be involved.

Despite a ventilatory limitation to exercise, arterial blood gas values did not change dramatically. The pH was slightly alkalotic at rest, which is consistent with hyperventilation. The pH fell with exercise but remained within a normal range. $PaCO_2$ remained constant. PaO_2, slightly low at rest, fell minimally. The subject used his remaining cardiopulmonary reserves to maintain normal blood gas levels.

4   Treatment

This subject demonstrated a marked reduction in exercise capacity based on his $\dot{V}O_{2max}$ of 57% of expected. This reduction was caused primarily by a ventilatory limitation but with possible evidence of deconditioning. His rehabilitation program subsequently included conditioning exercises within the limits of his pulmonary system.

CASE 7B

History

J.Y. is a 69-year-old woman with a history of chronic bronchitis who was referred for exercise evaluation. She complained of shortness of breath on exertion. Her smoking history is 56 pack/years, but she quit more than 1 year before this test. Her chest x-ray is consistent with chronic bronchitis, showing increased vascular markings and an enlarged heart. She had no significant family history or occupational exposure. She has a morning cough that produces thick white sputum.

Pulmonary Function Tests

Personal data

Sex: Female
Age: 69 yr
Height: 64 in
Weight: 128 lb

Spirometry

	Before drug	*Predicted*	%
FVC (L)	1.3	2.85	46
FEV_1 (L)	0.73	2.04	36
$FEV_{1\%}$ (%)	56	72	—
$FEF_{25\%-75\%}$ (L/sec)	0.43	2.32	18
$\dot{V}max_{50}$ (L/sec)	0.55	3.8	14
$\dot{V}max_{25}$ (L/sec)	0.25	1.27	20
MVV (L/min)	31	85	36
Raw (cm H_2O/L/sec)	2.77	0.6-2.4	—
SGaw (L/sec/cm H_2O/L)	0.09	0.15-0.60	—

Lung volumes (by plethysmograph)

	Before drug	Predicted	%
VC (L)	1.3	2.85	46
IC (L)	1.08	1.99	54
ERV (L)	0.23	0.86	26
FRC (L)	3.78	2.77	137
RV (L)	3.55	1.91	186
TLC (L)	4.85	4.76	102
RV/TLC (%)	73	40	—

Diffusing capacity (single-breath)

	Before drug	Predicted	%
DL_{CO} (ml CO/min/mm Hg)	8.3	17.4	48
$\dot{V}A$ (L)	4.7	—	—
DL/VA	1.77	3.77	—

Technologist's Comments

All spirometry maneuvers were performed acceptably. Postbronchodilator studies were not performed because the patient had used her inhaled medication (albuterol) immediately before testing. Lung volumes by body plethysmography were performed variably, but three acceptable maneuvers were obtained after eight efforts. DL_{CO} maneuvers were acceptable but not corrected for Hb or COHb.

A multistage exercise test was performed with a treadmill and an arterial catheter in place. Level 1 was a 10-minute baseline at rest (Table 7-7).

Questions

1. What is the interpretation of:

   a. Spirometry?

   b. Lung volumes and diffusing capacity?

2. What is the interpretation of:

   a. Ventilation during exercise?

   b. Gas exchange during exercise?

   c. Blood gas levels during exercise?

3. What is the cause of the patient's exercise limitation?

4. What treatment might be recommended based on these findings?

Discussion

1   **Interpretation (pulmonary function)**

   All spirometry data were acceptable, as were data for diffusing capacity. Several plethysmographic lung volume maneuvers had to be discarded before three acceptable measurements were obtained.

   Spirometry results are consistent with obstructive airway disease. Lung volumes indicate air trapping with a normal total lung capacity (TLC). The diffusing capacity is reduced. Blood gas analysis was deferred because this study immediately preceded the exercise test. Bronchodilator studies were not performed because the patient had used her usual regimen immediately before the pulmonary function study.

2   **Interpretation (exercise test)**

   The reason for termination of the test was a systolic BP of 250 mm Hg. The subject's respiratory rate increased from 12 to 33 breaths/min, with an increase in ventilation from 8 to 22 L/min. The VT was relatively fixed at approximately 700 ml. $\dot{V}A$ increased in proportion to $\dot{V}E$.

   Her $\dot{V}O_2$ rose to only 0.548 L/min, or 34% of her predicted maximum (1.634). Her ventilatory equivalent for O_2 ($\dot{V}E/\dot{V}O_2$) remained elevated throughout the test. Her O_2 pulse was low but elevated normally with exercise, although not to maximal levels.

TABLE 7-7 Exercise Test—Case 7B

Exercise level	1	2	3
Workload			
mph	0	1.5	3
Grade (%)	0	0	0
Duration (min)	10	3	3
METS	1	3.3	3.4
Ventilation			
f (breaths/min)	12	27	33
V_E (L/BTPS)	8.020	21.220	22.630
V_A (L/BTPS)	4.17	11.671	12.447
V_T (L/BTPS)	0.668	0.768	0.686
V_D (L/BTPS)	0.321	0.350	0.309
V_D/V_T	0.48	0.45	0.45
Gas exchange			
V_{O_2} (L/STPD)	0.160	0.530	0.548
V_{CO_2} (L/STPD)	0.149	0.489	0.498
RER	0.930	0.923	0.908
V_E/V_{O_2} (L/L)	50.14	40.04	41.28
V_{O_2}/HR (ml/beat)	2.459	5.047	5.221
Blood gases			
pH	7.48	7.42	7.41
Pa_{CO_2} (mm Hg)	34	39	37
Pa_{O_2} (mm Hg)	74	60	63
Sa_{O_2} (%)	94.9	89.9	91.0
$A-a_{O_2}$ (mm Hg)	39	48	45
Hemodynamics			
HR (beats/min)	65	105	105
Systolic BP (mm Hg)	160	212	250
Diastolic BP (mm Hg)	80	100	102

Blood gas studies indicate mild hypoxemia during exercise with an increased A-a gradient. Pa_{CO_2} rose slightly, and the pH changed accordingly but without evidence of anaerobic metabolism.

Her HR rose to 105 beats/min, which is only 72% of her age-related predicted maximum. The systolic BP rose dramatically from 160/80 to 250/102, at which point the test was terminated. There were no arrhythmias, ST-segment changes, or other evidence of ischemia noted.

Impression: (1) Exercise limited by marked hypertension, (2) ventilatory reserve is present despite moderately severe airway obstruction, and (3) mild impairment of oxygenation during exercise, but not significantly limiting.

3 **Cause of exercise limitation**

J.Y. is an example of an individual with well-documented airway obstruction in whom exercise limitation is primarily caused by an inappropriate cardiovascular response.

Comparison of her maximal ventilation of 22.6 L/min with her MVV of 31 L/min indicates very little ventilatory reserve. Because her MVV is so markedly reduced, there must be some ventilatory limitation to work. Her V_T (at rest and during mild exercise) remained relatively fixed near 700 ml. Because this volume was already 50% to 60% of her VC, she could increase her ventilation only by increasing her rate. Her V_D/V_T ratio decreased only slightly, probably as a direct result of the fixed V_T. In instances in which both the V_T and V_D increase proportionately, the VD/VT ratio does not decrease. This pattern may be consistent with pulmonary vascular disorders but is probably not in evidence here because neither the VT nor the VD increased significantly.

J.Y. has marked aerobic impairment as indicated by the low $\dot{V}o_2$ of 0.548 L/min, at 3.0 mph and 0% grade on the treadmill. Her RER appears to fall, perhaps because she was hyperventilating at the resting level. Her ventilation is inappropriately elevated for the workloads evaluated, as shown by the $\dot{V}E/\dot{V}o_2$ ratio. This pattern is consistent with the increased VD/VT ratio. High ventilation is required to maintain an adequate $\dot{V}A$.

Her O_2 pulse (i.e., $\dot{V}o_2$/HR) was low at rest and increased only slightly during mild exercise. The maximal O_2 pulse that might have been attained can be estimated by dividing her predicted $\dot{V}o_{2max}$ by her predicted maximum HR × 1000. In this case, the calculation would be 1.634/148 × 1000, or 11.

J.Y. failed to increase her O_2 pulse because she was limited by other factors at an HR significantly lower than her predicted maximum. An inappropriate rise in systolic BP to 250 mm Hg led to termination of the test. Peripheral vasodilatation normally redirects cardiac output to exercising muscles. The hypertensive response observed here indicates a failure of this mechanism. Local lesions (e.g., claudication) or diffuse disease (e.g., essential hypertension) can result in anaerobic metabolism in the exercising muscles. As a result, metabolic acidosis develops, with stimulation of respiration and dyspnea. Acidosis and dyspnea did not develop in J.Y. during the test (i.e., pH of 7.41). Her presenting complaint of increasing shortness of breath may have been related to both the hypertensive response and her pulmonary limitations.

4   Treatment

Based on the results of the exercise test, the subject was referred for further evaluation and treatment of her hypertension. She was maintained on bronchodilator therapy and asked to return in 6 months for reevaluation of possible need for supplemental oxygen.

CASE 7C

History

C.J. is a 53-year-old office worker who was referred for evaluation of shortness of breath. She has a 44 pack/year history of smoking and continued to smoke up to the time of her test. She has a morning cough that produces 50 to 100 ml of thick white sputum per day. Her chest x-ray shows increased vascular markings and mild hyperinflation. She was taking no medications at the time of this test. No familial history of lung disease or cancer was found, and she had no unusual environmental exposure.

Pulmonary Function Tests

Personal data

Sex: Female
Age: 53 yr
Height: 65 in
Weight: 131 lb

Spirometry

	Before drug	*Predicted*	*%*	*After drug*	*%*
FVC	3.24	3.35	97	3.34	100
FEV$_1$ (L)	1.49	2.53	59	1.56	62
FEV$_{1\%}$ (%)	46	75	—	47	—
FEF$_{25\%-75\%}$ (L/sec)	0.79	2.86	27	1.19	42
$\dot{V}max_{50}$ (L/sec)	1.99	4.24	47	2.25	53
$\dot{V}max_{25}$ (L/sec)	0.68	1.86	37	0.99	53
MVV (L/min)	52	97.9	53	55	56
Raw(cm H$_2$O/L/sec)	2.22	0.6-2.4	—	2.1	—
SGaw (L/sec/cm H$_2$O/L)	0.12	0.14-0.58	—	0.13	—

Lung volumes (by plethysmograph)

	Before drug	Predicted	%
VC (L)	3.27	3.35	98
IC (L)	1.80	2.31	78
ERV (L)	0.99	1.04	95
FRC (L)	3.54	2.88	123
RV (L)	2.55	1.84	136
TLC (L)	5.82	5.20	112
RV/TLC (%)	44	35	—

Diffusing capacity (single-breath)

	Before drug	Predicted	%
DL_{CO} (ml CO/min/mm Hg)	8.8	20	44
DL_{CO} (adj)	10.3	20	51
$\dot{V}A$ (L)	5.67	—	—
DL/VA	1.55	3.85	—

Blood gases (FIO_2 0.21)

pH	7.38
$PaCO_2$ (mm Hg)	43
PaO_2 (mm Hg)	59
SaO_2 (%)	85.1
Hb (g/dl)	11.7
COHb (%)	5.7

Technologist's Comments

All spirometric efforts were acceptable, both before and after bronchodilator administration. Lung volume and DL_{CO} testing were performed acceptably and corrected for an Hb of 11.7 and COHb of 5.7.

Three days later a treadmill exercise test was performed with an arterial catheter in place. The test was repeated with oxygen supplementation. Gas with an FIO_2 of 0.28 was prepared in a meteorologic balloon for the portion of the exercise test using O_2 (Table 7-8).

Questions

1. What is the interpretation of:
   a. Spirometry, prebronchodilator and postbronchodilator?
   b. Lung volumes and diffusing capacity?
   c. Room air blood gases at rest?
2. What is the interpretation of:
   a. Ventilation during exercise?
   b. Gas exchange during exercise?
   c. Blood gase levels during exercise?
3. What is the cause of the patient's exercise limitation?
4. What treatment might be recommended based on these findings?

Discussion

1 Interpretation (pulmonary function tests)

All spirometry, lung volume, diffusing capacity, and blood gas measurements were acceptable.

Spirometry results show an obstructive process with a well-preserved FVC. There is only a 5% improvement in the FEV_1 after bronchodilator administration. Lung volumes by plethysmography show increased FRC and RV consistent with air trapping. The TLC is close to normal so there is little hyperinflation. The DL_{CO}SB is reduced, even after correction for Hb and COHb. Arterial blood gases on air show hypoxemia that is complicated by an elevated COHb.

TABLE 7-8 Exercise Test–Case 7C

Exercise level	1	2	3	4	5
	Air		Oxygen		
Workload					
mph	0	1.5	0	1.5	2
Grade (%)	0	0	0	0	4
Duration (min)	10	3	10	3	3
METS	1.48	4.00	1.34	3.11	4.73
Ventilation					
f (breaths/min)	16	28	13	20	31
$\dot{V}_E$ (L/BTPS)	10.20	23.40	6.23	16.59	27.81
$\dot{V}_A$ (L/BTPS)	6.02	14.74	3.74	10.45	17.80
V_T (L/BTPS)	0.638	0.836	0.479	0.830	0.897
V_D (L/BTPS)	0.262	0.309	0.190	0.307	0.323
V_D/V_T	0.41	0.37	0.40	0.37	0.36
Gas exchange					
$\dot{V}_{O_2}$ (L/STPD)	0.310	0.835	0.279	0.649	0.986
$\dot{V}_{CO_2}$ (L/STPD)	0.303	0.743	0.251	0.617	0.976
RER	0.98	0.89	0.90	0.95	0.99
$\dot{V}_E/\dot{V}_{O_2}$ (L/L)	32.90	28.00	22.33	25.50	28.20
$\dot{V}_{O_2}$/HR (ml/beat)	3.44	7.59	3.29	6.18	8.57
Pulse oximeter					
Sp_{O_2} (%)	92	87	97	93	93
Blood gases					
pH	7.45	7.39	7.39	7.38	7.36
Pa_{CO_2} (mm Hg)	34	39	44	45	46
Pa_{O_2} (mm Hg)	61	47	84	71	66
Sa_{O_2} (%)	87.4	77.3	91.4	88.9	87.0
COHb (%)	5.1	4.7	4.8	4.7	4.6
$P(A-a)_{O_2}$ (mm Hg)	51	56	64	78	84
Hemodynamics					
HR (beats/min)	90	110	92	105	115
Systolic BP (mm Hg)	130	145	134	145	150
Diastolic BP (mm Hg)	85	88	90	90	90

Impression: Moderately severe obstructive disease with no significant response to bronchodilators. Air trapping is present, and the DL_{CO} is severely reduced. Exercise evaluation for oxygen desaturation is recommended.

2   **Interpretation (exercise test)**

The exercise test was performed in two parts; the first part of the test was stopped because the subject's Pa_{O_2} fell to 46 mm Hg with an Sa_{O_2} of 77.3%. The second phase, using oxygen, was terminated because of shortness of breath. The subject tolerated very low workloads even with supplemental O_2.

Ventilation was slightly elevated at rest but increased normally. When given O_2, the subject's ventilation was slightly lower both at rest and at similar workloads. The V_D/V_T ratio was mildly elevated but decreased with exercise, on both air and oxygen. The subject's minute ventilation was only 51% of her observed MVV after bronchodilator administration, indicating some ventilatory reserve.

The subject achieved a maximal $\dot{V}_{O_2}$ of only 0.986 L/min on oxygen, which is 53% of her age-related predicted value of 1.858 L/min. This is consistent with moderately severe exercise impairment. The ventilatory equivalent for O_2 is within normal limits, and the O_2 pulse increased normally, although not to maximal values.

Blood gas analysis during exercise shows borderline hypoxemia at rest resulting from PaO_2 of 61 mm Hg in combination with elevated COHb. The PaO_2 fell to 47 mm Hg with only slight exertion. On 28% oxygen, the PaO_2 improved to 84 mm Hg at rest but decreased as workload increased. Her $PaCO_2$ increased slightly during oxygen breathing, possibly as a result of respiratory depression. The COHb was elevated, likely resulting from the subject's continued smoking. Pulse oximetry (SpO_2) during exercise shows readings higher than the actual saturation, presumably as a result of the subject's COHb.

The HR and BP responses were appropriate for the workloads achieved breathing both air and oxygen. The low maximal HR suggests an exercise limitation other than cardiovascular pathology or deconditioning. The ECG was unremarkable.

Impression: Moderately severe exercise impairment primarily caused by desaturation during exercise. Some ventilatory limitation is probably present as well. The desaturation is aggravated by an elevated COHb.

3   **Cause of the patient's exercise limitation**
This patient characterizes the subject with obstructive lung disease in whom derangement of blood gases limits exercise more than impaired ventilation does. C.J.'s ventilation and gas exchange are close to normal at rest and at 1.5 mph, 0% grade. The PO_2 is low, however, and falls abruptly with just a small increase in workload. The decrease is severe enough that desaturation might occur with daily activities or during sleep. The elevated COHb further impairs O_2 delivery. Although a pulse oximeter was used during the exercise test, its readings were falsely high because of the elevated COHb. Even if pulse oximeter readings are corrected for COHb, a discrepancy often exists between SpO_2 and SaO_2 during exercise. This error in pulse oximeter readings may result from changes in blood flow at the sensor site or motion artifact during exercise (see also Case 7D, below). Desaturation might be expected because of her low DL_{CO}. There is some evidence that DL_{CO} values less than 50% of predicted values suggest exercise desaturation.

To evaluate the effect of oxygen therapy, a controlled trial of walking while breathing supplemental O_2 was performed. The subject breathed from a balloon containing gas blended to have an FIO_2 of 0.28. The most notable change was the increase in resting PaO_2 from 61 to 84 mm Hg. However, the pattern of desaturation persisted. Her O_2 tension fell dramatically, just as when she breathed room air. Because her PaO_2 was elevated by the supplemental O_2, it remained above 55 mm Hg. This is the level at which serious symptoms of hypoxemia begin to occur. Supplemental O_2 also may be responsible for the decrease in ventilation exhibited by the patient at rest and during exercise. The mild increase in $PaCO_2$ may be evidence of increased sensitivity to hypoxemia. When she breathes O_2, her respiratory drive decreases slightly, allowing CO_2 to rise. Abnormal $\dot{V}/\dot{Q}$ is the most likely explanation of desaturation observed in the subject. The bronchitic component of her obstructive disease results in shunting and venous admixture.

While breathing oxygen she did not desaturate to a level at which hypoxemia might be considered as a cause of the exercise limitation. She also did not increase her ventilation to her maximal level. This might suggest that deconditioning was responsible for the low maximal workload achieved. However, her HR and BP did not increase as typical in significant deconditioning. Other possible causes for the low workload achieved while breathing oxygen might be inadequate subject effort, the development of bronchospasm, or a greatly increased work of breathing.

4   **Treatment**
The patient began a formal effort to stop smoking and eventually quit. She was also referred for pulmonary rehabilitation which included bronchial hygiene, breathing retraining, and exercise with supplemental O_2. She began using nasal oxygen at 1 to 2 L/min for exertion. A follow-up evaluation was recommended 3 to 6 months after smoking cessation.

CASE 7D

History

E.E. is a 65-year-old man who was referred to the pulmonary function laboratory. He had spirometry testing in the referring physician's office which indicated obstruction. Because of his chief complaint of dyspnea on exertion, his physician recommended that he get full pulmonary function studies. The referring physician also requested a simple exercise test with pulse oximetry to determine whether E.E. required supplemental O_2. The patient was not currently taking any medications for heart or lung disease. He confirmed that he had been a smoker until approximately 6 months ago. He had smoked approximately 20 cigarettes per day for 30 years.

Pulmonary Function Tests

Personal data

Sex: Male
Age: 65 yr
Height: 69 in
Weight: 185 lb

Spirometry

	Before drug	Predicted	%	After drug	% Chg
FVC (L)	4.03	4.35	92	4.11	2
FEV_1 (L)	2.62	3.01	87	2.65	1
$FEV_{1\%}$ (%)	65	69	—	64	—
$FEF_{25\%-75\%}$ (L/sec)	1.75	2.83	62	1.85	6
$\dot{V}max_{50}$ (L/sec)	3.01	4.94	61	3.11	3
$\dot{V}max_{25}$ (L/sec)	1.56	1.8	87	1.47	−6
MVV (L/min)	92	118	77	89	−2
Raw (cm H_2O/L/sec)	2.01	0.6-2.4	—	1.71	−15
SGaw (L/sec/cm H_2O/L)	0.17	0.11-0.44	—	0.27	59

Lung volumes (by He dilution)

	Before drug	Predicted	%
VC (L)	4.03	4.35	93
IC (L)	3.01	2.96	102
ERV (L)	1.02	1.39	73
FRC (L)	4.11	3.81	108
RV (L)	3.09	2.42	128
TLC (L)	7.12	6.77	105
RV/TLC (%)	43	36	—

Diffusing capacity (single-breath)

	Before drug	Predicted	%
DL_{CO} (ml/CO/min/mm Hg)	19.3	25.7	75
$\dot{V}A$ (L)	6.8	—	—
$DL/\dot{V}A$	2.84	3.8	—

Technologist's Comments

All spirometry efforts before and after bronchodilator therapy were performed acceptably. Lung volumes by He dilution were acceptable (two tests were averaged). DL_{CO} maneuvers were also performed acceptably.

A cycle ergometer exercise test was performed. The subject was monitored using a modified 12-lead ECG system and a pulse oximeter attached to his finger (Table 7-9).

Questions

1. What is the interpretation of:

    a. Spirometry, prebronchodilator and postbronchodilator?

    b. Airway resistance and conductance?

    c. Lung volumes and diffusing capacity?

2. What is the interpretation of:

    a. Ventilation during exercise?

TABLE 7-9 Exercise Test—Case 7D

Exercise level	1	2	3	4
Activity (cycle)	Sit	Pedal	Pedal	Pedal
Watts	0	25	50	75
Duration (min)	5	3	3	2
Respiratory rate (breaths/min)	18	22	30	32
Spo_2 (%)	92	88	83	84
Heart rate (beats/min)	98	122	147	151
Systemic BP (mm Hg)	128	154	190	200
Diastolic BP (mm Hg)	80	88	100	100
pH	—	—	—	7.31
Pco_2 (mm Hg)	—	—	—	31
Po_2 (mm Hg)	—	—	—	77
Sao_2 (%)	—	—	—	90

    b. Gas exchange during exercise?

    c. Blood gas levels during exercise?

3. What is the cause of the patient's exercise limitation?

4. Why was the pulse oximeter reading different from the saturation measured by co-oximetry?

Discussion

1 **Interpretation (pulmonary function tests)**

All spirometry, lung volume, and diffusing capacity maneuvers were performed acceptably. All data were reproducible.

    Spirometry indicates slightly reduced FEV_1 consistent with mild obstruction. The $FEF_{25\%-75\%}$ and all other flows are also slightly reduced. There is no significant improvement after administration of inhaled bronchodilators. Airway resistance and conductance are within normal limits but improve significantly after inhaled bronchodilator therapy. Lung volumes show a slight elevation of the FRC and RV, indicating that there may be some air trapping. The DL_{CO} is also mildly reduced.

    Impression: There is mild obstruction and air trapping without significant response to bronchodilator therapy.

2 **Interpretation (exercise test)**

The patient exercised on a cycle ergometer for a total of 8 minutes. After 3 minutes at 50 watts, the patient's pulse oximeter reading was 83%. He gave no sign of distress as might have been expected with a low O_2 saturation. The ergometer resistance was advanced to 75 watts and the patient pedaled for two more minutes. When the patient signaled that he was becoming very short of breath, an arterial blood gas sample was obtained by radial puncture. The patient achieved an HR of 151 beats/min, or 89% of his predicted maximum. There were no arrhythmias, or ST- or T-wave changes. His blood pressure increased to 200/100 at peak exercise. His respiratory rate was 30 breaths/min. Arterial blood gas testing revealed metabolic acidosis consistent with anaerobic metabolism. Pao_2 was 77 mm Hg, with Sao_2 of 90% measured by co-oximeter. The co-oximeter saturation value did not support the value of 84% obtained by pulse oximeter.

    Impression: (1) Exercise was limited by cardiovascular system. Absence of arrhythmias and slight hypertensive response suggests deconditioning. (2) There was no O_2 desaturation at this time. A program of aerobic conditioning, including adequate warm-up and cool-down, is recommended. A target HR of 120 to 130 beats/min would be appropriate.

3 **Cause of the patient's exercise limitation**

This patient is typical of those referred to a full-function laboratory after spirometry and symptoms suggest pulmonary disease. In this case the subject had mild obstructive airways disease with little response to bronchodilators. The complaint of shortness of breath prompted the referring physician to suggest a simple exercise evaluation to assess possible O_2

desaturation. The exercise test revealed cardiovascular limitations rather than hypoxemia as the cause of the shortness of breath.

4   **Pulse oximetry versus co-oximetry**

The discrepancy between the pulse oximeter and measured blood saturation by co-oximeter is noteworthy. Pulse oximeters offer a simple, inexpensive means of assessing oxygen saturation of hemoglobin. The limitations of pulse oximetry should be considered, especially when used in conjunction with exercise tests. Motion artifact, incident light, local perfusion, and skin pigmentation have all been demonstrated to affect accuracy of pulse oximeters. COHb is also known to erroneously elevate readings (see Chapter 6). The reason why the pulse oximeter read lower than the co-oximeter in this case was not readily apparent. Motion and changes in local perfusion are the most likely factors during exercise. Because the patient exercised with an ergometer, his hand was relatively stable on the handle bar. Squeezing the handle bar may have caused the problem, even though the subject was coached to relax his hand.

To reduce the possibility of false-positive (as in this case) or false-negative results of pulse oximetry, several steps can be taken. Sensor placement should be chosen to minimize motion. The connecting cable between the sensor and oximeter should be stabilized to prevent pulling or twisting during exercise. A pulse oximeter capable of displaying pulse waveforms and HR is preferable. Visualization of the pulse waveform can help the physician or technologist judge validity of the saturation reading. If there is not a good pulse waveform or if the HR differs significantly from the ECG, saturation values should be monitored.

As was done in this case, an arterial blood gas sample at peak exercise may be necessary to completely answer the clinical question. A blood gas sample drawn at rest may correlate with pulse oximetry readings. The same may not be true during exercise. A radial puncture may be performed at peak exercise or within 15 seconds of termination of exercise. A modified Allen's test (see Chapter 6) should be performed to assess the sample site before exercise begins. A cycle ergometer provides a good platform for performing a radial puncture because there is minimal body movement. A blood gas sample at peak exercise can be obtained from a subject on a treadmill but may require the use of a side rail to stabilize the wrist. The specimen should be obtained within 15 seconds after the end of exercise, before recirculation occurs. If the co-oximeter saturation verifies the pulse oximeter reading, additional arterial specimens should not be necessary. If a significant discrepancy exists between blood and pulse oximeter values, further sampling may be required. If blood cannot be obtained within 15 seconds, the exercise session may need to be repeated. For patients in whom there is difficulty obtaining blood by radial puncture, an arterial catheter may be indicated. Radial artery cannulation may be less traumatic if multiple blood gases need to be obtained, as in titration of O_2 therapy for exercise.

SUMMARY

THIS CHAPTER HAS EXAMINED THE measurement of cardiopulmonary variables during exercise. Various protocols for assessing exercise responses have been described, including treadmill and cycle egrometry methods. Monitoring of the cardiovascular system with a special concern for patient safety has been discussed. Techniques for measuring ventilation, oxygen consumption, carbon dioxide production, and the associated variables during exercise have been delineated. Special emphasis has been given to criteria for acceptability and interpretive strategies for the various measurements described. Assessment of blood gases and CO have been covered as well. Case studies and self-assessment questions directed at the topic of cardio-pulmonary exercise testing have been included.

SELF-ASSESSMENT QUESTIONS

1 *To measure the maximum $\dot{V}O_2$ that can be achieved by a healthy adult man, which of the following exercise protocols could be used?*
   I.   Ramp test using a cycle ergometer
   II. 6-Minute walk test
   III. 8 minutes of treadmill walking at 2.5 mph, 12% grade
   IV. Bruce protocol
   a. I and III only
   b. I and IV only
   c. II and III only
   d. II, III, and IV

2 *Which of the following are true concerning exercise testing performed with a cycle ergometer?*
   a. A higher maximum $\dot{V}O_2$ can be achieved than with a treadmill.
   b. Workload can be changed only in 1-minute intervals.
   c. $\dot{V}O_2$ can be estimated from pedaling speed and resistance.
   d. Work performed depends on the subject's height and weight.

3 *In a healthy adult subject with a resting BP of 120/80, which of the following responses would be expected during a maximal incremental exercise test?*
   a. Systolic increases to 240, diastolic to 95
   b. Systolic increases to 300, diastolic to 130
   c. Systolic increases to 160, diastolic to 130
   d. Systolic remains at 120, diastolic decreases to 60

4 *Which combination of gases would be most appropriate to check the linearity of the oxygen analyzer used for exhaled gas analysis during exercise?*
   a. 100% O_2, room air
   b. 40% O_2, 5% CO_2
   c. Room air, 24% O_2, 7% CO_2
   d. Room air, 12% O_2, 24% O_2

5 *Which of the following is (are) indication(s) for terminating a cardiopulmonary exercise test?*
   I.   Progressive chest pain (angina)
   II. 2 mm downsloping ST depression
   III. Ventricular tachycardia
   IV. Monitoring system failure
   a. I and II only
   b. III and IV only
   c. I, II, and III
   d. I, II, III, and IV

6 *A patient with an MVV of 120 L/min has the following results of an exercise test (values in parentheses are percentages of predicted):*

$\dot{V}O_{2max}$ L/min (STPD)	2.81	(99%)
HR_{max} b/min	167	(94%)
$\dot{V}E_{max}$ L/min (BTPS)	37	

   Which statement best describes these results?
   a. Normal exercise response
   b. Mild exercise impairment, probably deconditioning
   c. Poor subject effort indicated by low maximal ventilation
   d. Moderate exercise impairment with ventilatory limitation

7 *The following values are obtained during exercise using a mixing chamber system:*

F_{IO_2}	0.2093
F_{EO_2}	0.166
F_{ECO_2}	0.035
$\dot{V}E$ (L STPD)	27.5

   What is the $\dot{V}O_2$ in L/min STPD?
   a. 0.96
   b. 1.25
   c. 3.60
   d. 4.85

8 *The following graph plots ventilation and CO_2 production against $\dot{V}O_2$:*

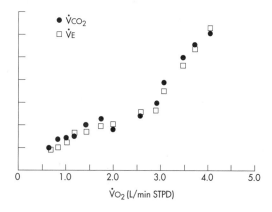

   At approximately what $\dot{V}O_2$ does the ventilatory threshold occur?
   a. 1.0 L/min
   b. 2.0 L/min
   c. 3.0 L/min
   d. 4.0 L/min

9 *A patient performs a symptom-limited maximal exercise test on a cycle ergometer; the ventilatory threshold is estimated at 37% of the subject's $\dot{V}_{O_{2max}}$. These findings are consistent with which of the following?*
   a. Hyperventilation because of anxiety
   b. Poor subject effort
   c. Primary ventilatory limitation to exercise
   d. Early onset of anaerobic metabolism

10 *A subject has the following results of an exercise test:*

	Maximal exercise	Predicted
HR (beats/min)	110	167
ST change (mm)	0.5	<1
$\dot{V}_{O_2}$ (ml/min/kg)	9.2	23
$\dot{V}_E$	23	26
S_{aO_2} (%)	85	>90

Which of the following clinical conditions is most consistent with these findings?
   a. Cardiomyopathy
   b. Chronic obstructive pulmonary disease
   c. Marked deconditioning
   d. Acute pulmonary embolism

11 *A subject who has severe dyspnea on exertion performs a maximal exercise test with arterial line and exhaled gas analysis. The following data are obtained:*

	Maximal exercise	Predicted
HR (beats/min)	163	171
$\dot{V}_{O_2}$ (L/min)	0.85	2.89
$\dot{V}_E$ (L/min)	23	96
Pa_{O_2}	72	>85
Pa_{CO_2}	41	<40
V_D/V_T	0.42	<0.25
Sp_{O_2} (%)	93	95

Which of the following diagnoses best fit these findings?
   a. Coronary artery disease
   b. Pulmonary hypertension
   c. Restrictive lung disease
   d. Poor subject effort

12 *Which of the following describe cardiac output in healthy adult subjects?*
   I.   At low workloads both SV and HR contribute to increased output.
   II. It can increase up to 10 to 15 L/min at maximal exercise.
   III. It increases linearly with increasing workload ($\dot{V}_{O_2}$).
   IV. It changes only slightly above the anaerobic threshold (AT).
   a. I and III only
   b. II and IV only
   c. I, II, and III
   d. II, III, and IV

SELECTED BIBLIOGRAPHY

General References

Hansen JE: Exercise instruments, schemes, and protocols for evaluating the dyspneic patient, *Am Rev Respir Dis* 129(suppl):S25, 1984.

Hansen JE, Sue DY, Wasserman K: Predicted values for clinical exercise testing, *Am Rev Respir Dis* 129(suppl): S49, 1984.

Hellerstein HK, Brock LL, Bruce RA: *Exercise testing and training of apparently healthy individuals: a handbook for physicians,* New York, 1972, Committee on Exercise American Heart Association.

Jones NL: *Clinical exercise testing,* ed 3, Philadelphia, 1988, WB Saunders.

McKelvie RS, Jones NL: Cardiopulmonary exercise testing, *Clin Chest Med* 10:277, 1989.

Wasserman K, Hansen J, Sue D, et al: *Principles of exercise testing and interpretation,* ed 2, Philadelphia, 1994, Lea & Febiger.

Wasserman K, Whipp BJ: Exercise physiology in health and disease, *Am Rev Respir Dis* 112:219, 1975.

Weber KT, Janicki JS: *Cardiopulmonary exercise testing: physiologic principles and clinical applications,* Philadelphia, 1986, WB Saunders.

Cardiovascular Monitoring During Exercise

Bruce RA: Value and limitations of the electrocardiogram in progressive exercise testing, *Am Rev Respir Dis* 129(suppl):S28, 1984.

Ellestad MH, Allen WA, Wan MCK, et al: Maximal treadmill stress testing for cardiovascular evaluation, *Circulation* 39:517, 1969.

Pollack ML, Bohannon RL, Cooper KH, et al: A comparative analysis of four protocols for maximal stress testing, *Am Heart J* 92:39, 1976.

Stone HL, Liang IYS: Cardiovascular response and control during exercise, *Am Rev Respir Dis* 129(suppl):S13, 1984.

Ventilation, Gas Exchange, and Blood Gases

Beaver WL, Wasserman K, Whipp BJ: A new method for detection of anaerobic threshold by gas exchange, *J Appl Physiol* 60:2020, 1986.

Eschenbacher WL, Mannina A: An algorithm for the interpretation of cardiopulmonary exercise tests, *Chest* 97:263, 1990.

Escourrou PJL, Delaperche MF, Visseaux A: Reliability of pulse oximetry during exercise in pulmonary patients, *Chest* 97:635-638, 1990.

Hansen J, Casaburi R: Validity of ear oximetry in clinical exercise testing, *Chest* 91:333-337, 1987.

Jones NL: Normal values for pulmonary gas exchange during exercise, *Am Rev Respir Dis* 129(suppl):S44, 1984.

Jones NL: Exercise testing in pulmonary evaluation: rationale, methods and the normal respiratory response to exercise, Parts I and II, *N Engl J Med* 293:541, 1975.

Neuberg GW, Friedman SH, Weiss MB, et al: Cardiopulmonary exercise testing: the clinical value of gas exchange data, *Arch Intern Med* 148:2221, 1988.

Sue DY, Hansen JE, Blais M, et al: Measurement and analysis of gas exchange during exercise using a programmable calculator, *J Appl Physiol* 49:456, 1980.

Wasserman K: The anaerobic threshold measurement in exercise testing, *Clin Chest Med* 5:77, 1984.

Weber KT, Janicki JS, McElroy PA, et al: Concepts and applications of cardiopulmonary exercise testing, *Chest* 93:843, 1988.

Whipp BJ, Ward SA, Wasserman K: Ventilatory responses to exercise and their control in man, *Am Rev Respir Dis* 129(suppl):S17, 1984.

Standards and Guidelines

American Association for Respiratory Care: Clinical practice guideline: exercise testing for evaluation of hypoxemia and/or desaturation, *Respir Care* 37:907-912, 1992.

American College of Sports Medicine: *Guidelines for graded exercise testing and exercise prescription,* ed 3, Philadelphia, 1986, Lea & Febiger.

Ellestad MH, Blomquist CG, Naughton JP: Standards for adult exercise testing laboratories, *Circulation* 59(suppl):421A-430A, 1979.

Fletcher GF, Froelicher VF, Hartley LH, et al: Exercise standards: a statement for health professionals from the American Heart Association, *Circulation* 82:2286-2322, 1990.

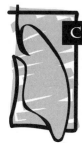

CHAPTER 8

Specialized Test Regimens

OBJECTIVES

After studying this chapter you should be able to do the following:

1 Describe at least two methods of performing bronchial challenge tests

2 Identify a positive response to a bronchial challenge test

3 List two indications for preoperative pulmonary function testing

4 Suggest appropriate tests to evaluate disability in either chronic obstructive pulmonary disease or pulmonary fibrosis

5 Contrast spirometry measurements in children to those performed on adults

6 Name two criteria for judging the acceptability of metabolic measurements

DIAGNOSIS OF SPECIFIC PULMONARY disorders requires that appropriate tests are performed. Specialized test regimens, such as those described in this chapter, often consist of standard tests performed under special conditions. For example, forced expiratory volume (FEV_1), may be analyzed after inhalation challenge, hyperventilation, or exercise to quantify airway reactivity. The clinical question asked regarding an individual patient may be whether he or she qualifies for disability or if it is safe for the patient to undergo surgery. Spirometry, lung volumes, diffusing capacity (DL_{co}), or blood gas analysis may be required to resolve these questions.

Pulmonary function tests are also performed on pediatric patients. Newborns, infants, and very young children cannot perform spirometry or related tests that require cooperation. Specialized testing techniques allow some tests to be adapted for children.

Metabolic measurements are widely used to assess caloric needs and nutritional support in a variety of patients. The methods used are similar to those used in gas exchange measurements during exercise. Specialized calculations allow very precise description of the nutritional status of the patient.

Bronchial Challenge Testing

Bronchial challenge testing is used to identify and characterize airway hyperreactivity. Challenge tests are performed in subjects with symptoms of bronchospasm who have normal pulmonary function studies or uncertain results of bronchodilator studies. Bronchial challenge can also be used to assess changes in hyperreactivity of the airways or to quantify its severity. Bronchial challenge tests are sometimes used to screen individuals who may be at risk from environmental or occupational exposure to toxins.

Several commonly used provocative agents can be used to assess airway hyperreactivity. These include the following:

- Methacholine challenge
- Histamine challenge
- **Eucapnic** hyperventilation (using either cold or room temperature gas)
- Exercise

Each of these agents may trigger bronchospasm, but in slightly different ways. Methacholine is a chemical stimuli that increases parasympathetic tone in bronchial smooth muscle. Histamine triggers a similar response producing bronchoconstriction. Hyperventilation, either at rest or during exercise, results in heat and water loss from the airway. This provokes bronchospasm in susceptible subjects. With each of these agents, pulmonary function variables are assessed before and after exposure to the challenge. FEV_1 is the variable most commonly used. Other flow measurements, as well as airway resistance (Raw) and conductance (SGaw) are also evaluated before and after challenge.

METHACHOLINE CHALLENGE

Bronchial challenge by inhalation of methacholine is performed by having the subject inhale increasing doses of the drug. Spirometry, and sometimes SGaw are measured after each dose. Most clinicians consider the test positive when inhalation of methacholine precipitates a 20% decrease in the FEV_1. The methacholine concentration at which this 20% decrease occurs is called the provocative dose or **$PD_{20\%}$**. In the doses usually employed (Table 8-1), normal subjects do not display decreases greater than 20% in the FEV_1. Therefore the methacholine challenge test is highly specific for airway hyperreactivity. Many subjects who have hyperreactive airways experience a 20% reduction in FEV_1 with doses of 8 mg/ml or less. Some subjects who have hyperreactive airways may display decreases in FEV_1 less than 20%, even at the highest dose of methacholine.

Subjects to be tested should be asymptomatic, with no coughing or obvious wheezing. Their baseline FEV_1 should be greater than 80% of their expected value. For subjects with known obstruction or restriction, the FEV_1 should exceed 80% of their highest previously observed value. Obvious airway obstruction (i.e., $FEV_{1\%}$ less than predicted, SGaw less than 0.09 L/sec/cm H_2O/L) are relative contraindications. Bronchial challenge may be indicated in obstructed patients if the clinical question is related to the degree of responsiveness.

If the subject has been taking bronchodilators, they should be withheld according to the schedule listed in Table 8-2. Other medications or substances can affect the validity of the challenge as well.

Baseline spirometry is performed to establish that the subject's FEV_1 is greater than 80% of

TABLE 8-1   Methacholine Dosing Schedules

0.025 mg/ml	0.075 mg/ml
0.250 mg/ml	0.150 mg/ml
2.50 mg/ml	0.310 mg/ml
5.00 mg/ml	0.620 mg/ml
10.0 mg/ml	1.25 mg/ml
25.0 mg/ml	2.50 mg/ml
	5.00 mg/ml
	10.0 mg/ml
	25.0 mg/ml

TABLE 8-2   Withholding Bronchodilators Before Bronchial Challenge

β-Adrenergic agents (oral or inhaled)	12 hours
Anticholinergic aerosols	12 hours
Sustained-action theophylline preparations	48 hours
Cromolyn sodium and related preparations	48 hours
Antihistamines	48 hours
Corticosteroids, inhaled or oral	Subjects should be challenged while taking a stable dosage
Antihistamines	72-96 hours
H_1-receptor antagonists	48 hours
Caffeine-containing drinks (cola, coffee)	6 hours
β-Blocking agents	May increase the response

predicted or the previously observed best value. Subjects who demonstrate obstruction based on reduced $FEV_{1\%}$ or other flows do not require challenge testing to document airway hyperreactivity. However, obstructed subjects may be tested to establish the degree of hyperreactivity. Subjects who have a restrictive process (i.e., reduced FEV_1, forced vital capacity [FVC], and total lung capacity [TLC]) may also be tested for hyperreactive airways. The FEV_1 measured before inhalation of the aerosolized drug is called the baseline value. Spirometric measurements should meet all the criteria for acceptability as for routine spirometry (see Chapter 2).

A small-volume, gas-powered nebulizer may be used to generate the methacholine aerosol. The nebulizer should generate an aerosol with a particle size in the range of 2 to 5 μm (mass median aerodynamic diameter). This particle range promotes deposition in the medium and small airways. A **dosimeter** may provide a true "quantitative" challenge test by delivering a consistent volume of drug. The dosimeter (or nebulizer) should be activated during inspiration, either automatically by a flow sensor or manually by the subject. A driving pressure of approximately 20 psi is used for most dosimeters. An activation time of 0.5 to 0.6 seconds allows a fixed volume of aerosol to be generated for each breath. By limiting the period of aerosol production, the last part of the inhalation carries the aerosol into the lung. Some dosimeters generate aerosol for a longer interval (5 to 6 seconds) so that the **agonist** is delivered throughout the vital capacity (VC) maneuver. Ideally the dosimeter or nebulizer should have an output sufficiently high so that 1 ml of solution can be aerosolized during the course of the inhalations at each level. If multiple nebulizers are used for the increasing dilutions, their outputs should be similar. Continuous low- or high-flow nebulization schemes may also be used. Aerosol output and flow rates should be kept as constant as possible to ensure reproducibility.

The delivered dose of methacholine is standardized by using a fixed number of breaths or breathing for a fixed length of time (2 minutes). In the first method the subject begins by inhaling five breaths of nebulized **diluent**, usually normal saline. The breaths should be slow and deep. The subject should inspire from functional residual capacity (FRC) to TLC, with a short (2 to 5 seconds) breath hold at TLC to maximize aerosol deposition. In the second method, normal relaxed breathing is used as the subject inhales the aerosol. After 3 minutes with either method, spirometry is repeated. The highest FEV_1 after inhalation of the diluent then becomes the "control." If FEV_1 is not reduced 10% from the baseline value, inhalation of methacholine is begun. Some subjects with highly reactive airways may have a positive response (i.e., a 10% decrease in FEV_1) to the diluent. As for routine spirometry, three acceptable FVC maneuvers should be obtained. The two best FEV_1 and FVC values should be within 200 ml. If the FEV_1 values are not reproducible (i.e., within 200 ml), the validity of further testing may be questionable. Because the test's objective is to detect a fall in FEV_1, results that cannot be reproduced may lead to a false-positive interpretation.

Two dosage protocols with slightly different methacholine dilutions are commonly used (see Table 8-1). The five-dilution set allows the test to be completed more quickly. The nine-dilution protocol uses smaller differences between concentrations at the lower levels. Each of these dilutions may be prepared from a 25 mg/ml stock solution. The stock solution is prepared by dissolving the powdered drug in an aqueous diluent containing 0.5% NaCl, 0.275% $NaHCO_3$, and 0.4% phenol. This diluent has a pH of 7.0 and helps sterilize the solution. Methacholine is stable after mixing and usually may be kept for up to 4 months if refrigerated at 4° C. The smallest dose (0.025 mg/ml) is the least stable and may need to be prepared immediately before testing.

Volumes of 1 ml are suitable for five inhalations or 2 minutes of quiet breathing using common nebulizers. Other dilutions may be used but should be arranged in such a way that doses approximately double, up to 25 mg/ml. An adequate number of intermediate concentrations should be used (five or more) so that a 20% decrease in FEV_1 can be detected without inducing a more severe response. A bolus technique may also be used. In this protocol the subject inhales multiple breaths of a fixed concentration, with spirometry performed after each five breaths.

The subject either inhales five breaths (as described for the diluent) or breathes aerosol for 2 minutes, beginning with the lowest concentration. Spirometry is repeated at 3 minutes, with the "best" test selected from duplicate or triplicate efforts. The percent of decrease is calculated as follows:

$$\% \text{ Decrease} = \frac{X - Y}{X} \times 100$$

where:

X = control FEV_1 (after diluent)

Y = current FEV_1 after methacholine inhalation

A 20% or greater decrease in the FEV_1 is considered a positive test. The decrease should be sustained. Additional spirometry efforts may be necessary to distinguish an actual decrease from variability in the maneuvers. If the test is negative, the next larger dose is administered and measurements repeated. If the test is borderline positive (i.e., a fall of 15% to 20%), a partial dose of the next dilution may be given.

At each concentration, the subject should be observed and questioned for the perception of symptoms such as chest tightness or wheezing. Auscultation should be routinely performed to help detect the beginning of bronchospasm. As soon as a 20% fall in FEV_1 is observed, administration of methacholine is terminated. Bronchospasm may be reversed by means of an appropriate inhaled bronchodilator. Spirometry should be performed after reversal to document the efficacy of bronchodilator therapy in reversing the effects of methacholine (Fig. 8-1).

Several methods of quantifying the results of the procedure are commonly used. The concentration of methacholine that produced the 20% decrease in FEV_1 is reported as the provocative dose (PD_{20}). The PD_{20} is interpolated from the doses of methacholine just before and after the greater than 20% fall (see Fig. 8-1). A second method totals the amount of methacholine inhaled to produce the 20% decrease by multiplying the number of breaths times the dilution. Table 8-3 lists cumulative amounts of methacholine delivered using the five-breath routine and the nine-dilution dosage schedule listed previously.

A number of physiologic factors may limit the sensitivity and **specificity** of methacholine challenge testing. Spirometry (i.e., FEV_1) may not detect a response in all subjects. Raw or SGaw may be more sensitive in detecting hyperreactive airways in some individuals. A decrease in SGaw of 35% to 40% is considered a positive methacholine response. A significant number of individuals with symptoms of asthma may have primarily large airway changes in response to methacholine. These changes may manifest themselves as a fall in SGaw or blunting of the inspiratory limb of the flow-volume loop. Subjects with vocal cord dysfunction (**VCD**) are commonly referred for evaluation of asthma symptoms but may show little response to bronchial challenge. Deep inspiration and repeated spirometric efforts may also affect bronchial muscle tone. This may cause either bronchodilatation or bronchoconstriction.

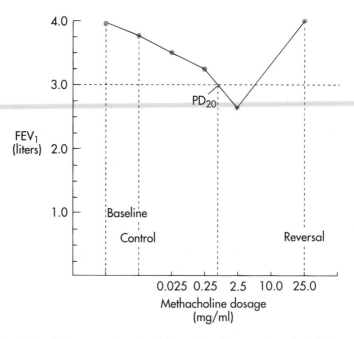

FIG. 8-1 *Methacholine challenge test.* Results of data gathered during a bronchial challenge test are shown. The dosage of the challenge agent (methacholine in this case) is plotted on a logarithmic scale on the X axis. FEV_1 (or other variable) is plotted on the Y axis. In this plot the first point represents a baseline FEV_1 of 4 L. The control (i.e., the FEV_1 after inhalation of the diluent) is plotted next. The FEV_1 after each dose of methacholine is plotted until a 20% decrease occurs. In this plot the FEV_1 fell by more than 20% with a dose of 2.5 mg/ml. A vertical line drawn from the point at which the dose response curve crosses the 20% line defines the PD_{20}. The subject was then given an inhaled bronchodilator to reverse the effect of the provocative agent, and this response is plotted.

Technical factors can also make methacholine challenge tests difficult, if not impossible, to interpret (Box 8-1). Variable efforts by the subject (FEV_1 values not within 200 ml or SGaw values not within 10%) may produce a false-positive test result. Different types of nebulizers and dosimeters affect the amount of agonist reaching the airways. Factors that should be controlled as much as possible include nebulizer output, particle size, inhaled volumes, breath-hold times, and inspiratory flow. Nebulizer driving pressure and/or flow should be consistent throughout the test. The spirometer used should meet the minimal standards set by the American Thoracic Society (see Chapter 10). It should provide spirometric tracings or flow-volume loops for later evaluation.

Methacholine challenge testing presents some risk to the subject, so a physician experienced in bronchial provocation should be immediately available. Technologists administering bronchial challenge tests should be thoroughly familiar with the procedure and with the signs and symptoms of bronchospasm. Medications for reversal of the bronchospasm (i.e., epinephrine) and for resuscitation should be immediately available in the event of an adverse reaction. Because of the risks involved, some laboratories require written consent from the subject. The test should be

TABLE 8-3   Units for Methacholine Challenge*

Methacholine concentration (mg/ml)	Cumulative number of breaths	Cumulative units/five breaths	Cumulative number of minutes
0.075	5	0.375	3
0.15	10	1.125	6
0.31	15	2.68	9
0.62	20	5.78	12
1.25	25	12.00	15
2.50	30	24.50	18
5.00	35	49.50	21
10.00	40	99.50	24
25.00	45	225.00	27

*One methacholine unit is arbitrarily defined as one inhalation of 1 mg/ml of methacholine in diluent. The quantity of drug required to provoke a 20% decrease in FEV_1 is expressed in X units/X minutes, for example, 12 methacholine units/15 minutes.

BOX 8-1
CRITERIA FOR ACCEPTABILITY—BRONCHIAL CHALLENGE TESTS

1   The subject should withhold all bronchodilators before the test. The subject should also be free of upper or lower respiratory infection, and not ingest any caffeinated beverages before the test.

2   Spirometric and/or plethysmographic efforts must meet standard criteria for acceptability and re-producibility. For adults, two FEV_1 measurements should be within 200 ml or 5% (depending on the criteria used by the laboratory) at each challenge level. SGaw measurements should be within 10% after each challenge level.

3   For methacholine and histamine challenges, a nebulizer that produces aerosol particles in the 2 to 5 μm range should be used. Nebulizer output, inspiratory flow, lung volume, and breath-hold time should be consistent for all levels (doses) of challenge.

4   For exercise challenge, the subject should attain at least 75% of the predicted maximal heart rate (or $\dot{V}O_{2max}$, if measured). This level should be maintained for 6 to 8 minutes. Measurement of $\dot{V}E$ is recommended.

5   For hyperventilation challenges (cold or room air), the target ventilation level should be maintained for the specified interval (dependent on protocol used). For EVH, a target ventilation of $30 \times FEV_1$ for 6 minutes is recommended.

6   For all challenge protocols, clinical signs and symptoms (e.g., presence or absence of coughing, wheezing) should be documented.

administered in a well-ventilated room to protect other patients and the technologist from exposure. Technologists with known sensitivity to methacholine should not perform this procedure.

HISTAMINE CHALLENGE

Aerosolized histamine extract (histamine phosphate) may be used for inhalation challenge in a manner similar to methacholine challenge. Histamine produces bronchoconstriction by an uncertain pathway. The response to histamine can be blocked by **antihistamines** or H_1-receptor antagonists. Histamine-induced bronchospasm is also partially blocked by most classes of bronchodilators. Histamine differs from methacholine in its side effects, **half-life,** and cumulative effects. Flushing and headache are two common side effects of histamine inhalation. The peak action of histamine occurs within 30 seconds to 2 minutes, which is similar to that observed in methacholine. Recovery of baseline function is significantly shorter for histamine than for methacholine. The action of histamine, unlike methacholine, is thought to be less cumulative.

Subject preparation for histamine challenge is similar to that used for methacholine (see Table 8-2). Antihistamines and H_1-receptor antagonists should be withheld for 48 hours before testing.

Table 8-4 lists the dosing protocol for histamine challenge. These increments approximately double the concentration of drug at each level. The same criteria as those used for baseline spirometry in methacholine challenge are observed. Diluent is administered first to determine a control value for FEV_1.

If FEV_1 does not fall by more than 10%, then five breaths of the first dilution are administered. Spirometric measurements are performed immediately, then repeated at 3 minutes. A response is considered positive if FEV_1 falls by 20% or more below the control at 3 minutes. If there is a negative response, the next dose is given and measurements repeated.

The results of histamine challenge are reported in a manner similar to that described for methacholine. The concentration of histamine that produced a 20% fall in FEV_1 is termed the PD_{20}. Response may also be reported by graphing the percentage of change in FEV_1 against the concentration (or its logarithm) of the drug. This type of plot is commonly called a dose-response graph. It permits interpolation of the precise concentration of drug that elicited the 20% decrease (see Fig. 8-1).

Histamine, like methacholine, is relatively safe if testing follows the procedures described. Baseline and control values should always be established (Box 8-2). Bronchial challenge should always begin with a low concentration of drug. The range of concentrations used should be appropriate for the subject tested. For adult subjects in whom airway hyperreactivity is the suspected diagnosis, the dosing schedules previously described are recommended. Subjects who have a positive response to histamine challenge recover more quickly than if tested with methacholine. Histamine challenge can be repeated within 2 hours after the subject has returned to baseline level of function.

EUCAPNIC HYPERVENTILATION

Airway hyperreactivity may also be assessed by having the subject breathe at a high level of ventilation. Heat or water loss from the upper airways has been demonstrated to provoke bronchospasm in susceptible individuals. These physiologic changes are most pronounced when the subject inhales cold, dry gas, but they can also be demonstrated with gas at room temperature.

TABLE 8-4	Histamine Dosing Schedule
	0.03 mg/ml
	0.06 mg/ml
	0.12 mg/ml
	0.25 mg/ml
	1.00 mg/ml
	2.50 mg/ml
	5.00 mg/ml
	10.00 mg/ml

To prevent respiratory alkalosis (i.e., true hyperventilation) carbon dioxide (CO_2) is mixed with inspired air. This gas mixture allows high levels of ventilation with little effect on pH.

Subjects to be tested using eucapnic hyperventilation should withhold bronchodilators as suggested in Table 8-2. Baseline spirometry is performed to ascertain that airway obstruction is not present. In ventilation challenges, the baseline is the control value with which subsequent measurements will be compared.

If cold air is to be used, the mixture is passed through a heat exchanger or over a cooling coil. These devices lower the temperature and remove water vapor from the gas. Gas temperatures are reduced to a subfreezing level in the range of $-10°$ to $-20°$ C. The relative humidity is usually very near 0%.

The subject breathes the gas at an elevated level of ventilation. In one method the subject breathes at a fraction of their maximal voluntary ventilation (MVV) (i.e., 30% to 70% of the MVV). CO_2 is added to the gas to maintain a stable $Petco_2$. This is accomplished either by titrating CO_2 into the mixture or by using a gas composed of 5% CO_2, 21% O_2, and the balance N_2. The subject maintains the specified level of ventilation for 4 to 6 minutes. Spirometry or SGaw is then measured at fixed intervals after the hyperventilation (e.g., 1, 5, and 10 minutes). A second method has the subject breathe at increasing levels of ventilation up to the MVV (e.g., 7.5, 15, 30, 60 L/min and MVV). Again CO_2 is added to the inspired gas to maintain isocapnia (i.e., $Paco_2$ of approximately 40 mm Hg).

Eucapnic voluntary hyperventilation (EVH) with room-temperature gas also provides a ready stimulus for bronchospasm. In this technique, the subject breathes a mixture of 5% CO_2, 21% O_2, and balance N_2 at room temperature. The gas is used to fill a "target" bag or balloon of approximately 5 L (Fig. 8-2). The subject breathes from the bag via a nonrebreathing valve (see Chapter 9) and large-bore tubing. A nose clip is worn by the subject. A high-output flow meter is used to fill the target bag. The flow meter is adjusted to deliver gas at approximately 30 times the subject's FEV_1. The subject breathes from the bag and tries to match ventilation to the bag to keep it partly deflated. The high level of ventilation is continued for 5 to 6 minutes. Spirometry is performed immediately after hyperventilation and then at 5-minute intervals.

For both the cold-air and room-temperature protocols, if no fall in FEV_1 occurs within 20 minutes after hyperventilation, the test may be considered negative. The percentage of decrease is calculated just as for methacholine challenge testing, described previously. A fall of 15% is

---

BOX 8-2
INTERPRETIVE STRATEGIES—BRONCHIAL CHALLENGE TESTS

1 Was the challenge agent administered appropriately?
   For methacholine or histamine, were the doses of agonist appropriate?
   Was nebulizer output, inspiratory flow, etc. consistent for each dose?
   For exercise, did the subject maintain an appropriate workload for 6 to 8 minutes?
   For hyperventilation, did the subject maintain the target level of ventilation?

2 Were there any pretest factors that might influence results? Failure to withhold bronchodilators? Respiratory infection? If so, interpret cautiously or not at all.

3 Were spirometric efforts acceptable and reproducible before and after challenge? If not, interpret very cautiously or not at all.

4 For methacholine or histamine challenge, was there a 10% decrease in FEV_1 after inhaling diluent? If so, test is positive. Was there a 20% decrease in FEV_1 after inhalation of the agonist? If so, test is positive. Was there a 35% decrease in SGaw (if measured)? If so, test is positive.

5 For exercise or hyperventilation challenge, was there a 15% to 20% decrease in FEV_1 after challenge? If so, test is positive.

6 Were there signs or symptoms of airway hyperreactivity (coughing, wheezing, shortness of breath)? If so, test suggests bronchial hyperresponsiveness.

7 Were the results borderline? If so, consider repeat testing in the future.

8 Were symptoms present despite little or no change in FEV_1? Consider additional measurements such as SGaw, or related conditions such as vocal cord dysfunction.

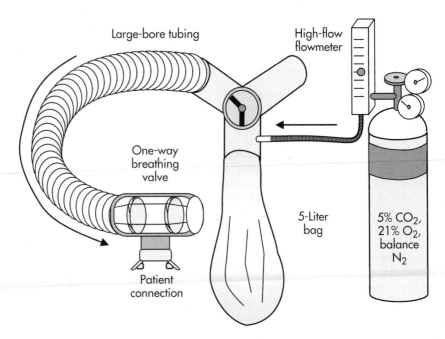

FIG. 8-2 *Breathing circuit for eucapnic voluntary hyperventilation (EVH).* A gas containing 5% CO_2, 21% O_2, and balance N_2 is directed through a precision high-flow flowmeter to a reservoir bag. Flow is adjusted to a target ventilation level, such as 30 times the subject's FEV_1. The subject then breathes from the bag via a one-way valve with large-bore tubing. The subject is coached to increase ventilation so as to keep the bag partially deflated. The test is continued for a predetermined interval, usually 6 minutes.

consistent with some degree of airway hyperreactivity (see Box 8-2). Some asthmatic subjects may experience decreases of FEV_1 greater than 20%. Bronchospasm should be reversed with inhaled bronchodilators, and the reversal documented with spirometry.

Hyperventilation tests can be used when SGaw is measured. Because the airway challenge is applied once, the subject can remain in the body plethysmograph for measurements at defined intervals. Cold-air testing requires specialized equipment to refrigerate and dry inspired gas. Testing with cold air is slightly more sensitive and specific than testing with room-temperature gas. Both techniques correlate well with the results of methacholine challenge tests, although they are slightly less specific. If multiple levels of ventilation are evaluated, a dose-response curve can be constructed. However, the single challenge is less complicated and can be used to evaluate subjects with airway hyperreactivity.

EXERCISE CHALLENGE

Exercise-induced asthma (**EIA**) is typified by bronchospasm during or immediately after vigorous exercise. EIA is related to heat and water loss from the upper airway that accompanies increased ventilation during exercise. Evaluation of exercise-induced bronchospasm (**EIB**) may be helpful in the following instances:

1. In subjects who have shortness of breath on exertion but exhibit normal resting pulmonary function
2. In symptomatic subjects in whom other bronchial provocation tests produce negative or ambiguous results
3. In subjects with known EIA in whom therapy is being evaluated
4. In screening subjects where some risk to asthmatics might be involved (e.g., athletics)

Subjects referred for exercise challenge should be evaluated by means of an appropriate history and physical examination. The evaluation should include a resting electrocardiogram (ECG) to ascertain potential contraindications to exercise testing (see Chapter 7). Bronchodilators should be withheld as for methacholine challenge testing, as described previously (see Table 8-2). Before exercise, the subject's FEV_1 should not be less than 65% of the predicted value. Subjects with overt obstruction do not require an exercise challenge to demonstrate airway hyperreactivity.

Either a treadmill or cycle ergometer may be used, depending on the type of physiologic measurements being made. Exercise should be vigorous enough to elicit work rates of 60% to 85% of the subject's predicted heart rate (HR) for 6 to 8 minutes. The subject's response to an increasing workload should be monitored via continuous ECG and blood pressure (BP). Measurement of variables such as minute ventilation ($\dot{V}E$) and tidal volume (VT) may be helpful in assessing the ventilatory load imposed by the exercise.

A spirometer that meets the American Thoracic Society requirements (see Chapter 10) is necessary. The spirometer should store data from multiple efforts with volume-time or flow-volume curves, or both. Some systems provide software specifically for challenge testing (either by inhalation or exercise) with capability for superimposing maximum expiratory flow-volume (MEFV) curves. Resuscitation equipment, as described in Chapter 7, should be available.

Low-intensity exercise for 1 to 2 minutes allows evaluation of ventilatory and cardiovascular responses to work. As soon as a normal cardiovascular response is observed, workload should be increased until the subject attains 85% of predicted maximum HR or predicted maximum oxygen consumption ($\dot{V}O_2$). In most instances, a short period (6 to 8 minutes) of moderately heavy work is all that is required to trigger exercise-induced bronchospasm. Bronchospasm usually occurs immediately after the exercise, not during it, unless the test is extended over a longer interval (see Box 8-2). Repeated testing within 2 hours may result in a **"refractory period"** during which the severity of the bronchoconstriction lessens. This response is presumably caused by the release of catecholamines. An extended warm-up period before the actual exercise may also protect the airways and lessen subsequent bronchoconstriction.

Baseline spirometry values are established before testing. As for hyperventilation challenge, the baseline value is also the control. After exercise, spirometry is performed at 1 to 2 minutes, then every 5 minutes as the selected variable (usually FEV_1 or SGaw) decreases to a minimum. The highest value of acceptable measurements is recorded. Testing is continued until the parameter returns to baseline. Maximal decreases are typically seen in the first 5 to 10 minutes after cessation of exercise. A fall in the FEV_1 of 10% to 20% is usually consistent with increased airway reactivity. Spontaneous recovery occurs within 20 to 40 minutes. Severe bronchospasm may be reversed using an inhaled bronchodilator. Ambient temperature, relative humidity, and barometric pressure (PB) should be recorded because of their influence on airway muscle tone.

Several methods of reporting the response to exercise are commonly used:

1. Maximum percent of decrease of baseline function:

$$\frac{X - Y}{X} \times 100$$

where:

$$X = \text{baseline value (such as } FEV_1)$$
$$Y = \text{lowest postexercise value}$$

2. Maximum decrease as a percentage of the predicted value:

$$\frac{X - Y}{P} \times 100$$

where:

$$X = \text{baseline value (such as } FEV_1)$$
$$Y = \text{lowest postexercise value}$$
$$P = \text{subject's predicted value}$$

3. Lowest value as a percent of predicted value:

$$\frac{Y}{P} \times 100$$

where:

$$Y = \text{lowest postexercise value}$$
$$P = \text{subject's predicted value}$$

The first method is the same as that described for inhalation or ventilation challenge tests. The advantage of this method is that the baseline (i.e., control) parameter is included in both numerator and denominator, providing a measure independent of absolute values. This makes it useful for comparison between subjects. The second method relates postexercise decreases to the subject's predicted value. The third method simply states the lowest value after the challenge as a percentage of the predicted value. Baseline values should always be reported, particularly if the third method is used.

One potential problem with using exercise to elicit EIB is that the level of exercise chosen may not mimic the real-world triggers. Subjects who are fit may not attain a level of ventilation high enough to trigger EIB, even though exercising at 85% of their maximum HR. Measurement of $\dot{V}_E$ during exercise may be needed to determine the level of ventilation attained. Similarly, subjects whose asthma is triggered by cold, dry air may not show a maximal response if tested under standard laboratory conditions. Exercise-induced bronchospasm may be evaluated using one of the hyperventilation techniques described previously. These techniques eliminate the need for more complicated exercise testing. EVH (using a target ventilation level) may be more sensitive in detecting airway hyperreactivity than exercise testing.

Preoperative Pulmonary Function Testing

Preoperative pulmonary function testing is one of several means available to clinicians to evaluate surgical candidates at risk for developing respiratory complications. Preoperative testing, in conjunction with history and physical examination, ECG, and chest x-ray examination, is indicated for any of the following reasons:

1. To estimate postoperative lung function in candidates for **pneumonectomy** or lobectomy
2. To plan perioperative care, including preoperative preparation, type and duration of anesthetic during surgery, and postoperative care to minimize complications
3. To enhance the estimate of risk involved in the surgical procedure (i.e., morbidity and mortality) derived from history and physical examination

The need for preoperative pulmonary function testing is determined by the type of surgical procedure and the individual's risk factors. Many investigations, both prospective and retrospective, have identified that the risk of postoperative pulmonary complications are highest in thoracic procedures, followed by upper and lower abdominal procedures. Increased incidence of complications occurs in both healthy subjects and those who have pulmonary disorders. Subjects who have pulmonary disease are at higher risk in proportion to the degree of pulmonary impairment.

Preoperative pulmonary function testing is indicated in subjects who have the following:

1. A smoking history
2. Symptoms of pulmonary disease (i.e., cough, sputum production, shortness of breath)
3. Abnormal physical examination findings, particularly of the chest (i.e., abnormal breath sounds, ventilatory pattern, respiratory rate)
4. Abnormal chest radiographs

Preoperative testing may also be indicated in the following:

1. Subjects who are morbidly obese (i.e., greater than 30% above ideal body weight)
2. Subjects advanced in age, usually greater than 70 years
3. Subjects who have current or recent respiratory infections or a history of respiratory infections
4. Subjects who are markedly **debilitated** or malnourished

In each of these subjects, the primary purpose of pulmonary function testing is to reveal preexisting pulmonary impairment. VC may decrease more than 50% from the preoperative value in thoracic or upper abdominal procedures. This places individuals with compromised function at risk of developing atelectasis and pneumonia. Postoperative decreases in the FRC and increases in closing volume (CV) may lead to ventilation-perfusion ($\dot{V}/\dot{Q}$) abnormalities and hypoxemia. Abnormal ventilatory function related to the central control of respiration or to the ventilatory muscles may also play a role in postoperative complications.

Certain tests of pulmonary function appear to be better predictors of postoperative complications. These tests should be used both for risk evaluation and to assist in planning the perioperative care of the individual.

1. *Spirometry.* FVC, FEV_1, $FEF_{25\%-75\%}$, MVV. Obstructive disease can be easily identified with simple spirometry. A significant percentage of subjects who might have postoperative problems develop can be detected with minimal screening. Subjects who have reduced FVC, with or without airways obstruction, typically have an impaired ability to cough effectively when the VC decreases further during the immediate postoperative period. The MVV, although dependent on subject effort, appears to be uniquely suited to detecting postoperative risk. This may result in part from the fact the MVV tests lung parenchyma, airway function, ventilatory muscle function, and subject cooperation. The measured MVV correlates better with the incidence of postoperative problems than the estimated MVV (i.e., $FEV_1 \times 35$ or 40). This may be attributable to measurement of both inspiratory and expiratory flow during the MVV, whereas the FEV_1 assesses just expiration. Because the ventilatory muscles may be involved in the development of postoperative complications, the MVV may be a more sensitive predictor than forced expiratory flows.

2. *Bronchodilator studies.* Operative candidates who have airway obstruction should also be tested with bronchodilators. Postbronchodilator values for FVC, FEV_1, $FEF_{25\%-75\%}$, and MVV may be used in estimating the surgical risk. There may be significantly less risk if the subject's airway obstruction is reversible. Bronchodilator studies are similarly helpful in planning perioperative care. Bronchodilator therapy may improve the subject's bronchial hygiene both before and after surgery.

3. *Blood gas analysis.* Arterial blood gas analysis is helpful in assessing subjects with documented lung disease to determine the response to pulmonary changes that occur postoperatively. The Pa_{O_2} itself is not a good predictor of postoperative problems. Individuals with hypoxemia at rest usually also have abnormal spirometry results, and hence are at risk. The Pa_{O_2} may actually improve postoperatively in subjects undergoing thoracotomy for lung resection, if the resected portion was contributing to $\dot{V}/\dot{Q}$ abnormalities. The Pa_{CO_2} appears to be the most useful blood gas indicator of surgical risk. If the Pa_{CO_2} is above 45 mm Hg, there is a marked increase in postoperative morbidity and mortality. Elevated Pa_{CO_2} values are most commonly encountered in subjects with significant airways obstruction.

4. *Exercise testing.* Exercise studies can accurately predict subjects at risk. Individuals who cannot tolerate moderate workloads typically have airways obstruction or similar ventilatory limitations. Subjects who can attain an oxygen uptake of greater than 20 ml/min/kg typically have a low incidence of cardiopulmonary complications. Those unable to attain a $\dot{V}_{O_2}$ of 15 ml/min/kg almost always have complications.

Lung volumes, even though they may be reduced dramatically in the immediate postsurgical phase, do not correlate well preoperatively with postoperative complications and do not enhance the estimate of complications. Diffusion studies, like lung volume determinations, do not appear to improve the prediction of postoperative complications.

In addition to routine pulmonary function studies, several other tests are used in predicting postoperative lung function in candidates for pneumonectomy or lobectomy. These procedures are normally used in addition to spirometry and blood gas analysis.

1. *Perfusion and $\dot{V}/\dot{Q}$ scans.* Lung scans are particularly useful in estimating the remaining lung function in patients who are likely to require removal of all or part of a lung. Split-function scans are performed. These allow partitioning of lungs into right and left halves, or into multiple lung regions. Although ventilation-perfusion scans give the best estimate of overall function, simple perfusion scans yield similar information. Lung scan data, in the form of regional function percentages, are used in combination with simple spirometric indices to calculate the patient's postoperative capacity. An example follows:

$$\text{Postoperative } FEV_1 = \text{Preoperative } FEV_1 \times \%\text{Perfusion to unaffected portions}$$

Subjects whose postoperative FEV_1 is calculated to be less than 800 ml are typically not considered surgical candidates. Resection of any lung parenchyma resulting in an FEV_1 less than 800 ml would leave the subject more severely impaired. One exception to this general guideline occurs in patients referred for lung volume reduction surgery. These candidates are usually end-stage chronic

| TABLE 8-5 | Preoperative Pulmonary Function | | |

Test	Increased postoperative risk	High postoperative risk	Candidate for pneumonectomy*
FVC	Less than 50% of predicted	Less than 1.5 L	
FEV_1	Less than 2.0 L or 50% of predicted	Less than 1.0 L	Greater than 2.0 L
$FEF_{25\%-75\%}$	Less than 50% of predicted		
MVV		Less than 50 L/min or 50% of predicted	Greather than 50 L/min or 50% of predicted
$Paco_2$		Greater than 45 mm Hg	
Vo_{2max}	15-20 ml/min/kg	Less than 15 ml/min/kg	
Predicted post-operative FEV_1			Greater than 0.8 L/min
Pulmonary artery occlusion			Less than 35 mm Hg

*Values in this column determine whether the subject is to be considered a candidate for lung resection (see text).

obstructive pulmonary disease (COPD) patients, often with FEV_1 values less than 800 ml. Removal of poorly ventilated lung tissue often results in an improvement in spirometry, with significant increases in both FVC and FEV_1.

2. *Pulmonary artery occlusion pressure.* In some candidates for pneumonectomy, the development of postoperative pulmonary hypertension may be a limiting factor. To estimate the effect of redirecting the entire right ventricular output to the remaining lung, a catheter is inserted into the pulmonary artery of the affected lung and blood flow occluded by means of a balloon. The resulting pressure increase in the remaining lung is then measured. A pressure increasing to less than 35 mm Hg is usually considered consistent with acceptable postoperative pressures. The effect of redirected blood flow on oxygenation may also be a consideration. This can also be examined during occlusion to estimate postoperative Pao_2.

These tests to predict the effects of resection on the remaining lung are normally used in series, with spirometry done first, followed by split-function lung scans if the spirometry results are acceptable, and then pulmonary artery occlusion pressure if the development of cor pulmonale is a concern. Table 8-5 summarizes some general ranges of values used for preoperative pulmonary function testing.

Pulmonary Function Testing for Disability

Pulmonary function tests are one of several means of determining a subject's inability to perform certain tasks. Respiratory impairment and disability, however, are not synonymous. Respiratory impairment relates to the failure of one or more of the functions of the lungs, as measured by pulmonary function studies. Disability is the inability to perform tasks required for employment and includes medically determinable physical or mental impairment. The impairment must be expected to either result in death or last for at least 12 months. Impairment in children must be comparable to that which would disable an adult.

Pulmonary function tests used to determine impairment leading to disability should characterize the type, extent, and cause of the impairment. Pulmonary function testing may not completely describe all the factors involved in the disabling impairment. Other factors involved may be the age, educational background, and the subject's motivation. The energy requirements of the task in question also affect a subject's level of disability.

Determination of the level of impairment caused by pulmonary disease usually includes history and physical examination, chest x-ray examination, other appropriate imaging techniques, and pulmonary function tests.

Physical examination does not allow measurement of disabling symptoms, but is useful in grading shortness of breath. Shortness of breath is the most prominent feature of respiratory impairment. Shortness of breath, like pain, is subjective. Tachypnea, cyanosis, and abnormal

TABLE 8-6   FEV₁ and FVC Values for Disability Determinations

Height without shoes (in)	FEV_1 equal to or less than (L/BTPS)	FVC equal to or less than (L/BTPS)
60 or less	1.05	1.25
61 to 63	1.15	1.35
64 to 65	1.25	1.45
66 to 67	1.35	1.55
68 to 69	1.45	1.65
70 to 71	1.55	1.75
72 or more	1.65	1.85

Adapted from Disability Evaluation under Social Security, US Department of Health and Human Services, Publication No. 64-039, 1994.

respiratory patterns are not indicative of the extent of impairment but may be helpful in interpretation of pulmonary function studies.

Chest x-ray studies do not correlate well with shortness of breath or pulmonary function studies, except in advanced cases of pneumoconioses (i.e., "dust" diseases). Absence of usual findings in the pneumoconioses may be helpful in excluding occupational exposure to toxins as part of the impairment.

Pulmonary function studies should be objective and reproducible, and most important, specific to the disorder being investigated. Impairments caused by chronic respiratory disorders usually produce irreversible loss of function because of ventilatory impairment, gas exchange abnormalities, or a combination of both.

FORCED VITAL CAPACITY AND FORCED EXPIRATORY VOLUME

Spirometry is the most useful index for the assessment of impairment caused by airway obstruction. The test should not be performed unless the subject is stable. The three largest FVC values and FEV_1 values should be within 5% or 0.1 L, whichever is greater. Each maneuver should be continued for 6 seconds or until there is no detectable change in volume for the last 2 seconds of the maneuver. The largest FVC and FEV_1 of three acceptable maneuvers is reported. FEV_1 reported when only a flow-volume curve is recorded is not acceptable. A volume-time tracing from which the FEV_1 can be measured is required. Spirometry is normally repeated after bronchodilator therapy. All lung volumes and flows must be reported at BTPS. Standing height, without shoes, should be used for comparison of measured values with limits for disability (Table 8-6). In case of marked spinal deformity, arm-span measurement should be used (see Chapter 1).

Volume calibration of the spirometer should agree to within 1% of a 3-L syringe. If spirometer accuracy is less than 99% but within 3% of the calibration syringe, a calibration correction factor should be used (see Chapter 10). If a flow-sensing spirometer is used, linearity should be documented by performing calibration at three different flows (3 L/6 sec, 3 L/3 sec, and 3 L/1 sec). The volume-time tracing should have the time sensitivity marked on the horizontal axis and the volume sensitivity marked on the vertical axis. The paper speed should be at least 20 mm/sec and the volume excursion at least 10 mm/L. The manufacturer and model of the spirometer should be stated in the report (Box 8-3).

DIFFUSING CAPACITY

The DL_{CO} is useful in determining impairment in restrictive disorders such as pulmonary fibrosis. The single-breath method should be used. The standard criteria for acceptability for the DL_{CO} maneuver should be applied (see Chapter 5). The reported value should be uncorrected for hemoglobin (Hb), but abnormal Hb or carboxyhemoglobin (COHb) values should be reported as well. If the DL_{CO} is greater than 40% of predicted but less than 60%, resting blood gas analysis is indicated.

ARTERIAL BLOOD GAS ANALYSIS

Although blood gas results are objective, they are largely nonspecific in determining impairment. The $A\text{-}aO_2$ gradient may not be reliable because it can be affected by hyperventilation (Table 8-7). Blood gas analysis may be required in diffuse pulmonary fibrosis and should include both the PaO_2 and the $PaCO_2$. Blood gases (and A-a gradient) may also be assessed during exercise. The require-

BOX 8-3
CRITERIA FOR ACCEPTABILITY—DISABILITY TESTING

1 Spirometer must show a 3-L calibration that is within 1% or corrected within 3%. Flow-based spirometers should be calibrated at three different flows to demonstrate linearity. The manufacturer and model of spirometer should be stated.

2 All FVC maneuvers should be recorded before and after bronchodilator challenge. Time scale must be at least 20 mm/sec, volume scale at least 10 mm/L. FEV_1 may *not* be calculated from a flow-volume tracing.

3 There must be at least three acceptable FVC maneuvers before bronchodilator; the two largest values (FVC, FEV_1) should be within 5% or 0.1 L, whichever is greater.

4 The spirogram must show peak flow early in expiration with a smooth, gradually decreasing flow. The maneuver is acceptable if the effort continues for 6 seconds or if there is a plateau with no change in volume for 2 seconds. The FEV_1 should be measured using back-extrapolation; the back-extrapolated volume should be less than 5% of FVC or 0.1 L, whichever is greater.

5 Postbronchodilator studies should be performed if FEV_1 is less than 70% of predicted. Postbronchodilator testing should be done 10 minutes after administration of the drug. The name of the drug should be included.

6 DL_{CO} testing (if performed) should meet all current American Thoracic Society recommendations. DL_{CO} uncorrected for Hb is reported.

7 Exercise testing (if performed) should be for 6 to 8 minutes at a workload of approximately 5 METS. Blood gas samples should be obtained at rest and during exercise.

8 Statements regarding the subject's ability to understand directions, as well as effort and cooperation, should be included with all tests.

TABLE 8-7   Arterial Oxygen Tension for Disability Determinations

	Less than 3000 ft above sea level	3000 to 6000 ft above sea level	Over 6000 ft above sea level
P_{CO_2} (mm Hg)	P_{O_2} (mm Hg)	P_{O_2} (mm Hg)	P_{O_2} (mm Hg)
30 or below	≤ 65	≤ 60	≤ 55
31	≤ 64	≤ 59	≤ 54
32	≤ 63	≤ 58	≤ 53
33	≤ 62	≤ 57	≤ 52
34	≤ 61	≤ 56	≤ 51
35	≤ 60	≤ 55	≤ 50
36	≤ 59	≤ 54	≤ 49
37	≤ 58	≤ 53	≤ 48
38	≤ 57	≤ 52	≤ 47
39	≤ 56	≤ 51	≤ 46
40 or above	≤ 55	≤ 50	≤ 45

Adapted from Disability Evaluation under Social Security, US Department of Health and Human Services, Publication No. 64-039, 1994.

ment for supplemental oxygen (O_2) may also be quantified by exercise blood gas analysis. Pulse oximetry or capillary blood gas analysis is not an acceptable substitute for arterial blood gas analysis.

EXERCISE TESTING

Subjects considered for exercise evaluation should first have resting blood gas evaluation, either sitting or standing. A steady-state exercise test (see Chapter 7) is then performed, preferably using a treadmill. The subject should exercise for 4 to 6 minutes at an O_2 consumption rate of

BOX 8-4
INTERPRETIVE STRATEGIES—DISABILITY TESTING

1 Were spirometry, diffusing capacity, blood gases, and exercise tests performed acceptably? If not, interpret very cautiously or not at all.

2 Was the FEV_1 less than the predicted limit for the subject's height? If so, disabling obstruction is very likely.

3 Was the FVC less than predicted limits for the subject's height? If so, disabling restrictive disease is likely.

4 Was the DL_{CO} (if measured) less than 10.5 ml/min/mm Hg or less than 40% of predicted? If so, the subject has a marked gas exchange abnormality.

5 Was the subject's Pao_2, measured while clinically stable on two occasions at least 3 weeks apart but within 6 months, equal to or less than published limits (adjusted for Pco_2 and altitude)? If so, disabling hypoxemia is present.

6 Was Pao_2 equal to or less than published limits during steady-state exercise (less than or equivalent to 5 METS) breathing air? If so, disabling hypoxemia is present.

7 Are the lung function measurements consistent with history, physical examination, chest x-ray study, and other imaging techniques?

approximately 17.5 ml/min/kg (approximately 5 METS) breathing room air. An equivalent workload should be used for cycle ergometry (e.g., 75 watts for a 175-lb subject). Blood gas samples should be drawn at this workload to determine whether significant hypoxemia is present (see Table 8-7). If the patient does not desaturate at this level, a higher workload can be used to determine exercise capacity. If the patient cannot achieve a workload of 5 METS, a lower workload can be selected to determine exercise capacity. Blood gas samples obtained after completion of exercise are unacceptable.

ECG should be monitored continuously throughout the exercise evaluation, and blood gases drawn during the final 2 minutes of the test. It may be helpful to measure $\dot{V}o_2$, $\dot{V}co_2$, and $\dot{V}E$. The altitude of the test site and barometric pressure should be included in the report to assist with interpretation of blood gas values.

In reporting impairment for the purpose of determining disability, the remaining functional capacity is as important in determining the subject's ability to perform a certain task as the percentage of lost function. Some statement of the subject's ability to understand and cooperate during pulmonary function measurements should accompany the tabular and graphic data.

Limits for determining disability on the basis of respiratory impairment have been set for the United States by the Social Security Administration. Criteria are set according to the disease category (Box 8-4). COPD is evaluated by comparing the FEV_1 to the values listed in Table 8-6. Restrictive ventilatory disorders are evaluated by comparing FVC with the respective values in Table 8-6. Impaired gas exchange is evaluated by comparing the subject's Pao_2 with the appropriate value in Table 8-7. Disability caused by asthma is also evaluated using FEV_1. Episodes of asthma (requiring emergency treatment or hospitalization) occurring at least every 2 months or at least six times per year may also be evidence of disability.

Pulmonary Function Testing in Children

Pulmonary function testing in children uses many of the same basic tests as employed for testing adults. Differences between adult and pediatric testing exist not only in the absolute dimensions of the pulmonary system but in two main areas concerned with the testing regimens themselves:

1. Newborns, infants, and very young children cannot strictly perform those tests that require and depend on subject cooperation. Such tests include VC, FVC maneuvers, MVV, and $DL_{CO}SB$.

2. Young children may perform variably on those tests that are effort dependent or that require considerable cooperation.

TESTING INFANTS AND YOUNG CHILDREN

Tests of lung function in infants and very young children are used to assess lung volumes, flows, and mechanical factors, including compliance and resistance. Inability to perform maximal efforts eliminates such parameters as FVC, FEV_1, or MEFV curves. Techniques have been developed that are particularly applicable to young children.

Partial Expiratory Flow Volume Curves

The partial expiratory flow volume (PEFV) curve is a record of the maximal flow developed over a portion of the VC. Infants and small children cannot voluntarily breathe in to TLC to perform an FVC maneuver. PEFV techniques attempt to measure maximal flow, or flow limitation, over only part of the subject's VC. In infants the forced exhalation is obtained by applying either a positive pressure to the thorax and abdomen or a negative pressure to the airway.

Forced Deflation Technique

An infant who is intubated and sedated can have the lungs manually inflated to TLC using approximately $+40$ cm H_2O. This inflation is performed four times with a 2 to 3 second breath-hold at TLC. The airway is then connected to a source of negative pressure (usually approximately -40 cm H_2O). Air is evacuated for a maximum of 3 seconds or until expiratory flow ceases (i.e., residual volume [RV] is reached). As the lungs empty, expiratory flow is plotted versus volume to obtain a flow-volume curve. The lungs are then reinflated with 100% O_2. This technique is usually reserved for flow measurements in infants in the critical care setting and is not performed routinely in the laboratory.

This technique produces an MEFV curve because the lungs can be inflated to near TLC. The test is repeated until reproducible curves are obtained. A number of factors influence flow measurements using the forced deflation technique. The size of the endotracheal tube, as well as its ability to seal the airway, affects maximal flow. The infant's sedation level may alter the lung volume (i.e., FRC) or the tone of the bronchial smooth muscle.

Rapid Thoracoabdominal Compression

In infants who are not intubated, the pressure necessary to produce a forced exhalation may be generated by an inflatable jacket that encircles the infant's chest and abdomen. This technique is called rapid thoracoabdominal compression (**RTC**) or more commonly the "squeeze" or "hug" technique. A PEFV curve is obtained by rapidly applying pressure around the thorax and abdomen at the end of inspiration. This increases pleural pressure and generates a forced expiration. The pressure jacket must reach 95% of the peak pressure within 50 to 100 msec. To do this, the jacket is connected to a pressure reservoir with a volume ten times greater than the jacket. This reservoir ensures a relatively constant pressure. Jacket pressure is increased during repeated maneuvers until flow limitation is achieved. That is, increasing the squeeze pressure does not result in any further increase in flow at a specific lung volume.

The infant is evaluated after falling asleep spontaneously or after sedation. The most commonly used sedative is chloral hydrate (50 to 100 mg/kg). Larger doses may be required for older infants or toddlers. Chloral hydrate should be used with caution if the child has clinical signs of wheezing. Barbiturates such as pentobarbital may be administered intravenously by a nurse or physician. Guidelines for sedation should be established by each laboratory in accordance with the guidelines of the Joint Commission for Accreditation of Healthcare Organizations.

Flow is measured using an infant face mask sealed with lubricant and attached to a low dead space pneumotachometer. The flow-volume curve may be displayed on either a storage oscilloscope or a computer display (Fig. 8-3). The tracing usually includes a display of tidal breathing as well as the RTC curve. The end-expiration point of the tidal breathing curve represents the child's FRC. Flow is commonly related to this point as the $\dot{V}_{max}FRC$.

Raised Volume Rapid Thoracoabdominal Compression

PEFV curves measured using RTC do not measure flows over the entire VC of the infant. To measure flow over a wider range of lung volume, two adaptations of RTC can be used. In one method the airway is occluded, or "clamped," using a cuff with variable pressures (20 to 90 cm H_2O). Rapid chest compression is then performed. Higher flows are generated, presumably as a result of increased lung volume. A second method uses a pump to increase lung volume before the squeeze is performed. During inspiration flow is augmented (by the pump) to increase intrathoracic pressure and lung volume. This technique is called raised volume rapid thoracic

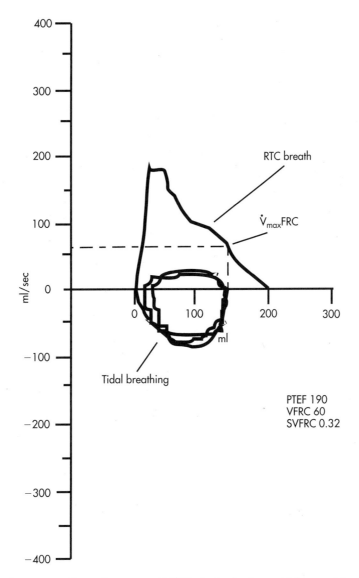

FIG. 8-3 *Partial expiratory flow-volume curve (PEFV) obtained using rapid thoracoabdominal compression (RTC or "squeeze").* The term *partial* refers to the fact that flow is plotted only over a portion of the vital capacity, rather than over the entire VC. The PEFV curve is obtained by applying positive pressure to the thorax and abdomen at end-inspiration using a pressure jacket. Jacket pressure is increased until no further increase in flow is achieved (see text). The primary flow measurement is the $V_{max}FRC$ (in this example, 60 ml/sec). Flow at FRC is determined by recording tidal breathing (smaller loops) to identify the end-expiratory point. Maximal flow at that volume is read from the PEFV tracing. Peak flow (PTEF) can also be read. If FRC has been determined, the specific flow at FRC (SVFRC) can be calculated (see text). A similar maneuver can be performed in young children who may not be able to inspire to TLC or exhale completely to RV by having them exhale forcefully after a normal inspiration.

compression (RVRTC). A pressure of 15 to 20 cm H_2O is all that may be required to significantly increase lung volumes. This technique allows FEV_t measurements, even in infants (where t = 0.5, 0.75, and even 1.0 seconds). These FEV_t measurements appear less variable than the V_{max} measured at FRC. FEV_t measured from RVRTC may also be more sensitive in detecting airway obstruction.

Flow measured by the squeeze technique may also be affected by numerous factors. Increased upper airway resistance, reflex glottic closure, and head and neck position can all alter measured flows. The infant's FRC may change during testing, thus influencing maximal flow. Sleeping or sedation may also affect flow measurements. Flow-limited curves have been demonstrated in infants with airway obstruction. Flow limitation in normal infants has not been clearly documented. In normal infants, high intrathoracic pressures are required to produce flow limitation at FRC. Another potential source of error may be gas compression in obstructed infants, so that volume measured (from flow) at the mouth may be less accurate than volume measured by plethysmograph.

In young children (ages 3 to 6 years) cooperation is essential to obtain reliable PEFV curves. Some children in this age group who have a good attention span and coordination may be capable of performing full MEFV curves. The child must be relaxed and able to follow instructions. The technologist's ability to elicit cooperation and to motivate the child is very important. Several attempts may be necessary to generate an adequate, reproducible effort.

The young child performs the PEFV maneuver breathing through a mouthpiece with a nose clip in place. Flow is measured by a pneumotachometer. Volume is determined by integration of the flow signal. The tracing may be displayed on a storage oscilloscope or computer screen. Tidal breathing is recorded to obtain a consistent end-expiratory point (FRC) on the volume axis. The child is then instructed to exhale forcefully from end-inspiration and to continue exhaling past the end-expiratory level to produce the PEFV curve.

The primary variable derived from the PEFV curve is flow at FRC (see Fig. 8-3). The highest flow obtained from multiple efforts is reported as the $\dot{V}_{max}FRC$. In infants, the pressure in the reservoir attached to the inflatable jacket is increased with each maneuver until a maximal flow is reached. Theoretically, when no further increase in flow results from increasing jacket pressure, flow limitation has been reached. However, it is unclear whether the applied pressure can be directly related to the pleural pressure under dynamic conditions. Flow limitation may not be achieved in a reproducible fashion. PEFV curves in young children probably represent maximal flows (i.e., flow limitation) if two or more reproducible curves can be obtained.

Infants with obstructive disease (i.e., severe airflow limitation) have intrathoracic obstruction which suggests that true flow limitation is reached during external compression. In healthy infants, inspiratory efforts or upper airway resistance such as closure of the glottis may impede forced expiratory flow. This causes flow at FRC to appear less than it would if true flow limitation occurred. Flow limitation occurs but not in an effort-independent manner.

To standardize measurements the $\dot{V}_{max}FRC$ may be divided by the absolute FRC determined either by helium (He) dilution, by nitrogen (N_2) washout, or by plethysmograph (V_{TG}). Maximal flow at FRC is then expressed as $\dot{V}_{max}FRC/FRC$ (or FRC/sec). This ratio in healthy infants is approximately 1.1 to 1.6. The $\dot{V}_{max}FRC$ displays a variability similar to flow measurements at low lung volumes ($\dot{V}max_{50}$, $\dot{V}max_{25}$) in older children or adults. Intersubject variability (approximately 30%) makes $\dot{V}_{max}FRC$ less sensitive than FEV_1 for detecting differences between healthy children and those with asthma.

PEFV curves in infants and young children have been used to assess normal lung growth and development. Asthma, cystic fibrosis, and bronchopulmonary dysplasia all cause reduced $\dot{V}_{max}FRC$ values. Bronchial challenge studies using methacholine, histamine, or cold air as the stimulus and $\dot{V}_{max}FRC$ as the dependent variable have shown that a significant number of infants and young children have nonspecific airway hyperreactivity. Because young children and infants typically cannot perform a forced expiratory maneuver to determine FEV_1, the $\dot{V}_{max}FRC$ may be helpful in tracing effectiveness of bronchodilators or related therapies. The FEV_1 is still the parameter of choice for detecting airway reactivity in older children and adolescents.

Lung Volumes

Lung volume determinations, specifically FRC, in infants and young children are usually accomplished using the closed-circuit He dilution, open-circuit N_2 washout, or body plethysmograph techniques. Special equipment is required to adapt the general methods for each of these techniques to the pediatric patient. For the He dilution technique, a small-volume spirometer is used for infants. System volume and dead space components must be reduced to accommodate the small FRC volumes encountered in children. FRC determination by N_2 washout must also be adjusted for infants and small children. Analyzer response time, phase delay between flow and gas concentrations, and sampling rate may affect accuracy. For both gas dilution methods, small leaks have a major impact on the accuracy of results because of the small absolute volumes being measured. Multiple FRC measurements (five to six) are recommended, with highest and lowest values discarded and the remaining results averaged (Box 8-5).

BOX 8-5
CRITERIA FOR ACCEPTABILITY—PFTs IN CHILDREN*

1   Volume displacement spirometers should be calibrated using a syringe volume appropriate for the child to be tested. Flow-based spirometers should be calibrated using flows that approximate the range over which measurement will be made. Flow-measuring devices should maintain accuracy with various compositions of test gases (He, N_2).

2   Gas analyzers should have a 2-point calibration before each test; linearity should be checked at least every 6 months.

3   PEFV curves generated using a squeeze technique should include tidal breathing tracings and notations of the pressures applied. Repeated flows should be related to lung volume, preferably FRC. If FRC is measured, maximal flow may be expressed as FRC/sec.

4   Lung volume determination (FRC) should be repeated at least 6 times; after discarding the highest and lowest values, the remaining results should be averaged. Those averaged results should have a coefficient of variation (i.e., SD/mean) 8% or less. The interval between repeated lung volume determinations should be equal to the test time; a 5-minute delay is acceptable.

5   For respiratory mechanics measurements, the method used should be documented (passive flow-volume, multiple occlusion, esophageal balloon).

Adapted from American Association for Respiratory Care: Clinical practice guideline; infant/toddler pulmonary function tests, *Respir Care* 40:761-768, 1995.
*These criteria refer to infants and small children. For older children and adolescents, criteria similar to those for adults may be used (except for reproducibility of spirometry).

Infant plethysmography is accomplished using a small, constant-volume chamber in which the infant reclines. The infant's nose and mouth rest against a cuffed opening in the plethysmograph. Flows can be measured by a close-fitting face mask as is done for PEFV curves. The airway is occluded at end-expiration for determination of VTG and Raw. In some instances the airway may be occluded at end-inspiration. The volume above end-expiration is then subtracted from the measured volume to obtain FRC. This technique improves the signal-to-noise ratio in infants. It also reduces the occurrence of glottic closure. At least five tidal breaths should be recorded to fix the end-inspiratory and end-expiratory points. The infant is then allowed to make two to four respiratory efforts against the shutter. Infants cannot "pant" (as do adult subjects) but breathe spontaneously at a rate of 30 breaths/min or less. The mean of three to five acceptable measurements should be reported.

Plethysmographic lung volume recordings are possible in young children by allowing a parent to hold the child on the lap while sitting in the plethysmograph. The adult is instructed to hold his or her breath while the child breathes through a pneumotachometer, and the mouth shutter is closed at end-expiration. Nonpanting VTG maneuvers are normally obtained, but some children can be coached to perform the closed-shutter panting acceptably. Corrections for the gas displacement of both the child and parent based on their combined weights are used in the calculation of the VTG (see Appendix F).

Because VC may not be obtained in infants or young children, FRC is often the only reproducible lung volume that can be determined (Box 8-6). The FRC in infants not only is a function of the recoil forces of the lung and chest wall but is dynamically maintained by the laryngeal "braking" (of flow) and by shortening of expiratory time. Because of these mechanisms, FRC may change rapidly from breath to breath, confounding measurements by gas dilution techniques. This variability of the FRC may lead to errors in calculation that use lung volumes such as $\dot{V}_{max}FRC$ or specific compliance. The problem of variability of the FRC may occur in young children as well as infants. Despite the mechanisms by which the FRC can change dynamically, the FRC has been shown to be reproducible in sedated children.

Pulmonary Mechanics

Measurements of lung compliance and resistance are of greatest importance in infants with abnormal pulmonary physiology. The respiratory system compliance (C_{rs}) and resistance (R_{rs}) can be determined noninvasively by several methods. These methods measure the mechanics of the

---

BOX 8-6
INTERPRETIVE STRATEGIES—PFTs
(INFANTS, VERY YOUNG CHILDREN)

1   Were acceptable data obtained?
    Forced deflation or RTC: Is there evidence of flow limitation (reproducible loops)? Was the coefficient of variation for repeated measures less than 8% to 10%?
    Respiratory mechanics: Are the data consistent for the method used (multiple occlusion, passive flow-volume)?
    Lung volumes: Were repeated measurements reproducible (plethysmography approximately 5%, gas dilution 10% or less)?

2   Were reference values selected appropriately (similar test methods and similar age/weight/length of infants)?

3   Is the $V_{max}FRC/FRC$ less than 1.1? If so, there is probably airway obstruction. Consider repeat measurements (flows, lung volumes) after bronchodilator.

4   Is FRC less than 15 ml/kg (by gas dilution methods)? If so, significant reduction of lung volume is probably present. If FRC is greater than 25 ml/kg, consider overinflation. (A higher range of lung volumes should be considered if measured by body plethysmography.)

---

chest wall, lungs, and airways. For these techniques, it is assumed that the respiratory muscles are completely relaxed during the measurements. Two techniques require occlusion of the infant airway. Both of these methods are based on eliciting the Hering-Breuer reflex. This reflex in infants causes complete relaxation of inspiratory and expiratory muscles when the airway is occluded. This allows alveolar pressure to be estimated so that compliance ($\Delta V/\Delta P$) and resistance ($\Delta P/\dot{V}$) can be calculated.

Multiple occlusion. Pressure is measured at the infant's mouth (or endotracheal tube) while the airway is momentarily occluded. Airway occlusion is performed at different lung volumes during multiple breaths. A pressure-volume curve is constructed using a least-squares linear regression technique to measure C_{rs}.

Passive flow-volume. Airway pressure may be measured by occluding the airway at end-inspiration and recording the pressure as the respiratory muscles relax (Hering-Breuer reflex). Using the difference between the relaxed volume of expiration and the volume at end-inspiration, a pressure-volume slope (i.e., compliance) can be determined. Resistance can be measured as well. The slope of the flow-volume curve must be linear over the volume range measured for the results to be valid.

Two problems that interfere with these measurements are long time constants and the effects of changes in the upper airway. Measurement of a stable pressure during airway occlusion may be impossible in infants with marked differences in the compliance-resistance characteristics in different lung units (i.e., long time constants). This phenomenon occurs if equilibration of pressures within the lung is incomplete when a subsequent breath begins. Because the infant chest wall is extremely compliant, distortion of pleural pressure within the thorax may occur during inspiration, also affecting measurements of esophageal pressure. Similarly, the upper airway (i.e., the larynx) may influence the time constants because of its contribution to the total resistance. To make these measurements, the infant or child must be heavily sedated or paralyzed.

Other methods. Dynamic compliance or resistance determinations require measurement of flow, volume, and esophageal pressure. These tests are usually reserved for infants requiring ventilatory support. If esophageal pressure is measured, the compliance and resistance of the respiratory system can be subdivided into the lung and chest wall components.

Compliance (CL) can also be estimated using a weighted spirometer. The infant or child performs tidal breathing into a closed-circuit spirometer. Weights may then be added to the spirometer bell to increase end-expiratory pressure and FRC. CL is calculated as the change in volume versus the change in pressure, after correcting for (subtracting) spirometer compliance.

TESTING IN OLDER CHILDREN AND ADOLESCENTS

Pulmonary function testing in older children and adolescents is often directed toward diagnosis and evaluation of common pediatric respiratory diseases. Among these are asthma, cystic fibrosis, and chest deformities. In each of these diseases, the tests used are basically the same as might be used in adults with obstructive or restrictive disorders.

The presence and severity of asthma in children is evaluated using a method similar to that used for testing the extent of reversible obstructive lung disease in adults.

---

1. *Spirometry and peak flow measurements* (FEF_x, FEV_T, $FEV_{T\%}$, MEFV curves, and peak expiratory flow [PEF]) help quantify the degree of obstruction and determine the effectiveness of bronchodilators. PEF may be particularly useful because it can be measured conveniently at the bedside with a portable peak-flow meter, providing serial measurements for planning and evaluating therapy. PEF should be correlated with the FEV_1 or other flow measurements to detect changes that may be caused by obstruction and not just effort.

2. *Lung volume measurements* (VC, TLC, RV, FRC, RV/TLC) provide information about air trapping and hyperinflation, particularly in acute asthmatic episodes.

3. *Blood gas analysis* may be indicated in acute asthmatic episodes to detect hypoxemia and hypercapnia. Impending respiratory failure may be signaled by worsening hypoxemia that is accompanied by hypocapnia progressing to hypercapnia.

4. *Exercise or bronchial challenge testing* may be used to determine the presence of airway hyperreactivity and to evaluate the effectiveness of particular therapeutic regimens.

The alterations in lung function in children who have cystic fibrosis may be monitored using the same group of tests as used in adults with COPD.

---

1. *Lung volumes* (VC, FRC, RV, TLC, RV/TLC) are most useful in detecting increases in FRC and RV associated with air trapping typical of advanced obstruction.

2. *Flow measurements* (FEF_x, FEV_T, $FEV_{T\%}$, MEFV curves, and PEF) assess the extent of obstruction caused by mucous plugging, bronchospasm, and edema. The efficacy of bronchodilators, aerosol therapy, chest physical therapy, and other therapeutic modalities aimed at management of secretions can be assessed by measuring FEV_1 and FVC before and after treatment.

3. *Arterial blood gas analysis* may provide information concerning the degree of respiratory insufficiency, particularly the effects of $\dot{V}/\dot{Q}$ mismatching on oxygenation.

Chest deformities that are commonly evaluated by pulmonary function studies include kyphoscoliosis and pectus excavatum. Measurements include those parameters that are useful in assessing restrictive ventilatory patterns (e.g., lung volumes and DL_{CO}). Flow studies such as FEV_1 and MEFV curves may provide additional information if the chest deformity contributes to large airway abnormalities. Spirometry, lung volumes, and blood gas analysis may all be used to assess postoperative changes if surgical intervention is used. Calculation of predicted values based on height should be performed using arm span if it is greater than standing height.

Normal values of lung function for children in all cases depend on height (length in infants), sex, and age. Lung function reference values in children vary mainly with height. Some variables change dramatically at the onset of puberty. For spirometric variables (i.e., FVC, FEV_1) lung function increases up to approximately 18 years of age in boys and approximately 16 years of age in girls. After these ages, volumes and flows plateau and then begin to decline. Because of this "peaking" of lung function in the late teens to early twenties, separate regression equations are often used for young children, adolescents, and adults. Problems can arise if gaps occur in the ranges over which reference values were derived. For example, regressions from a study of children might include ages 6 to 17 years, and regressions from a study of adults from 20 to 80 years. It is not valid to extrapolate either set of equations to determine expected values in 18- or 19-year-old persons. Rather, reference equations should be selected that eliminate these gaps. Nomograms and regression equations for lung volumes and flows in children are included in Appendix B.

Metabolic Measurements (Indirect Calorimetry)

DESCRIPTION

Measurements of $\dot{V}O_2$ and $\dot{V}CO_2$, and their ratio (RER), may be used to determine the resting energy expenditure (REE). REE is usually expressed in kilocalories/day (kcal/day). These measurements allow nutritional assessment and management. In combination with measurements of urinary nitrogen (UN), indirect **calorimetry** allows calories to be partitioned among various substrates (i.e., fat, carbohydrate, protein).

TECHNIQUE

Indirect calorimetry may be performed using either an open- or closed-circuit system to measure O_2 consumption, CO_2 production, and RER.

Open Circuit Calorimetry

Exchange of O_2 and CO_2 may be measured by recording $\dot{V}E$ and the fractional differences of O_2 and CO_2 between inspired and expired gas. These measurements are accomplished using either a mixing chamber, dilution system, or breath-by-breath system similar to those used for expired gas analysis during exercise (see Chapter 7). $\dot{V}O_2$ and $\dot{V}CO_2$ are measured as described for exercise testing using mixing chamber and breath-by-breath systems. The $\dot{V}E$, V_T, and f (respiratory rate) may also be measured. In systems that use the dilution principle, a constant flow of gas is mixed

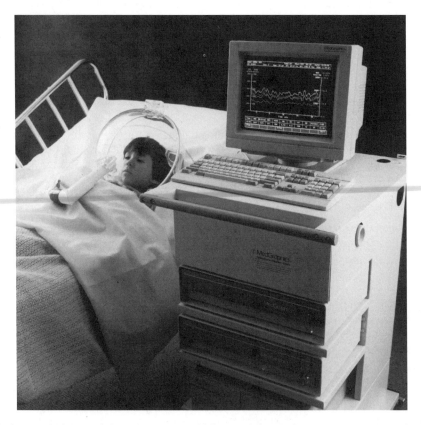

FIG. 8-4 *Canopy for metabolic measurements (indirect calorimetry).* Resting energy expenditure (REE) may be measured from changes in gas flow and fractional concentrations of expired air drawn from a hood or canopy. A continuous or "bias" flow of gas is drawn through the canopy. Changes (i.e., increases or decreases) in the bias flow are measured to determine ventilation. Fractional gas concentrations are determined from the gas drawn from the hood. The canopy offers the advantage of not requiring direct connection to the subject's airway, which may affect ventilation and the measurement of REE. For patients requiring mechanical support of ventilation, the measuring apparatus samples gas from the ventilator circuit. (Courtesy Medical Graphics Corporation, St. Paul, MN.)

with expired air. The dilution of CO_2 is then used to calculate ventilation. Connection to the subject may be made by a standard unidirectional valve with mouthpiece and nose clips. A ventilated hood or canopy (Fig. 8-4) may also be used. Almost all metabolic measurement systems provide for connection to a mechanical ventilator circuit.

A hood or canopy allows long-term measurements without direct connection to the patient's airway. The hood is ventilated by drawing a flow of gas through it that exceeds the patient's peak inspiratory demand (40 L/min is usually adequate). Ventilation can be calculated by measuring the change in flow into and out of the hood during breathing ("**bias**" flow).

Connection to a ventilator requires a means of measuring exhaled volume along with fractional concentrations of both inspired and expired gas. Breath-by-breath metabolic measurement systems usually sample gas at the patient-ventilator connection.

Closed Circuit Calorimetry

The simplest type of closed circuit calorimeter is one which volumetrically measures $\dot{V}O_2$. The subject rebreathes gas from a closed system that contains a spirometer that has been filled with oxygen. CO_2 is scrubbed from the circuit and a recording of the decrease in spirometer volume equals the rate of O_2 uptake of $\dot{V}O_2$. A similar approach uses a closed spirometer system that allows measured amounts of oxygen to be added as the subject rebreathes and removes oxygen. $\dot{V}O_2$ is then equal to the volume of O_2 that must be added per minute to maintain a constant volume. CO_2 production cannot be measured using a closed-circuit system unless a CO_2 analyzer is added to the device. $\dot{V}E$, $\dot{V}I$ and respiratory rate may all be determined from volume excursions of the spirometer. Closed-circuit systems may be used with spontaneously breathing patients by means of a simple breathing valve and mouthpiece. Use of a closed-circuit calorimeter with a mechanical ventilator requires that the spirometer system be connected between the patient and ventilator. The ventilator then "ventilates" the spirometer, which ventilates the patient. This technique usually requires a bellows-type spirometer in a fixed container so that the bellows can be compressed by the positive pressure generated by the ventilator. The volume delivered by the ventilator (i.e., $\dot{V}I$) must be increased to compensate for the volume of gas compressed in the closed-circuit spirometer during positive pressure breaths.

Performing Metabolic Measurements

The primary purpose of indirect calorimetry is to estimate REE over an extended period, usually 24 hours. To extrapolate the values obtained during the sampling period, the subject's condition during the measurement is critical (Box 8-7). The following guidelines help ensure that measurements are made under steady-state conditions:

---

1. The subject should be recumbent or supine for 20 to 30 minutes before beginning measurements and should stay quiet during the test. Ideally, the subject should be awake and aware during testing. The testing apparatus should not cause discomfort or exertion for the subject. Breathing valves, mouthpieces, and nose clips may alter the subject's breathing pattern.

2. The subject should fast for 2 to 4 hours before the test starts. If the subject is receiving either **enteral** or **parenteral** feedings, the feedings should be continuous rather than in bolus form. Information about the type and amount of nutritional support in the previous 24 hours may be helpful in interpreting test results.

3. The subject should be in a neutral thermal environment. Special corrections may be required for subjects who are **febrile** or **hypothermic.** The subject's temperature at the time of the test should be recorded along with a temperature history of the previous 24 hours.

4. Drugs or substances that alter metabolism should be avoided. Substances related to caffeine and nicotine are particularly common stimulants. Theophylline-based drugs may also increase metabolic rate.

5. Data collection should continue for long enough that a stable baseline is established and steady-state conditions can be verified (Fig. 8-5). From 10 to 15 minutes of stable readings for $\dot{V}O_2$ and $\dot{V}CO_2$ is recommended. Common indicators of steady-state conditions are the parameters assessed as part of the metabolic study itself. The $\dot{V}O_2$ should not vary more than 10% from the mean value measured during the test interval. $\dot{V}CO_2$ measurements should

be within 6% of the mean during the same interval. RER (RQ) values should be within the normal physiologic range (i.e., 0.67 to 1.30). If the subject does not achieve steady-state conditions, a longer test interval may be required to average representative periods of metabolic activity.

BOX 8-7
CRITERIA FOR ACCEPTABILITY—INDIRECT CALORIMETRY

1   Appropriate calibration of gas analyzers and volume transducers should be documented daily, preferably before each test.

2   The RQ should be within the normal physiologic range of 0.67 to 1.30.

3   Measured $\dot{V}o_2$ values should vary by no more than ±10% around the mean; $\dot{V}co_2$ values should vary by less than ±6% of the mean.

4   Data should be collected for a minimum of 10 to 15 minutes with minimal variability.

5   RQ values should be consistent with the patient's current nutritional intake.

6   Documentation should include the patient's medications, nutritional support, body temperature at time of test, and ventilatory support settings (if applicable).

7   The patient should be resting; no bolus feedings or pharmacologic stimulants or depressants. There should be no physical therapy, airway care, or major ventilator changes immediately before assessment.

8   If a 24-hour urinary urea nitrogen (UUN) is collected for substrate use, it should be concurrent with the metabolic study.

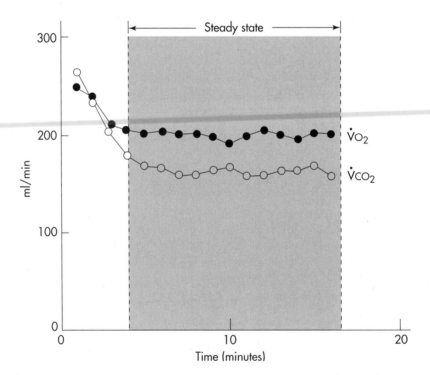

FIG. 8-5 *Indirect calorimetry.* Typical tracing of continuous measurement of $\dot{V}o_2$ and $\dot{V}co_2$ as performed during open-circuit indirect calorimetry. The subject's expired gas is analyzed to determine O_2 consumption, CO_2 production, and RQ during a resting state. The measurements are observed until a metabolic steady state can be determined (usually 10 to 15 minutes). During the steady-state interval, values representative of resting energy expenditure (REE) can be measured. From these measurements the daily caloric requirements can be estimated. If a 24-hour urinary urea nitrogen (UUN) sample is obtained, the percentages of energy derived from fats, carbohydrates, and proteins can be calculated (see text).

6. Patients on ventilators should be in a stable condition. No ventilator adjustments should be made for 1 to 2 hours before the test period. Modifications in minute ventilation or FiO_2 settings can cause gross changes in the patterns of gas exchange, particularly in subjects with pulmonary disease. The ventilator must have a stable delivered oxygen concentration; FiO_2 settings greater than 0.60 may result in erroneous measurements of $\dot{V}O_2$. Appropriate valving may need to be used for ventilator modes that involve continuous gas flow.

7. The calorimeter or metabolic cart should be calibrated at least daily, preferably before each test. Gas analyzers should be calibrated using gas concentrations appropriate for the clinical situation. Sample lines and gas conditioning devices (absorbers) should be checked before each test. If calibration or testing produces questionable values, the device should be checked against a known standard. Burning ethanol or other material with a fixed RQ can be used. A large-volume syringe can be used to simulate a subject with $\dot{V}O_2$ and $\dot{V}CO_2$ values near zero.

Metabolic Calculations

1. Harris-Benedict equations for estimating REE:
   Men:

$$REE \text{ (kcal/24 hr)} = 66.47 + 13.75W + 5.00H - 6.76A$$

   Women:

$$REE \text{ (kcal/24 hr)} = 655.10 + 9.56W + 1.85H - 4.68A$$

   where:

$$W = \text{weight in kilograms}$$
$$H = \text{height in centimeters}$$
$$A = \text{age in years}$$

   The REE by these formulas was originally described as the basal metabolic rate (BMR). These equations may be used to estimate the caloric expenditure in normal subjects under conditions of minimal activity. The BMR in these circumstances is related to lean body mass. To determine the optimum level of caloric intake, the BMR must be adjusted upward because trauma, surgery, infections, and burns all cause the REE to increase.

2. Weir equation for calculating REE from respiratory gas exchange and urinary N_2:

$$REE \text{ (kcal/24 hrs)} = 1.44(3.941\dot{V}O_2 + 1.106\dot{V}CO_2) - 2.17(UN)$$

   where:

$$\dot{V}O_2 \text{ is expressed in ml/min}$$
$$\dot{V}CO_2 \text{ is expressed in ml/min}$$
$$UN = \text{urinary nitrogen (g/24 hr)}$$
$$1.44 = \text{correction from ml/min to L/24 hr}$$

   Indirect calorimetry by the open-circuit method provides measures of both oxygen consumption and CO_2 production. The RER is the ratio of $\dot{V}CO_2/\dot{V}O_2$. Under steady-state conditions, the RER approximates the mean respiratory quotient (RQ) at the cell level. RQ normally varies from 0.71 to 1.00, depending on the substrates being metabolized. Carbohydrate oxidation produces an RQ near 1.0, fat oxidation produces an RQ near 0.71, and protein oxidation produces an RQ of 0.82. The RQ attributable to carbohydrates and fats may be determined by subtracting the $\dot{V}O_2$ and $\dot{V}CO_2$ derived from protein. This form of the RQ is termed the nonprotein RQ or RQ_{NP} and is calculated as follows:

$$RQ_{NP} = \frac{(\dot{V}_{CO_2} \text{ (in L/24 hr)} - 4.8 \text{ UN})}{(\dot{V}_{O_2} \text{ (in L/24 hr)} - 5.9 \text{ UN})}$$

   where:

$$\dot{V}CO_2 \text{ (in L/24 hr)} = 1.44 \, \dot{V}CO_2 \text{ (in ml/min)}$$
$$\dot{V}O_2 \text{ (in L/24 hr)} = 1.44 \, \dot{V}O_2 \text{ (in ml/min)}$$
$$UN = \text{urinary nitrogen (g/24 hr)}$$

Because CO_2 production varies with O_2 uptake, deviations of the RQ from the average value of 0.85 result in differences of less than 5% in the calculation of REE if the $\dot{V}_{O_2}$ and RQ are used. Indirect calorimetry by the closed-circuit (volumetric) method takes advantage of this small difference by assuming a fixed RQ (usually 0.85) and measuring only $\dot{V}_{O_2}$. UN is obtained from a 24-hour collection. Because protein metabolism accounts for only a small proportion of the total calories per day (approximately 12%), omission of the UN in the Weir equation changes the calculated REE by only 2%.

3. Consolazio equations for determination of energy expenditure from gas exchange ($\dot{V}_{O_2}$, $\dot{V}_{CO_2}$), UN, and the caloric equivalents of carbohydrates, fats, and proteins:

$$\text{Carbohydrates (in g)} = (5.926\dot{V}_{O_2}) - (4.189\dot{V}_{CO_2}) - (2.539UN)$$
$$\text{Fat (in g)} = (2.432\dot{V}_{O_2}) - (2.432\dot{V}_{CO_2}) - (1.943UN)$$
$$\text{Protein (in g)} = (6.25UN)$$

From the grams of each substrate used, the kilocalories derived from that source can be computed:

$$\text{Carbohydrates (in kcal)} = 4.18 \text{ carbohydrates (in g)}$$
$$\text{Fat (in kcal)} = 9.46 \text{ fat (in g)}$$
$$\text{Protein (in kcal)} = 4.32 \text{ protein (in g)}$$
$$\text{Total (in kcal)} = \text{carbohydrate} + \text{fat} + \text{protein (in kcal)}$$

The percentage of calories attributable to each of the substrates may also be calculated by dividing the kilocalories derived from the substrate by the total kilocalories. Because the Consolazio equations are intended for analysis of normal substrate partitioning, RQ values outside of the range of 0.71 to 1.00 will result in negative values for either carbohydrates or lipids (fat). These negative values are erroneous if the RER does not equal the RQ (i.e., the patient is not in a metabolic steady state).

SIGNIFICANCE AND PATHOPHYSIOLOGY

See Box 8-8 for interpretive strategies. Indirect calorimetry is often used to assess nutritional status in patients whose daily energy needs are altered by disease, injury, or therapeutic interventions. REE accounts for approximately two thirds of the daily energy requirements in healthy subjects. The Harris-Benedict equations, or similar predictive equations, are commonly used to estimate the REE. Various factors can be used to adjust estimated REE to account for additional caloric needs imposed by the patient's clinical status. This approach works well in many patients. However, metabolic requirements of critically ill patients vary widely. Indirect calorimetry is indicated for

---

> **BOX BOX 8-8**
> **INTERPRETIVE STRATEGIES—INDIRECT CALORIMETRY**
>
> 1 Were metabolic data collected acceptably? Did $\dot{V}_{O_2}$ values vary by less than 10%? Did $\dot{V}_{CO_2}$ value vary by less than 6%? If not, interpret cautiously. Was RQ between 0.67 and 1.30? If not, interpret very cautiously or not at all.
>
> 2 Was measured REE less than that predicted (Harris-Benedict equation)? If so, consider technical error or hypometabolic state.
>
> 3 Was RQ less than 0.70? If so, consider ketosis or starvation.
>
> 4 Was RQ greater than 1.00? If so, consider lipogenesis or nonsteady state (hyperventilation).
>
> 5 Is the measured REE significantly greater than the patient's intake in the previous 24 hours? If so, the patient is probably being underfed or may be febrile.
>
> 6 Is the measured REE significantly less than the patient's intake in the previous 24 hours? If so, the patient is probably being overfed.
>
> 7 Is the nonprotein RQ near 1.00? If so, the main substrate being used is carbohydrate. Is the nonprotein RQ near 0.70? If so, the main substrate is fat.
>
> 8 Are the metabolic measurements consistent with the patient's clinical status? Is nutritional support (if provided) appropriate for metabolic needs?

patients who do not respond favorably to traditional methods of nutritional assessment and support. Indirect calorimetry can be used to detect undernourishment, overnourishment, or use of inappropriate substrates (Table 8-8).

Undernourishment or starvation can occur during illness. It may be detected by caloric expenditure in excess of caloric intake (negative energy balance). Both fat stores and protein from muscle breakdown may contribute to metabolism during periods of undernourishment. Indirect calorimetry is often used along with measurement of body weight, triceps skinfold measurements, and other approximations of energy reserves. These measurements allow planning of nutritional therapy to replenish diminished reserves.

Overnourishment occurs when any substrate is supplied in excess of the energy requirements. Overfeeding is most deleterious when the patient's nutritional status is already adequate. Excess lipid or carbohydrate calories are stored as fat, which may place stress on one or more organ systems.

Patients with pulmonary disease present a special dilemma. Excessive carbohydrate intake results in increased CO_2 production because the RQ of carbohydrates is 1.00. In patients who have respiratory failure, excess production of CO_2 increases the ventilatory load on the respiratory system. Adjustments in substrate use can be made after the nonprotein RQ is determined by indirect calorimetry. Lipids (i.e., fats) are typically substituted for glucose so that the RQ can be reduced while the caloric intake is maintained. Patients with respiratory failure may also experience atrophy of ventilatory muscles. Substrate analysis can be used to assess N_2 balance related to the breakdown of muscle protein. Substrate analysis permits measurement of nutritional requirements necessary to maintain N_2 balance.

Technical considerations involved in indirect calorimetry include the accuracy of gas analysis and measurement of expired volume during the test. The most common problem during metabolic measurements is attainment of a true steady state. Only if the measurements are made under steady-state conditions is the metabolic rate representative of caloric expenditure over 24 hours. Hyperventilation resulting from connection to a mask or mouthpiece or from ventilator manipulation is a frequent occurrence. Head hoods or continuous-flow canopies can eliminate much of the stimulation associated with connection to the metabolic measurement system (see Fig. 8-4) but cannot be used for patients on mechanical ventilators. An RER greater than 1.00 should always be evaluated in relation to the $\dot{V}E$ and end-tidal CO_2. Abnormally high $\dot{V}E$ and low end-tidal CO_2 values may indicate hyperventilation. RER values in excess of 1.00 that cannot be explained as hyperventilation may be caused by storage of excess calories as fat (lipogenesis). RER values between 0.67 and 0.70 may occur in **ketosis** caused by extreme fasting or diabetic ketoacidosis. However, more commonly low RER values (less than 0.67) signal improper calibration of the gas analyzers. Inaccurate calibration or improper performance of either the CO_2 or O_2 analyzers can result in RER values outside of the usual metabolic range of 0.70 to 1.00.

Special problems may be encountered in performing metabolic measurements on patients requiring mechanical ventilatory support. A common difficulty relates to measurements of O_2 consumption in patients receiving supplemental O_2. Measurement of $\dot{V}O_2$ by respiratory gas exchange requires analysis of the difference between inspired and expired O_2 along with $\dot{V}E$. In subjects breathing room air, inspired FIO_2 is constant. Many oxygen-blending systems,

TABLE 8-8 Indications for Indirect Calorimetry*

Head trauma or paralysis
COPD
Multiple trauma
Acute pancreatitis
Patients in whom height or weight is indeterminate
Poor response to enteral or parenteral support
Patients receiving total parenteral nutrition at home
Transplant patients
Morbidly obese patients
Patients with demonstrated hypermetabolism or hypometabolism
Patients on prolonged mechanical ventilation who are unable to eat

*Risk and/or stress factors known to interfere with calculation of energy expenditure.

such as those used on ventilators, may not provide a constant fraction of inspired O_2. Large differences in the calculated $\dot{V}_{O_2}$ can result from small fluctuations in the F_{IO_2}, even if F_{EO_2} remains relatively constant. Small differences in the inspired and expired volumes (resulting from the RER) are corrected by adjusting the inspired fraction of oxygen according to the following equation:

$$\frac{(1 - F_{EO_2} - F_{ECO_2})}{(1 - F_{IO_2})} \times F_{IO_2}$$

The correction of inspired F_{IO_2} for gas balance in the lung (i.e., the Haldane transformation; see $\dot{V}_{O_2}$, Chapter 7) limits the accuracy of the open-circuit method of determining $\dot{V}_{O_2}$. As the F_{IO_2} is increased, the value in the denominator of the equation becomes smaller. Even with very accurate gas analyzers, measurement of differences between the F_{IO_2} and F_{EO_2} when the F_{IO_2} is above 0.60 is variable. Indirect calorimetry by the volumetric method (i.e., a closed system) avoids this problem by measuring the actual volume of O_2 removed during rebreathing. Measurement of $\dot{V}_{O_2}$ and $\dot{V}_{CO_2}$ in spontaneously breathing patients who require supplemental O_2 can usually be accommodated by allowing the subject to breathe from a reservoir bag containing increased F_{IO_2}.

Other considerations involved in metabolic measurements of ventilated patients include the effects of positive pressure on gas analysis and on volume determination. Analysis of O_2 and CO_2 in the ventilator circuit must take into account the effect of positive pressure breaths on the gas analyzers. Depending on the sampling method used, positive pressure swings during each breath may generate falsely high partial pressure readings. Closed-circuit calorimetry places a volumetric device in the breathing circuit between the ventilator and the patient. The volume delivered by the ventilator must be increased to accommodate the higher compressible gas volume in the circuit, approximately 1 ml/cm H_2O for each liter of added volume.

CASE STUDIES

CASE 8A

History

M.M. is a 39-year-old secretary who has recently begun experiencing episodes of "choking and coughing." She was referred by an industrial health specialist who suspected reactive airways involvement. She relates that cigarette smoke and strong odors seem to bring on the episodes. She has never smoked and has no history of lung disease. She had some childhood allergies that disappeared at puberty. There is no history of lung disease in any of her immediate family. She is not currently taking any medications.

Pulmonary Function Tests

Personal data

Sex: Female
Age: 39 yr
Height: 66 in
Weight: 130 lb

Spirometry

	Before drug	Predicted	%
FVC (L)	3.71	3.8	98
FEV_1 (L)	2.96	2.97	99
$FEV_{1\%}$ (%)	80	78	—
$FEF_{25\%-75\%}$ (L/sec)	2.99	3.34	90
$Vmax_{50}$ (L/sec)	3.93	4.62	85
$Vmax_{25}$ (L/sec)	1.01	2.36	43
MVV (L/min)	106.4	109.7	97
Raw (cm H_2O/L/sec)	2.37	0.6-2.4	—
SGaw (L/sec/cm H_2O/L)	0.14	0.14-0.56	—

Methacholine challenge*

Methacholine (mg/ml)	FEV₁	% Control	SGaw	Cumulative breaths	Cumulative units/five breaths
Baseline	2.96	—	0.14	—	—
Control	2.92	100	0.14	—	—
0.075	2.93	100	0.13	5	0.375
0.150	2.90	99	0.11	10	1.125
0.310	2.75	94	0.11	15	2.68
0.62	2.41	83	0.09	20	5.78
1.25	1.99	68	0.08	25	12.00

*One methacholine unit is arbitrarily defined as 1 mg/ml of methacholine in diluent.

Technologist's Comments

All spirometry and body box efforts were acceptable and reproducible.

Questions

1. What is the interpretation of:
   a. Spirometry?
   b. Airway resistance and conductance?
2. What is the interpretation of the methacholine challenge?
3. What is the cause of the patient's symptoms?
4. What treatment might be recommended based on these findings?

Discussion

1 **Interpretation (prechallenge pulmonary function)**
Spirometry before and during the inhalation challenge was performed acceptably, as were maneuvers in the body plethysmograph.
  Spirometry results are within normal limits, except for the $\dot{V}max_{25}$, which is reduced. The Raw and SGaw are close to the limits of normal, consistent with some airflow obstruction.

2 **Interpretation (methacholine challenge)**
The methacholine challenge test is positive with a PD_{20} of approximately 0.64 mg/ml (interpolated). This represents a total dose of between 5 and 12 cumulative breath units. The test was terminated because the subject's FEV_1 fell below 80% of the control value. The SGaw fell in a similar fashion, with 57% decrease at the maximal inhaled dose. Wheezing was present on auscultation for the last two methacholine doses, and the subject experienced symptoms similar to her chief complaint when the test became positive.
  Impression: Normal lung function with a positive methacholine challenge, consistent with hyperreactive airway disease.

3 **Cause of symptoms**
This subject is an ideal candidate for an inhalation challenge test. Her baseline pulmonary function studies are normal, with possible small airway involvement. Her complaint of episodic coughing and choking suggests some form of hyperreactive airways abnormality. Many subjects who develop an asthmatic response to inhaled irritants complain of cough as the primary symptom, whereas wheezing may or may not be present.
  If obvious airway obstruction were present on the baseline spirometry, the challenge test would have been contraindicated. A simple before- and after-bronchodilator trial may have been sufficient to demonstrate reversible obstruction. Methacholine challenge testing may be used in subjects with known obstruction to quantify the degree of airway hyper-reactivity. In this case, the objective of the test was to determine whether the subject had hyperreactivity.
  The FEV_1 is commonly used as the index of obstruction for inhalation challenge tests because it is simple to perform and highly reproducible. Other parameters may also be evaluated because the forced expiratory maneuver is repeated at each dosage. The $FEF_{25\%-75\%}$, $\dot{V}max_{50}$, $\dot{V}max_{25}$, Raw, and SGaw are sometimes used to define the extent of airway reactivity. The SGaw is sensitive and reproducible and is often used to quantify changes occurring during challenge testing. A fall of 35% to 40% in the SGaw is usually considered indicative of a positive

response. As in this patient, SGaw may actually fall at a more rapid rate than FEV_1. The variability of the $FEF_{25\%-75\%}$, $\dot{V}max_{50}$, and $\dot{V}max_{25}$ make interpretation of changes during challenge testing somewhat difficult. In some instances the PEF may fall as the challenge is performed, particularly if the large airways are involved.

Results of a methacholine challenge test should be interpreted cautiously. The subject should be free of symptoms at the time of the test. β-Adrenergic, anticholinergic, or methylxanthine bronchodilators that might influence the results must be withheld before testing (see Table 8-2). These conditions were met in this subject. Because both FEV_1 and SGaw fell markedly after a moderate methacholine dose, the test can be interpreted as positive with some certainty.

4   Treatment

To better manage this patient, a portable peak-flow meter was used (see Chapter 9). The subject was instructed in its use, and her PEF while using it correlated well with that measured during spirometry. She was told to use the device every morning and evening or when symptoms appeared. Any significant change in PEF was treated using a β-adrenergic bronchodilator via metered-dose inhaler. Subsequent reports indicated that her peak flow fell in excess of the level demonstrated on the challenge, but the symptoms were promptly relieved with use of the inhaler.

CASE 8B

History

R.I. is a 38-year-old woman whose presenting complaint is shortness of breath while jogging or playing tennis. She has been physically active for several years but recently had a "chest cold" that took 4 weeks to resolve. She smoked for approximately 2 years while in high school. She works as a teacher and has no unusual environmental exposures. Family history includes an older sister who has chronic bronchitis. She is not currently taking any medications. Her HMO referred her for evaluation of possible exercise-induced bronchospasm.

Pulmonary Function Tests

Personal data

Sex: Female
Age: 38 yr
Height: 62 in
Weight: 119 lb

Eucapnic voluntary hyperventilation

	Baseline	5 min	10 min	15 min	Postbronchodilator
FEV_1 (Pred: 2.64 L)	1.97	1.25			1.92
% Predicted	75	47			73
% Change	0	−37			−3
FVC (Pred: 3.37 L)	2.71	2.07			2.8
% Predicted	81	61			83
% Change	0	−24			3
PEF (Pred: 6.03 L/sec)	5.48	2.77			3.65
% Predicted	91	46			61
% Change	0	−49			−33

Technologist's Comments

All spirometry maneuvers were performed acceptably before and after hyperventilation. The patient hyperventilated at 60 L/min for 6 minutes. There were audible wheezes immediately after hyperventilation.

Questions

1.   What is the interpretation of:
    a. Baseline spirometry?

    b. Response to eucapnic voluntary hyperventilation?

    c. Response to bronchodilator?

2. What is the cause of the patient's symptoms?

3. What other tests might be indicated?

4. What treatment might be recommended based on these findings?

Discussion

1 Interpretation

All spirometric maneuvers were performed acceptably. Baseline spirometry results are within normal limits although FEV_1 is mildly reduced. After eucapnic voluntary hyperventilation, there is a significant fall in FEV_1, FVC, and peak flow at 5 minutes. After bronchodilator therapy, FEV_1 returned to prechallenge levels and FVC increased. Peak-flow recovery was somewhat slower.

    Impression: Borderline normal spirometry results with a positive eucapnic voluntary hyperventilation test consistent with hyperreactive airways.

2 Cause of symptoms

This patient is typical of an adult who begins experiencing breathlessness with increased physical activity and seeks medical attention. Her complaints suggest exercise-induced bronchospasm. The development of this problem may or may not be related to her recent chest infection.

    EVH is an excellent way to challenge the airways in cases such as this. The subject breathed a mixture of 5% CO_2, 21% O_2, and balance N_2 for 6 minutes. The target level of ventilation was set at 30 times her FEV_1, or approximately 60 L/min. Spirometry was repeated 5 minutes after hyperventilation. In this case, the patient experienced a significant decrease in FEV_1, FVC, and PEF (Fig. 8-6). Two inhalations of an albuterol metered-dose inhaler reversed the obstruction, although PEF recovered only partially.

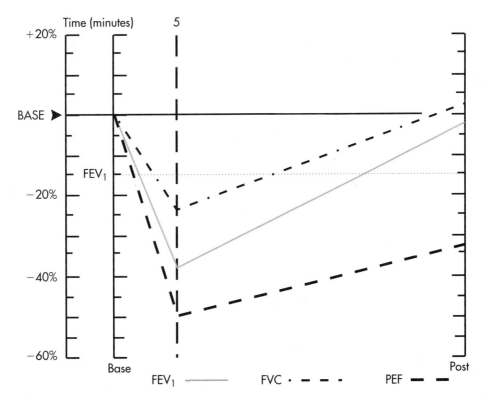

FIG. 8-6 *Eucapnic voluntary ventilation (EVH) graph for Case 8B.* FVC, FEV_1, and PEF are plotted after the bronchial challenge maneuver. In this subject there was a marked decrease in all three variables at 5 minutes (i.e., a positive test). The graph also plots the reversal of the induced bronchospasm by inhaled bronchodilator.

3   **Other tests**

Eucapnic hyperventilation challenges the airways by inducing heat and water loss by elevating the level of ventilation. This is the same physical stimulus that may be responsible for exercise-induced bronchospasm. The patient in this case could have been tested using either methacholine or exercise as the challenge agents. However, EVH is simpler and takes less time.

EVH may be more sensitive in detecting exercise-induced asthma than exercise testing itself. Exercise tests are often performed with the subject working at 60% to 80% of their maximal HR for 6 to 8 minutes. In many subjects this workload may not induce a high enough level of ventilation to provoke bronchospasm.

4   **Treatment**

The patient was given inhaled bronchodilators and reported significant improvement in her symptoms. A trial regimen of cromolyn sodium also reduced the occurrence of symptoms associated with athletic activities.

CASE 8C

History

C.K. is a female child whose presenting problems include failure to thrive, an unknown neuromuscular disorder, and documented gastroesophageal reflux with probable aspiration. She was referred to a pediatric pulmonologist for evaluation of lung volumes and flows. She was sedated in the pulmonary function laboratory with chloral hydrate. Multiple FRC measurements were made using an N_2-washout technique. Although she was 5 years old, PEFV curves were obtained using RTC with reservoir pressures from 30 to 100 cm H_2O. A nebulized solution of 0.5 ml albuterol in 2 ml of normal saline was administered and all measurements were repeated 15 minutes after bronchodilator administration.

Pulmonary Function Tests

Personal data

Sex: Female
Age: 5 yr
Length: 91 cm
Weight: 10.3 kg

Lung volumes and spirometry

	Prebronchodilator	Postbronchodilator
FRC (ml, mean)	344	321
SD (ml)	10	14.4
CV (%)	5.7	4.5
FRC (ml/kg)	33.4	31.2
$\dot{V}_{max}$FRC (ml/sec)	272	340
SD (ml/sec)	19.8	7.2
$S\dot{V}_{max}$FRC (sec)	0.79	1.06
SD (sec)	0.06	0.02
CV (%)	6.7	2.1

Technologist's Comments

All trials were acceptable with coefficients of variation of less than 8%.

Questions

1. What is the interpretation of:
    a. Lung volumes and flows before bronchodilator?
    b. Lung volumes and flows after bronchodilator?
2. How do the flow-volume curves differ from those performed on an adult subject?
3. Is there a significant response to bronchodilator?
4. Why is it important to calculate standard deviation (SD) and coefficient of variation (CV)?

Discussion

1   Interpretation

This child has an elevated FRC (normal range 15 to 25 ml/kg) suggesting overexpansion. There is mild obstruction on forced flows. This is evidenced by reduced specific flow at FRC of 0.79 second (normal range: 1.0 to 1.6). After bronchodilator administration, raw and specific flows significantly increase.

2   Flow-volume curves

C.K. appears to have an elevated FRC based on her weight and length. Repeated measurements of FRC by N_2 washout (five trials) produced a CV of 8.9%. This is an acceptable level of reproducibility. Flow-volume loops (Fig. 8-7) are "squeezed" breaths following successive tidal breaths at a consistent FRC. Because the infant is not at TLC when the squeeze occurs, a different lung volume must be used to reference forced flow. The end-expiratory level (i.e., FRC) is fairly consistent from breath to breath. FRC is also lower than TLC, making it a useful reference point for evaluating smaller airways. When the raw flow at FRC (V_{max}FRC) is divided by the measured FRC, a specific flow ($S\dot{V}_{max}$FRC) can be calculated. The flow-volume loop (Fig. 8-7, A) produced with increased jacket pressure suggests that flow limitation is being achieved. When the $\dot{V}_{max}$FRC of 272 ml/sec is divided by the FRC of 344 ml, a reduced $S\dot{V}_{max}$FRC of 0.79 is obtained.

3   Bronchodilator response

The postbronchodilator loop (Fig. 8-7, B) shows a marked change. The convex shape of the curve is typical of forced expiratory flow in a normal child. Forced flows increased from 272 ml/sec to 340 ml/sec. $S\dot{V}_{max}$FRC increased from 0.79 to 1.06, approaching the normal range. Both of these changes are considered positive responses, evidenced by a greater than two-fold change in the SD of each measurement. The increase in specific flow is caused by both an improvement in absolute flow and a reduction in the FRC. Although FRC decreased from 344 to 320 ml, the variability of the repeated measurements (postbronchodilator) also increased. The SD of these measurements is greater (i.e., 14.4 versus 10.0), making the change in FRC fall slightly below a statistically significant level. Overall, study of this infant supports an impressive response to inhaled bronchodilators.

4   Importance of SD and CV for reproducibility

Reproducibility of infant pulmonary function tests continues to be the subject of much controversy. The child must be sedated for testing because of stimulation of mask placement

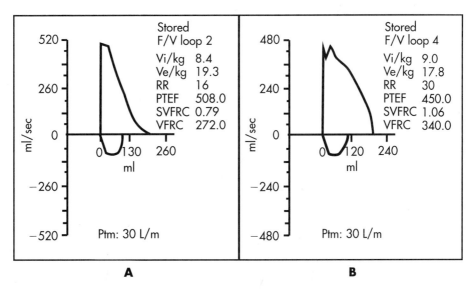

FIG. 8-7 *Flow-volume curves for Case 8C.* Both tracings are partial flow-volume curves produced by rapid thoracoabdominal compression (RTC). **A,** Prebronchodilator, the flow at FRC (VFRC) was approximately 272 ml/sec with a specific flow (SVFRC) of 0.79 sec. The curve has a concave appearance consistent with reduced flows. **B,** Postbronchodilator, VFRC has increased significantly to 340 ml/sec, and SVFRC is almost normal at 1.06. (Other abbreviations shown: *Vi/kg,* inspired volume per kg of body weight; *Ve/kg,* expired volume per kg; *RR,* respiratory rate during tidal breathing; *PTEF,* peak expiratory flow during compression; *Ptm,* pneumotach flow range.)

and thoracoabdominal squeeze. Sedation, as well as sleep state and degree of hypoxia, can change the child's FRC. Gas dilution measurements of FRC, although standard, may derive lung volumes that err on the low side in airway obstruction. Body plethysmography produces higher volumes, even in healthy infants, but is not widely available. Partial forced flows are more difficult to reproduce than spirometry in older subjects. There are several reasons why this is the case: (1) technical aspects of performing RTC on chest walls with varying compliance, (2) partial forced flows obtained over a tidal breathing range that is variable, (3) reference values that are not well established in the infant age groups, and (4) the pressure exerted during RTC may not be sufficient to produce true flow limitation. Despite these difficulties, FRC and forced flow measurements are helpful in assessing infants with the types of problems this child displays.

CASE 8D

History

J.P. is a 53-year-old woman who received multiple abdominal injuries in a motor vehicle accident. After surgical repair of a perforated bowel, acute renal failure developed and then respiratory failure. She was placed on mechanically supported ventilation and became increasingly dependent on the ventilator. After 13 days, a metabolic study was requested to assess the adequacy of parenteral nutrition.

Metabolic Assessment

Personal data

Age: 53 yr
Height: 157 cm
Weight: 50 kg

Nutritional information

	Total calories	Nonprotein calories	Protein (g)
Parenteral	1717	1393	75
Enteral	(none)	—	—
24-Hour UN	9 g	—	—

Basal metabolic rate 1176 kcal/24 hours (estimated)

Ventilator settings

FIO_2	0.35
V_T	750 ml
Rate	10
Mode	SIMV*
Status	Awake, resting

*Synchronized intermittent mandatory ventilation.

Metabolic measurements

$\dot{V}CO_2$ (ml/min)	205
$\dot{V}O_2$ (ml/min)	200
RER (RQ)	1.03
$\dot{V}E$ (L/min)	10.2
REE	1442 kcal/day
RQ_{NP}*	1.07

*Nonprotein RQ, see text.

Energy substrate use:
Carbohydrate (kcal/day)	1480
Fat (kcal/day)	−280
Protein (kcal/day)	243

Blood gases

pH	7.37
Pa_{CO_2}	51
Pa_{O_2}	71
HCO_3^-	29

Questions

1. What is the interpretation of:
   a. Resting energy expenditure (REE)?
   b. Substrate utilization?
2. Why does this patient have an RER (RQ) greater than 1.00?
3. Are the data representative of the patient's caloric requirements?
4. What changes in therapy (ventilator settings, nutritional support) are indicated?

Discussion

1   Interpretation

Data for this study were collected over 26 minutes and appear to represent a steady state. A UN sample was collected for 24 hours before the test. The patient was receiving 1717 kcal/day of parenteral nutrition. Estimated energy expenditure as determined by metabolic assessment indicates a requirement of 1442 kcal/24 hours. Substrate utilization showed carbohydrate oxidation (104%). The negative value for fat utilization is consistent with lipogenesis. Recommended replacement of glucose with lipids, and reduction of total calories to approximately 1450 kcal/day. Patient should be reassessed within 24 hours.

2   Cause of elevated RER (RQ)

This study involves factors commonly encountered in the nutritional support of critically ill patients. These elements include the patient's clinical status, estimated and actual caloric requirements, and the role of nutritional status in ventilatory support.

This patient was critically ill and required ventilatory support. Parenteral nutrition was being supplied approximately 45% above the estimated resting caloric requirements. Estimation of caloric requirements is often performed by calculating the basal rate using the Harris-Benedict equations (see "Indirect Calorimetry," p. 229). The BMR is then adjusted using factors that consider the clinical status of the patient (i.e., disease state, trauma).

The metabolic assessment indicated that the patient required fewer calories per day than were currently being given. In addition, carbohydrates were supplying the entire caloric need. The negative value calculated for fat utilization indicates that some of the carbohydrates were probably being stored as fat (i.e., lipogenesis). When carbohydrates are oxidized, CO_2 is produced. The RER of 1.03 supports an excess CO_2 production in relation to metabolic demands.

The metabolic assessment was performed with the patient on a ventilator. The patient's $\dot{V}E$ during the assessment was 10.2 L, slightly higher than the ventilator settings. Difficulty weaning this patient from mechanically supported ventilation may have been caused by the CO_2 load induced by parenteral nutrition in excess of metabolic demand. The arterial blood gas analysis supports increased CO_2 production. Pa_{CO_2} is increased in spite of mechanical support of ventilation. The patient was unable to ventilate enough to return her Pa_{CO_2} to near 40 mm Hg. Excess CO_2 apparently contributed to the difficulty weaning the patient from mechanical ventilation.

3   Valid data (steady state)

The interpretation notes that the data were representative of a steady state. Steady-state measurements are essential to estimate caloric requirements for an entire 24-hour period. Each metabolic assessment should include adequate data so that steady-state conditions can be verified. The length of the study should be appropriate to establish that a steady state existed. Analysis of the variability of the $\dot{V}O_2$ and $\dot{V}CO_2$ may be helpful. The O_2 consumption and CO_2 production ideally should vary during measurements less than 10% and 6%, respectively. RER values outside the normal range of 0.70 to 1.00 should be carefully evaluated to ensure that measurement errors did not occur. Difficulty measuring $\dot{V}O_2$ in subjects receiving supplemental O_2 is well documented. Calorimetry using open-circuit methods is usually limited to measurements when the F_{IO_2} is 0.60 or less.

4   **Changes in therapy**
J.P. was switched to a 50/50 mixture of lipid and carbohydrate. The total caloric intake was also reduced to 1450 kcal/day. Her ventilation decreased, and ventilatory support was gradually reduced. An additional metabolic study indicated agreement between the prescribed nutritional support and her metabolic demands. Her RER on the subsequent study was 0.79 with an REE of 1395 kcal/day. This RER value compares favorably with 0.82, which is a target value for metabolism of appropriate amounts of carbohydrate, fat, and protein. She was successfully weaned from the ventilator 4 days after the initial assessment.

SUMMARY

THIS CHAPTER HAS DISCUSSED application of pulmonary function tests for specific purposes. Each of these special regimens use tests previously discussed. Spirometry is used for bronchial challenge tests, preoperative testing, tests designed to evaluate disability, and pediatric pulmonary function evaluation. Other tests (e.g., lung volumes, blood gases) are used because they have been shown to answer specific clinical questions. Metabolic studies that use techniques associated with exhaled gas analysis during exercise have become an additional tool for managing critically ill patients.

Bronchial challenge tests can be done using several different agents, all of which test the responsiveness of the airways in slightly different ways. Methacholine challenge is the most commonly used and best standardized test of airway hyperreactivity. Histamine and antigenic agents are also sometimes used. Exercise testing can be specifically used to evaluate exercise-induced bronchospasm. Hyperventilation tests, with either cold or room temperature air, mimic the ventilatory load that occurs with exercise.

Preoperative and disability testing use spirometry, lung volumes, diffusing capacity, blood gases, and exercise testing. Each of these tests can be used to examine a specific aspect of either preoperative risk or respiratory impairment that prevents work.

Pediatric pulmonary function tests in older children and adolescents (6 to 18 years old) are performed in a manner similar to adult tests. For infants and young children, highly specialized tests have been developed to assess respiratory function without dependence on subject effort. These include rapid thoracoabdominal compression, forced deflation, and partial flow-volume curves to assess airway function. Airway occlusion and passive flow-volume techniques can be used for noninvasive assessment of respiratory mechanics. Gas dilution and body plethysmography can be applied to measure lung volumes, specifically the FRC.

Metabolic measurements, notably indirect calorimetry, provide a means of assessing nutritional status and support. Indirect calorimetry has been shown to be more accurate than simple estimates of resting energy expenditure in mechanically ventilated patients. It may be particularly useful in the evaluation of those patients who do not respond adequately to estimated nutritional needs.

SELF-ASSESSMENT QUESTIONS

1 *Which of the following should be withheld for 48 hours before bronchial challenge testing?*
   a. Cromolyn sodium
   b. β-Adrenergic agents
   c. Anticholinergic preparations
   d. Beverages containing caffeine

2 *A subject performing a methacholine challenge test has the following reproducible results:*

FEV_1 (baseline)	3.3 L
FEV_1 (control)	3.2 L
FEV_1 (0.075 mg/ml)	3.2 L
FEV_1 (0.150 mg/ml)	2.6 L

   The technologist should do which of the following?
   a. Repeat methacholine 0.150 mg/ml dose.
   b. Administer methacholine 0.310 mg/ml.
   c. Give 10 breaths of the next dose.
   d. Stop; the test is positive.

3 *A patient has an eucapnic voluntary hyperventilation (EVH) test to evaluate bronchial hyperreactivity. If the subject FEV_1 is 3.3 L, which of the following is an appropriate target ventilation for this test?*
   a. Is 50 times the FEV_1 for 1 minute
   b. Is 30 times the FEV_1 for 6 minutes
   c. Starts at 2 times the FVC for 6 minutes
   d. Cannot be determined without the MVV

4 *Which of the following changes in SGaw is consistent with increased airway reactivity?*
   a. Increase of 20% after inhalation of histamine
   b. Decrease of 15% after inhalation of methacholine
   c. Decrease of 35% after inhalation of histamine
   d. Increase of 12% after cold air inhalation challenge

5 *PEFV curves may be obtained in infants by using which of the following?*
   a. Forced tidal breathing
   b. Voluntary hyperventilation
   c. Multiple occlusion technique
   d. Rapid thoracoabdominal compression

6 *A 3.0-kg infant has her $\dot{V}_{max}FRC$ measured using a squeeze technique and FRC measured by He dilution with the following results:*

$\dot{V}_{max}FRC$ 80 ml/sec
FRC   90 ml

These findings are consistent with which of the following:
   a. Airway obstruction
   b. Marked restrictive disease
   c. Normal lung function
   d. Improperly calibrated pneumotachometer

7 *Which of the following patients would be at greatest risk for postoperative complications after lung resection?*
   a. A patient with FEV_1 of 1.65 L
   b. A patient with MVV of 74% of predicted
   c. A patient with $Paco_2$ of 35 mm Hg
   d. A patient with $\dot{V}o_{2max}$ of 9 ml/min/kg

8 *A patient referred for exercise testing for disability determination should have which of the following?*
   a. 6-minute walk with pulse oximetry to document hypoxemia
   b. 5 minutes of treadmill exercise at 1.7 mph, 10% grade
   c. 4 to 6 minutes of treadmill exercise at 5 METS with blood gases
   d. Cycle ergometer exercise at 85% predicted maximum HR with pulse oximetry

9 *An indirect calorimetry system uses a dilution technique that mixes a constant flow of entrained air with expired gas; this technique allows determination of which of the following?*
   a. Exhaled ventilation
   b. End-tidal CO_2
   c. Nonprotein RQ
   d. Feo_2

10 *Which of the following findings indicates that indirect calorimetry data may be unacceptable?*
   I.   Data were collected for 5 minutes
   II.   RQ of 1.01
   III. $\dot{V}co_2$ varies by 10%
   IV. $\dot{V}o_2$ varies by 6%
   a. I and III only
   b. II and IV only
   c. I, II, and III
   d. II, III, and IV

SELECTED BIBLIOGRAPHY

Bronchial Challenge

Argyros GJ, Roach JM, Hurwitz KM, et al: Eucapnic voluntary hyperventilation as a bronchoprovocation technique, *Chest* 109:1520-1524, 1996.

Assoufi BK, Dally MB, Newman-Taylor AJ, et al: Cold-air test: a simplified standard method for airway reactivity, *Clin Respir Physiol* 22:349-357, 1986.

Cockcroft DW, Killian DN, Mellon JJA et al: Bronchial reactivity to inhaled histamine: a method and clinical survey, *Clin Allergy* 7:235-243, 1977.

Cropp GJA: The exercise bronchoprovocation test: standardization of procedures and evaluation of response, *J Allergy Clin Immunol* 64:627-633, 1979.

Eliasson AH, Phillips YY, Rajagopal KR, et al: Sensitivity and specificity of bronchial provocation testing: an evaluation of four techniques in exercise induced bronchospasm, *Chest* 102:347, 1992.

Haas F, Axen K, Schicchi JS: Use of maximum expiratory flow-volume curve parameters in the assessment of exercise induced bronchospasm, *Chest* 103:64-68, 1993.

Hargreave FE, Ryan A, Thomson NC, et al: Bronchial responsiveness to histamine or methacholine in asthma: measurement and clinical significance, *J Allergy Clin Immunol* 68:345-347, 1981.

Irvin CG: Bronchial challenge testing, *Respir Clin North Am* 1:265-285, 1995.

Pepys G, Hutchcroft BJ: Bronchial provocation tests in etiologic diagnosis and analysis of asthma, *Am Rev Respir Dis* 112:829, 1975.

Phillips YY, Jaeger JJ, Laube BL, et al: Eucapnic voluntary hyperventilation of compressed gas mixture, *Am Rev Resp Dis* 131:31-35, 1985.

Preoperative Pulmonary Function Testing

Boysen PG: Preoperative pulmonary function tests and complications after coronary artery bypass, *Anesthesiology* 57:A499, 1982.

Cain HD, Stevens PM, Adaniya R: Preoperative pulmonary function and complications after cardiovascular surgery, *Chest* 76:130, 1979.

Olsen GN, Block AJ, Swenson EW, et al: Pulmonary function evaluation of the lung resection candidate: a prospective study, *Am Rev Respir Dis* 111:379, 1975.

Reichel J: Assessment of operative risk of pneumonectomy, *Chest* 62:570, 1972.

Tisi GM: Preoperative evaluation of pulmonary function: Validity, indications, and benefits, *Am Rev Respir Dis* 119:293, 1979.

Respiratory Impairment for Disability

Gaensler EM, Wright GW: Evaluation of respiratory impairment, *Arch Environ Health* 12:146, 1966.

Harber P, Schnur R, Emery J, et al: Statistical 'biases' in respiratory disability determinations, *Am Rev Respir Dis* 128:413, 1983.

Morgan WKC: Pulmonary disability and impairment: can't work? won't work? basics of RD, *Am Thoracic Soc* 10:No. 5, 1982.

Disability evaluation under social security. US Department of Health and Human Services, SSA Pub No. 64-039, 1994.

Pulmonary Function Testing in Children

Dundas I, Dezateux CA, Fletcher ME, et al: Comparison of single-breath and plethysmographic measurements of resistance in infancy, *Am J Respir Crit Care Med* 151: 1451-1458, 1995.

England SJ: Current techniques for assessing pulmonary function in the newborn and infant: advantages and limitations, *Pediatr Pulmonol* 4:48, 1988.

Gappa M, Fletcher ME, Dezateux CA, et al: Comparison of nitrogen washout and plethysmographic measurement of lung volume in healthy infants, *Am Rev Respir Dis* 148:1496-1501, 1993.

Hanrahan JP, Tager IB, Castile RG, et al: Pulmonary function measures in healthy infants: variability and size correction, *Am Rev Resp Dis* 141:1127, 1990.

Lebowitz MD, Sherrill DL: The assessment and interpretation of spirometry during the transition from childhood to adulthood, *Pediatr Pulmonol* 19:143-149, 1995.

LeSouef PN, Hughes DM, Landau LI: Shape of forced expiratory flow-volume curves in infants, *Am Rev Respir Dis* 138:590, 1988.

Morgan WJ, Geller DE, Tepper RS, et al: Partial expiratory flow-volume curves in infants and young children, *Pediatr Pulmonol* 5:232, 1988.

Panitch HB, Kekklian EN, Motley RA, et al: Effect of altering smooth muscle tone on maximal expiratory flows in patients with tracheomalacia, *Pediatr Pulmonol* 9:170-176, 1990.

Polgar G, Promadhat V: *Pulmonary function testing in children: techniques and standards,* Philadelphia, 1971, WB Saunders.

Pfaff JK, Morgan WJ: Pulmonary function in infants and children, *Pediatr Clin North Am* 41:401-423, 1994.

Rosenthal M, Bain SH, Cramer D, et al: Lung function in white children ages 4 to 19 years: I—Spirometry, *Thorax* 48:794-802, 1993.

Stocks J, Nothen U, Sutherland P, et al: Improved accuracy of the occlusion technique for measuring total respiratory compliance in infants, *Pediatr Pulmonol* 3:71, 1987.

Taussig LM, Landou LI, Godfrey S, et al: Determination of forced expiratory flows in newborn infants, *J Appl Physiol Respir Environ Exercise Physiol* 53:1220-1227, 1982.

Tepper RS, Asdell S: Comparison of helium dilution and nitrogen washout measurements of functional residual capacity in infants and very young children, *Pediatr Pulmonol* 13:250-254, 1992.

Tepper RS, Pagtakhan RD, Taussig LM: Noninvasive determination of total respiratory compliance in infants by the weighted spirometer method, *Am Rev Respir Dis* 130:461, 1984.

Turner DJ, Stick SM, LeSouef KL, et al: A new technique to generate and assess forced expiration from raised lung volume in infants, *Am J Respir Crit Care Med* 151:1441-1450, 1995.

Metabolic Measurements (Indirect Calorimetry)

Askanazi J, Nordenstrom J, Rosenbaum SH, et al: Nutrition for the patient with respiratory failure: glucose vs fat, *Anesthesiology* 54:373, 1981.

Branson RD: The measurement of energy expenditure: instrumentation, practical considerations and clinical application, *Respir Care* 35:640-659, 1990.

Consolazio CF, Johnson RE, Pecora LJ: *Physiological measurements of metabolic functions in man,* New York, 1963, McGraw-Hill.

Ferrannini E: The theoretical bases of indirect calorimetry: a review, *Metabolism* 37:287-301, 1988.

Harris JA, Benedict FG: *Biometric studies of basal metabolism in man,* Carnegie Institute of Washington, Publication #279, 1919.

Kemper MA: Indirect calorimetry equipment and practical considerations of measurements. In Weissman C, ed: *Problems in respiratory care: nutrition and respiratory disease,* Philadelphia, 1989, JB Lippincott.

Makita K, Nunn JF, Royston B: Evaluation of metabolic measuring instruments for use in critically ill patients, *Crit Care Med* 18:638-644, 1990.

Weir JB: New methods for calculating metabolic rate with special reference to protein metabolism, *J Physiol* 109: 1-9, 1949.

Weissman C, Kemper M, Elwyn D, et al: The energy expenditure of the mechanically ventilated critically ill patient—an analysis, *Chest* 89:2, 254, 1986.

Weissman C, Kemper MA, Askanazi J, et al: Resting metabolic rate of the critically ill patient: measured versus predicted, *Anesthesiology* 64:673-679, 1986.

Guidelines and Standards

American Association for Respiratory Care: Clinical practice guideline: infant/toddler pulmonary function tests, *Respir Care* 40:761-768, 1995.

American Association for Respiratory Care: Clinical practice guideline: metabolic measurement using indirect calorimetry during mechanical ventilation, *Respir Care* 39:1170-1175, 1994.

American Association for Respiratory Care: Clinical practice guideline: bronchial provocation, *Respir Care* 37: 902-906, 1992.

American Thoracic Society/European Respiratory Society: Respiratory function measurements in infants: measurement conditions, *Am J Respir Crit Care Med* 151: 2058-2064, 1995.

American Thoracic Society/European Respiratory Society: Respiratory mechanics in infants: physiologic evaluation in health and disease, *Am Rev Respir Dis* 147:474-496, 1993.

Chai H, Farr RS, Froelich LA, et al: Standardization of bronchial inhalation challenge procedures, *J Allergy Clin Immunol* 56:323, 1975.

Cropp GJA, Bernstein IL, Boushey HA, et al: Guidelines for bronchial inhalation challenges with pharmacologic and antigenic agents, *ATS News* Spring, 11-19, 1980.

Eggleston PA, Rosenthal RR: Guidelines of the methodology of exercise challenge testing of asthmatics, *J Allergy Clin Immunol* 64:642, 1979.

CHAPTER 9

Pulmonary Function Testing Equipment

OBJECTIVES

After studying this chapter and reviewing its tables and figures, you should be able to do the following:

1 Describe at least three types of volume displacement spirometers

2 Explain how flow-sensing spirometers measure volume

3 State how different types of gas analyzers are used in the pulmonary function laboratory

4 Explain the causes of common blood gas electrode problems

5 Contrast and compare the measurement of oxygen saturation by multiwavelength and pulse oximeters

6 Describe the three basic signals used by the body plethysmograph to measure thoracic gas volume and airway resistance

7 Define the basic components of an interface between pulmonary function equipment and a computer

8 List the advantages of a relational database for storing pulmonary function records

THE PRECURSOR OF THE MODERN spirometer was introduced by Hutchinson in the mid-1800s. Some aspects of the original device are still evident in today's spirometers. Analysis of respiratory gases by volumetric methods was pioneered by Haldane in the early part of the twentieth century. Modern gas analyzers use indirect means of assessing the partial pressures of gases. Many of the instruments in the pulmonary function laboratory today combine physical transducers, analog signal generators, and computerized representations of those signals. Some devices, such as the pulse oximeter, are based almost entirely on electronic components. The use of microcomputers has eliminated many tedious calculations. Sophisticated data processing is available, even at the bedside.

This chapter describes pulmonary function equipment used for common testing applications. Included are volume-displacement and flow-sensing spirometers, peak flow meters, gas analyzers, blood gas electrodes and oximeters, body plethysmographs, breathing valves, and computers.

Volume Displacement Spirometers

WATER-SEALED SPIROMETERS

For many years, the basic tool in the determination of lung volumes and flow rates was the water-sealed spirometer. The water-sealed spirometer consists of a large bell (7 to 10 L) suspended in a container of water with the open end of the bell below the surface of the water. (Fig. 9-1). A system of breathing tubes into the interior of the bell allows for the accurate measurement of gas volumes. The subject breathes into the spirometer and in so doing moves the bell up or down proportionately. Each spirometer bell has a "bell factor" relating the vertical distance moved to a specific volume (milliliters or liters). The movement of the bell can be used to move a pen across a rotating drum or kymograph. Volumes can be measured directly from the kymograph tracing by using paper that incorporates the bell factor for the spirometer.

The spirometer bell can also activate a **potentiometer** to produce an analog DC voltage signal. A potentiometer is a device that produces a variable voltage depending on its position, much like

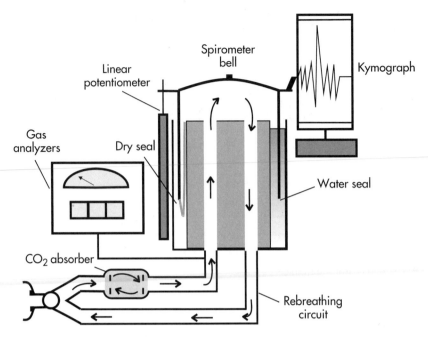

FIG. 9-1 *Water-seal type spirometer.* Typical water-seal or dry-seal spirometer is shown cut away; the spirometer bell "floats" in a well. On the right side a water seal is shown, on the left a dry rolling seal (see text). Also included is a rebreathing breathing circuit with CO_2 absorber and gas analyzers, as might be used for the closed circuit FRC determination. A kymograph can be attached so that excursions of the bell trace a volume-time spirogram on moving graph paper. A linear potentiometer provides analog outputs for volume and flow.

a dimmer switch connected to a light. The analog output provided by the potentiometer (in volts) is proportional to the position of the bell. The analog signal can be used to drive a mechanical recorder such as a strip-chart recorder. However, more commonly the analog signal is digitized using an analog-to-digital (A/D) converter (see "Computer Systems," p. 283). The digitized signal from the spirometer can then be stored and processed by computer.

For simple spirometry, a single large-bore tube can be used for both inspiration and expiration. For rebreathing studies the breathing circuit incorporates a CO_2 absorber (soda lime). Inspiratory and expiratory circuits are separated, with one-way valves to eliminate dead space. Water-seal spirometers are typically used for spirometry. They may also be used for measurements of ventilation, including minute ventilation ($\dot{V}E$), tidal volume (VT), and respiratory rate. In conjunction with an appropriate potentiometer and recording device, water-sealed spirometers can be used to obtain flow-volume curves. By including the rebreathing apparatus described, lung volumes by helium dilution can be obtained. In combination with an appropriate reservoir for the test gas, water-sealed spirometers can be used to perform diffusing capacity tests, both single breath and rebreathing. The water-sealed spirometer can itself be used as a reservoir for special gas mixtures such as those used for diffusing capacity tests.

The Stead-Wells water- or dry-seal spirometer is still commonly used. The Stead-Wells spirometer uses a lightweight plastic bell (Fig. 9-2). The water-sealed bell "floats" in the water well, rising and falling with breathing excursions. In the dry-seal version, a rubberized seal connects the bell to the internal wall of the spirometer well. The rubber seal then "rolls" much the same as the dry rolling-seal spirometer. The spirometer bell can carry a recording pen mounted against a variable-speed (i.e., 32, 160, and 1920 mm/min) kymograph. Respiratory excursions deflect the pen in the same direction as the bell. Expiration is traced upward on the volume-time graph (see Fig. 2-1). For manual measurements from kymograph tracings, corrections from ATPS to BTPS are necessary. The Stead-Wells bell can also be directly attached to a linear potentiometer. The linear potentiometer provides analog signals proportional to volume and flow. These signals can be passed to an analog recorder or to an **A/D converter**. The Stead-Wells design is capable of meeting the minimum requirements for flow and volume accuracy recommended by the American Thoracic Society (ATS) (see Chapter 10).

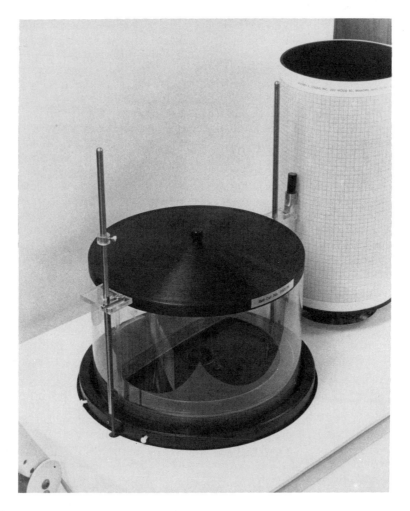

FIG. 9-2 *Stead-Wells dry-seal spirometer.* The conventional Stead-Wells spirometer uses a lightweight plastic bell that floats in water. This version of the Stead-Wells uses a silicon seal similar to that found in the dry rolling-seal spirometer. The spirometer bell carries a pen that traces directly on a rotating kymograph. With appropriate circuitry and gas analyzers, He dilution FRC determinations and DL_{CO} measurements are easily performed. (Courtesy Warren E. Collins, Inc., Braintree, MA.)

The primary advantages of the water-sealed spirometer are its simplicity and its accuracy. Because the spirometer bell can be used to directly drive a pen against the chart drum, direct mechanical tracings can be obtained. These tracings can be used for manual calculation of volumes and flows. The tracings can also be used for comparison with results derived by computer or from the analog recordings. Measurements of volumes and flows can be taken from the kymographic tracings if the bell factor and paper speed are known. Although most laboratories use computer-derived measurements, the capability to perform tests manually may be useful for quality assurance or for calibration. The "waterless" version of this type of spirometer allows the device to be transported more easily. In addition, periodic draining is eliminated and cleaning of the spirometer is simplified.

Problems with water-sealed spirometers are usually caused by leaks in the bell or in the breathing circuit. Gravity causes the spirometer to lose volume in the presence of leaks. Leaks in the spirometer, tubing, or valves can be detected by raising the bell and plugging the patient connection. Any change in volume can be detected easily by recording the spirometer volume over several minutes. Small weights can be added to the top of the bell to enhance detection of small leaks.

During patient testing, improper positioning of the spirometer can cause inaccurate measurements. If positioned too high, the bell can rise out of the water or reach the top of its travel range. This causes the volume-time tracing to appear abruptly flattened. The pattern observed may be mistaken for a normal end of expiration. If a Stead-Wells spirometer is positioned too low, it may empty completely. This may result in water being drawn into the breathing circuit, gas analyzer, or other system components. Inadequate water in the device may also lead to erroneous readings that are sometimes difficult to detect. The size of the water-sealed spirometer and its weight when filled with water make it somewhat difficult to transport. The waterless version of the spirometer eliminates the last consideration.

Maintenance of water-sealed spirometers includes routine draining of the water well. Both wet and dry versions of the Stead-Wells spirometer must be checked for cracks or leaks in the bell itself. Chemical absorbers for water vapor must be routinely checked. Water absorbers are rapidly exhausted because the gas in the spirometer is almost completely saturated with water vapor.

Infection control of water-sealed spirometers typically involves replacing breathing hoses and mouthpieces after each subject. Although the subject's expired gas comes into direct contact with the water in the spirometer, cross-contamination is not common. Some systems allow the use of low-resistance bacteria filters to protect those parts of the breathing circuit not changed after each patient use from contamination. Such filters should be used with caution for flow-dependent maneuvers. Water condensation in the filter element may significantly alter its resistance. The volume of these filters may need to be considered when calculating system volume or system dead space.

DRY ROLLING-SEAL SPIROMETERS

Another type of volume-displacement spirometer is the dry rolling-seal spirometer. A typical unit consists of a lightweight piston mounted horizontally in a cylinder. The piston is supported by a rod that rests on frictionless bearings (Fig. 9-3). The piston is coupled to the cylinder wall by a flexible plastic seal. The seal rolls on itself rather than sliding as the piston moves. A similar type of rolling-seal may also be used with a vertically mounted, lightweight piston that rises and falls with breathing. The maximum volume of the cylinder with the piston fully displaced is usually 10 to 12 L. The piston has a large diameter so that excursions of just a few inches are all that is necessary to record large volume changes. The piston is normally constructed of lightweight aluminum to reduce inertia. Mechanical resistance is kept to a minimum by the bearings supporting the piston rod and by the rolling seal itself.

Some dry rolling-seal spirometers use a mechanical recorder in which the piston rod has a pen attached. The pen moves across graph paper or a strip chart recorder as the subject inspires and expires. Most dry rolling-seal spirometers, however, use linear or rotary potentiometers. The potentiometer responds to piston movement to produce DC voltage outputs for volume and flow. For example, a 10-V potentiometer attached to a 10-L spirometer might produce an output of 1 V/L. On a separate channel, a flow of 1 L/sec might produce an output of 1 V. Flow in this case is

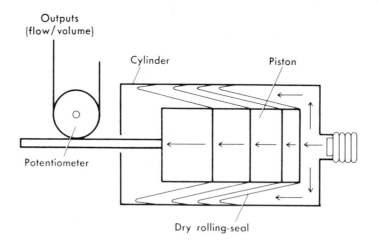

FIG. 9-3 *Cutaway view of a dry rolling-seal spirometer.* The figure gives an exaggerated view of the rolling-seal, which actually fits closely between the piston and cylinder wall. The piston has a large surface area, so horizontal movement is minimized. This allows recording of normal breaths and maximal respiratory excursions with little resistance. The piston is supported by a rod that activates a rotary potentiometer. Rotation of the potentiometer generates analog signals for flow and volume. (From Form 370, Ohio Medical Products, Madison, WI.)

proportional to the speed of the moving piston. These analog outputs for volume and flow are usually directed to an A/D convertor (see "Computer Systems," p. 283) so that the data can be stored by computer.

The piston of the standard dry rolling-seal spirometer (Fig. 9-4) travels horizontally, eliminating any need for counterbalancing. The vertically mounted version depends on the lightweight piston and the rolling seal to reduce resistance to breathing. Temperature corrections (i.e., from ATPS to BTPS) may be made by either adjusting the analog signal or applying a correction factor to the digital value stored in the computer. A one-way breathing circuit and CO_2 scrubber may be added so that dry rolling-seal spirometers can be used for rebreathing tests in much the same way as water-sealed spirometers.

To perform studies in which gas volumes larger than the spirometer itself are measured, such as the open-circuit nitrogen (N_2)-washout test, a "dumping" mechanism is attached to the spirometer. The dumping device empties the spirometer after each breath or after a predetermined volume has been reached. Addition of an automated valve and alveolar sampling device allows the dry rolling-seal spirometer to be used for single-breath diffusion studies. Dry rolling-seal spirometers are typically capable of meeting the minimum standards recommended by the ATS (see Chapter 10).

As with other volume displacement spirometers, dry rolling-seal spirometers can be adapted for manual or computerized testing. Manual testing using a mechanical recorder may be used for bedside or screening tests or for quality assurance checks. Despite their large size, most dry rolling-seal spirometers can be transported rather easily. However, addition of a computer, gas analyzers, or recorder may make the system too bulky for bedside testing.

Common problems encountered with dry rolling-seal spirometers are sticking of the rolling-seal and increased mechanical resistance in the piston-cylinder assembly. These difficulties can usually be avoided by adequate maintenance of the spirometer. Infection control of the dry

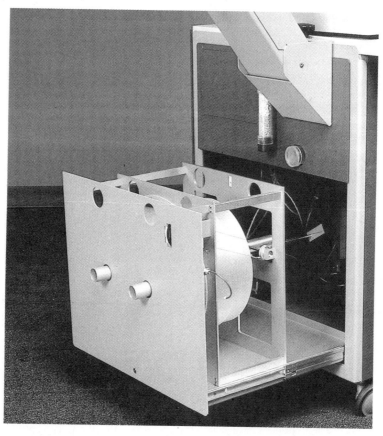

FIG. 9-4 *Dry rolling-seal spirometer.* A typical dry-seal spirometer consisting of a large aluminum piston mounted in a cylinder, with two ports to accommodate simple spirometry, as well as rebreathing maneuvers with a CO_2 absorber (see Fig. 9-3).

rolling-seal involves disassembling the piston-cylinder. The interior of the cylinder and the face of the piston are usually wiped with a mild antibacterial solution. The rolling-seal itself is also wiped with disinfectant. Alcohol or similar drying agents may cause deterioration of the seal and should not be used. The seal may be lubricated with cornstarch to prevent sticking, but care must be taken to avoid excessive powder being left in the spirometer. The seal should be routinely checked for leaks or tears. After reassembly the piston should be positioned at the maximum volume position. When the rolling-seal is extended completely, the material of the seal is less likely to develop creases that can result in uneven movement of the piston. With the previously described reservations, filters may be used to avoid contamination of the spirometer.

BELLOWS-TYPE SPIROMETERS

A third type of volume-displacement spirometer is the bellows or wedge bellows. Both of these devices consist of collapsible bellows that fold or unfold in response to breathing excursions. The conventional bellows design is a flexible accordion-type container. One end is stationary and the other end is displaced in proportion to the volume inspired or expired. The wedge bellows operates similarly except that it expands and contracts like a fan (Fig. 9-5). One side of the bellows remains stationary; the other side moves with a pivotal motion around an axis through the fixed side. Displacement of the bellows by a volume of gas is translated either to movement of a pen on chart paper or to a potentiometer. For mechanical recording, chart paper moves at a fixed speed under the pen while a spirogram is traced. For computerized testing, displacement of the bellows is transformed into a DC voltage by a linear or rotary potentiometer. The analog signal is routed to an A/D converter and then to a computer.

The conventional and wedge bellows may be mounted either horizontally or vertically. Horizontal bellows are mounted so that the primary direction of travel is on a horizontal plane. This design minimizes the effects of gravity on bellows movement. Horizontal bellows, either conventional or wedge, with a large surface area offer little mechanical resistance. This type of bellows is normally used in conjunction with a potentiometer to produce analog volume and flow signals. Several types of small (approximately 7 to 8 L), vertically mounted bellows are currently available and may be used for portable spirometry and bedside testing. Most of these bellows offer simple mechanical recording and/or digital data reduction by means of a small, dedicated **microprocessor.**

Both types of bellows (Fig. 9-6) can be used to measure vital capacity and its subdivisions, as well as forced vital capacity (FVC), forced expiratory volume (FEV_1), expiratory flows, and maximal voluntary ventilation (MVV). Some bellows-type spirometers, especially those that are mounted vertically, are designed to measure expiratory flows only. These types expand upward when gas is injected, then empty spontaneously under their own weight. Horizontally mounted bellows can usually be set in a mid-range to record both inspiratory and expiratory maneuvers. This

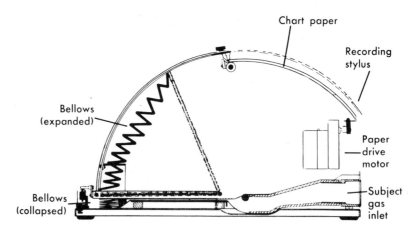

FIG. 9-5 *Cross-sectional diagram of a wedge-bellows type of spirometer.* The fanlike movements of the wedge bellows cause the recording stylus to move across graph paper. Some manufacturers suspend the bellows so that the primary movement is in a horizontal rather than vertical plane. Large wedge-bellows offer little resistance and are comparable to dry-seal or water-seal spirometers in accuracy and linearity. (Modified from Vitalograph Medical Instrumentation, Product Brochure, Lenexa, KS.)

allows measurements such as flow-volume loops to be made. With appropriate gas analyzers and breathing circuitry, bellows systems may be used for lung volume determinations and diffusing capacity (DL_{CO}) measurements. Most bellows-type spirometers meet ATS recommendations for flow and volume accuracy.

One problem that may occur with bellows spirometers is inaccuracy resulting from sticking of the bellows. The folds of the bellow may adhere because of dirt, moisture, or aging of the bellows material. Some bellows-type spirometers require the bellows to be partially distended when not in use. This technique allows moisture from exhaled gas to evaporate and prevents deterioration of the bellows. Leaks may also develop in the bellows material or at the point where the bellows is

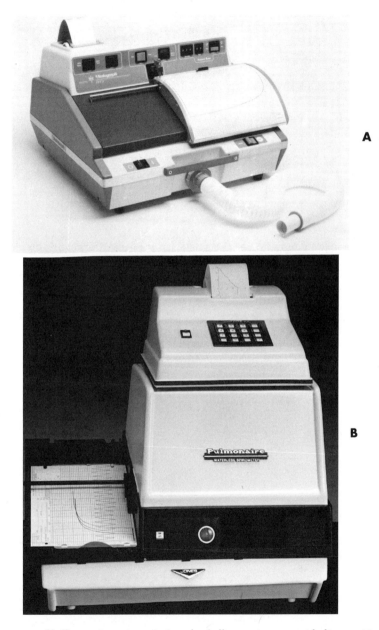

FIG. 9-6 *Two types of bellows spirometers.* **A,** A wedge-bellows spirometer with direct writing recorder, digital displays, and built-in printer for automated data reduction. (Courtesy Vitalograph Medical Instrumentation, Lenexa, KS.) **B,** A conventional bellows-type spirometer, with the bellows mounted horizontally and driving a pen across moving graph paper. A potentiometer allows analog output to a dedicated microprocessor with built-in printer for automatic data reduction. (Courtesy Jones Medical Instrument Co., Oakbrook, IL.)

mounted. Leaks can usually be detected by filling the bellows with air, plugging the breathing port, and attaching a weight or spring to pressurize the gas inside.

Infection control of bellows-type spirometers depends on the method of construction. In some instruments the bellows can be entirely removed, whereas in others the interior of the bellows must be wiped clean. Many bellows are made from rubberized or plastic-based material that can be cleaned with a mild detergent and dried thoroughly before reassembly. Filters may be used to avoid contamination of the bellows, with the reservations described previously.

Flow-Sensing Spirometers

In contrast to volume-displacement spirometers is the flow-sensing spirometer, or pneumotachometer. The term *pneumotachometer* describes a device that measures gas flow. Flow-sensing spirometers use various physical principles to produce a signal proportional to gas flow. This signal is then integrated to measure volume in addition to flow. Integration is a process in which flow (i.e., volume per unit of time) is divided into a large number of small intervals (i.e., time). The volume from each interval is summed (Fig. 9-7). Integration can be performed easily by an electronic circuit or by computer software. Accurate volume measurement by flow integration requires an accurate flow signal, accurate timing, and sensitive detection of low flow.

One type of device that responds to bulk flow of gas is the turbine or impeller. Integration is unnecessary because the turbine directly measures gas volumes. Some flow-sensing spirometers produce volume pulses in which each "pulse" equals a fixed volume. These spirometers incorporate very accurate counters to count the pulses. The remaining types of flow-sensing spirometers all use tubes through which laminar airflow is possible (see Appendix E). Although a wide variety of flow-sensing spirometers is presently available, four basic types are commonly used: turbines, pressure-differential, heated-wire, and **Pitot tube** flow sensors.

TURBINES

The simplest type of flow-sensing device is the turbine or **respirometer.** This instrument consists of a vane connected to a series of precision gears. Gas flowing through the body of the instrument causes the vane to rotate, registering a volume (Fig. 9-8). The respirometer can be used to measure vital capacity. It can also be used for ventilation tests such as VT and VE. One such device is the

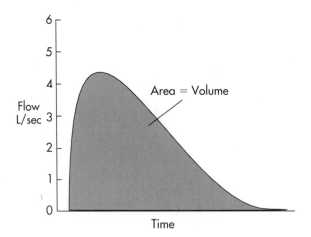

FIG. 9-7 *Volume measurement by flow integration.* The flow signal from many types of flow-sensing spirometers is integrated to compute volume. Flow is measured against time. The area under the flow-time curve is subdivided into a large number of small sections. Each section represents a small time interval. Volume is equal to the sum of the areas of all these sections. By dividing the curve into a large number of sections, even irregular flow curves can be accurately integrated. Integration is usually performed by a dedicated electronic circuit or by software.

Wright respirometer. This respirometer can measure volumes at flows between 3 and 300 L/min. At flows above 300 L/min (5 L/sec) the vane is subject to distortion. Because of this limitation, it should not be used to measure FVC when the subject is capable of flows greater than 300 L/min. At low flows (less than 3 L/min), inertia of the vane-gear system may underestimate volume.

The special advantage of this type of respirometer is its compact size and usefulness at the bedside. Most respirometers can register a wide range of volumes, from 0.1 to 1 L on one scale, and up to 100 L on another scale. Turbine devices are also widely used for bulk measurements in various dry gas meters.

An adaptation of the turbine flow device includes a photo cell and light source that is interrupted by the movement of the vane or impeller (Fig. 9-9). Rotation of the vane interrupts the light beam between its source and the photo cell. This produces a pulse, with each pulse equivalent to a fixed gas volume. The pulse count is summed to obtain the volume of gas flowing through the device. The signal produced may not be linear across a wide range of flows because of inertia or distortion of the rotating vane.

The accuracy of turbine flow devices is usually limited by the factors described. For this reason, most turbine devices do not meet the ATS minimum recommendations for diagnostic spirometers. However, most do meet the recommendations for monitoring devices (see Chapter 10). Because of their simplicity and small size, several such devices are marketed for home use. This type of spirometer allows FVC, FEV_1, and peak expiratory flow (PEF) to be monitored outside the usual clinical setting.

Infection control of turbine-type respirometers depends on their construction and intended use. Devices such as the Wright respirometer usually must be gas sterilized. Water condensation from exhaled gas can damage the vane-gear mechanisms. Some turbine spirometers use disposable impellers. This avoids cross-contamination, but accuracy is limited by the quality of the disposable sensor.

PRESSURE-DIFFERENTIAL FLOW SENSORS

The most common type of flow-sensing device consists of a tube containing a resistive element. The resistive element allows gas to flow through it but causes a pressure drop. The pressure difference across the resistive element is measured by means of a sensitive pressure transducer. The transducer usually has pressure taps on either side of the element. The pressure differential across the resistive element is proportional to gas flow as long as flow is laminar (see Fig. 9-9). This flow signal is integrated to measure volume. Turbulent gas flow upstream or downstream of the resistive element

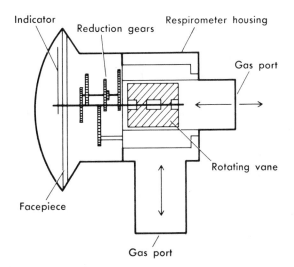

FIG. 9-8 *Turbine-type flow sensor.* A cutaway diagram of the Wright respirometer. A rotating vane mounted on jeweled bearings drives reduction gears connected to the main indicator arm. Two gas ports allow flow through the housing for measurement of volume. Although the vane turns in only one direction, inspired or expired volumes can be measured by attachment to the appropriate port. Not pictured is a small indicator arm, which marks volumes larger than 1 L on the face, so that accumulated volumes can be measured. The instrument also features controls for engaging or disengaging the vane and for resetting the indicators to zero. (From the British Oxygen Co., Ltd. Operating Instructions, Wright Respirometer, print No. 630207, Issue 3:6, Aug., 1971.)

may interfere with development of true **laminar flow.** Most pneumotachometers attempt to reduce turbulent flow by tapering the tubes in which the resistive elements are mounted.

Two types of resistive elements are commonly used. The Fleisch-type pneumotachometer uses a bundle of capillary tubes as the resistive element. Laminar flow is ensured by size and arrangement of the capillary tubes. The cross-sectional area and length of the capillary tubes determines the actual resistance to flow through the Fleisch pneumotachometer. The dynamic range of the Fleisch device must be matched to the range of flows to be measured. Different sizes (i.e., resistances) of pneumotachometers may be used to accurately measure high or low flows.

The other common type of pressure differential flow sensor is the Silverman, or Lilly, type. The Silverman pneumotachometer uses one or more screens to act as a resistive element. A typical arrangement has three screens mounted parallel to one another. The middle screen acts as the resistive element with the pressure taps on either side, whereas the outer screens protect the middle screen and help ensure laminar flow. The Silverman pneumotachometer has a somewhat wider dynamic flow range than the Fleisch type. As a result, it is somewhat better suited for measuring widely varying flows. Most Fleisch and Silverman pneumotachometers use a heating mechanism to warm the resistive element to 37° C or higher. Heating the resistive element prevents condensation of water vapor from exhaled gas on the element. Condensation or other debris lodging in the resistive element changes the resistance across it, thus changing its calibration.

Some flow-sensing spirometers use resistive elements such as porous paper, rendering the flow sensor disposable. These devices usually have a single pressure tap upstream of the resistive element. Pressure measured in front of the resistive element is referenced against ambient pressure. This technique requires that the flow sensor be carefully "zeroed" before making any flow measurements. The accuracy of these types of spirometers often depends on how carefully the disposable resistive elements are manufactured. If the resistance varies widely from sensor to sensor, each unit may need to be calibrated before use to ensure accuracy. Some manufacturers

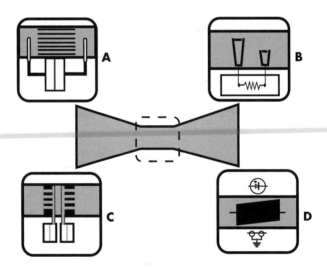

FIG. 9-9 *Common flow-sensing devices (pneumotachometers).* Each flow sensor is mounted in a tube that promotes laminar flow *(center).* **A,** Pressure-differential pneumotachometer in which a resistive element causes a pressure drop proportional to the flow of gas through the tube. A sensitive pressure transducer monitors the pressure drop across the resistive element and converts the differential into an analog signal. The resistive element may be a mesh screen or capillary tube; it is usually heated to 37° C or higher to prevent condensation of water from expired gas. **B,** A heated-wire type of pneumotachometer in which heated elements of small mass respond to gas flow by heat loss. An electrical current heats the elements. Gas flow past the elements causes cooling. In one element current is increased to maintain a constant temperature; the other element acts as a reference (see Fig. 9-10). The current change is proportional to gas flow, and a continuous signal is supplied to an integrating circuit as for the pressure differential flow sensor. **C,** A Pitot tube flow sensor in which a series of small tubes are placed at right angles to the direction of gas flow. Changes in gas velocity are detected by sensitive pressure transducers. The Pitot tubes are mounted in struts in the flow tube; separate devices face either way so that bidirectional flow can be measured (see Fig. 9-11). **D,** An electronic rotating-vane type of flow sensor. A vane or impeller is mounted in the flow tube. A light emitting diode (LED) is mounted on one side of the vane, a photodetector on the other side. Each time the vane rotates it "chops" the light from the LED reaching the detector. These pulses are counted and summed to calculate gas volume.

calibrate disposable sensors and provide a calibration code. This code is then used to identify a particular sensor by the software that makes the measurements.

Systems that use permanent pressure-differential flow sensors usually meet or exceed the ATS minimal recommendations for diagnostic spirometers. Spirometers that use disposable sensors can meet or exceed the minimal requirements depending on the quality of the sensor and the application software responsible for signal processing. Some pressure-differential flow sensors may meet only the less stringent recommendations for monitoring devices. Gas composition affects the accuracy of flow measurements in pressure-differential pneumotachometers. Correction factors for gases other than air can be applied by software so that these types of flow sensors can be used for most types of pulmonary function tests.

Infection control of pressure-differential flow sensors depends on their placement in the spirometer. In open-circuit systems in which only exhaled gas is measured, only the mouthpiece needs to be changed between subjects. If inspiratory and expiratory flow are measured, the flow sensor may need to be disinfected between patients. Disassembly and cleaning of flow sensors usually require that the spirometer be recalibrated. Disposable or single-use sensors avoid this problem. In-line filters may be used to isolate the pneumotachometer from potential contamination. The spirometer should meet all ATS requirements for range, accuracy, and flow resistance with the filter in place (see Chapter 10). If a filter is used, calibration with the filter in-line may be required. The effect of bacteria filters on spirometric measurements has not been well defined.

HEATED-WIRE FLOW SENSORS

A third type of flow-sensing spirometer is based on the cooling effect of gas flow. A heated element, usually a thin platinum wire, is situated in a laminar flow tube (see Fig. 9-9). Gas flow past the wire causes a temperature drop so that more current must be supplied to maintain a preset temperature. The current needed to maintain the temperature is proportional to flow. The heated element usually has a small mass so that very slight changes in gas flow can be detected. The flow signal is integrated electronically or by software to obtain volume measurements. The heated wire is protected behind a screen to prevent impaction of debris on the element. Debris or moisture droplets on the element can change its thermal characteristics. Some systems use two wires (Fig. 9-10). One measures gas flow and the second serves as a reference. Most heated wire flow-sensors maintain a temperature in excess of 37° C. This prevents condensation from expired air from interfering with sensitivity of the element.

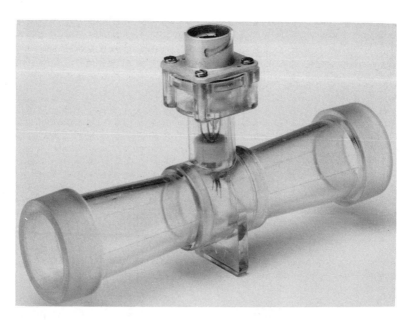

FIG. 9-10 *A heated-wire flow sensor.* A tube contains very thin, paired stainless steel wires. The wires are maintained at two different temperatures exceeding body temperature connected by a Wheatstone bridge. The tube streamlines gas flow into laminar flow. The temperature of the wires decreases in proportion to the mass of the gas and its flow. Two wires are used, one measuring expiratory flow and the other serves as a reference. (Courtesy SensorMedics, Corp., Yorba Linda, CA.)

Most heated-wire flow sensors meet or exceed ATS recommendations for accuracy and precision. Gas composition may affect the accuracy of flow measurements. Correction factors for gases other than room air can be applied via software. This allows heated-wire devices to accurately measure gases for pulmonary function tests using helium, oxygen, and other gases. Infection control for heated-wire sensors is similar to that for pressure-differential devices. Disposable or single-use devices avoid cross-contamination even when the sensor is located proximal to the patient's airway.

PITOT TUBE FLOW SENSORS

A fourth type of flow sensor uses the Pitot tube principle. The pressure of a gas flowing against a small tube is related to the gas's density and velocity. Flow can be measured by placing a series of small tubes in a flow sensor and connecting them to a sensitive pressure transducer (see Fig. 9-9). The pressure signal must be linearized and integrated as described for other flow-sensing devices. In practice, two sets of Pitot tubes are mounted in the same device so that bidirectional flow can be measured (Fig. 9-11). A wide range of flows can be accommodated by using two pressure transducers with different sensitivities. Because this type of flow-sensing device is affected by gas density, software correction for different gas compositions is necessary. This is accomplished by actually sampling the gas, analyzing O_2 and CO_2, and applying the necessary correction factors. Software corrections for test gases used for various pulmonary function tests (e.g., DL_{CO}) can be easily applied.

Pitot tube flow sensors easily meet or exceed ATS recommendations for accuracy and precision. Their practical applications include routine pulmonary function tests, metabolic measurements, and exercise testing. Infection control for this type of device includes single-use or disposable flow meters.

Pulmonary function testing using flow-based spirometers has some advantages over volume-displacement systems. When combined with appropriate gas analyzers and breathing circuits, flow-sensing spirometers can be used to perform lung volume determinations by the open- or closed-circuit methods. Diffusing capacity can be measured with flow-sensing spirometers as well. Pressure-differential and Pitot tube pneumotachometers are used to measure flow and volume in body plethysmographs, exercise testing systems, and metabolic carts. Because of their small size, flow-sensing devices are often incorporated into spirometers designed for portability. Because flow sensors require electronic circuitry to integrate flow or sum volume pulses, flow-based spirometers are usually microprocessor controlled. Some flow-sensing spirometers provide their analog signal (flow, volume, or both) to a strip chart or X-Y recorder. However, most flow-sensors use computer-generated graphics to produce volume-time or flow-volume tracings.

Many flow-sensing spirometers interface directly with small personal computers (Fig. 9-12). Many of these systems use an interface (see "Computer Systems," p. 283), which plugs directly into the user's personal computer (PC). With the appropriate software installed on the PC, spirometry can be performed. Other spirometers contain the electronic hardware in the flow sensor head. This implementation allows the flow sensor to be connected to a **serial port,** which is standard on most computers. Still other flow sensors use dedicated microprocessors that can be incorporated in a

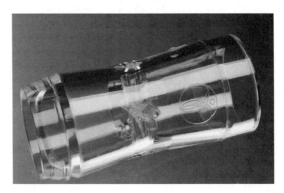

FIG. 9-11 *Pitot tube flow sensor.* A series of small tubes is mounted on struts in the flow tube. The tubes are connected to very sensitive pressure transducers (not shown). Using a series of transducers allows a wide range of flows to be accurately measured. Pitot tubes are mounted with struts facing both directions so that inspiratory and expiratory flow can be detected. (Courtesy Medical Graphics Inc., St. Paul, MN.)

very small package. This allows the unit to be hand-held and portable. Interfacing a flow sensor to a PC or laptop computer makes spirometry available in a variety of clinical settings. Hand-held or PC-based systems provide a relatively inexpensive way to perform spirometry, both before and after bronchodilator studies and bronchial challenge.

Most flow-based spirometers can be easily cleaned and disinfected. Some flow sensors can be immersed in a disinfectant without disassembly. As noted, many systems use inexpensive, disposable sensors that can be discarded after one use. The use of in-line bacteria filters to prevent contamination of flow-based spirometers may result in changes in the operating characteristics of the spirometer. Any resistance to airflow through the filter will be added to the resistance of the spirometer itself. For this reason, the spirometer may need to be calibrated with the filter in place. Although the resistance offered by most filters is low, it may change with use. This may occur if water vapor from expired gas condenses on the filter media. Use of barrier filters does not eliminate the need for routine decontamination of spirometers.

Most flow-based spirometers operate on the premise that a given flow will generate a proportional signal. However, across a wide range of flows, the signal generated may not be proportional (i.e., not linear). Almost every type of flow-sensing device displays some nonlinearity. Some systems use two separate flow sensors to accommodate both low and high flows. Better accuracy can be obtained for flow and volume by matching the flow range of the sensor to the physiologic signal. Most flow-based spirometers "linearize" the flow signal electronically or by means of software corrections. In many systems, a "look-up table" is stored in the computer. The flow signal is continuously checked against the table and corrected. By combining a calibration factor (see Chapter 10) with the look-up table corrections, very accurate flow and integrated volume measurements are possible. Flow and volume are corrected before variables such as FEV_1 are measured.

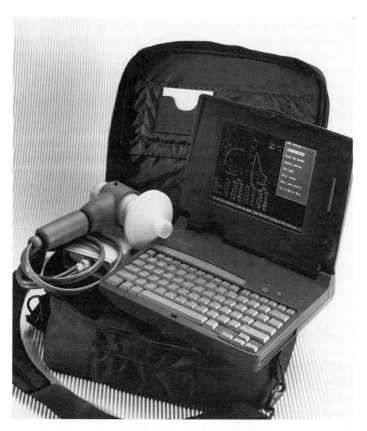

FIG. 9-12 *Flow-sensing spirometer interfaced to personal computers.* A pressure-differential pneumotachometer with its interface electronics connects to the serial port of the PC. The laptop or portable computer runs software that provides calculations, data storage, and printing of results. (Courtesy Pulmonary Data Service Instrumentation, Louisville, CO.)

Turbines, pressure-differential, heated-wire, and Pitot tube flow-sensing spirometers are all affected by the composition of the gas being measured. Changes in gas density or viscosity require correction of the transducer signal to obtain accurate flows and volumes. In most systems these corrections are performed by computer software using a stored table. A flow-sensing spirometer may be calibrated with air, but then used to measure mixtures containing helium, neon, oxygen, or other test gases. Some gases cause a linear shift in flow depending on their concentration. Correction in this case is usually made by applying a simple multiplier to the signal.

Results from flow-based spirometers depend on the electronic circuitry that converts the raw signal into flow or volume. Pulmonary function variables measured on a time base (e.g., FEV_1 or MVV) require precise timing as well as accurate flow measurement. The timing mechanism in flow-based spirometers is critical in the detection of the start or end of test. Timing is usually triggered by a minimum flow or pressure change. Integration of the flow signal begins when flow through the spirometer reaches a threshold limit, usually 0.1 to 0.2 L/sec. Instruments that initiate timing in response to volume pulses usually have a similar threshold that must be achieved to begin recording. Contamination of resistive elements, thermistors, or Pitot tubes by moisture or other debris can alter the flow-sensing characteristics of the transducer and interfere with the spirometer's ability to detect the start or end of test.

Problems related to electronic "drift" require flow sensors to be calibrated frequently. Many systems "zero" the flow signal immediately before a measurement. Zeroing corrects for much of the electronic drift that occurs. A true zero requires no flow through the flow sensor. Hence the flow sensor must be held still or occluded during the zero maneuver. Most flow-based systems use a 3-L syringe for calibration. By calibrating with a known volume signal, the accuracy of the flow sensor and the integrator can be checked with one input. Calibration and quality control techniques for volume-displacement and flow-sensing spirometers are included in Chapter 10.

Peak Flow Meters

PEF can be measured easily with most types of spirometers, either volume-displacement or flow-sensing types. Many devices are available that measure PEF exclusively. PEF has become a recognized means of monitoring patients who have asthma (see Chapter 2). By incorporating a simple measurement into an inexpensive package, portable peak flow meters allow monitoring of airway status in a variety of settings.

Most of the peak flow meters available use similar designs. The subject expires forcefully through a resistor or flow tube that has a movable indicator attached (Fig. 9-13). The resistance in most devices is provided by an orifice. The movable indicator is deflected in proportion to the velocity of air flowing through the device. PEF is then read directly from a calibrated scale. Because these devices are nonlinear, different flow ranges are usually available. High-range peak flow meters typically measure flows as high 850 L/min. Low-range meters measure up to 400 L/min (Table 9-1). Low-range peak flow meters are useful for small children or for subjects who have marked obstruction.

The absolute accuracy of portable peak flow meters is less important than precision of the device. Repeated measurements with the same PEF meter should be reproducible within 5% or 10 L/min, whichever is greater. These devices are intended to provide serial measurements of peak flow as a guide to treatment. Normal subjects who are carefully instructed should be able to reproduce their peak flow measurements within 10%. PEF meters must be easy to use and easy to read. Scale divisions of 5 L/min for low-range devices and 10 L/min for high-range devices allow small changes in PEF to be detected. The scale should be calibrated to read flow in BTPS units. Corrections for altitude should be included because PEF meters tend to underestimate flow as altitude increases (i.e., approximately 7% per 100 mm Hg change in barometric pressure).

TABLE 9-1   Peak Flow Meter Recommended Ranges

	Children	Adults
National Asthma Education Program	100-400 L/min ± 10%	100-700 L/min ± 10%
American Thoracic Society	60-400 L/min ± 10% or 20 L/min, whichever is greater	100-850 L/min ± 10% or 20 L/min, whichever is greater

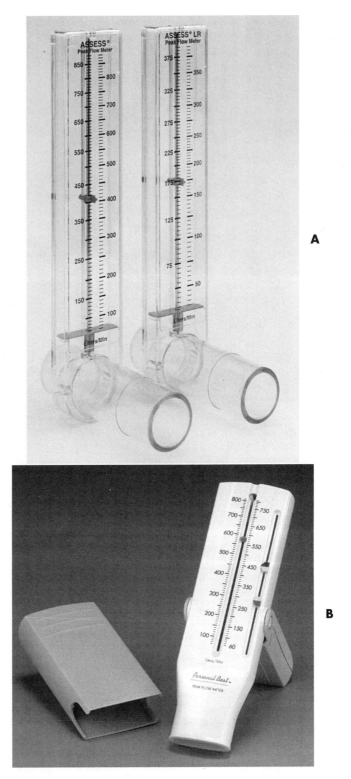

FIG. 9-13 *Portable peak-flow meters.* **A,** Portable peak-flow meters for measuring PEF outside of the pulmonary function laboratory. The subject exhales forcefully through the mouthpiece at the bottom. Pressure generated by the flow of gas deflects the movable indicator up the scale. Two flow ranges are available, for normal and reduced peak flows. **B,** Portable peak-flow meter in which exhaled flow is directed against a movable indicator. Two separate flow ranges are provided in the same device. (Both courtesy HealthScan Products Inc., Cedar Grove, NJ.)

Although their simple design allows them to be used repeatedly, moisture or other debris can cause sticking of the movable indicator. Some instruments can be cleaned but may require periodic replacement. Because portable peak flow meters may have a limited life span, reproducibility between same model instruments should be 5% (ATS recommendations suggest 10% or 20 L/min). This allows the patient to continue monitoring with a new device. Clear instructions on how to use and maintain the PEF meter should come with each device. Most peak flow meters comply with the National Asthma Education Program's "color zone" scheme for identifying clinically significant changes (see Chapter 2).

Breathing Valves

Various types of valves are commonly used with both volume-displacement and flow-sensing spirometers. These valves direct inspired or expired gas through the spirometer or provide a means of sampling for gas analysis.

FREE BREATHING VALVES

The simplest type of valve allows the subject to be switched from breathing room air to breathing gas contained in a spirometer or special breathing circuit. Free breathing valves are routinely used in both open- and closed-circuit FRC determinations. The free breathing valve is designed so that the subject can be "switched in" to the system either manually or by computer control at any point in the breathing cycle.

The typical free breathing valve consists of a body with two or more ports. A drum in the valve body rotates to connect different combinations of ports. Because these types of valves are used mainly for tidal breathing or slow vital capacity (VC) maneuvers, resistance to flow is not critical. Most have ports with diameters of 1.5 to 3 cm. For studies involving gas analysis, such as the FRC determination, the valve must be free of leaks.

Some systems use a "breathing manifold" that consists of multiple ports and valves. The ports allow inspired or expired gas to be directed to the spirometer or gas sampling devices. The valves may be electrical or gas-powered **solenoids**, or balloon valves that inflate with compressed air. With computer control, different combinations of valves and ports are opened and closed. This type of manifold permits spirometry, gas dilution lung volumes, and diffusing capacity tests to be performed with the same breathing circuit.

Infection control for free breathing valves and multiple-port manifolds involves disassembly, cleaning, and disinfection or sterilization. Because cleaning between patients may not be practical, in-line filters may be used to prevent contamination of these devices.

DIRECTIONAL (ONE-WAY, TWO-WAY) VALVES

Directional valves are used in many types of breathing circuits. The simplest type consists of a flap or diaphragm that opens in only one direction. The valve is then mounted in a rigid tube that can be inserted in a breathing circuit. Because gas is only permitted to flow in one direction, these valves are called one-way valves.

A more common design is that used to separate inspired from expired gas, often called a two-way nonrebreathing valve. This type of directional valve consists of a T-shaped body with three ports and two separate diaphragms (Fig. 9-14). The diaphragms allow gas to flow in only one direction. The subject connection is between the diaphragms, effectively separating inspired from expired gas. Two-way nonrebreathing valves are used in exercise testing, metabolic studies, or any procedure requiring collection, measurement, or analysis of exhaled gas. The valve body may contain a tap for connection of gas sample tubing. This tap is typically placed between the diaphragms so that both inspired and expired gas can be sampled.

Two factors must be considered in the selection of appropriate directional valves: dead space volume and flow resistance. In one-way valves, only flow resistance is a concern. In two-way nonrebreathing valves, dead space is the volume contained between the two diaphragms along with the volume of any connectors (i.e., mouthpiece). Most manufacturers supply information on the dead space of individual valves. Sometimes the dead space value is printed on the valve body. Unknown dead space can be determined by blocking two of the three ports and measuring the water volume required to fill the dead space portion of the valve.

Low-dead space valves (less than 50 ml) may be required if the patient already has increased dead space, particularly if only tidal breathing is being assessed. Valves with large-bore ports and low-resistance diaphragms usually have larger dead space volumes. To minimize resistance at high

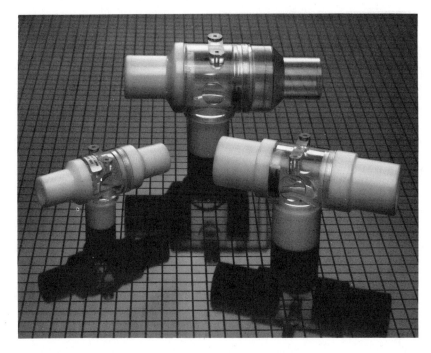

FIG. 9-14 *Two-way nonrebreathing valves.* Three differently sized valves used for measurement of expired gas are shown. Each valve consists of a T-shaped body containing two diaphragms that separate inspired and expired gas. The smaller valves have less dead space but higher resistance to flow; the large valve has low flow resistance but more dead space. The small and medium valves are used for studies in which low flows are encountered, such as metabolic measurements. The large valve is appropriate for high flow rates such as those occurring during maximal exercise testing. (Courtesy Hans Rudolph Inc., Kansas City, MO.)

flows during exercise testing, large-bore nonrebreathing valves are used. These valves usually have a large dead space volume. Selection of the appropriate-size nonrebreathing valve should be based on the maximal flow anticipated during the test. For example, a maximal exercise test for a healthy adult subject may include flows greater than 100 L/min. A large-bore valve would be selected to accommodate the high flow. Valve dead space would be less of a concern because large tidal volumes are necessary to generate the increased flow. Mechanical (i.e., valve) dead space must be accurately determined for use in calculations involving gas analysis, such as physiologic dead space measurements.

Low resistance to flow is also a critical characteristic of both one-way and two-way valves. Resistance to flow through most valves is nonlinear and depends on the cross-sectional area of valve leaflets or diaphragms (Fig. 9-15). Resistance is usually not critical for tests during which flows less than 1 L/sec are developed. Small-bore directional valves can be selected on the basis of an appropriate dead space volume. Most small-bore nonrebreathing valves have resistances in the range of 1 to 2 cm H_2O/L/sec at flows up to 1 L/sec (60 L/min). If the subject breathes through the valve for long intervals, even small resistances may result in respiratory muscle fatigue and changes in the ventilatory pattern. Applications such as exercise testing often involve increased flows. Large-bore two-way valves are indicated when flows greater than 1 L/sec (60 L/min) can be expected to develop. Pressures lower than 3 cm H_2O can be maintained even at flows of 5 L/sec (300 L/min) with large-bore valves. Saliva may build up in valves during prolonged tests (e.g., exercise or eucapnic hyperventilation). Valves with "saliva traps" may be needed for these types of procedures. Any valves used in a spirometry circuit must have very low resistance to meet the ATS recommendation of less than 1.5 cm H_2O/L/sec at flows of 12 L/sec.

Even appropriately selected valves can cause increased resistance if not properly maintained. Rubber, plastic, or silicon leaflets and diaphragms can stick or become rigid with age. Valves should be disassembled and cleaned according to the manufacturers' directions after each use and allowed to dry thoroughly before reassembly. Care must be taken when reassembling valves to ensure that all diaphragms are oriented properly. Valves should be visually inspected to make sure diaphragms open and close correctly before being used.

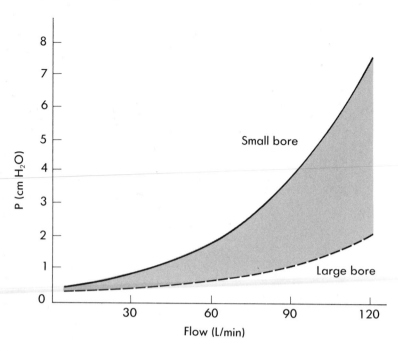

FIG. 9-15 *Breathing valve resistance.* A graph plotting pressure developed across two differently sized valves in relation to gas flow through them. For small-bore valves (see Fig. 9-14), pressures less than 1 cm H_2O are generated up to approximately 60 L/min (1 L/sec). Large-bore valves have less resistance (i.e., pressure per unit of flow) and are typically used for studies in which the subject develops high flow rates. Other factors affecting resistance include the design and material used for the diaphragms in the valve and whether the diaphragms move freely. Resistance increases nonlinearly in all types of valves; high resistance can occur even in large-bore valves at very high flows.

GAS SAMPLING VALVES

Specialized valves may be used to sample gas during tests such as the single-breath DL_{CO}. Many gas sampling valves use electrical or pneumatically powered solenoids to direct flow to a spirometer or sample bag. The primary concern with gas sampling valves is smooth operation with appropriate direction of the gas to be sampled. Electrically activated solenoids may deteriorate with age, particularly if exposed to high-humidity conditions (e.g., expired air). Replacement of O-rings or similar types of seals may be necessary to ensure uncontaminated gas samples. Some sampling valves use balloons that inflate to block or direct the gas flow. These balloons require periodic replacement because a small leak in a balloon can prevent the balloon from "seating." As a result, gas may not be directed to the appropriate device.

Infection control for sampling valves usually requires disassembly and cleaning. Some complex valve manifolds may be difficult or impossible to disassemble. In these devices, an in-line filter may be needed to avoid cross-contamination.

Pulmonary Gas Analyzers

Various types of gas analyzers are used in pulmonary function testing. O_2 and CO_2 are analyzed during metabolic studies and exercise testing. Helium analysis is used for closed-circuit functional residual capacity (FRC) determinations and for several types of DL_{CO} tests. N_2 analysis is used in the open-circuit FRC method. CO measurements are integral to all of the diffusion capacity methods currently used. Analyses of neon, argon, methane, and acetylene are used in specialized tests for diffusion, lung volume measurements, and cardiac output determination.

How rapidly a gas analyzer can detect and display a change in gas concentration is termed response time. Response time is commonly measured in seconds or milliseconds (thousandths of a second). Manufacturers of gas analyzers list response time as the interval required for an analyzer to measure some fraction of a step change in gas concentration. For example, an O_2 analyzer might require 2 seconds to respond to an increase in O_2 concentration from 21% to 100%. The response time would be listed as the time required for 90% of the total change to be detected. Response time

TABLE 9-2 Oxygen Analyzers

Type	Applications	Advantages/Disadvantages
Paramagnetic	Monitoring	Discrete sampling only
Polarographic electrode	Monitoring, exercise testing, metabolic studies	Discrete or continuous sampling; requires special electronic circuitry for fast response (200 msec)
Galvanic cell (fuel cell)	Monitoring	Continuous sampling; similar to polarographic but does not require polarizing voltage
Zirconium cell	Breath-by-breath exercise and metabolic studies	Heated (700° to 800° C) fuel cell; fast response useful for continuous sampling; thermal stabilization required
Gas chromatograph	Exercise testing, monitoring, metabolic measurements	Discrete sampling; response time ~30 seconds; very accurate; multiple gas analysis

of an analyzer often depends on the size of the change in gas concentration. Another important factor is transport time. Transport time is how long it takes to move the gas from the sample site to the analyzer itself. How rapidly a gas (e.g., O_2) can be analyzed depends on both the response time and the transport time of the instrument.

OXYGEN ANALYZERS

Oxygen analysis can be performed by several different methods. Table 9-2 lists some of the types of O_2 analyzers available. Two types are used for rapid analysis of O_2 (e.g., in breath-by-breath exercise tests): the polarographic electrode and **zirconium** fuel cell. The other O_2 analyzers listed are used for specialized applications, including patient monitoring.

Polarographic Electrodes

The polarographic electrode is similar to the blood gas O_2 electrode (see "Blood Gas Electrodes," p. 268). For gas analysis, a platinum cathode is used without a membrane covering the tip. A gas pump draws the sample past the polarized electrode at a constant flow. Oxygen is reduced in proportion to its partial pressure. The electrode is calibrated by exposing it to known fractional concentrations of O_2 at a known barometric pressure. A response time of approximately 200 msec can be attained by using special electronic circuitry. Rapid response allows continuous analysis for breath-by-breath measurements. Contamination of the electrode can degrade its response time and cause difficulty with calibration.

Zirconium Fuel Cells

An electrode is formed by coating a zirconium element with platinum. The zirconium, when heated to 700° to 800° C acts as a solid electrolyte between the platinum coating on either side. When the two sides of the electrode are exposed to different partial pressures of O_2, gas traverses the electrode, creating a voltage proportional to the difference in concentrations. Sample gas is drawn past the element at a constant low flow. This allows rapid, continuous analysis without altering the temperature of the electrode. Electrode temperature must be held constant so the electrode requires adequate insulation. A warm-up period of 10 to 30 minutes is typically required to reach thermal equilibrium at the elevated temperature. Response times of less than 200 msec are possible with the zirconium fuel cell, making it useful for breath-by-breath measurements.

The zirconium fuel cell, like the polarographic electrode, measures partial pressure of oxygen. Changes in the pressure in the sampling circuit can affect the concentration measurement. Such pressure changes can be caused by gas flow in a breathing circuit or by positive pressure in a mechanical ventilator circuit. The presence of water vapor in the sample affects both of these electrodes similarly (see "Gas Conditioning Devices," p. 268). Oxygen concentration is measured accurately but is diluted in proportion to the water vapor pressure present in the sample. Zirconium fuel cells eventually degrade in relation to the volume of O_2 analyzed. The cell may be refreshed by passing a current through it, thus reversing the oxygen uptake process.

INFRARED ABSORPTION (CO_2, CO)

Various respiratory gas analyzers are based on absorption of infrared radiation to measure gas concentrations. Infrared absorption is used in CO analyzers for the DL_{CO} tests. Infrared CO_2 analyzers are used for exercise testing, metabolic studies, and bedside monitoring (capnography) in critical care (Fig. 9-16).

Certain gases (e.g., CO_2 and CO) absorb infrared radiation. Two beams of infrared radiation are directed through parallel cells. One cell contains sample gas, the other contains a reference gas. The two beams converge on a single infrared detector (Fig. 9-17). A small motor rotates an interrupter or "chopper" between the infrared source and the cells. The chopper blades alternately interrupt the infrared radiation passing through the sample and reference cells. If the sample and reference gases have the same concentration, the radiation reaching the detector is constant. However, when a sample with a different gas concentration is introduced, the radiation reaching the detector varies in a rhythmic fashion. This causes a vibration in the detector that is translated into a pulsatile signal proportional to the difference between the two beams.

Infrared analyzers can measure small changes in gas concentrations such as differences between inspired and expired CO in tests of diffusing capacity. Gas can be sampled either continuously or discretely with infrared analyzers. For continuous sampling, the gas flow must be constant. The analyzer must be calibrated using the same flow at which measurements are made. Pump settings and the sample line itself should not be altered after calibration. Condensation of water in the sample line can significantly alter the flow rate and affect the accuracy of the measurement. Water vapor in the sample will dilute the gas being analyzed. Water vapor can be removed if response time is not critical. For rapid response times, as required for breath-by-breath analysis, the effects of water vapor can be corrected mathematically by assuming that expired gas is fully saturated.

The most common problems occurring with infrared analyzers involve the chopper motor, sample cell, and infrared detector. Motors turning the chopper blades may wear out or work intermittently. Some analyzers use a nonmechanical means of alternating the infrared beams, thus

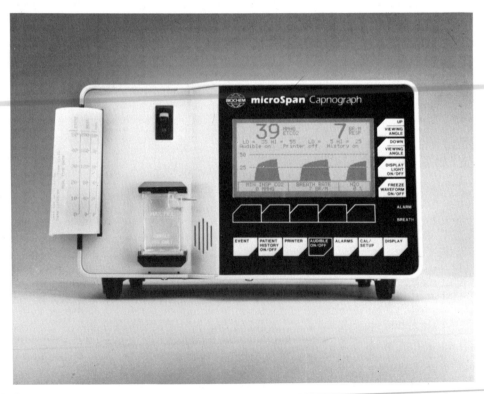

FIG. 9-16 *Infrared CO_2 monitor.* A microprocessor-controlled infrared CO_2 analyzer as used for critical care monitoring. A liquid crystal display allows presentation of end-tidal CO_2 values, breathing rate, and CO_2 waveforms. This capnograph includes a printer and alarms, along with a water trap to remove condensation from the sample line. (Courtesy Biochem International Inc., Waukesha, WI.)

eliminating this problem. The sample cell can easily become contaminated. Water condensation or other debris can contaminate the cell "window," interfering with transmission of the infrared beam. Infrared detector cells degrade over time and become less sensitive. Both contamination of the sample cell and detector aging can alter response time or make the analyzer impossible to calibrate.

EMISSION SPECTROSCOPY

The single-breath and multiple-breath N_2-washout tests, as well as the open-circuit FRC determination (see Chapter 3) use N_2 analysis. The Giesler tube ionizer is an N_2 analyzer based on the principle of emission spectroscopy (Fig. 9-18). This instrument consists of an enclosed

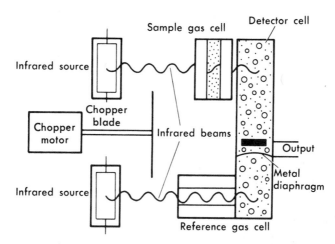

FIG. 9-17 *Infrared absorption gas analyzer.* Components of an infrared analyzer used to measure CO_2 are depicted. Infrared sources emit beams that pass through parallel cells. One cell contains a reference gas, the other a gas sample to be analyzed. A rotating blade "chops" the infrared beams in a rhythmic fashion. When both the reference and sample cells contain the same gas, radiation reaching either half of the detector cell does not vary. When the gas to be sampled is introduced, it absorbs some infrared radiation. Different amounts of radiation reach the two halves of the detector cell, causing the diaphragm separating the compartments of the detector to oscillate. This oscillation is transformed into a signal proportional to the difference in gas concentrations. The infrared analyzer is ideal for determination of small changes in concentration in gas samples. (From Beckman Instruments, Inc., Medical gas analyzer LB-2: operating instructions, FM-149997-301, Schiller Park, IL, 1972.)

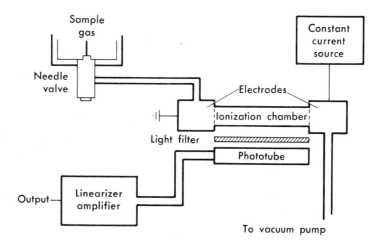

FIG. 9-18 *Emission spectroscopy-type gas analyzer.* The optical emission analyzer (Giesler tube) is commonly used for N_2 analysis. A vacuum pump draws a gas sample into an ionization chamber, where the ionized gas emits light. All light except that from the desired gas is filtered out, and the remaining light is monitored by a phototube. The phototube transmits a signal proportional to the intensity of the light, allowing rapid gas analysis. (From Hewlett-Packard, Application note AN 729, San Diego, CA, 1973.)

ionization chamber that contains two electrodes and a photocell. A vacuum pump creates a constant pressure in the ionization chamber by bleeding gas through a needle valve. The needle valve draws gas to be sampled from a breathing circuit. When a current is supplied to the electrodes, the N_2 between them is ionized and emits light. After being filtered, this light is monitored by a photodetector. The intensity of the light is directly proportional to the concentration of N_2 in the sample. The current, distance between electrodes, and gas pressure must remain constant. The photodetector converts the light signal into a DC voltage. This analog signal is then amplified, linearized, and directed to an appropriate meter or computing circuit. The Giesler tube ionizer allows continuous and rapid analysis of N_2 with response times less than 100 msec.

Analyzers using emission spectroscopy usually require a vacuum pump. Vacuum pressure must be maintained at a stable level to ensure accuracy and linearity. Leaks in the seals around the needle valve or in the pump itself may occur. Inability to zero and **span** the analyzer may be the first sign of a leak or faulty vacuum source. The photodetector, ionizing electrodes, and light filter all degrade over time. Periodic linearity checks allow adjustment for small changes in any of these components.

THERMAL CONDUCTIVITY ANALYZERS

Measurement of FRC by the closed-circuit method and the single-breath DL_{CO} each require He analysis. Thermal conductivity analyzers measure gas concentrations in a sample by detecting the rate at which different gases conduct heat. Heated wires or beads (thermistors) are exposed to the gas sample. The concentration of a specific gas can be detected by measuring the change in electrical resistance of the thermistors. Two glass-coated thermistors serve as sensing elements connected by a **Wheatstone bridge** circuit (Fig. 9-19). Thermistors change temperature and electrical resistance as a function of the molecular weight of the gases surrounding them. One thermistor serves as a reference. A difference in the concentration of gases between two thermistors can be detected because the differences in heat conducted away alters the electrical resistance in the circuit. He analyzers use a reference cell containing no helium (He). Other gases can be analyzed by means of thermal conductivity if no interfering gases are present. Thermal conductivity analyzers are used in conjunction with gas chromatography (see "Gas Chromatography," p. 267). Water vapor and CO_2 are usually scrubbed before He analysis. Thermal conductivity analyzers can be used for

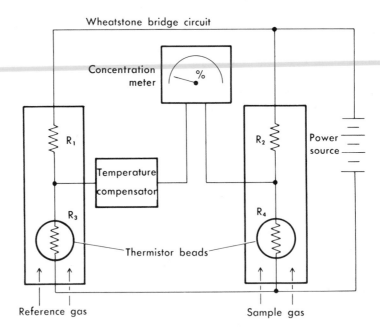

FIG. 9-19 *Thermal conductivity analyzer.* Thermal conductivity gas analyzer, such as used for He analysis or gas chromatography, is depicted. Two thermistor beads (temperature-sensitive electrical resistors) are connected in a Wheatstone bridge circuit. When the thermistors are subjected to the same gas concentrations, their electrical resistances are equal and the meter registers zero (by calibration). When a gas is applied to the sample thermistor (R_4 in the diagram) and the reference thermistor submitted to a reference gas, a potential occurs. This deflects the concentration meter by a proportional amount. (From Bourns, Inc., Life systems operations instruction manual, Model LS114-5, Riverside, CA.)

continuous or discrete measurements but have a response time in the range of 10 to 20 seconds. Thermal conductivity analyzers cannot be used to detect rapid changes in gas concentration.

   Thermal conductivity analyzers are very stable. Unless the thermistor in the sampling chamber is contaminated or physically damaged, the analyzer remains accurate for an extended period. Water vapor or CO_2 in the sample circuit (caused by malfunctioning absorbers) are common causes of errors with this type of analyzer. Some He analyzers use a water absorber in line with the reference thermistor. This allows dry room air to be used to zero the analyzer. Exhaustion of this absorber can result in calibration errors.

GAS CHROMATOGRAPHY

   Gas chromatography combines a means of separating a sample into component gases and a detector mechanism. The detector is usually a thermal conductivity analyzer as previously described. Most chromatographs use the principle of column separation to segregate the component gases of the sample (Fig. 9-20). A column contains material that impedes movement of gas molecules depending on their size. Some columns also use materials that combine chemically with specific gases. A combination of columns allows a wide range of gases to be analyzed with a single detector. He is used as a carrier gas because of its high thermal conductivity. The sample gas, along with the He carrier gas, is injected into the column. Component gases exit the column at varying rates and are detected by a thermal conductivity analyzer. The concentrations of each gas can be determined by comparing the output of the thermal conductivity analyzer with a known calibration gas. Because He is used as the carrier gas, it cannot be used as an inert indicator for lung volume determinations or diffusing capacity measurements. Neon, which is relatively insoluble, may be substituted for He in these tests. Water vapor and CO_2 are usually scrubbed from the sample to prevent contamination of the separator column.

   Gas chromatographs are well suited to applications requiring analysis of multiple gases, such as DL_{CO} determinations. Chromatography is very accurate and is widely used for analysis of certified reference gases. Gas chromatographs can be used for discrete or continuous measurement. However, their response times are from 15 to 90 seconds, depending on the gas to be detected.

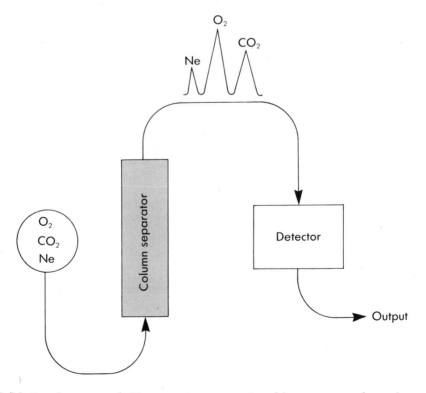

FIG. 9-20 *Gas chromatograph.* Diagrammatic representation of the components of a gas chromatograph for analyzing respiratory gases. The gas sample moves through a separator column via a carrier gas, usually He. Gases of different molecular sizes pass through the column at different rates and are monitored sequentially by a thermal conductivity-type detector. Gases can be analyzed very accurately by means of appropriate columns.

Gas chromatographs that are properly maintained are very accurate. Column material must be replaced when exhausted to maintain accuracy. Some chromatographs heat the column to enhance separation. Failure of the heating mechanism can lead to inaccurate analyses. Exhaustion of water or CO_2 absorbers can also cause the column to become contaminated.

GAS CONDITIONING DEVICES

Interference from water vapor or CO_2 in expired gas is common to many types of gas analyzers. These two gases are usually removed by chemical "scrubbers."

CO_2 may be absorbed by passing the sample through granules containing either barium hydroxide ($Ba(OH)_2$) or sodium hydroxide ($NaOH$). Granules containing $NaOH$ have a light brown appearance that changes to white when saturated with CO_2. The $Ba(OH)_2$ (Baralyme) scrubber is usually supplied with an indicator (ethyl violet), which changes from white to purple when saturated with CO_2. $NaOH$ and $Ba(OH)_2$ are mildly corrosive and may generate heat if exposed to high concentrations of CO_2. Both generate water as a product of combination with CO_2. Therefore they should be placed upstream of any water vapor absorber used in the same circuit.

Water vapor is absorbed by passing the humidified gas over granules of anhydrous calcium sulfate ($CaSO_4$) or silica gel. These substances are called **desiccants.** $CaSO_4$ usually contains an indicator that changes from blue to pink when saturated with water vapor. Some analyzers use silica gel to remove water vapor.

Conditioning of gas containing water vapor may also be accomplished using special sample tubing (Permapure). This tubing is permeable to water vapor. Sample gas passing through the tubing equilibrates its water vapor pressure with that of the surrounding atmosphere. Water vapor is not removed but remains constant at a known level. This allows corrections for water vapor pressure to be accurately applied when other gases are analyzed. Failure to adequately scrub water vapor or CO_2 from a gas sample results in dilution of the remaining gases. Dilution lowers the fractional concentration of the gas being analyzed. Chemical scrubbers or permeable tubing should always be replaced according to the manufacturers' recommendations.

Blood Gas Electrodes, Oximeters, and Related Devices

Measurements of arterial or mixed venous blood gases include determination of Po_2, Pco_2, and pH. Calculation of arterial oxygen concentration (SaO_2), bicarbonate (HCO_3^-), total CO_2, base excess, and other variables depend on measurements derived from one or more of the three primary electrodes. Oxyhemoglobin saturation is measured using a multiwavelength oximeter; it may also be estimated using a pulse oximeter. Other methods of assessing blood gases rely on transcutaneous electrodes, intraarterial and extraarterial **optodes,** and reflective spectrophotometry.

pH ELECTRODE

The glass pH electrode contains a solution of constant pH on one side of a glass membrane. The sample to be analyzed is brought into contact with the other side of the pH-sensitive glass (Fig. 9-21). The difference in pH on either side of the glass causes a potential difference, or voltage. To measure this potential, two half-cells are used: one for the constant solution and one for the sample. The constant solution half-cell (i.e., the measuring electrode) is usually a silver-silver chloride wire. The external half-cell is usually a saturated calomel (i.e., approximately 20% KCl) electrode called the reference electrode. The reference electrode makes contact with the unknown solution by means of a permeable membrane or a liquid junction. These half-cells are connected to a voltmeter calibrated in pH units. The voltage difference between the two electrodes is proportional to the pH difference of the solutions. Because the pH of one solution is constant, the developed potential is a measure of the pH of the sample.

Protein contamination of the pH-sensitive glass is a common problem and increases with the number of specimens analyzed. Routine cleaning with a proteolytic agent (e.g., bleach) reduces buildup of protein on the electrode tip. KCl depletion or blockage of the reference junction can also cause pH electrode malfunction. Contamination of reagents used for pH electrode calibration may also result in measurement errors. Daily (or more frequent) use of suitable quality control materials can detect these and other problems (see Chapter 10).

Pco_2 ELECTRODE

The Pco_2 electrode (Severinghaus electrode) measures Pco_2 potentiometrically using an adaptation of the pH electrode (Fig. 9-22). A combined pH-reference electrode is placed inside of a

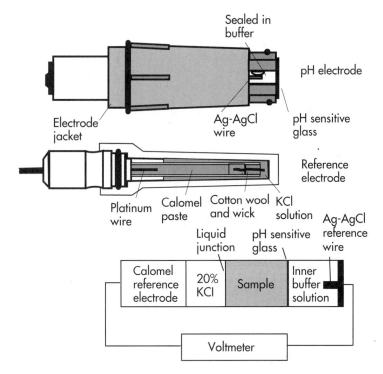

FIG. 9-21 *pH and reference electrodes.* The pH electrode is a microelectrode, shown here with its plastic jacket. At the tip is a silver-silver chloride wire in a sealed-in buffer behind pH-sensitive quartz glass. The reference electrode contains a platinum wire in calomel paste that rests in a 20% KCl solution. The blood sample is introduced in such a way that it contacts the measuring electrode tip and the KCl; a voltmeter measures the potential difference across the sample which is proportional to the pH.

membrane-tipped plastic jacket. The jacket is filled with a bicarbonate electrolyte. The membrane is usually Teflon or a similar material permeable to CO_2 molecules. A spacer or wick made of nylon is usually placed between the pH-sensitive glass and the membrane. The spacer ensures that a thin layer of bicarbonate electrolyte is in contact with the electrode. When the sample is introduced at the tip of the electrode, CO_2 diffuses across the membrane. CO_2 is hydrated in the electrolyte according to the following equation:

$$CO_2 + H_2O \rightleftarrows H_2CO_3 \rightleftarrows H^+ + HCO_3^-$$

The higher the P_{CO_2}, the more the equation is driven to the right. The change in H^+ concentration is proportional to the change in P_{CO_2}. The electrode detects the change in P_{CO_2} as a change in pH of the electrolyte. The voltage developed is exponentially related to P_{CO_2}. A tenfold increase in P_{CO_2} is approximately equal to a decrease of 1 pH unit. Partial pressure of CO_2 can be determined by calibrating the pH change when the electrode is exposed to gases with known P_{CO_2} values.

The most common problem with the P_{CO_2} electrode is degradation or contamination of its membrane. Protein or debris deposited on the membrane slows diffusion of CO_2. Equilibrium between the sample and electrode may not be achieved. Electrolyte depletion or exhaustion in the jacket around the electrode may also occur with extended use. Careful attention to shifts in electrode performance, either during calibration or control runs, can detect these common problems. Routine maintenance includes replacing the membrane and refilling the electrode with fresh electrolyte. Guidelines for quality control of blood gas electrodes are included in Chapter 10.

P_{O_2} ELECTRODE

The P_{O_2} electrode (Clark electrode) consists of a platinum cathode which is usually a thin wire encased in plastic or glass, together with a silver-silver chloride (Ag-AgC1) anode (see Fig. 9-22). Both anode and cathode are placed inside a plastic jacket that is tipped with a polypropylene or polyethylene membrane. This membrane is semipermeable and allows diffusion of oxygen molecules. The jacket is filled with phosphate-potassium chloride buffer. A polarizing voltage of approximately −630 mV is applied to the electrode. The cathode is slightly negative with respect to the anode. Because the electrode is polarized it is often called a polarographic electrode. Oxygen is reduced (i.e., takes up electrons) at the cathode according to the following equation:

$$O_2 + 2H_2O + 4e^- \rightarrow 4OH^-$$

Electrons (i.e., e in the equation above) are supplied by the Ag-AgCl anode. Electrons flow from the anode to the cathode with a current proportional to the number of molecules of O_2 reduced. Each O_2 molecule can take up four electrons, and the greater the number of O_2 molecules present, the greater the current. The membrane causes a diffusion limitation to the number of molecules reaching the electrode. The greater the partial pressure on the sample side of the membrane, the higher the rate of diffusion. The measurement of the current developed within the electrode is therefore proportional to P_{O_2}.

As with the P_{CO_2} electrode, contamination or degradation of the membrane alters diffusion of O_2 and can result in erratic measurements. Most polarographic electrodes use a platinum wire of small diameter to reduce the actual consumption of O_2 at the tip of the electrode. The exposed surface of the platinum cathode gradually becomes plated with metal ions and must be periodically polished to maintain its sensitivity. The platinum wire can be polished by brushing or by abrading with a coarse substance such as pumice.

Because the membrane causes a diffusion limit to O_2 molecules reaching the cathode, the electrode performs differently when exposed to liquid versus gas samples. Some blood gas systems use gas to calibrate the P_{O_2} electrode. Noticeable differences may result when the electrode is then

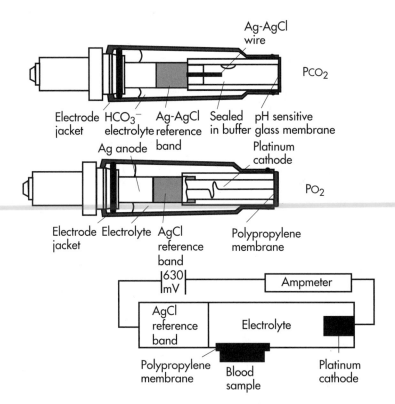

FIG. 9-22 ***P_{CO_2} and P_{O_2} electrodes.*** The P_{CO_2} (Severinghaus) electrode is actually a modified pH electrode. The pH electrode has a sealed-in buffer; an Ag-AgCl reference band is the other half-cell. The entire electrode is encased in a Lucite jacket filled with a bicarbonate electrolyte. The jacket is capped with a Teflon membrane that is permeable to CO_2. A nylon mesh (not shown) covers the pH-sensitive glass, acting as a spacer to maintain contact with the electrolyte. CO_2 diffuses through the Teflon membrane, combines with the electrolyte, and alters the pH (see text). The change in pH is displayed as partial pressure of CO_2. The P_{O_2} (polarographic or Clark) electrode contains a platinum cathode and a silver anode. The electrode is polarized by applying a slightly negative voltage of approximately 630 mV. The tip is protected by a polypropylene membrane that allows O_2 molecules to diffuse but prevents contamination of the platinum wire. O_2 migrates to the cathode and is reduced by picking up free electrons that have come from the anode through a phosphate-potassium chloride electrolyte. Changes in the current flowing between the anode and cathode result from the amount of O_2 reduced in the electrolyte and are proportional to partial pressure of O_2.

used to analyze the tension of O_2 dissolved in a liquid (e.g., blood). These differences are usually compensated for by correcting the Po_2 with an empirically determined gas-to-liquid factor (see Chapter 10).

BLOOD GAS ANALYZERS

Laboratory Analyzers

Although the gas measuring (Po_2 and Pco_2) electrodes and the pH electrode system can each be used separately, all three are usually implemented together in a blood gas analyzer (Fig. 9-23). The three electrodes are mounted in a single measuring chamber. This allows a small blood sample (200 μL or less) to be analyzed. Most blood gas analyzers are microprocessor controlled. Sample aspiration, rinsing, and calibration can all be done automatically with program control. Standardization of these functions, especially calibration, reduces measurement error and improves precision. The microprocessor can calculate a wide variety of parameters derived from pH, Pco_2, and Po_2, as well as from data received from other instruments. In addition, computerized analyzers can monitor automated calibrations and electrode performance to alert the technologist of existing or impending problems.

Point-of-Care Analyzers

To provide rapid results of critical analytes (i.e., blood gases and electrolytes), several portable or bedside analyzers are available (Fig. 9-24). These devices are designed for use in the emergency department or critical care unit. Most can be battery operated, but some point-of-care (POC) instruments require standard power. The blood gas measurement techniques differ slightly between models. Some POC blood gas analyzers use microelectrodes, similar to those described previously. Others use electrochemical film methods or fluorescence optode technology (see "Blood Gas Optodes," p. 272). Reagents and calibration materials are contained in disposable packages. Some POC systems use cartridges that allow a fixed number of analyses. Others use a single-patient sample chamber. Calibrations for POC systems that use multiple specimen cartridges are usually performed in the traditional manner (see Chapter 10). Single-use devices often have the sample chamber precalibrated by the manufacturer. Some POC instruments use aqueous buffers in the single-patient chamber to perform calibration immediately before sample analysis.

The accuracy and precision of most POC blood gas analyzers appear comparable with that

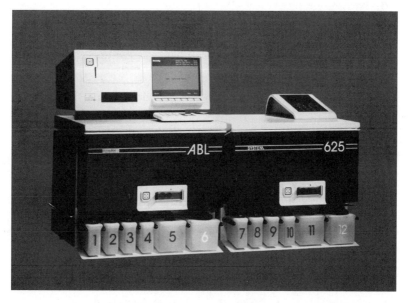

FIG. 9-23 *Automated blood gas analyzer, including spectrophotometric oximeter.* This system provides automatic sample handling, flushing, and calibration. Results of sample analysis and calibrations are displayed using an integrated computer and display terminal. pH, Pco_2, and Po_2 are measured; HCO_3^-, total CO_2, standard bicarbonate, and many other variables can be calculated. This system also incorporates a spectrophotometric oximeter for analysis of Hb, O_2Hb, COHb, and MetHb. Base excess is calculated using the HCO_3^- from the blood gas analysis and the Hb measured by the oximeter. Electrolytes and glucose can be measured by an interfaced module. (Courtesy Radiometer America, Westlake, OH.)

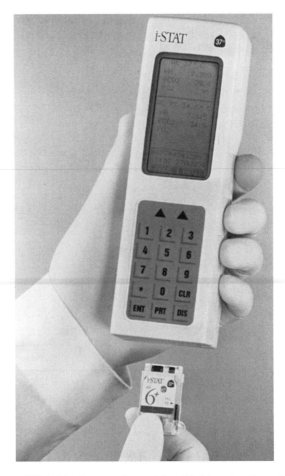

FIG. 9-24 *Point-of-care (POC) blood gas analyzer.* A hand-held, point-of-care blood gas analyzer. This device uses microelectrodes and is battery powered so it can be used in a variety of clinical settings. (Courtesy I-Stat Corp., Princeton, NJ.)

obtained with standard laboratory instruments. Routine analysis of multiple levels of quality control material is required to assess precision. Analysis of unknown specimens and comparison to other instruments or laboratories **(proficiency testing)** is required to determine accuracy. Many POC instruments include ion-specific electrodes for analysis of potassium (K^+), sodium (Na^+), and calcium (Ca^{++}).

BLOOD GAS OPTODES

Devices capable of measuring pH, Pco_2, and Po_2 in vivo are available. These sensors are called optodes because of their principle of operation. Optodes for pH and blood gas measurements are based on the concept of **luminescence quenching**.

When light strikes a photoluminescent dye, certain wavelengths are absorbed and electrons are excited to an elevated energy state. When the light source is removed the electrons decay to a lower energy level and emit light at a different wavelength than was originally absorbed. The light emitted from the dye (fluorescence) is altered by the presence of CO_2 or H^+. Certain photoluminescent dyes are inhibited from emitting light by the presence of O_2. This mechanism is called luminescence quenching. Optical electrodes may be created by using dyes that respond to O_2 and CO_2 molecules and to hydrogen ions (i.e., change with pH).

A fluorescent optode is composed of a fiberoptic element with a fluorescent dye at the tip (Fig. 9-25). A membrane permeable to O_2, CO_2, or H^+ separates the dye from the subject's blood. An intermittent light source transmits light at an appropriate wavelength down the optical fiber. The resulting photoluminescence intensity is transmitted back up the fiber. The optode measures the difference between the excitation and emission energy of the light. If the excitation energy is kept constant, the light emitted from the dye is altered by the presence of the specific analyte (i.e., O_2, CO_2, or pH).

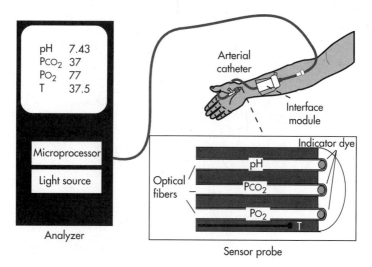

FIG. 9-25 *Intraarterial blood gas monitor.* A diagrammatic representation of an in-dwelling blood gas monitor using optode technology. The sensor probe is small enough to be placed into an artery. It contains optodes (see text) for measuring pH, P_{CO_2} and P_{O_2}, along with a temperature probe. The analyzer contains a microprocessor and light source for the optodes themselves. Optical fibers transmit the light to the sensor. The microprocessor performs all calculations to display blood gas variables continuously.

The H^+ and P_{CO_2} optodes agree very closely with measurements using conventional electrodes. Differences in pH or P_{CO_2} measurements between optodes and a blood gas analyzer do not appear to be clinically significant. The accuracy of the P_{O_2} optode varies with the absolute value of the Pa_{O_2}. Optode luminescence and P_{O_2} appear to be inversely related. Low O_2 values produce higher optode signal intensities. The O_2 optode is potentially most accurate at low P_{O_2} levels. This is in contrast to the polarographic electrode, in which the current produced by reduction of O_2 is directly proportional to partial pressure of the gas present. Optode technology is used in both POC blood gas analyzers and blood gas monitors.

Intraarterial Monitors

All three optodes can be combined into a probe small enough to be inserted through a 20-gauge arterial catheter. The probe itself is coated with a special form of heparin to inhibit intravascular clotting. The probe assembly connects to an interface that routes the light beam and signals to an electronics module (see Fig. 9-25). Blood gas parameters are displayed digitally. The optode system requires approximately 15 seconds to compute a new set of blood gas data. During nonsteady-state conditions, the monitor simply indicates that the desired parameter is changing in a certain direction. The bias (i.e., mean difference) of these optodes compares favorably with laboratory analysis of blood gases. However, intermittent inaccuracies have been reported. These fluctuations in accuracy of optode-derived blood gas values may be caused by the intraarterial site itself.

Extraarterial Monitors

Optode-based blood gas monitoring may also be performed without inserting the device into the artery. Extraarterial monitors place the optodes in an interface located near the arterial catheter (Fig. 9-26). Arterial blood is then withdrawn into a reservoir in the interface. The blood remains in contact with the optodes long enough for the measurements to be made. The sample is then reinfused using a heparinized flush solution. This technique produces acceptable bias and precision compared with laboratory analysis. In addition, extraarterial monitoring appears to be unaffected by intermittent inaccuracies encountered with intraarterial monitoring. The only disadvantage of extraarterial monitors is that they provide intermittent data (updates take approximately 2 to 3 minutes).

TRANSCUTANEOUS P_{O_2} ELECTRODE

The transcutaneous O_2 electrode (tcP_{O_2}) operates on a principle similar to the polarographic electrode. The tcP_{O_2} electrode consists of a ring-shaped silver anode heated by a coil to increase blood flow at the skin placement site. Inside the circular anode is a series of thin platinum cathodes (Fig. 9-27). All elements are enclosed in a plastic case. The face of the sensor is covered by a Teflon

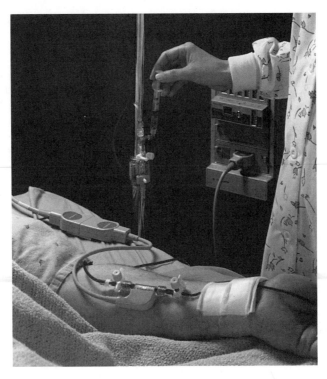

FIG. 9-26 *Extraarterial blood gas monitor.* An extraarterial blood gas monitor that uses optode technology to measure blood gas variables is shown. In this instrument a sample is "withdrawn" from an in-dwelling arterial catheter, bringing blood into contact with the optodes. After analysis, the blood is infused back into the patient with a standard flush solution. This type of system avoids the artifact associated with an in-dwelling optode. Blood loss is minimized and blood gas analysis is available at the bedside as often as required. (Courtesy Marquette Medical Systems, Milwaukee, WI.)

membrane. Electrolyte (KCl) is placed between the membrane and the sensor. A second layer of electrolyte and a cellophane membrane are added to form a double membrane. The current between the silver anode and platinum cathodes is proportional to the P_{O_2} diffusing through the skin and membrane. A feedback controller keeps the temperature constant at the skin site. This also compensates for changes in capillary blood flow and stabilizes the measurement.

The gradient between tcP_{O_2} and Pa_{O_2} is relatively constant in subjects with normal cardiac output. In neonates there is a close correlation between transcutaneous and Pa_{O_2}. In hemodynamically stable adults, tcP_{O_2} is approximately 80% of Pa_{O_2}. Measurement of tcP_{O_2} can trend oxygenation when this gradient has been established. In subjects with reduced cardiac output, the gradient between tcP_{O_2} and Pa_{O_2} widens. Conditions that affect perfusion to the skin may also alter the gradient between arterial and transcutaneous P_{O_2}.

Most transcutaneous monitors heat the skin site from 40° to 45° C. The increased temperature "arterializes" capillary blood flow. However, this necessitates moving the electrode every 3 to 4 hours to prevent burns. Changing sensor sites is particularly important in neonates because of the reduced thickness of their epidermis. Periodic recalibration of the electrode is necessary even if the sensor site has not been changed. After placement of the electrode, an interval from 5 to 30 minutes may be required for equilibration to be reached.

SPECTROPHOTOMETRIC OXIMETER

The spectrophotometric oximeter uses light absorption to analyze saturation of hemoglobin (Hb) with O_2. The concentration of carboxyhemoglobin (COHb) or other forms of Hb (e.g., methemoglobin, sulfhemoglobin) can also be determined. This type of spectrophotometer is sometimes called a co-oximeter.

The blood oximeter analyzes the absorption of light in a blood sample at multiple wavelengths. At certain wavelengths, two or more forms of Hb have similar **absorbances** (Fig. 9-28). These common wavelengths are called isobestic points. A wavelength that is isobestic for oxyhemoglobin (O_2Hb), reduced Hb (RHb), and COHb is 548 nm. At this wavelength, absorbance of a mixture of

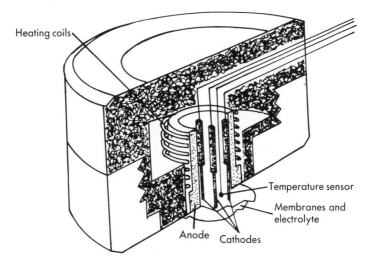

FIG. 9-27 *Transcutaneous* Po_2 *electrode.* A cross-sectional diagram of the components of the $tcPo_2$ electrode shows a circular anode around a series of cathodes and a temperature sensor. A heating coil causes local hyperemia so that skin Po_2 closely resembles Pao_2. A double membrane separates the electrode proper from the skin.

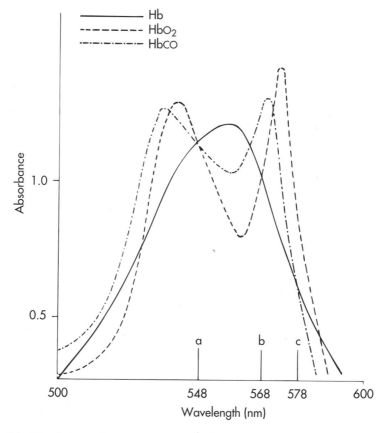

FIG. 9-28 *Principle of spectrophotometric oximetry.* Absorbance measurements are made at three or more distinct wavelengths (548, 568, 578 nm in this example) as light passes through a sample of hemolyzed blood. At 548 nm, all three forms of Hb (Hb, O_2Hb, and COHB) have identical absorbances. At 568 nm only Hb and HbO_2 coincide, whereas at 578 nm, Hb and COHb coincide. The solution of simultaneous equations provides the relative proportions of each species, as well as the total Hb (see text).

the three pigments is directly proportional to the total concentration of Hb. An isobestic point for O_2Hb and RHb is 568 nm. The absorbance of COHb at this point is considerably higher. A change in absorbance at 568 nm compared with 548 nm indicates a change in the concentration of COHb relative to the sum of the concentrations of the other two species. The isobestic point for RHb and COHb is 578 nm, with O_2Hb absorbance being considerably greater. The difference in absorbance at 578 nm indicates the concentration of O_2Hb relative to the other two pigments. The total Hb concentration, O_2Hb, COHb, and methemoglobin (MetHb) saturation can be determined by analyzing absorbances and solving simultaneous equations.

The spectrophotometric oximeter provides the true O_2Hb saturation. This is particularly important if increased concentrations of COHb, MetHb, or other abnormal hemoglobins are present. Most automated blood gas analyzers calculate O_2Hb saturation. Calculated saturation is based on the measured Po_2 and pH at 37° C and assumes that the Hb has a normal P_{50} (see Chapter 6). Calculated O_2Hb significantly overestimates true saturation in the presence of COHb or methemoglobin. The co-oximeter provides the most accurate estimate of the actual O_2 saturation of the blood. Combination blood gas analyzers and co-oximeters are available. These instruments combine conventional pH and blood gas electrodes with spectrophotometric measurements of Hb saturation, all performed with the same blood sample.

A co-oximeter may give erroneous Hb, O_2Hb, or COHb readings if forms of hemoglobin are present that the instrument does not recognize. For example, blood from a newborn (i.e., containing fetal Hb) will give erroneous values if analyzed by an oximeter set up for adult blood. Substances that cause light scattering in the specimen (e.g., lipids resulting from lipid therapy) also may cause false readings. To function properly, the blood oximeter must hemolyze the sample so that Hb molecules are suspended in solution rather than contained within the red cells. **Hemolysis** is accomplished by chemical or mechanical disruption of red cell membranes. Incomplete hemolysis results in light scattering within the sample rather than simple absorption. Sickle cells are not easily disrupted, particularly by chemical lysis, and may result in false readings for O_2Hb and COHb. Incomplete hemolysis may be difficult to detect unless whole blood quality control or proficiency testing is performed (see Chapter 10).

Some co-oximeters feature microprocessor control so that errors such as incomplete hemolysis or light scattering can be detected. Microprocessor-controlled oximeters also provide options so that fetal or animal Hb can be analyzed. In addition to measurements of O_2Hb, COHb, and MetHb saturations, the blood oximeter can calculate oxygen content and P_{50}. The P_{50} can be estimated by measuring the actual saturation of a specimen (usually a venous sample with a saturation less than 90%) and comparing this value with the calculated saturation based on Po_2 and pH of the same blood. This simplified method compares favorably with tonometering of the blood sample with various low-oxygen concentrations and constructing a dissociation curve.

PULSE OXIMETERS

Pulse oximeters (Fig. 9-29) are commonly used to assess oxygenation noninvasively. The pulse oximeter's immediate predecessor was a fiberoptic oximeter that passed multiple wavelengths of light through the earlobe and measured the absorption to derive oxygen saturation of Hb.

Pulse oximeters treat Hb as a filter that allows only red and near-infrared light to pass. Beer's law relates to total absorption in a system of absorbers to the sum of their individual absorptions:

$$A_{total} = E_1C_1L_1 + E_2C_2L_2 + \ldots E_nC_nL_n$$

where:

A_{total} = the absorbance of a mixture of substances at a specific wavelength

E_n = the extinction of substance n

C_n = the concentration of substance n

L_n = the length of the light path through substance n

In principle, the pulse oximeter measures absorption of a mixture of two substances, O_2Hb and RHb. The concentration of either can be determined if their extinction is measured while the path length stays constant. The wavelengths of light used in pulse oximetry are near 660 nm in the red region of the spectrum, and near 940 nm in the near-infrared. Extinction curves for O_2Hb and RHb show that reduced Hb has an absorption 10 times higher than oxyhemoglobin at 660 nm, whereas O_2Hb has a higher absorbance (2 to 3 times) at 940 nm. Calculating all the possible combinations of the two forms of Hb (i.e., varying the saturation from 0% to 100%) allows the ratio

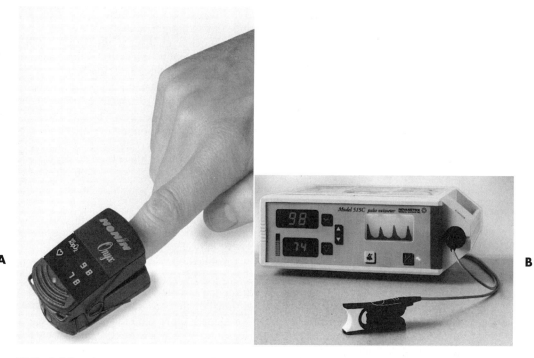

FIG. 9-29 *Pulse oximeters.* Two different types of pulse oximeters, each providing a digital display of oxygen saturation and pulse rate. **A,** A small, portable pulse oximeter that fits over the subject's finger. Miniaturized components allow a device of this size to be easily transported. (Courtesy Nonin Medical Inc., Plymouth, MN.) **B,** A liquid crystal display included with this oximeter allows the user to visualize pulse waveforms and monitor signal quality, both of which may be helpful in detecting conditions that interfere with accurate saturation determinations. Alarms for high and low saturations or pulse rates may be set. (Courtesy Novametrix Medical Systems Inc., Wallingford, CT.)

of absorbances at the two wavelengths to be determined. As a result, a calibration curve can be constructed. The capillary bed does not follow the optical principles exactly as described by Beer's law, so the calibration curve is derived empirically. The ratio of absorbances at the two distinct wavelengths is expressed as follows:

$$R = A_{660nm}/A_{940nm}$$

A series of R values (i.e., the calibration curve) is determined by relating the ratio to actual saturation measurements. Unlike the spectrophotometric oximeter, which measures absorption in a hemolyzed blood sample, the pulse oximeter measures light passing through living tissue. The transmitted light is not only absorbed but refracted and scattered. This causes the absolute accuracy of the pulse oximeter to be less than the blood oximeter.

The transmitted light at each wavelength consists of two components, the AC and DC components (Fig. 9-30). The AC component varies with the pulsation of blood. The DC component represents light absorbed by tissue and venous blood. The DC component is larger than the AC and is relatively constant. The amplitude of both the AC and DC levels depends on the intensity of the incident light. The AC component represents the arterial blood because the arterioles pulsate in the light path. By dividing the AC level by the DC level at each of the two wavelengths, the AC component is effectively corrected. The AC component then becomes a function of the extinction of O_2Hb and RHb. The ratio just described then becomes as follows:

$$R = \frac{(AC_1/DC_1)}{(AC_2/DC_2)}$$

where:

1 = the red wavelength (660 nm)

2 = the near-infrared wavelength (940 nm)

Correcting the pulsatile component (AC) in this manner allows the pulse oximeter to "ignore" absorbances caused by venous blood, tissue, and skin pigmentation.

The light source used in pulse oximetry is the light emitting diode (**LED**). LEDs are capable of emitting a very bright light near the 660- and 940-nm wavelengths required for analysis of Hb saturation. Light intensity is controlled by a feedback circuit that regulates the driving current to the LED. The greater the DC component resulting from pigmentation or venous blood, the greater the current supplied to the LED. One problem with LEDs is that the exact wavelength of light emitted varies with individual diodes. Each LED has its own center wavelength that may differ from 660 or 940 nm by as much as 15 nm. To overcome this variation, each oximeter must have a series of calibration curves programmed into it so that it can accommodate a range of LEDs. The extinction curves for RHb and O_2Hb are steep and quite different at 660 nm, so 10 or more calibration curves are typically required for the red light range. Slight variations in center wavelength are less critical in the 940-nm region because the extinction characteristics of O_2Hb and RHb are the same from 800 to 1000 nm.

A photo diode detects transmitted light in the pulse oximeter. A single photo diode senses both the red and near-infrared light. The microprocessor that controls the oximeter cycles the LEDs on and off separately 400 to 500 times per second. The oximeter also turns both LEDs off during each cycle. This allows the photo diode to detect ambient light caused by scattering and to offset the LED signals.

Pulse oximeter accuracy tends to decrease at low saturations. Low saturations occur as the concentration of RHb increases. RHb has a much higher absorbance at 660 nm than does O_2Hb. Therefore, slight variations in the center wavelength of the red LED (as described) exaggerate the error in measured saturation. This is one reason why pulse oximeters exhibit decreasing accuracy at lower saturations.

Because the AC, or pulsatile component, is usually much smaller than the DC component, detecting it can sometimes cause problems. Low perfusion or poor vascularity can cause the oximeter to be unable to measure the pulsatile component. Most oximeters display a warning message if the photo detector senses light levels that are inadequate. Motion artifact can also cause inaccuracy with pulse oximeters. Movement, especially shivering, often occurs in the same frequency range as the signal to be detected (i.e., arterial pulsations). If the motion is consistent and

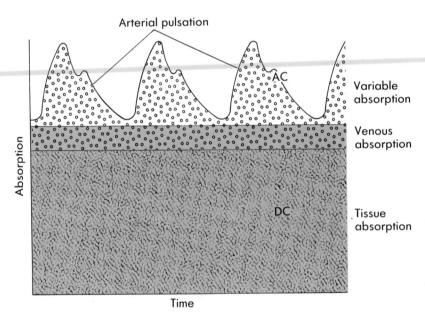

FIG. 9-30 *Measurement principle of pulse oximetry.* Transmitted light (at wavelengths of 660 and 940 nm) consists of an AC and DC component. A large fixed component, the DC component, represents light passing through tissue and venous blood without being absorbed. A smaller portion is pulsatile in nature and changes absorption as blood pulses through the arterioles; this is represented as the AC component. The pulse oximeter divides the AC signal by the DC signal at each wavelength, effectively cancelling the DC component. The ratio of the AC signals at the two wavelengths is then a function of the relative absorptions of O_2Hb and RHb (see text).

lasts long enough, it introduces a signal of approximately the same amplitude into both the red and infrared channels. The pulse oximeter senses motion artifact as part of the DC component. This adds a large value to both the numerator and the denominator of the ratio (R). The motion signal forces R toward a value of 1, which is equal to a saturation of 85% on the typical oximeter calibration curve.

Most pulse oximeters use the AC signal from one channel (either 660 or 940 nm) to calculate pulse rate. An algorithm implemented by the microprocessor locates peaks in the waveform of the AC signal and counts them (see Fig. 9-30). Some oximeters use this signal to display graphic representations of pulse waveforms. Pulse detection may be enhanced by the addition of a single electrocardiograph (ECG) lead. The additional input may allow the microprocessor to distinguish motion artifact or noise from the true signal.

REFLECTIVE SPECTROPHOTOMETERS

Reflective spectrophotometry is based on the variable reflection of light by O_2Hb and RHb at different wavelengths. Just as the light absorbed by oxygenated and RHb is a function of wavelength, so is the intensity of reflected or back-scattered light. Carefully spaced optical fibers can be used as transmitting and receiving paths for light. Reflective spectrophotometry can be used to monitor arterial saturation in a manner similar to pulse oximetry. It can also be incorporated into a pulmonary artery catheter to measure mixed venous oxygen saturation ($S\bar{v}O_2$).

A specially designed pulmonary artery (Swan-Ganz) catheter contains fiberoptic bundles (Fig. 9-31). The catheter has the regular pressure-sensing ports, a balloon tip for flotation through the right side of the heart, and a thermistor for thermodilution cardiac output determinations. Three LEDs, similar to those used in pulse oximeters, illuminate blood flowing past the tip of the catheter via one of the optical fibers. A photo detector senses the reflected light and converts its intensity into a signal. A microprocessor calculates two independent ratios of reflected light intensities from the three wavelengths. Combining two reflected light intensity ratios reduces the instrument's sensitivity to pulsatile blood flow or changing hematocrit. This design also minimizes changes caused by light scattering from red cell surfaces and the walls of the blood vessel. The $S\bar{v}O_2$ is calculated from the light ratios using programmed calibration curves, such as for the pulse oximeter. As in a pulse oximeter, saturation measured is the saturation of functional Hb (see Chapter 6). $S\bar{v}O_2$ determination by this method will be higher than that measured by a co-oximeter, especially if large amounts of COHb or MetHb are present. The $S\bar{v}O_2$ is then displayed and may be printed using a trend recorder (Fig. 9-32).

The reflective spectrophotometer must be routinely calibrated to ensure that observed changes in $S\bar{v}O_2$ are the result of physiologic phenomena rather than instrument drift. The catheter is usually standardized by calibrating it against an absolute color reference before insertion. After the catheter is in place, calibration is accomplished by adjusting the output to match saturation measured by a co-oximeter. This type of calibration is accurate at the time it is performed but may change if there

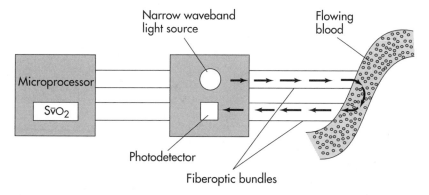

FIG. 9-31 *Principle of reflective spectrophotometry.* A diagrammatic representation of the components of the optical pulmonary artery catheter used for continuous monitoring of $S\bar{v}O_2$. Light emitting diodes (LEDs) provide a narrow-waveband light source. Light is transmitted along one fiberoptic filament to blood flowing past the tip of the catheter. Light reflected from the blood is transmitted back to a photodiode by the second fiberoptic bundle. The light intensity signals are then evaluated by a microprocessor to calculate light intensity ratios. These ratios (usually two ratios are determined from three wavelengths) determine the $S\bar{v}O_2$. The principle of reflective absorption has also been implemented as a pulse oximeter.

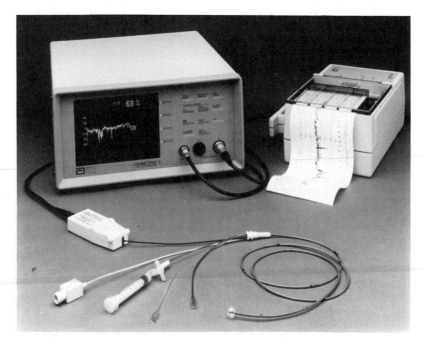

FIG. 9-32 *Reflective spectrophotometer and pulmonary artery catheter.* A microprocessor-controlled reflective spectrophotometer. The pulmonary artery catheter contains fiberoptic bundles for continuous measurement of $S\bar{v}o_2$, as well as the usual pressure-measuring ports and thermistor for thermodilution cardiac output. The instrument displays mixed venous saturation digitally and as a trend graph that can be printed. High and low saturation alarms are included along with a "light intensity" alarm to detect artifact caused by catheter motion or problems with the fiberoptics. (Courtesy Abbott Critical Care Systems, Mountain View, CA.)

are shifts in the pH or hematocrit. Because reflective spectrophotometers measure reflected light in whole blood that is flowing rather than transmitted light in a hemolyzed blood sample, their absolute accuracy is less than that of a co-oximeter.

Body Plethysmographs

Whole body plethysmographs are used in many pulmonary function laboratories. Two types of body plethysmographs are commonly used: the constant-volume, variable-pressure plethysmograph and the flow or variable-volume plethysmograph. These are sometimes called the pressure and flow plethysmographs, respectively. Whole body plethysmographs are also called body-boxes. Both designs are used to measure thoracic gas volume (VTG) (see Chapter 3) and airway resistance (Raw) and its derivatives (see Chapter 2).

PRESSURE PLETHYSMOGRAPHS

The pressure plethysmograph is based on an adaptation of Boyle's law (see Appendix E). Volume changes in a sealed box can be determined by measuring pressure changes if temperature is constant. A sensitive pressure transducer monitors box pressure changes. Pressure change is related to volume change by calibration (see Chapter 10 for calibration techniques). Pressure changes result from compression and decompression of gas within both the subject's chest and the box. If box temperature remains constant, each unit of pressure change equals a specific volume change. For example, 15 ml of volume change might result in a pressure change of 1 cm H_2O.

The pressure plethysmograph must be free of leaks. A solenoid valve can be used to vent the pressure box to maintain thermal equilibrium. Making VTG and Raw measurements with the subject panting reduces pressure changes caused by thermal drift, leaks, or background noise. Some pressure plethysmograph systems use a "slow" leak to facilitate thermal equilibrium. A leak to allow thermal equilibration may be created by connecting a long length of small-bore tubing to the box. Similarly, connecting the atmospheric side of the box pressure transducer to a glass bottle within the box dampens the effects of thermal drift. Both methods reduce the effect of temperature changes within the box and maintain good **frequency response.** Pressure plethysmographs are best suited to maneuvers that measure small volume changes (i.e., 100 ml or less). Measurements of VC or FVC can usually be made only with the door open or the box adequately vented to the atmosphere.

FLOW PLETHYSMOGRAPHS

The flow plethysmograph uses a flow transducer in the box wall to measure volume changes in the box. Gas in the box is compressed or decompressed causing flow through the opening in the box wall. Flow through the wall is integrated, corrections applied, and the volume change recorded as the sum of the volume passing through the wall and the volume compressed. In one implementation, the subject breathes through a pneumotachometer connected to the room (transmural breathing). The transmural pneumotachometer allows larger gas volumes (i.e., the VC or maximal expiratory flow volume [MEFV] curves) to be measured while the subject is enclosed in the plethysmograph. The transmural flow is redirected to the plethysmograph for Raw measurements, so that the ratio of flow to box volume can be plotted. For VTG measurements, the flow transducer in the plethysmograph wall is blocked so that the device works like a pressure box. The flow-type plethysmograph requires computerization so that the pressure, volume, and flow signals can be measured in phase. Although thermal changes must be accounted for, the flow plethysmograph does not need to be rigorously airtight. The flow box's primary advantage is the ability to measure flows at absolute lung volumes (i.e., corrected for gas compression).

In both types of plethysmographs, a pneumotachometer is needed to measure airflow at the mouth (Fig. 9-33). Flow measurement is required to compute Raw. The integrated flow signal (i.e., volume) is also used to determine end-expiration for shutter closure in VTG measurements. The pneumotachometer must be linear across the range of flows encountered in spontaneous breathing and panting (−2 to +2 L/sec). Heated Fleisch or Silverman types of pressure-differential pneumotachometers are usually implemented in the plethysmograph. Pitot tube flow transducers can also be used.

A mouth pressure transducer is normally coupled to an electronic shutter mechanism. The transducer records mouth pressures in the range of −20 to +20 cm H_2O when the airway is occluded. Some systems require the technologist to close the shutter by remote control at end-expiration. This is accomplished by observing the tidal breathing maneuver on a display and actuating the shutter at end-expiration. Computerized systems automatically close the shutter at a preselected point in the breathing cycle. The technologist initiates a sequence in which the computer monitors flow and closes the shutter when expiratory flow becomes zero.

Recording of plethysmographic maneuvers may be accomplished by one of several techniques. Some older plethysmograph systems use a storage oscilloscope to record the breathing maneuvers. The scope may be erased as often as necessary until an acceptable tracing is obtained. These tracings may be photographed or transferred to an X-Y plotter. Measurement of tangents from an oscilloscope is performed by rotating a graticule to align it with the tracing. The angle (or tangent) may then be read directly from the graticule.

Most commercially available systems are computerized. Breathing maneuvers are stored in memory, analyzed, then displayed on the screen. Computerized plethysmographs allow the technologist to select a "best-fit" line drawn by the computer or to manipulate the tangent via the computer keyboard or mouse. Computerized plethysmographs offer the advantage of providing lung volume and Raw information immediately after completion of the maneuver. This aids in selecting appropriate maneuvers to report. In addition, the test can be repeated as required when questionable values are obtained. Comparison of lung volumes by alternate methods (i.e., He dilution or N_2 washout) to plethysmographically determined volumes is easily accomplished with computer-stored data. Computerization also allows panting frequency to be calculated and displayed. Using computer-displayed panting frequency, the technologist can coach the subject to maintain a desired rate.

Most plethysmographs include the hardware to perform physical calibration (see Chapter 10). This equipment includes three signal-generating devices. A pressure manometer or U-tube may be mounted on the box for calibration of the mouth pressure transducer. A flow generator and rotameter (i.e., a flow meter) is included for pneumotachometer calibration. A volume-displacement device such as a 30- to 50-ml syringe driven by an electric motor allows box pressure, or flow, calibration. The motorized pump usually produces a sine-wave flow with frequency that can be varied. This allows checking of box calibration at various frequencies.

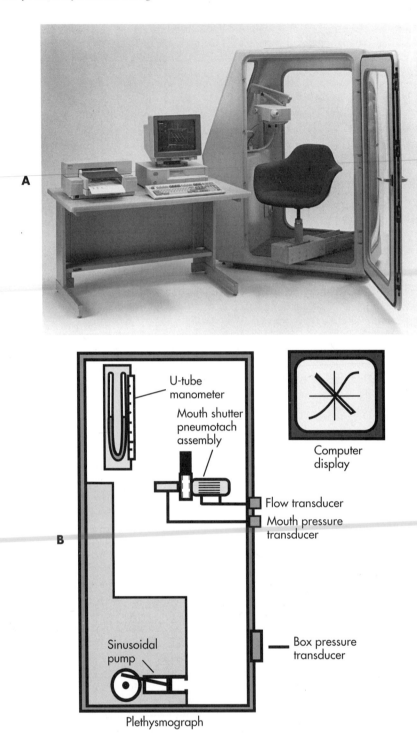

FIG. 9-33 *Body plethysmograph.* **A,** Modern plethysmograph setup, with a highly transparent box, self-contained calibration equipment, and computerized data reduction and display. (Courtesy SensorMedics Corp., Yorba Linda, CA.) **B,** Diagram of plethysmograph components. A pneumotachometer with automatic shutter mechanism is mounted at a height that is comfortable for a patient sitting in the plethysmograph. Pressure transducers for flow, mouth pressure, and box pressure provide signals that are digitized and processed by a computer. A sinusoidal pump allows calibration of the box pressure signal; a small, known volume change can be repeatedly generated. A pressure manometer (U-tube) is used to calibrate the mouth pressure transducer. A 3-L syringe is used to calibrate the pneumotachometer.

Computerized plethysmograph systems support automated calibration of transducers. In conventional calibration techniques, a signal such as pressure or flow is applied to a transducer. The output of the transducer (i.e., its amplified signal) is then adjusted to match the known calibration input. Computerized systems often bypass the physical adjustment of the output of the transducer. Instead of adjusting an amplifier zero or gain, the computer generates a software correction factor. This correction is then applied to every measurement made with the calibrated transducer. A few manufacturers also supply quality control devices such as the **isothermal lung analog** (see Chapter 10). These devices provide quality control to verify calibration of transducers and software correction factors as well.

The ease with which the subject can enter the plethysmograph and perform the required maneuvers is an important feature. Some subjects may experience claustrophobia when inside the plethysmograph. Older boxes relied on materials such as plywood to provide the necessary rigidity for the cabinet, so that pressure changes were not attenuated. Boxes made of durable plastics are largely transparent and less confining for the subject (see Fig. 9-33) while maintaining the necessary rigidity. Equally important is a communication system that allows both voice and visual contact with the subject. Panting against a closed shutter may be difficult for some individuals and continuous coaching is often necessary to elicit valid maneuvers.

Computer Systems

Computerized pulmonary function systems allow very sophisticated data handling and storage, accurate calculations, and enhanced reporting capabilities. Most pulmonary function equipment is interfaced to a dedicated microprocessor (Fig. 9-34) or to a PC (Fig. 9-35). Some laboratories use minicomputers or mainframe computers interfaced to spirometers and gas analyzers, or networked with PC-based systems. Both dedicated microprocessor systems and PC-based systems use similar components.

COMPONENTS OF COMPUTERS

Microprocessors

The microprocessor refers to the "brain" of the computer. Microprocessors are sometimes called the central processing unit (CPU). The microprocessor performs most, if not all, of the instructions provided by a software program. These instructions include performing calculations and storing or retrieving data in memory. The CPU also controls peripheral devices such as the display, printers, and disk drives.

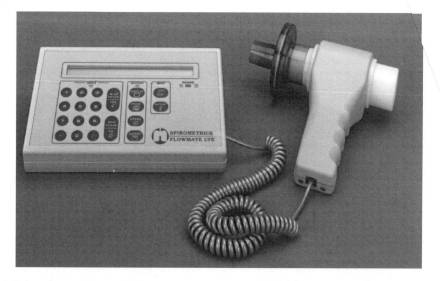

FIG. 9-34 *Spirometer with dedicated microprocessor.* A flow-based spirometer that uses a pressure differential pneumotachometer interfaced with a dedicated microprocessor. The computer executes instructions stored in read-only memory (ROM). A simple keypad provides user access to various functions. Stored data may be downloaded to another computer or to a printer. The entire unit is small enough to be easily transported to the bedside. (Courtesy Spirometrics, Auburn, ME.)

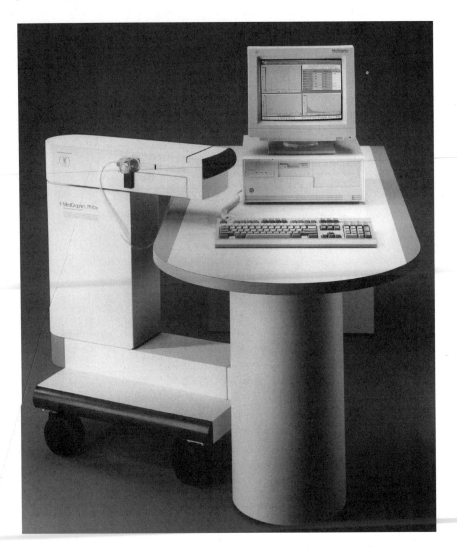

FIG. 9-35 *Computerized pulmonary function system.* An automated pulmonary function system including Pitot tube flow sensor, gas analyzers and computer-controlled breathing circuit. This system for performing spirometry, lung volumes, and DL_{CO} is interfaced to desktop PC. The PC allows rapid processing of data, including calculation of test variables, calibration, BTPS and STPD corrections, and display of graphs. Data is stored on a high capacity hard disk and may be transferred to other media for archiving. The computer's capacity to store large volumes of data allows trending and recall of individuals or groups of patients. (Courtesy Medical Graphics, Inc., St. Paul, MN.)

Microprocessors are classified by the number of "bits" of information that can be handled at one time. A bit is a 0 or 1 in the binary number system. Laboratory computer systems use 8-, 16-, and 32-bit CPUs. Early microprocessors were 8-bit devices capable of addressing 65,536 memory locations. More advanced processors (i.e., 32- or 64-bit) are capable of addressing more than a billion memory addresses. In general, 32-bit and larger processors can perform calculations more rapidly than smaller microprocessors. Their size allows manipulation of large numbers without breaking the number into smaller parts. They can also directly address large blocks of memory and are capable of operating at faster clock speeds.

Clock speed refers to the rate at which the microprocessor operates. Speed is usually measured in megahertz (millions of cycles per second, or MHz). The fastest microprocessors operate at speeds greater than 200 MHz. How quickly a computer can store a file on disk or retrieve information from memory depends on the speed of other computer components as well as the CPU. Fast microprocessors require equally fast input-output devices (see "Input-Output Devices," p. 286).

In addition to faster clock speeds, microprocessors such as the Pentium* are capable of multitasking, or simultaneously running multiple programs. Multitasking requires a special operating system. Multitasking permits the user to perform one task in the foreground, while the computer performs other tasks in the background. For example, a multitasking testing system could allow spirometry to be performed on one patient while the report from another patient is being printed. The same types of processors allow multiple users, as well as peripheral devices such as printers or disk storage, to share the computer. This arrangement is called a network. The network typically consists of a primary computer or server. Other microcomputers are then linked by one of several types of networks. Data can be transferred between any two computers linked by the system. The server usually maintains programs and data that all of the networked users need.

The combination of multitasking and multiuser capabilities offers numerous possibilities to enhance laboratory data management. Some multitasking systems permit the user to perform diagnostic testing in real time while the computer prints reports or transmits data to another system in the background. A network allows pulmonary function testing to be performed at one terminal, while blood gas data are entered at a second terminal, physicians review test results at a third station, and clerical staff print final reports at a fourth work station.

Most commercially available computerized pulmonary function testing systems use PCs. Although many laboratories do not require multitasking or networking, the availability of microprocessors and software that support these functions permits expansion of the system.

Memory

Memory may be classified as read-only memory **(ROM)** or random access memory **(RAM).** Both RAM and ROM are quantified in terms of memory units or bytes. Each byte contains 8 bits (either 0 or 1). A byte can take on 256 distinct values. Two bytes taken together form a word that contains a 16-bit number. Each memory byte or word can be used to store either data or instructions. A kilobyte **(kb)** is the equivalent of 1024 bytes. A megabyte **(Mb)** is 1024 kb of memory.

A computer's ROM usually contains programs such as the Basic Input-Output System (BIOS). The BIOS provides common instructions for controlling input and output from various devices such as the video display. Simple ROM cannot be changed by an application program, but it can be altered if the chip containing the instructions is replaced.

PROMs (programmable ROM chips) or EPROMs (erasable programmable ROM chips) are often used in pulmonary function testing systems. Changing to different equipment is simplified by placing instructions for a particular piece of equipment on a PROM—just install a new PROM. PROMs and EPROMs are often included in the interface between a computer and pulmonary function testing hardware (see "Data Acquisition and Instrument Control," p. 289). The most advanced type of ROM is flash ROM. This type of memory works like an EPROM chip but can be reprogrammed while in the computer. Flash ROM allows basic computer functions (e.g., the BIOS) to be **upgraded** easily.

The RAM available in a computer refers to the amount of memory that is available for user programs. RAM is normally occupied by the computer's operating system and the user's application programs. Both operating system and application software are loaded from an external source such as a disk. Many computers maximize memory use by breaking application programs into modules. Only segments required for a certain test are loaded. This technique conserves RAM but may slow down overall program execution if many modules are loaded and unloaded. Advances in chip technology have made large amounts of RAM relatively inexpensive, so that even PCs can manage extremely large and complicated programs. Operating systems such as Windows 95† can use 16 Mb or more of RAM.

Most pulmonary function application programs do not require large amounts of memory to run. However, more data can be held in memory and complex functions can be performed with more available RAM. High-resolution display of multiple spirometry efforts, such as MEFV curves, may require considerable amounts of RAM. The amount of available RAM may determine how efficiently different applications run in a multitasking system.

The storage capacity of diskettes, hard drives, and CD-ROMs (see "Mass Storage Devices," p. 286) is often classified in units of either kb or Mb.

---

*Pentium is a registered trademark of Intel, Inc., Ft. Worth, Texas.
†Windows 95 is a trademark of Microsoft, Inc., Redmond, Washington.

Input-Output Devices (Keyboards and Monitors)

Input-output (I/O) devices are components of the computer system through which data are either entered or displayed. These include the monitors, keyboards, pointing devices (e.g., a mouse), disk drives, printers, and fax modems, as well as special interfaces between computer and analog instruments. Some I/O devices (e.g., disk drives, modems, and special interfaces) function for both input and output. Other I/O devices are for input only, such as the keyboard or mouse. Monitors and printers are examples of output only devices.

Most I/O devices use specialized integrated circuits (i.e., chips), or even their own microprocessor, to perform various tasks. Most PCs are modular, using a main circuit board (i.e., mother board) into which various I/O cards may be plugged. This open design is flexible. It allows systems to meet very specific needs such as those found in the pulmonary function laboratory. Upgrading a computer system (e.g., adding more memory) is enhanced by being able to replace individual components rather than the entire system. Advanced chip technologies now allow many of the functions previously assigned to specific I/O cards to be placed directly on the mother board. Although this limits flexibility somewhat, the overall size of the computer can be reduced dramatically.

Mass Storage Devices

Mass storage devices include magnetic tape systems, floppy and hard disks, and optical disks. Magnetic tape systems are usually used on large, multiuser systems such as mainframe computers, where a large amount of data must be maintained. Small tape drive units are sometimes used for data storage when a large volume of data is recorded but does not require rapid retrieval. Some tape units are used as inexpensive backups to floppy or hard disk systems.

All PCs include at least one floppy disk drive. The most common diskette size is $3\frac{1}{2}$ inches, which can hold approximately 1.44 Mb of data. How much pulmonary function data can be stored on a diskette depends on the software that creates the data files. A large number of tests (including numeric data and graphs) can be stored if compression is used. The chief advantages of floppy disks for program and data storage are that they are inexpensive, lightweight, and portable. The primary disadvantages of diskettes are that they can be damaged rather easily, are very slow compared to hard disks, and eventually wear out.

The hard disk, or fixed drive, uses technology similar to that of the floppy disk, except that instead of a flexible plastic disk, a solid metal platter is used. A hard disk allows a larger volume of data to be stored in the same space as a floppy disk. Data on a hard disk can be accessed much more quickly. Hard disks are commonly described by the total storage space provided. Hard disks of more than 2 gigabytes (2000 Mb) are commonly available. The advantages of the fixed disk over floppy disks are the large volume of data contained on a single device and the speed with which the data can be accessed. Some disadvantages of the hard disk include the necessity of backing up large amounts of information (on floppy disks or tape) and managing thousands of files on a single device.

Advances in hard disk technology have reduced mechanical failure rates as well as the cost per megabyte. Sophisticated software tools are usually required to manage hard disks. Most of these programs feature file management, diagnostics, and backup features. Several manufacturers offer drives that feature removable media. These devices store large amounts of data but can be physically moved from one computer to another or can be removed for security purposes.

An optical drive (i.e., laser drive) is a high-capacity storage device that uses a laser to write information on a plastic disk. The simplest type of optical disk is not erasable. Data can be written to the disk only once. These types of devices are commonly called Write Once Read Many (WORM) drives. A more sophisticated type of optical drive uses a combination of laser and magnetic pulses to write data on the plastic disk. The data may then be erased or modified by altering the state of the magnetic pulses. Either type of optical disk is ideally suited for storage of large amounts of data such as spirometric tracings. Optical drives are also useful for storage of reference information or for archiving data that must be retained. Nonerasable optical disks are capable of holding approximately 900 Mb of data, so several thousand routine pulmonary function tests can be archived on a single disk. Erasable optical disks can hold slightly less, approximately 600 Mb. The drive itself is approximately the size of a conventional hard drive, and the laser disk is about the size of a $5\frac{1}{4}$-in floppy.

The CD-ROM is a read-only version of the laser disk. CD-ROMs are most commonly used to store reference material or to distribute programs. The capacity of the CD-ROM is similar to the erasable optical drive. The hardware for the drive is less complex because data are only read from the disk. CD-ROMs that provide access to large medical databases such as Medline are available. Because of their large capacity, CD-ROMs can be used for audiovisual data (i.e., sound and video).

Printers, Plotters, and Recorders

Computerized pulmonary function systems can provide hard copy output of high-resolution graphs. Volume-time spirograms, flow-volume loops, and plethysmograph curves can be printed rapidly. Tabular data can be presented in a variety of fonts and formats to produce concise and meaningful reports. Table 9-3 lists some of the peripheral devices commonly used with pulmonary function testing systems.

Programs and Data

Software refers to all of the instructions contained in a program. Programs are loaded into the computer's ROM and RAM memory. PC-based computers use an operating system (e.g., Windows 95) that controls various operations, such as loading files and executing programs. Application programs perform tasks that the user selects, such as pulmonary function testing, word processing, or database management. Most application programs are loaded into the computer from disk, but many basic functions are contained on ROM chips. This implementation is used in portable spirometry units that feature a dedicated microprocessor (see Fig. 9-34). These devices contain all software on chips (PROMs or EPROMs); the program is immediately available when the unit is powered on.

The format in which test data is stored depends on (1) complexity of the data, (2) how many tests will be done per month or year, and (3) how data will be accessed. Three methods for data management are used with computerized pulmonary function systems:

---

1. *Temporary or no data storage.* Some portable spirometers provide only temporary storage of patient data. In these systems a microprocessor performs calculations and then provides printed output; patient data are not stored. Some microprocessor-based spirometers use battery powered RAM to store tests in memory for viewing and printing. These instruments permit tests from multiple patients to be stored; data can be recalled whenever the system is operating. Data can usually be transferred to a host computer or to a printer. Some monitoring

---

TABLE 9-3   Pulmonary Function Output Devices

Device	Description	Advantages/Disadvantages
Kymograph	Rotating drum with chart paper and pen	Volume-time mechanical recording only; useful for quality control (QC) of spirometer
Strip-chart	Constant speed recorder; thermal or pressure-sensitive paper	Volume-time mechanical recording only; may be used for QC
X-Y plotter	Servo controlled or computerized 2-axis recorder with or without color pens	Volume-time or flow-volume tracings; may be driven by analog signals or by computer output (digital plotter)
Dot matrix printer	Uses 9-24 pins to print characters and graphics; can use color ribbons	Fast, computer driven, can print any digitalized data; letter-quality or color output may be slow
Thermal printer	Use heat-sensitive paper to transfer images	Output similar to dot-matrix but slower; inexpensive and small; paper may discolor or curl with age
Ink jet printer	Small nozzles paint characters and graphics	High-quality output; can print in color for text and graphics; inexpensive; not as fast as dot-matrix or laser printers
Laser printer	Laser transfer of toner to paper at 300-600 dpi	Fast, highest quality output of text and graphics; 12 ppm; may be expensive; color very expensive

dpi, Dots per inch; *ppm,* pages per minute.

devices (e.g., pulse oximeters) also provide limited data storage with interfaces for host computers or printers.

2. *Permanent patient data files.* Most pulmonary function systems use PCs. Patient data are stored by creating individual files, usually on the PC's hard disk. The volume of data stored in files of this type is limited only by the computer's operating system and the physical capacity of the storage device. A commonly used format stores patient data and test results in one file, with graphic data (e.g., flow-volume curves) in a separate file. Graph data often require more disk space than tabular data, depending on the format in which it is stored.

3. *Database storage.* Some pulmonary function systems use a relational database format. Tests from different patients are stored as individual records in a file. Files (sometimes called tables) are then "linked" to form a database. One file may contain all spirometry records, a second file all lung volume records, a third file DL_{CO} measurements, and so on. Individual patient data are linked across files by an index using patient number or test date. A database structure allows sorting, selecting, searching, and editing of patient data. Some applications of a database system for pulmonary function data include the following:

- Serial comparisons of multiple tests on a single subject may be extracted to plot a trend. Data from longitudinal studies on groups of subjects may be handled similarly.

- Queries may be performed to extract data that match selected criteria.

- Special reports may be generated in addition to those supported by the application software.

- Reference equations may be stored in a database format. This structure allows input of user-defined equations for predicting normal values.

Relational database systems support a special command language called Structured Query Language (SQL). SQL databases provide a standardized means for the user to enter and retrieve data, generate reports, and perform functions such as importing or exporting records. SQL databases can be easily restructured.

Interpretation Programs (Pulmonary Function and Blood Gases)

Pulmonary function software often includes an interpretation program. Interpretation programs use algorithms for identifying obstructive, restrictive, combined, or normal patterns of pulmonary function. The algorithms can evaluate spirometry, lung volumes, and DL_{CO}, comparing measured and reference values. Although algorithms use logic similar to that of a clinician, they are unable to consider the patient's clinical history or other laboratory findings. Some programs are very sophisticated and can diagnose obstruction or restriction reasonably well. An incorrect computer interpretation may occur if test data are invalid because of poor patient effort or technical problems. Computer interpretation in no way substitutes for evaluation by a qualified clinician. It may be helpful when an immediate report of abnormalities is necessary, such as for screening purposes. Computer interpretation can also be used in an educational setting. If a computer interpretation is included in the final report, it should be clearly labeled as such.

Blood gas interpretation by computer uses algorithms to evaluate acid-base and oxygenation status. Computerized blood gas interpretation may be useful when rapid interpretation to exclude abnormal findings is required. Because a computer can routinely evaluate all measured and calculated blood gas variables, it may suggest abnormalities that a casual interpreter might overlook. Computer-assisted blood gas interpretations should be considered preliminary until verified by a qualified interpreter.

A related area in which computer-assisted interpretation may be useful is quality control of blood gas analyzers. Evaluation of controls requires statistical calculations involving large volumes of data (see Chapter 10). Most quality control programs compute means and standard deviations (see Appendix G) for multiple levels of pH, PCO_2, PO_2, and Hb. Controls may be run daily or more often on multiple instruments. Computerized management of data and statistics can simplify record keeping in a busy laboratory. An added advantage is that a computer can interpret quality control data in real time. This allows the technologist to quickly determine the status of individual blood gas electrodes (see Chapter 10).

DATA ACQUISITION AND INSTRUMENT CONTROL

The main advantage of computerized pulmonary function systems is the ability to process analog signals from spirometers, pneumotachometers, and gas analyzers. Equally important is the computer's capacity to control instrument functions, such as switching valves or recording signals. Computer control allows the technologist to manage complex test maneuvers. Data acquisition and instrument control are implemented with an interface (Fig. 9-36) between the computer and pulmonary function equipment.

Analog-to-Digital Converters

A key component of the pulmonary function equipment interface is the A/D converter. An A/D converter accepts an analog signal and transforms it into a digital value. The analog signal is usually a DC voltage in the range of either 0 to 10 V or −5 to +5 V. A/D converters are classified by the number of bits (binary digits) into which they convert the signal. The higher the number of bits, the greater the resolution of the input signal in the resulting digital value. A 12-bit converter can transform a voltage into a number represented by 000000000000 to 111111111111 as a binary number. In the decimal notation this corresponds to a range of 0 to 4096, or 2^{12}. For example, a 10-L spirometer might produce an analog signal ranging from 0 to 10 V (i.e., 1 V = 1 L). If this spirometer is connected to a 12-bit converter, the signal can be divided into 4096 parts. This provides a resolution of approximately 0.0024 V or 2.4 ml over the 10-L volume range. The smallest volume change that could be detected by the computer would be 2.4 ml for this spirometer system. Some transducers (e.g., a flow sensor that measures bidirectional flow) have a voltage range of ±5 V. A 12-bit converter connected to this transducer would have a similar resolution of 0.0024 V, because the full-scale input range is still 10 V. However, the actual flow resolution would depend on the sensitivity of the transducer or the range of flows that produce a −5 to +5 voltage. For most volume and flow sampling applications, 12-bit converters are recommended. Sometimes 8- and 10-bit converters are used for functions that do not require high resolution.

The rate at which data are sampled also affects accuracy. Most A/D converter systems use 8 to 16 distinct channels. Each channel is capable of accepting a separate analog input. For tests such as an FVC maneuver, conversions may be performed on just one channel. High-speed converters can perform more than 20,000 conversions per second on a single channel. As more channels are

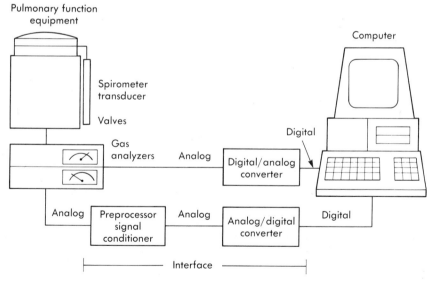

FIG. 9-36 *Computer interface for pulmonary function equipment.* Components of a typical interface between a spirometer, gas analyzers, and a personal computer are represented. Analog signals from the pulmonary function equipment are preprocessed and then passed to an A/D converter. The A/D converter transforms a voltage (usually DC) into digital data in the form of binary or hexadecimal numbers. Digital data are then processed by the computer for calculations, display, and storage. For the computer to control various instrument functions, a D/A converter transforms digital data into appropriate analog signals to control system functions such as opening valves in the breathing circuit.

included in the conversion, the rate for each channel is reduced. Most computerized pulmonary function systems sample data 100 times/sec (i.e., 100 Hz) or greater. These high rates exceed the frequency bandwidth of breathing maneuvers by a factor of more than two. Accuracy is attained by matching the analog output of a device such as a spirometer to an A/D converter with appropriate sampling rate and voltage resolution.

Encoders

Another means of sampling volume or flow signals is measuring the time required for a known change in volume or flow. For example, the number of clock ticks that occur for a volume change of 100 ml can be counted and flow calculated. This technique requires a spirometer that uses a position encoder or that generates pulses for each volume increment. The accuracy of encoder-pulse systems depends on clock resolution and volume increment, especially when measuring high flows.

Signal Processors

Some analog signals require special handling before A/D conversion. Signal conditioning functions are often performed in the interface between the test instrument and the computer. Signal conditioning is also called preprocessing. Most transducers include amplifiers that allow setting of offsets and gains. Amplifiers permit the analog signal to be adjusted to match an input such as volume or flow. Another example of signal preprocessing is transformation of resistance into a voltage so that A/D conversion is possible. Other preprocessing functions of an interface include peak signal detection, counters, and timers.

Many instruments (e.g., pulse oximeters or capnographs) use a dedicated microprocessor and A/D board to process data. These instruments often include a communication port so that data can be sent to an external computer or printer. Serial data ports are often used, but other types (e.g., infrared) are becoming common. Most computers have serial ports that can be used to interface various instruments. Some laboratory instruments support **parallel ports.** Parallel ports transmit entire bytes of data at one time rather than in bits (i.e., serially). Parallel ports are typically used for interconnection with printers.

Instrument Control

Another function of the interface is conversion of digital information from the computer into analog signals. This allows the computer to "control" the test equipment (e.g., spirometer, valves). A digital-to-analog (D/A) converter provides this ability. In its simplest form, the D/A converter acts as a relay switch between the computer and an instrument. A nonzero value sent from the computer can be used to activate an electrically operated valve or solenoid. D/A conversion allows the computer to control functions such as activating kymographs or recorders, switching valves in automated circuits, and opening solenoids to add O_2, He, or other gases.

Some pulmonary function systems provide an alternate means of controlling functions that are normally computer controlled. Manual controls allow use of the spirometer, gas analyzers, and associated equipment, even if the computer becomes unavailable. Manual operation of system components is also useful for quality assurance checks and trouble-shooting.

SUMMARY

THIS CHAPTER HAS EXAMINED various types of devices commonly found in the pulmonary function laboratory, as well as in other clinical settings. These include spirometers that use either volume-displacement or flow-sensing principles. Spirometers are used in many different types of pulmonary function tests. Peak flow meters are also common. The development of small portable peak flow devices has resulted in their widespread use both in clinical settings and by patients at home. Body plethysmographs are also more widely used than in the past; their design and methodology has benefited from advances in electronics and computerization.

Different types of pulmonary gas analyzers have been described. Their principles of operation have been outlined along with how they are used for pulmonary function testing. Breathing valves and related devices have also been outlined, with particular attention to selection and maintenance. Blood gas electrodes, oximeters, and related monitors have been reviewed. The use of technology such as blood gas optodes has been detailed. Some of the advantages and disadvantages of various methods of blood gas monitoring have been considered.

Computers, especially PC-based systems and dedicated microprocessors, have become a primary component of almost every type of pulmonary function system. Monitoring devices such as pulse oximeters rely almost completely on computerization. Information on the components of computer systems, programs (software), and specific interfaces to pulmonary function equipment has been presented.

SELF-ASSESSMENT QUESTIONS

1 *To interface a water-sealed spirometer to a computer, which of the following is required?*
   a. An X-Y plotter with analog input
   b. A variable-speed kymograph
   c. A small pneumotachometer
   d. A linear potentiometer

2 *A dry rolling-seal spirometer is checked by injecting 3 L volumes at different flows (high, medium, low) with the following results:*

   High: 2.60 L
   Medium: 2.62 L
   Low: 2.61 L

   Which of the following explains this data?
   a. An improperly functioning bacteria filter is in the circuit.
   b. The rolling-seal is sticking or leaking.
   c. The spirometer has not been calibrated.
   d. The 3 L volume is being corrected to BTPS.

3 *Dead space volume is a factor that must be considered when selecting which of the following?*
   I.   Free breathing valves
   II. One-way directional valves
   III. Two-way nonrebreathing valves
   IV. In-line bacteria filters
   a. I and II only
   b. III and IV only
   c. I, II, and IV
   d. II, III, and IV

4 *To measure volume using a flow-sensing spirometer, which of the following is necessary?*
   a. A low resistance bacteria filter
   b. An X-Y plotter or strip-chart recorder
   c. Integration of flow versus time
   d. A 3-L calibration syringe

5 *Which of the following can alter the calibration of a spirometer that uses a pressure-differential pneumotachometer?*
   a. Development of laminar flow in the pneumotachometer
   b. Allowing a healthy adult subject to exhale maximally through it
   c. Exhaustion of the water absorber (dessicant)
   d. Water droplet condensation in the resistive element

6 *Which of the following correctly describes flow-sensing spirometers?*
   I.   Corrections must be made for different gas compositions
   II. The flow transducer must be heated
   III. Nonlinearity is corrected electronically or by software
   IV. Water vapor must be removed using a chemical absorber
   a. I and III only
   b. II and IV only
   c. I, II, and III
   d. II, III, and IV

7 *Portable peak flow meters for small children should be able to measure flows up to how many liters per minute?*
   a. 100
   b. 400
   c. 700
   d. 850

8 *Which of the following types of analyzers can be used for breath-by-breath measurements of CO_2?*
   a. Infrared
   b. Polarographic
   c. Zirconium fuel cell
   d. Thermal conductivity

9 *Which type of gas analyzer uses a vacuum pump to allow ionization of gas to take place?*
   a. Gas chromatograph
   b. Emission spectroscopy
   c. Infrared absorption
   d. Thermal conductivity

10 *Which of the following can be used to analyze multiple gases simultaneously?*
   a. Gas chromatograph
   b. Polarographic electrode
   c. Zirconium fuel cell
   d. Paramagnetic sensor

11 *The P_{CO_2} electrode uses which of the following principles?*
   a. A pH electrode in a bicarbonate electrolyte
   b. A platinum cathode in a phosphate buffer
   c. Luminesence quenching
   d. Optical absorption at two wavelengths

12 *Which of the following problems affect the performance of P_{O_2} and P_{CO_2} electrodes?*
I.   Electrolyte depletion
II. Protein contamination of the membrane
III. Holes in the membrane
IV. Reference electrode malfunction
a. I and III only
b. II and III only
c. I and IV only
d. I, II, and III

13 *The polarographic electrode measures partial pressure of O_2 by which of the following methods?*
a. Measuring the intensity of polarized light
b. Reducing O_2 molecules with a platinum cathode
c. Binding O_2 molecules to ceramic disk
d. Detecting magnetic force lines generated by O_2 molecules

14 *Which of the following devices can be used to measure Hb concentration?*
a. Spectrophotometric oximeter
b. Pulse oximeter
c. Transcutaneous P_{O_2} sensor
d. Reflective spectrophotometer

15 *Fluorescent optodes are used for which of the following?*
I.   Expired gas analysis
II. Intraarterial blood gas monitoring
III. Extraarterial blood gas monitoring
IV. Point-of-care blood gas analysis
a. I and II only
b. III and IV only
c. II, III, and IV
d. I, II, III, and IV

16 *Pulse oximeters measure which of the following forms of Hb?*
a. RHb, total Hb
b. RHb, O_2Hb
c. O_2Hb, COHb
d. COHb, MetHb

17 *Which of the following can cause a pulse oximeter to display an inaccurate saturation?*
a. Total Hb greater than 17 g/dl
b. Total Hb less than 10 g/dl
c. Heart rate greater than 150/min
d. Low perfusion at the sensor site

18 *The flow-type plethysmograph differs from the constant volume (pressure) plethysmograph in which of the following ways?*
a. Forced expiratory maneuvers can be performed with the door closed.
b. Flow boxes must be rigorously air-tight.
c. Thoracic gas volume cannot be measured directly.
d. Airway resistance can be measured in small children.

19 *The number of complete pulmonary function tests that can be permanently stored by a computer depends on which of the following?*
a. Whether the computer uses PROMs or EPROMs
b. The amount of RAM available (in megabytes)
c. The presence of a built-in CD-ROM device
d. The capacity of the hard disk

20 *To interface a pressure differential pneumotachometer to a computer, which of the following devices are required?*
I.   Pressure transducer with amplifier
II. Linear potentiometer
III. A/D converter
IV. D/A converter
a. I and III only
b. II and III only
c. II and IV only
d. I, II, III, and IV

SELECTED BIBLIOGRAPHY

Spirometers

American Thoracic Society: Standardization of spirometry—1994 update, *Am J Respir Crit Care* 152:1107-1136, 1995.

Finucane KE, Egan BA, Dawson SV: Linearity and frequency response of pneumotachographs, *J Appl Physiol* 32:121, 1972.

Gardner RM, Hankinson JL, West BJ: Evaluating commercially available spirometers, *Am Rev Respir Dis* 121:73-78, 1980.

Hankinson JL: Pulmonary function testing in the screening of workers: guidelines for instrumentation, performance, and interpretation, *J Occup Med* 28:1081-1092, 1986.

Hankinson JL: Instrumentation for spirometry. In Eisen JE, ed: *Occupational medicine: state of the art reviews,* Philadelphia, 1993, Hanley and Belfus.

Johns DP, Ingram C, Booth H, et al: Effect of a microaerosol barrier filter on the measurement of lung function, *Chest* 107:1045-1048, 1995.

Nelson SB, Gardner RM, Crapo RO, et al: Performance evaluation of contemporary spirometers, *Chest* 97:288, 1990.

Porszaz J, Barstow TJ, Wasserman K: Evaluation of a symmetrically disposed Pitot-tube flowmeter for measuring gas flow during exercise, *J Appl Physiol* 77:2659-2665, 1994.

Pulmonary Function Standards for Cotton Dust. 29 Code of Federal Regulations; 1910.1043 Cotton Dust, Appendix D. Occupational Safety and Health Administration, 1980.

Sullivan WJ, Peters GM, Enright PL: Pneumotachographs: theory and clinical applications, *Respir Care* 29:736, 1984.

Townsend MC: The effects of leaks in spirometers on measurement of pulmonary function, *J Occup Med* 26:835-841, 1984.

Peak Flow Meters

Gardner RM, Crapo RO, Jackson BR, et al: Evaluation of accuracy and reproducibility of peak flowmeters at 1400 m, *Chest* 101:948-952, 1992.

Jackson AC: Accuracy, reproducibility, and variability of portable peak-flow meters, *Chest* 107:648-651, 1995.

Jensen RL, Crapo RO, Berlin SL: Effect of altitude on hand-held peak flowmeters, *Chest* 109:475-479, 1996.

Shapiro SM, Hendler JM, Ogirala RG, et al: An evaluation of the accuracy of Assess and miniWright peak flow meters, *Chest* 99:358-362, 1991.

Gas Analyzers

Norton AC: Accuracy in pulmonary measurements, *Respir Care* 24:131, 1979.

Rebuck AS, Chapman KR: Measurement and monitoring of exhaled carbon dioxide. In Nochomovitz ML, Cherniack NS, eds: *Non-invasive respiratory monitoring,* New York, 1986, Churchill Livingstone.

Sodal IE, Bowman RR, Filley GF: A fast-response oxygen analyzer with high accuracy for respiratory gas measurement, *J Appl Physiol* 25:181, 1968.

Wilson RS, Laver MB: Oxygen analysis: advances in methodology, *Anesthesiology* 37:112, 1972.

Blood Gas Electrodes, Oximeters, and Related Devices

Barker SJ, Tremper KK: Pulse oximetry: applications and limitations. In Tremper KK, Barker SJ, eds: *International anesthesiology clinics,* Boston, 1987, Little, Brown.

Brown LJ: A new instrument for the simultaneous measurement of total hemoglobin, % oxyhemoglobin, % carboxyhemoglobin, % methemoglobin, and O_2 content, *IEEE Trans Biomed Engr* 27:132, 1980.

Divertie MB, McMichan JC: Continuous monitoring of mixed venous saturation, *Chest* 85:423, 1984.

Huch A, and Huch R: Transcutaneous, noninvasive monitoring of Po_2, *Hosp Pract* 11:43, 1976.

Mahutte CK, Holody M, Maxwell TP, et al: Development of a patient-dedicated, on-demand, blood gas monitor, *Am J Respir Crit Care Med* 149:852-859, 1994.

Peruzzi WT, Shapiro BA, eds: Blood gas measurements, *Respir Care Clin North Am* 1:1-157, 1995.

Pologue JA: Pulse oximetry: technical aspects of machine design. In Tremper KK, Barker SJ, eds: *International anesthesiology clinics,* Boston, 1987, Little, Brown.

Severinghaus JW, Bradley AF: Electrodes for blood Po_2 and Pco_2 determination, *J Appl Physiol* 13:515, 1958.

Severinghaus JW, Astrup PB: History of blood gas analysis. V. Oxygen measurement, *J Clin Monit* 2:174, 1986.

Tremper KK, Waxman KS: Transcutaneous monitoring of respiratory gases. In Nochomovitz ML, Cherniack NS, eds: *Noninvasive respiratory monitoring,* New York, 1986, Churchill Livingstone.

Wahr JA, Tremper KK: Continuous intravascular blood gas monitoring, *J Cardiothorac Vasc Anesth* 8:342-353, 1994.

Plethysmographs

American Association for Respiratory Care: Clinical practice guideline: body plethysmography, *Respir Care* 39:1184-1190, 1994.

Bargeton D, Barres G: Time characteristics and frequency response of body plethysmographs. International Symposium on Body Plethysmography, Nijmegen, *Prog Respir Res* 4:2, 1969.

DuBois AB, Bothello SY, Bedell GN, et al: A rapid plethysmographic method for measuring thoracic gas volume: a comparison with nitrogen-washout method for measuring functional residual capacity in normal subjects, *J Clin Invest* 35:322, 1956.

DuBois AB, Bothello SY, Comroe JH: A new method for measuring airway resistance in man using a body plethysmograph: values in normal subjects and in patients with respiratory disease, *J Clin Invest* 35:327, 1956.

Lourenco RV, Chung SYK: Calibration of a body plethysmograph for measurement of lung volume, *Am Rev Respir Dis* 95:687, 1967.

Quanjer PH, Tammeling GJ, Cotes JE, et al: Lung volumes and forced ventilatory flows: report of the Working Party for Standardization of Lung Function Tests, European Community for Steel and Coal, *Eur Respir J* 16(suppl):5-40, 1993.

Computers

American Thoracic Society, Committee on Proficiency Standards for Clinical Pulmonary Laboratories: Computer guidelines for pulmonary laboratories, *Am Rev Respir Dis* 134:628, 1986.

Crapo RO, Gardner RM, Berlin SL, et al: Automation of pulmonary function equipment—user beware! *Chest* 90:1, 1986 (editorial).

Ellis JH, Perera SP, Levin DC: A computer program for the interpretation of pulmonary function studies, *Chest* 68:209, 1975.

Mellichamp D, ed: *Real-time computing—with applications to data acquisition and control,* New York, 1983, Van Nostrand Reinhold.

Scanlan C, Ruppel GL: Computer applications in respiratory care. In Scanlan, ed: *Egan's fundamentals of respiratory care,* St Louis, 1995, Mosby.

Tompkins WJ, Webster JG, eds: *Design of microcomputer-based medical instrumentation,* Newark, NJ, 1981, Prentice-Hall.

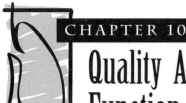

CHAPTER 10

Quality Assurance in the Pulmonary Function Laboratory

OBJECTIVES

After studying this chapter and reviewing its tables and figures, you should be able to do the following:

1 Give examples of accuracy and precision as they apply to measurements of pulmonary function tests and blood gas analysis

2 List at least three of the minimal requirements of an acceptable spirometer for diagnostic testing

3 Use results obtained from biologic control subjects to troubleshoot pulmonary function equipment

4 Determine whether a blood gas analyzer is "in control" using standard rules

5 Suggest appropriate technologist comments to include with a pulmonary function report

6 Describe universal precautions to be applied during blood gas specimen collection and analysis

THIS FINAL CHAPTER DISCUSSES issues related to quality assurance. General concepts include standards for equipment such as spirometers and blood gas analyzers. Instrument maintenance and calibration are the foundation for obtaining data that are acceptable and reproducible. This chapter deals with quality control for different types of equipment used for pulmonary function testing and blood gas analysis. Problems that are commonly encountered with various types of equipment are listed to guide in troubleshooting.

Special attention is given to methods by which the pulmonary function technologist can assess data quality. Documentation of pulmonary function data is discussed. Those who perform pulmonary function tests must make decisions during testing that often determine the quality of data obtained.

Safety and infection control are discussed as they relate to patients and to those performing pulmonary function tests. As in previous chapters, self-assessment questions are included.

Elements of Laboratory Quality Control

Quality control is essential to the operation of the pulmonary function laboratory to obtain valid and reproducible data. There are four general elements to consider in regard to a quality assurance program:

---

1. *Methodology.* The type of equipment used (e.g., volume versus flow-based spirometer) often determines which procedures are required for calibration and quality control. The equipment used may also determine how often quality control procedures must be performed. The number and complexity of the tests performed may dictate which equipment and methods are used. Methods and equipment that have been validated in the scientific literature should be used whenever possible. Quality control is usually easier to perform when standardized techniques are used.

2. *Equipment maintenance.* The type and complexity of instrumentation for a specific test will determine the long-term and short-term maintenance that will be required. Preventive maintenance is scheduled in anticipation of equipment malfunction to reduce the possibility

of equipment failure. Corrective maintenance or repair is unscheduled service that is required to correct equipment failure. This failure is often signaled by quality control procedures or extreme test results. Familiarity with the operating characteristics of spirometers, gas analyzers, plethysmographs, and computers, requires manufacturer support and thorough documentation. A procedure manual (Table 10-1) and accurate records are essential to a comprehensive maintenance program. Documentation of procedures and repairs is required by most accrediting organizations.

3. *Control methods.* A "control" is any known test signal for an instrument that can be used to determine its accuracy and precision. Control signals or materials must be available for spirometers, gas analyzers, blood gas analyzers, and other instruments. Because many laboratories use computerized pulmonary function or blood gas analyzers, control signals are required to ensure that both software and hardware are functioning within acceptable limits. Control methods may vary from use of 3-L syringes for spirometers to tonometered blood for blood gas analyzers. "Biologic" controls are test subjects for whom specific variables have been determined.

4. *Testing technique.* A primary means of ensuring quality of data is to rigidly control the procedures by which data are obtained. For pulmonary function testing, this refers to the technologist's ability to conduct the procedure and to elicit subject cooperation in the test maneuvers. Technologist and subject performance, as well as proper equipment function, must be evaluated on a test-by-test basis. This may be accomplished by using appropriate criteria to judge the acceptability of results.

Each pulmonary function laboratory should have a written quality assurance program that includes the following:

- The methods used for specific tests
- The limitations of the procedure (if any)
- Indications or schedules for maintenance
- Quality control materials or signals to be used
- Action to be taken if controls exceed specified limits
- Specific guidelines as to how tests are to be performed

TABLE 10-1   Pulmonary Function Procedure Manual

Items to be included in a typical procedure manual for a pulmonary function laboratory. For each procedure performed, the following should be present:

1. *Description* of the test and its purpose
2. *Indications* for ordering the test and contraindications, if any
3. Description of the *general method(s)* and any specific equipment required
4. *Calibration* of equipment required before testing (manufacturer's documentation may be referenced)
5. *Patient preparation* for the test, if any (e.g., withholding medication)
6. Step-by-step procedure for both computerized and manual *measurement/calculation* of results
7. *Quality control* guidelines with acceptable limits of performance and corrective actions to be taken
8. *Safety precautions* related to the procedure (e.g., infection control, hazards) and alert values that require physician notification
9. *References* for all equations used for calculating results and for predicted normals, including a bibliography
10. Documentation of *computer protocols* for calculations and data storage; guidelines for computer downtime
11. Dated *signatures* of the medical and technical directors

The quality assurance program should be included as part of the laboratory procedure manual (see Table 10-1).

Two concepts that are central to quality assurance are accuracy and precision. *Accuracy* may be defined as the extent to which measurement of a known quantity results in a value approximating that quantity. For most laboratory tests, repeated measurements of a control are made and the "mean" or average calculated. If this mean value approximates the "known" value of the control, the instrument is considered accurate.

Precision may be defined as the extent to which repeated measurements of the same quantity can be reproduced. If a variable is measured repeatedly and the results are similar, the instrument may be considered precise.

Accuracy and precision may not always be present together in the same instrument. For example, a spirometer that consistently measures a 3-L test volume as 2.5 L is precise, but not very accurate. A spirometer that evaluates a 3-L test volume as 2.5, 3.0, and 3.5 L on repeated maneuvers produces an accurate mean of 3.0 L, but the individual measurements are not precise. Determining both the accuracy and precision of instruments such as spirometers is important because many pulmonary function variables are effort dependent. The largest observed value, rather than the mean, is often reported as the "best test" (see Chapter 2). Reporting the largest result observed is based on the rationale that the subject cannot overshoot on a test that is effort dependent.

Calibration and Quality Control of Pulmonary Function Equipment

Calibration is the process in which the signal from an instrument is adjusted to produce a known output. This may be accomplished by one of several methods:

---

1. Adjustment of the analog output signal from the primary transducer (i.e., spirometer bell, flow sensor, gas analyzer)
2. Adjustment of the sensitivity of the recording device
3. Software correction or compensation

Calibration involves adjustment of the instrument (or its signal) and should not be confused with verification or quality control. Quality control assesses function of the instrument after it has been calibrated.

SPIROMETERS

Spirometers that produce a voltage signal by means of a potentiometer (see Chapter 9) normally allow some form of "gain" adjustment so that the analog output can be matched to a known input of either volume or flow. For example, a 10-L volume-displacement spirometer may be equipped with a 10-V potentiometer. This potentiometer amplifier would be adjusted so that 0 V equals 0 L (zero), and 10 V equals 10 L (gain). The calibration could be verified by setting the spirometer at a specific volume and noting the analog signal (i.e., 5 L should equal 5 V).

A second technique is adjustment of the sensitivity of the recording device. This method is used for spirometers equipped with X-Y plotters or strip chart recorders. In these devices a known volume is injected into the spirometer and deflection of the recording device is adjusted to match the volume. For example, a strip chart recorder is turned on and has its pen adjusted to read 0 L when the spirometer is empty. A 3-L volume is then injected. The gain of the recorder is adjusted so that the tracing deflects to the 3-L mark on the graph paper. This method is appropriate when the recorded tracing is to be manually measured. The ability to evaluate a spirometer's accuracy using a mechanical recorder is also useful for computerized systems.

Most spirometer systems are computerized (see Chapter 9). In computerized systems, the signal produced by the spirometer is often corrected by applying a software calibration factor. A known volume, or flow, is injected into the spirometer using a large-volume syringe, usually 3 L. A correction (i.e., calibration) factor is calculated based on the measured versus expected values:

$$\text{Correction factor} = \frac{\text{Expected volume}}{\text{Measured volume}}$$

The correction factor derived by this method is then stored, usually in memory and on disk. The correction is applied to all subsequent volume measurements. For example, if a syringe with a volume of 3 L is injected into a spirometer and a volume of 2.97 L recorded, the correction factor would be as follows:

$$1.010 = \frac{3.00 \text{ L}}{2.97 \text{ L}}$$

The correction factor 1.010 would then be used to adjust subsequent measured volumes. This method assumes that the spirometer's output is linear and that the same factor would be correct for any volume, large or small. Most automated spirometers allow the correction factor to be verified by reinjecting a known volume, usually 3 L. After calibration, the spirometer should display an accuracy of 3% or 50 ml, whichever is larger. Three percent of a standard 3-L syringe means that the spirometer should read 3.00 ± 0.09 L (range, 2.91 to 3.09 L).

Care should be taken that the gas in the syringe, which is at ambient temperature (ATPS) is not "temperature corrected" by the software. Many computerized spirometers provide software specifically for calibration and verification. This allows the use of a large-volume syringe without applying corrections that are necessary when patients are tested. Inappropriate temperature correction would produce an erroneously high measured value, and a low correction factor. Correct temperature should be available from an accurate thermometer, both for calibration and for testing. If the ambient temperature changes, recalibration may be needed. The calibration syringe should be maintained at the same environmental conditions as the spirometer itself.

Other factors that might influence establishment of the software correction value include the accuracy of the large-volume syringe and the speed with which the injection is performed. An inaccurate syringe or leaks in the connection to the spirometer may produce erroneous software corrections. Accuracy of calibration syringes should be verified annually. Syringes can be checked for leaks simply by occluding the port and trying to empty the syringe. Some laboratories use two syringes: one to calibrate and another to verify volume accuracy.

Some spirometers, particularly those that are flow-based, may require that the calibration volume be injected within certain flow limits. Volume calibration at different flows can be accomplished by injecting 3 L at flows between 2 and 12 L/sec. Varying the flow at which 3 L is injected permits the software to generate correction factors to accommodate a range of flows. Similarly, volume-displacement spirometers may be calibrated (or verified) using a range of flows. Ideally, volume accuracy (i.e., 3% or 50 ml) should be maintained across the flow range of the spirometer. Flow-based spirometers that measure both inspiratory and expiratory volumes require the syringe volume to be injected and withdrawn. This allows separate correction factors for inspired and expired gas to be generated. If an in-line bacteria filter will be used for testing, calibration should be performed with the device in place.

Quality control of spirometers is closely related to calibration, and the two are sometimes confused. An important distinction is that calibration (i.e., adjustment) may or may not be needed, but quality control must be applied on a routine basis. Calibration, whether it includes the output of the spirometer, recorder sensitivity, or generation of a software correction factor, involves *adjusting* of the device to perform within certain limits. Quality control is a *test* performed to determine the accuracy and/or precision of the device using a known standard or signal. Various control methods (i.e., signal generators) are available for spirometers.

Simple Large-Volume Syringe

A syringe of at least 3-L volume (Fig. 10-1) should be used to generate a control signal for checking spirometers. A 3-L syringe can be used to verify volume-displacement spirometers and associated deflection of mechanical recorders. A large-volume syringe may also be used to check the volume accuracy of flow-based spirometers. The 3-L syringe itself should be accurate to within 15 ml, or 0.5% for other volume syringes.

Quality control for spirometer volume measurements should be performed at least once each day that the device is to be used. For field studies, accuracy should be checked every 4 hours that the device is used. Frequent checks are recommended for industrial applications or epidemiologic research, especially if the spirometer is moved or used for a large number of tests.

Spirometer linearity should be verified at least quarterly. Volume-displacement spirometers should be checked in 1-L increments across their volume range. A 3-L syringe injection performed when the spirometer is nearly empty or nearly full should yield comparable results. The linearity of flow-sensing spirometers should be tested over a range of flows. Different flows can be generated

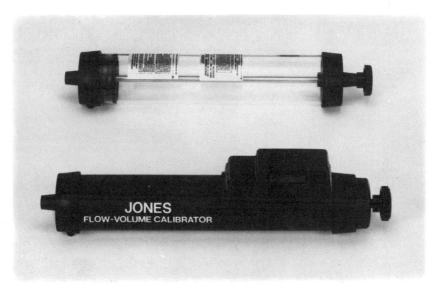

FIG. 10-1 *Calibration syringes. Top,* Standard 3-L syringe used for volume calibration of both volume- and flow-based spirometers. The same syringe may be used for FRC and DL_{CO} quality control. A 3-L syringe is recommended for both calibration and quality control. *Bottom,* Computerized FVC simulator that uses a microprocessor to measure FEV_1 and other flows during injection of a 3-L volume. The volumes and flows delivered can be compared with those reported by the spirometer. (Courtesy Jones Medical Instrument Co., Oakbrook, IL.)

by varying the speed at which the syringe is emptied. Applying different flows and measuring the resulting volumes may indicate if the spirometer (and its software) is accurate at low and high flows. For example, three different injection times, 0.5 to 1.0 seconds, 1.0 to 1.5 seconds, and 5.0 to 6.0 seconds, may be used with a 3-L syringe to simulate a wide range of flows.

Computerized syringes (see Fig. 10-1) are available for assessing the accuracy of commonly measured parameters such as forced expiratory volume (FEV_1) and $FEF_{27\%-75\%}$. These syringes use a built-in microprocessor that times volume injection and calculates the flows. The microprocessor displays volume and flows for comparison with those produced by the spirometer. A computerized syringe provides a 3-L volume for calibration or volume checks and also tests accuracy for commonly reported flows.

Quality control for spirometers should be performed as if a subject were being tested. The 3-L syringe should be connected to the patient port, with whatever circuitry is used for the actual test. Spirometer temperature correction should be set to 37° C (i.e., no correction applied). Most computerized spirometers provide a specific routine for volume checks or calibration that disables temperature corrections. In some systems temperature correction cannot be disabled. In these spirometers, injection of 3 L at ATPS results in a reading greater than 3 L because the system attempts to "correct" the volume to body temperature (BTPS). For water-seal spirometers, the syringe should be filled and emptied several times to allow equilibration with the humidified air in the device. Some flow-sensing spirometers require a length of tubing between the flow sensor and syringe to reduce artifact caused by turbulent flow in the syringe. If an in-line bacteria filter is used, volume verification should be performed with it in place.

The accuracy of any spirometer can be calculated as follows:

$$\% \text{ Error} = \frac{\text{Expected volume} - \text{Measured volume}}{\text{Expected volume}} \times 100$$

where:

expected volume = known syringe volume (usually 3 L)

measured volume = volume recorded for the test

The maximum acceptable error for diagnostic spirometers, according to the American Thoracic Society (ATS) recommendations, is ±3% or ±50 ml, whichever is larger (Table 10-2). For monitoring spirometers, maximum allowable error is ±5% or ±100 ml, whichever is greater (Table 10-3). If the percentage of error exceeds the allowable limits, careful examination of the spirometer,

TABLE 10-2 Minimal Recommendations for Spirometers (Diagnostic)

Test	Range/accuracy (BTPS)	Flow range (L/sec)	Time (sec)	Resistance/back pressure
	A 3-L calibration syringe is recommended for testing VC and FVC. Twenty-four standardized waveforms are available for validating FVC, FEV_1, and $FEF_{25\%-75\%}$. Twenty-six standard flow waveforms are available for validating PEF. Other flows require manufacturer's proof of performance. A sine wave pump is recommended for MVV validation.			
VC	0.5-8 L ± 3% of reading or ±0.05 L, whichever is greater	0-14	30	N/A
FVC	0.5-8 L ± 3% of reading or ±0.05 L, whichever is greater	0-14	15	<1.5 cm H_2O/L/sec
FEV_1	0.5-8 L ± 3% of reading or ±0.05 L, whichever is greater	0-14	1	<1.5 cm H_2O/L/sec
Time zero	Time point for calculating all FEV_T values, using back-extrapolation	N/A	N/A	N/A
PEF	Accuracy: ±10% of reading or ±0.4 L/sec, whichever is greater Precision: ±5% of reading or ±0.2 L/sec, whichever is greater	0-14	N/A	<1.5 cm H_2O/L/sec
$FEF_{25\%-75\%}$	7.0 L/sec ± 5% of reading or ±0.2 L/sec, whichever is greater	−14-+14	15	<1.5 cm H_2O/L/sec
$\dot{V}$	±14 L/sec ± 5% of reading or ±0.2 L/sec, whichever is greater	0-14	15	<1.5 cm H_2O/L/sec
MVV	250 L/min at V_T of 2 L ± 10% of reading or ±15 L/min, whichever is greater	−14-+14 ±3%	12-15	<(±)10 cm H_2O at V_T of 2 L at 2.0 Hz

Adapted from Standardization of spirometry—1994 update, *Am J Respir Crit Care Med* 152:1107-1136, 1995.
VC, Vital capacity; *FVC*, forced vital capacity; *PEF*, peak expiratory flow; *MVV*, maximal voluntary ventilation.

TABLE 10-3 Minimal Recommendations for Monitoring Spirometers and Peak Flow Meters

Requirement	FVC, FEV_1 (BTPS)*	PEF (BTPS)
Range	High: 0.50-8 L Low: 0.50-6 L	High: 100 L/min to ≥700 L/min but ≤850 L/min Low: 60 L/min to ≥275 L/min but ≤400 L/min
Accuracy	±5% of reading or ±0.1 L, whichever is greater	±10% of reading or ±20 L/min, whichever is greater
Precision	±3% of reading or ±0.05 L, whichever is greater	Intradevice: ≤5% of reading or ≤10 L/min, whichever is greater Interdevice: ≤10% of reading or ≤10 L/min, whichever is greater
Linearity	Within 3% over range	Within 5% over range
Resolution	High: 0.05 L Low: 0.025 L	High: 10 L/min Low: 5 L/min
Resistance	<2.5 cm H_2O/L/sec, from 0-14 L/sec	<2.5 cm H_2O/L/sec, from 0-14 L/sec

Adapted from Standardization of spirometry—1994 update, *Am J Respir Crit Care Med* 152:1107-1136, 1995.
*High and low refer to spirometers or peak flow meters with either a high or low range.

BOX 10-1
COMMON SPIROMETER PROBLEMS

Some problems detected by routine quality control of spirometers include the following:
- Cracks or leaks (in volume-displacement spirometers)
- Low water level (in water-seal spirometers)
- Sticking or worn bellows
- Inaccurate or erratic potentiometers
- Obstructed or dirty flow tubes (flow-sensors)
- Mechanical resistance (in volume-displacement spirometers)
- Leaks in tubes and connectors
- Faulty recorder timing
- Inappropriate signal correction (BTPS)
- Improper software calibration (corrections)
- Defective software or computer interface

---

recording device, software, most recent calibration, and the testing technique should be performed (Box 10-1).

Biologic Controls

Biologic controls are test subjects who are available for repeated tests. These controls can be laboratory personnel or other subjects who can be tested repeatedly. Using biologic controls does not eliminate other control devices such as large-volume syringes. Although a 3-L syringe can verify volume and flow accuracy of a spirometer, biologic controls can evaluate an entire system, including spirometers, gas analyzers, plethysmographs, and software. A disadvantage of using biologic controls is that pulmonary function varies from day to day. However, by establishing means and measures of variability from repeated tests, real problems with most pulmonary function equipment can be identified (Box 10-2).

Control subjects should have normal lung function (i.e., no asthma or other respiratory symptoms) and span a range of values. For example, a 64-in-tall woman and a 72-in-tall man will provide a wide range of values for most pulmonary function parameters. Pulmonary function studies on control subjects should be performed on a regular basis (weekly or monthly). All tests should use the same protocols applied to the patient population. Control measurements should meet all criteria for acceptability. Tests should be performed at the same time of day to minimize diurnal variation. If the laboratory has multiple pulmonary function systems, control subjects should be tested on each instrument on the same day.

To provide useful statistics, at least 10 sets of measurements should be recorded. However, means and standard deviations (SDs) from controls with fewer sets may be used. Pulmonary function variables that are not derived from other measurements should be recorded. These include forced vital capacity (FVC), FEV_1, functional residual capacity (FRC), and diffusing capacity (DL_{CO}). Calculated values such as total lung capacity (TLC) or DL/VA can be used as controls; however, if subsequent tests show significant differences, it may be unclear which component test is at fault. A calculator or a computer **spreadsheet** may be used to perform the simple statistics required (Table 10-4). Most spreadsheets have built-in functions to calculate mean ($\overline{X}$) and SD, and to allow data to be graphed. The coefficient of variation (CV) is calculated by dividing one SD by the mean. Separate statistics should be calculated for each control subject and for separate instruments. Data more than 1 year old should be replaced with more recent measurements to account for changes in pulmonary function that occur over time.

Other Calibration/Quality Control Tools

---

1. *Sine-wave rotary pump.* This device produces a biphasic volume signal. A biphasic or sine-wave signal may be useful for checking volume and flow accuracy for both inspiration and expiration. A rotary-drive syringe is ideal for checking frequency response of a spirometer or to evaluate a spirometer's ability to adequately record tests such as the MVV. **Sine-wave pumps** are also commonly used in the calibration of body plethysmographs.

BOX 10-2
HOW TO USE BIOLOGIC CONTROLS

1   *Performance of a single instrument.* Test biologic control subjects on a regular basis. Compare variables (e.g., FEV_1) to the established mean. Control values should fall within a range of ±2 SDs of the mean (at least 95% of the time). If the value is outside of this range, the cause of the change should be identified. Was the last calibration performed correctly? Have any modifications been made to the spirometer hardware? Have any software upgrades or modifications been made? If the source of the problem is found and corrected, the control subject should be retested to confirm that the instrument performs as expected.

2   *Establish precision of the system.* Include data in the control database that falls within the 2-SD limit. Data outside of 2 SDs may be included if it is clearly caused by variability and not an equipment problem. This may be verified by repeating the test. If the second test produces another result more than 2 SDs from the mean, there is likely an equipment or procedural error. By calculating SDs from repeated measures, the precision of a particular instrument or system can be established.

3   *Use CV to reduce variability.* The CV for most pulmonary function variables should be approximately 5% or less. Some measures, such as $FEF_{25\%-75\%}$ are variable even in healthy subjects and may show CV values closer to 10%. If the CV is greater than 10%, calibration and testing procedures should be reviewed to see if sources of error can be eliminated.

4   *Compare instruments or laboratories.* Biologic controls can be used to perform interinstrument or interlaboratory evaluation. Similar devices should produce similar control results. However, if different instruments (i.e., a flow-based and a volume-based spirometer) are compared, slightly different values for the same control subject may be obtained. This difference is termed bias. The true value (e.g., FVC) may be considered the average of the means for the two instruments or labs. Alternatively, one instrument may be considered the "gold standard"; the other instrument can be described as having a negative or positive bias, depending on whether its measurement is less than or greater than the gold standard.

5   *Compare methods.* Biologic controls may also be used to compare different methodologies within the same laboratory. For example, FRC might be measured using a gas dilution technique and by plethysmograph. The means, SDs, and CVs of each method can then be compared.

6   *Troubleshooting.* Biologic controls can be used to troubleshoot a problem instrument. For example, if a system produces low DL_{CO} values on several otherwise normal patients, a problem might exist. Test a biologic control; if the control value is within expected limits, the low DL_{CO} values may be valid.

TABLE 10-4   Example Spreadsheet for a Biologic Control*

Control subject: J.S.

Date	FVC	FEV_1	FRC	DL_{CO}
1/15/97	4.51	3.93	3.51	25.1
2/15/97	4.61	3.99	3.55	26.2
3/14/97	4.49	3.95	3.65	27.2
3/19/97	4.40	3.90	3.50	25.5
4/21/97	4.57	3.89	3.60	26.0
5/1/97	4.50	3.94	3.66	27.2
5/15/97	4.55	3.95	3.65	27.0
Mean	4.52	3.94	3.59	26.3
SD	0.06	0.03	0.06	0.78
CV	1.38%	0.79%	1.77%	2.97%

*Most spreadsheet programs have built-in functions to calculate means and standard deviations; additional calculations, such as coefficient of variation, can be entered by the user. Additional data can be entered by inserting more lines. Quality control charts may be constructed using the mean and standard deviation data for each variable.

2. *Computer-driven syringes.* These devices incorporate large-volume syringes with a computer-controlled motor drive. Computerized syringes are usually used only by equipment manufacturers or for research applications.

3. *Explosive decompression devices.* **Explosive decompression** simulates the exponential flow pattern of a forced expiratory maneuver. Such devices use compressed gas, such as CO_2, released through an orifice. The primary advantage of these devices is that they allow flow and volume signals to be reproduced. When the control signal can be reproduced, both accuracy and precision can be assessed.

In addition to checking the volume and flow accuracy of spirometers, several other important aspects of quality control require routine evaluation:

---

1. *Leak checks.* For volume-displacement spirometers, a check for leaks should be performed daily before assessing volume accuracy. Fill the device with air to approximately half of its volume range and apply a constant pressure by means of a weight or spring. No change in the volume tracing should be noted while the pressure is applied. The spirometer should return to its original volume baseline when the pressure is removed.

2. *Flow resistance.* The "back pressure" from a spirometer should be less than 1.5 cm H_2O up to a flow of 14 L/sec. Resistance to flow is measured by placing an accurate manometer or pressure transducer at the subject connection and applying a known flow. This is easily accomplished with flow-sensing devices but somewhat difficult with volume-displacement devices. Measurement of flow resistance is normally performed only when there is some reason to suspect that the spirometer is causing undue resistance. The total resistance requirement must be met with all tubing, valves, and filters in place.

3. *Frequency response.* Frequency response refers to the spirometer's ability to produce accurate volume and flow measurements across a wide range of frequencies. Frequency response is most critical for peak expiratory flow (PEF) and maximal voluntary ventilation (MVV) maneuvers. Frequency response is usually evaluated by means of a sine-wave pump or computer-driven syringe. It should be measured as part of the manufacturer's validation and rechecked if the spirometer is suspect.

4. *Flow.* Flow-sensing spirometers directly measure flow and indirectly calculate volume by integration or counting volume pulses. It is sometimes necessary to assess the flow accuracy of such devices. Inaccurate measurement of flow almost always results in inaccurate volume determinations. A rotameter may be used in conjunction with an adjustable compressed gas source to supply a gas at a known flow to the device. A weighted volume-displacement spirometer, such as a water-seal type, can also be used to generate a known flow. Many flow-sensing spirometers use a volume signal to perform software calibration as previously described. It may be useful to check the flow signal from the spirometer at different known flows if the volume accuracy is observed to vary with flow.

5. *Recorder/displays.* Printed records or computer-generated display of spirometry signals are required for diagnostic functions, validation, or when waveforms are to be measured manually. Table 10-5 lists recommended scale factors for recorders and displays. Hard-copy recordings of volume-time or flow-volume tracings should be available for diagnostic spirometry. Flow-volume curves should be plotted with expired flow upwards on the vertical axis and

TABLE 10-5   **Minimum Recommended Scale Factors for Recorders and Displays**

	Resolution	Scale factor
Volume	0.025 L	10 mm/L
Flow	0.100 L/sec	5 mm/L/sec
Time	0.20 sec	2 cm/sec

Adapted from Standardization of spirometry—1994 update, *Am J Respir Crit Care Med* 152:1107-1136, 1995.

expired volume from left to right on the horizontal axis. A flow-to-volume scales ratio of $2:1$ should be maintained. Accurate recorder speed and volume sensitivity are particularly important if results are calculated manually. Recorder accuracy should be checked at least quarterly. Paper speed of strip chart recorders can be easily checked with a stopwatch. Kymographs and similar mechanical recording devices may require repair or replacement of drive motors if paper speed is determined to be inaccurate.

GAS ANALYZERS

Accurate analysis of inspired and expired gases is required to measure lung volumes, DL_{CO}, and gas exchange during exercise or metabolic testing. The validity of these tests depends on accuracy of both the spirometer and gas analyzers used. Various types of gas analyzers are commonly used in pulmonary function testing (see Chapter 9). Calibration refers to the process of adjusting analyzer output to meet certain specifications. Quality control refers to a method for routinely checking the accuracy and precision of the gas analyzer. Calibration techniques for gas analyzers include the following:

1. *Physiologic range.* Many gas analyzers are not linear or exhibit poor accuracy over a wide range of gas concentrations. Analyzers should be calibrated to match the physiologic range over which measurements will be made. Oxygen analyzers may be used to measure fractional concentrations from 0.21 to 1.00, representing a wide physiologic range. If the O_2 analyzer is to be used for exercise tests in subjects breathing room air, its calibration range should be from 0.12 to 0.21. This narrow interval represents the physiologic range of expired O_2 likely to be encountered during an exercise test. Reducing the physiologic range of an analyzer generally allows greater accuracy and precision. Some types of analyzers provide range adjustments just for this purpose. Calibration gases should represent the extremes of the physiologic range.

2. *Sampling conditions.* Gas analyzers must be calibrated under the same conditions that will be encountered during the test. Analyzers that are sensitive to partial pressure (see Chapter 9) may be affected by the sample flow rate. For certain tests gas is sampled continuously from the breathing circuit using a pump. Sample flow through the pump must be adjusted *before* calibration, then left unchanged during sampling. If gas flow stops before analysis is actually performed, sample flow is not critical. This type of analyzer must be calibrated under conditions of zero flow. Measurement errors may occur if an analyzer is calibrated and then configuration of the sampling circuit is changed. This may happen with the addition of tubing, valves, or stopcocks. Any absorbers, such as those used for CO_2, H_2O, or dust, should be in place during calibration as well.

3. *Two-point calibration.* The most common technique for analyzer calibration involves introducing two known gases. If the test gas is not normally present in expired air (e.g., helium [He], CO, or neon [NE]), room air may be used to zero the analyzer. Calibration gas representing the other end of the physiologic range may be used to span the analyzer. The He dilution FRC and $DL_{CO}SB$ are examples of such tests. He and CO analyzers are zeroed by drawing room air into the measuring chambers. He and CO are assumed to be absent from the atmosphere. Calibration gas containing a known concentration of the gas to be analyzed is then introduced. The analyzer gain is adjusted to match the known concentration. The test gas approximates the concentration to be analyzed during the test. The analyzer may then be re-zeroed, and the entire process repeated to verify the calibration. A similar technique may be used with two gases of known concentration if the expirate normally contains varying concentrations of the gas. For example, room air and 12% oxygen might be used to perform a two-point calibration of an O_2 analyzer for exercise testing. Depending on the stability of the analyzer, calibration may need to be repeated before each test or measurement. Gas analyzers should be calibrated before each patient for lung volumes, DL_{CO}, exercise tests, and metabolic studies. Gas analyzers used for monitoring (e.g., capnographs) should be calibrated on a schedule appropriate for the extent of use. Calibration should be performed according to the manufacturer's recommendations. The accuracy of the calibration gas should reflect the necessary accuracy of the measurements involved. For exercise or metabolic studies, calibration gases should be accurate to at least two decimal places (i.e., hundredth of a percent). Calibration gases may require verification by an independent method.

4. *Multiple-point (linearity) calibration.* An assumption made by a two-point calibration is that analyzer output is linear between the points used. To verify linearity or to determine the pattern

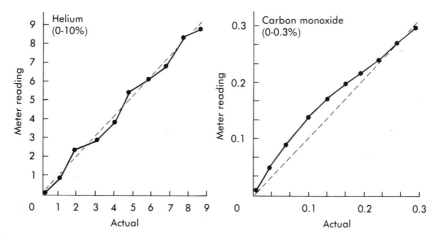

FIG. 10-2 *Calibration and linearity check of gas analyzers.* Two plots of varying gas concentrations (for He and CO) are shown. Each graph plots the meter reading of the analyzers against the actual concentration of the gas. Different dilutions of each gas are prepared and then analyzed. In the example, the He analyzer shows good linearity in the comparison of measured versus expected concentrations. The CO analyzer shows a nonlinear pattern, typical of an infrared analyzer. If enough points are determined a calibration curve can be generated to correct meter readings. Computerized systems often use an equation or a table of points representing a calibration curve. This allows an analyzer to be calibrated using only two points. Three or more points (gas concentrations) are required to demonstrate linearity.

of nonlinearity, three or more calibration points must be determined (Fig. 10-2). A multiple-point calibration is performed in a manner similar to the two-point calibration except that concentrations of known gases across the range to be analyzed are checked and plotted. If multiple points are determined, **linear regression** may be used to determine the slope of the line relating the measured gas concentrations to the expected gas concentrations. Most statistics textbooks describe calculation of simple linear regression. If the analyzer is linear, the points plotted fall in a straight line. If the analyzer is nonlinear, a calibration curve must be constructed to correct the results. In most instances an equation describing a nonlinear curve can be generated. This equation can then be used either manually or by software to correct analyzer readings. Many nonlinear analyzers incorporate electronics that linearize their output. Linearity of analyzers used for DL_{CO}, lung volumes, exercise, and metabolic studies should be assessed at least quarterly.

Quality control of gas analyzers can be performed by submitting known concentrations of gases to the analyzer, by testing a lung analog, or by using biologic controls. Several gases with concentrations spanning the range of the analyzer can be maintained. This can be a costly means of quality control for most pulmonary function laboratories. A simpler technique is to prepare serial dilutions of a known gas using a large-volume syringe. The syringe may be the type used for volume calibration. For example, 100 ml of He and 900 ml of air may be mixed in a syringe to produce a 10% He mixture, then injected into the analyzer. Subsequently 100 ml of He might be diluted in 1000 ml, then 1100 ml, and so on, with the expected concentrations calculated as follows:

$$\text{Expected \% test gas} = \frac{\text{Volume of test gas}}{\text{Total volume of gas}} \times 100$$

where:

$$\text{total volume of gas} = \text{test gas} + \text{added air} + \text{syringe dead space}$$

As each dilution is analyzed the meter reading is recorded and plotted against the expected percentage (see Fig. 10-2). This method is simple and available in most laboratories. Care must be taken when preparing samples so that air does not leak into the syringe, further diluting the test gas. The volume of air in the syringe connectors (i.e., dead space) must be included when calculating the dilution of the test gas. Some calibrated syringes include their dead space volume.

A second method of verifying analyzer performance involves simulating either lung volume or DL_{CO} tests. This may be accomplished using a lung analog. A lung analog is simply an air-tight container of known volume. The lung volume simulator is attached at the patient connection with

---

BOX 10-3
COMMON GAS ANALYZER PROBLEMS

Some of the problems occurring with gas analyzers that can be detected during calibration or by quality control:
- Leaks in sample lines or connectors
- Blockage of sample lines
- Exhausted water vapor or CO_2 absorbers
- Contamination of photocells or electrodes
- Improper mechanical zeroing (taut band display)
- Inadequate warm-up time
- Deterioration or contamination of column packing material (gas chromatographs)
- Poor vacuum pump performance (emission spectroscopy analyzers)
- Chopper motor malfunction (infrared analyzers)
- Electrolyte or fuel cell exhaustion (O_2 analyzers)
- Aging of detector cells (infrared analyzers)
- Poor optical balance (infrared analyzers)

---

the system set up for a lung volume or DL_{CO} test. A large-volume syringe is used to "ventilate" the lung analog, mimicking the patient's breathing. The resulting lung volume (e.g., FRC) is compared with the known volume of the analog system. A calibrated syringe alone may also be used as the lung analog. With a known volume of air in the syringe, the test is performed by filling and emptying the syringe to the starting volume.

Simulation of the $DL_{CO}SB$ maneuver using a lung analog can check analyzer linearity. Both He and CO are diluted equally in the lung analog, and their relative concentrations should be identical. This causes the calculated $DL_{CO}SB$ to be near zero. If the two analyzers are not linear in relation to one another, the ratio of He to CO will not equal 1.0. Calculated $DL_{CO}SB$ will be either above or below zero. This method tests not only the gas analyzers, but also the volume transducer, breathing circuit, and software. Temperature or gas corrections should be disabled. A linearity check at different dilutions can be performed by varying the volume of the lung analog.

Some computerized systems do not allow lung simulators to be used. The software may be designed to make all necessary corrections for human subjects, giving erroneous results when a simulator is used. However, if the software reports gas analyzer values, the accuracy and linearity of various dilutions can be checked.

Testing biologic controls (see Box 10-2) is a third means of evaluating gas analyzers. This method may not detect small changes in analyzer performance because of day-to-day variability of lung volumes, DL_{CO}, or resting energy expenditure. Despite variability as high as 10% for DL_{CO} or exercise parameters in healthy subjects, gas analyzer malfunctions can be detected. Biologic controls may be the simplest means of checking automated exercise/metabolic systems that depend on accurate gas analysis. Abnormal results from biologic controls can suggest more specific tests of suspect components (Box 10-3).

BODY PLETHYSMOGRAPHS

The calibration techniques described here apply primarily to variable-pressure, constant-volume plethysmographs. Flow-based plethysmographs need different calibration procedures for the box transducer. Mouth pressure and pneumotachometer calibration are similar for both types of plethysmographs.

---

1. *Mouth pressure transducer.* Calibration is done by connecting the pressure transducer to a water manometer. The manometer is a U-shaped tube with a calibration scale that allows very accurate pressures to be generated. The range of the mouth pressure transducer should be ±20 to 50 cm H_2O. Air is injected into one port of the manometer. For example, a small volume of air may be introduced to cause a deflection of 5 cm. In effect, this creates a difference of 10 cm between the two columns of the manometer. The gain of the mouth pressure amplifier is then adjusted so that its signal display deflects by an amount equivalent to 10 cm H_2O per

centimeter. The display device may be an oscilloscope, a plotter, or most commonly a computer screen. This deflection then becomes the calibration factor for the mouth pressure transducer. In the previous example, a pressure change of 10 cm H_2O results in a 1-cm deflection on the display. In computerized systems the analog output of the transducers is measured and a software correction factor determined. The correction (or calibration) factor is calculated in a manner similar to that used for spirometer output (see "Spirometers," p. 297). The correction factor is then applied by the software as the signals are acquired.

2. *Box pressure transducer.* Calibration of the box pressure transducer is accomplished by closing the plethysmograph's door and applying a volume signal comparable to that which occurs during subject testing. In a 500 to 600 L plethysmograph, a volume signal of 25 to 50 ml is typical. The box pressure transducer (for a 500-L pressure box) should have a range of ±2 cm H_2O. An adjustable sine-wave pump connected to a small syringe is ideal for box calibration (see Fig. 9-33). The volume is pumped in and out of the box. With the pump operating, the gain of the box pressure transducer is adjusted so that volume change in the box causes a specific deflection on the display. For example, the pressure signal generated by a 30-ml volume might be adjusted to cause a 2-cm deflection on the display. The box pressure calibration factor would then become 15 ml/cm. This procedure may be repeated by adjusting the pump speed from 0.5 to 5.0 cycles/sec (i.e., Hz). Varying the frequency allows the frequency response of the box and transducer to be checked. The volume deflection should not change at different frequencies. Flow-based plethysmographs may be calibrated similarly. The output of the box flow transducer is adjusted rather than that of a pressure transducer. The plethysmograph is normally calibrated empty. A volume correction for the patient is then applied in the calculation of results (see Appendix F).

3. *Flow transducer.* The pneumotachometer may be calibrated by applying either a known flow or volume. A precise flow may be generated using a rotameter or similar calibrated flow meter. Most systems, however, calibrate the pneumotachometer using a 3-L syringe. The flow is integrated, and the gain of the flow signal is then adjusted until the output of the integrator matches the 3-L volume. A software calibration factor, or table of factors, may be used rather than a physical adjustment of the flow signal. Either pressure-differential or Pitot-tube pneumotachometers may be used (see Chapter 9). The pneumotachometer signal is adjusted so that a known flow causes a specific deflection on the display. For example, a flow of 2 L/sec may cause a 2-cm deflection. This results in a flow calibration factor of 1 L/sec/cm. If an adjustable rotameter is used, linearity of the pneumotachometer can be verified by checking the deflections at various flows.

Quality control of body plethysmographs may be accomplished using an isothermal lung analog, known resistors, biologic controls, and comparison with gas dilution or radiologic lung volumes.

An isothermal volume analog can be constructed from a 4- or 5-L glass bottle filled with metal wool, usually copper or steel. The metal wool acts as a heat sink (Fig. 10-3). The mouth of the bottle is fitted with two connectors. One connector attaches to the mouth shutter. The other is attached to a rubber bulb of 50- to 100-ml volume (i.e., the bulb from a blood pressure cuff). The actual volume of the lung analog can be determined by subtracting the volume of the metal wool from the volume of the bottle. The volume occupied by metal wool is calculated from its weight times its density. Alternately, the gas volume of the bottle may be measured by filling it with water from a volumetric source. The volume of the connectors and rubber bulb should be added to the total volume.

The accuracy check is performed with an assistant seated in the sealed plethysmograph. The isothermal volume device is connected to the mouthpiece. The mouth shutter is then closed. While the patient is breatholding, the assistant squeezes the bulb. A P_{MOUTH}/P_{BOX} tangent is recorded just as would be done testing a patient. Thoracic gas volume (V_{TG}) is calculated as usual, except that PH_2O is not subtracted (see Appendix F). The V_{TG} calculated should equal the volume of the isothermal lung analog (as measured previously) within ±5%. Correction for the patient's volume (based on body weight) should include the assistant plus the known volume of the isothermal lung analog. The procedure may be repeated at frequencies from 0.5 to 5.0 cycles/sec to check the frequency response of the box. If the box's frequency response is "flat," tangents should not change when the bulb is squeezed at different rates. The lung analog must contain a sufficient volume of metal wool to act as a heat sink (i.e., isothermal). The metal wool "absorbs" changes in temperature

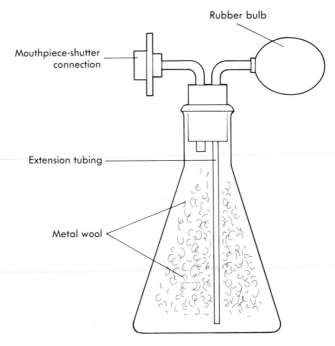

Rubber bulb

Mouthpiece-shutter
connection

Extension tubing

Metal wool

FIG. 10-3 *Isothermal lung analog.* A schematic of an isothermal lung analog for quality control of the body plethysmograph. A 3- to 4-L jar or flask is fitted with a stopper with two openings. One opening connects to the mouthpiece shutter apparatus of the plethysmograph. The other opening is connected to a rubber hand bulb with an extension tube to the bottom of the jar. Copper or steel wool is used to fill the container. The metal wool acts as a heat sink so that pressure changes in the bottle cause only minimal changes in gas temperature. A subject sits in the plethysmograph, holds his or her breath, and squeezes the bulb. This simulates a VTG maneuver. The P_{MOUTH}/P_{BOX} angle may be recorded and the volume of the jar calculated. The measured volume should be within 5% of the actual volume. The true volume is determined by filling the container with water and subtracting the volume of the metal wool. The volume of metal wool may be calculated from its density times its weight. The volumes of the connectors and rubber bulb should be considered as well.

that would result from the compression and decompression of gas in the bottle. If there is not enough metal wool, small temperature changes affect the volume determination.

The accuracy of the box for measuring airway resistance (Raw) can be assessed using known resistances. A resistor can be made using a plug with a small-diameter orifice. Alternately, a resistor can be constructed from capillary tubes arranged lengthwise in a flow tube. In either case, the pressure drop across the resistor is measured at a known flow rate. Some manufacturers supply resistors with known resistances. The resistor is then inserted in front of the pneumotachometer/mouth shutter assembly. A subject whose Raw has been previously measured then has the Raw measured with the resistor in place. The increase in measured Raw should approximate that of the resistor.

Another means of checking plethysmograph function is to measure VTG and/or Raw from a biologic control (see Box 10-1). A series of 10 box measurements provides an adequate mean value for comparison with subsequent results. Day-to-day variability in trained subjects is usually less than 10%. This method allows checking of the box itself, the transducers, the recording devices, and the software. A discrepancy between the established mean and an individual quality control trial may not indicate which component is causing the problem. For example, a control subject whose VTG has been established as 3.0 L is measured again and the VTG is calculated to be 2.0 L. The biologic control establishes that there is a problem, but the cause of the discrepancy requires further investigation. In this example, either incorrect calibration of box or mouth pressure transducers, or a leaky door seal, might be the cause (Box 10-4).

A third method of checking plethysmograph accuracy is to compare the VTG with FRC determined by gas dilution. Correlations greater than 0.90 have been demonstrated between gas dilution and plethysmograph lung volumes in healthy subjects. Differences greater than 10% (in healthy subjects) for volumes measured by plethysmograph and gas dilution are not specific, but may indicate equipment malfunction. This method, as well as use of biologic controls, is based on

---

BOX 10-4
COMMON PLETHYSMOGRAPH PROBLEMS

Problems that may be identified by routine quality control of body plethysmographs include the following:
- Leaks in door seals or connectors (pressure boxes)
- Improperly calibrated pressure transducers
- Obstructed or perforated pneumotachometers
- Excessive thermal drift
- Poor frequency response
- Excessive vibration (poorly mounted transducers)
- Inappropriate software calibration factors
- Procedural errors (e.g., testing before thermal equilibrium reached)

---

measurements of healthy subjects with day-to-day variability. It is important that control subjects perform the breathing maneuvers correctly (see Chapter 3).

Calibration and Quality Control of Blood Gas Analyzers

Most modern blood gas analyzers rely on computer control of functions such as calibration. The user selects a "calibration schedule" appropriate for the complexity and number of tests performed. For example, in a laboratory that performs many blood gas analyses, automated calibration may be performed every 30 minutes. Some older instruments may require manual calibration, in which the user selects reagents or gases and adjusts electrode response.

Calibration of blood gas electrodes involves exposing the gas electrodes (i.e., Po_2, Pco_2) to one or two gases with known partial pressures of O_2 and CO_2. One or two known buffers are used to calibrate the pH electrode. Calibration gases spanning the physiologic ranges of the Po_2, and Pco_2 electrodes are used just as for gas analyzers. Typical combinations would include one calibration gas with a fractional O_2 concentration of 0.20 (20%) and a fractional CO_2 concentration of 0.05 (5%). A second calibration gas would have a CO_2 concentration of 0.10 (10%) with an O_2 concentration close to zero. If blood with a very high Po_2 is to be analyzed (e.g., shunt studies), the analyzer may be calibrated with a gas of similar fractional concentration. This requires an analyzer that allows manual calibration.

Calibration gases are usually bubbled through water at 37° C to saturate them with water vapor. Calibration gases then flow into the measuring chamber. The partial pressures of O_2 and CO_2 in the calibration gases depend on local barometric pressure. For each gas the partial pressure is calculated as follows:

$$P_{gas} = F_{gas} \times (P_B - 47)$$

where

P_{gas} = partial pressure of calibration gas

F_{gas} = fractional concentration of the same gas

P_B = local barometric pressure

47 = partial pressure of water vapor (P_{H_2O}) at 37° C

As with gas analyzers, a "low" gas is used to zero (sometimes called balancing) each electrode. A "high" gas is used to adjust the gain (also called the slope) of the electrode's amplifier. Zeroing the electrode may be done without exposing it to a gas with a partial pressure of zero ("electronic" zeroing). Some blood gas analyzers use this method to zero the Po_2 electrode.

Calibration may consist of either a one-point or two-point calibration. One-point calibration exposes the gas electrodes to a single partial pressure of calibration gas and brings one buffer into contact with the pH electrode. Two-point calibration doubles the number of calibration gases and buffers. Most automated blood gas analyzers use a combination of one- and two-point calibrations. Computerized systems allow the user to select how frequently and what type of calibration is performed on the gas and pH electrodes. The Po_2 electrode is usually calibrated over a range of 0 to 150 mm Hg. The P_{CO_2} electrode is usually calibrated for the range of 40 to 80 mm Hg. The pH electrode is usually calibrated using buffers with pH values of 6.840 (low) and 7.384 (high).

Most blood gas analyzers use precision gases to calibrate the gas electrodes, even though gas tensions are measured in liquid (i.e., blood). Some difference may exist when partial pressure of gas is analyzed in gaseous versus liquid medium, especially for O_2. The reduction of O_2 at the tip of the polarographic electrode occurs more rapidly in a gaseous medium than in a liquid. If the electrode is calibrated with a gas, its response when measuring a liquid will be to read slightly lower. This difference is termed the gas-liquid factor. Gas-liquid corrections may be clinically important when measuring high partial pressures of O_2, particularly above 400 mm Hg. Some blood gas analyzers use tonometered solutions for routine calibration of the gas electrodes. Computerized blood gas analyzers often include a software correction for the difference in electrode response to gas and liquid. This allows the analyzer to be used to measure both liquid and gas specimens.

Computerized calibration of blood gas analyzers differs slightly from manual calibration. The computer brings calibration gases or buffers into contact with the electrodes. Electrode responses to the calibration gas or buffer are then stored. The microprocessor compares the measured responses to expected calibration values. The computer then "corrects" the zero and gain (for a two-point calibration) so that measured and expected values match. Most computerized blood gas analyzers compare the current calibration results with the previous calibration. The difference between calibrations is *drift* and indicates an electrode's stability.

Some computerized systems create solutions for calibration of the gas and pH electrodes. Calibration gases are bubbled through buffers in a process called "tonometering." The microprocessor calculates partial pressures of calibration gases based on an internal barometer. When the P_{CO_2} of the tonometered solution is calculated, pH of the solution can be determined. The built-in tonometer allows calibration materials for all three electrodes to be produced.

Automatic calibrations can be programmed to occur at predetermined intervals. Adjustments are performed automatically, based on the response of the electrodes. Because of this, all conditions for an acceptable calibration must be met before the procedure actually begins. Automated blood gas analyzers check most conditions that might affect accurate results, such as temperature of the measuring chamber. During automatic calibration, inadequate buffer or the wrong calibration gas may cause the microprocessor to correct an electrode inappropriately. A similar problem arises if protein contaminates the electrode tip, altering its sensitivity. The microprocessor adjusts the electrode's output in an attempt to bring it into range. This process works well for minor changes in electrode sensitivity. However, electrodes cannot be properly calibrated if they are contaminated with protein, if membranes are damaged, or if the electrolyte is depleted. The user must maintain reagents, calibration gases, and electrodes themselves so that automatic calibration can occur successfully. Systematic errors can sometimes be marked by automatic calibration. Contamination of the calibration gases or buffers is a common example. If the microprocessor adjusts electrodes to match a contaminated calibration standard, the calibrations appear normal but analysis of control samples will show differences. Detection of these errors usually requires appropriate quality control and proficiency testing (described later in this section). Automated blood gas analyzers reduce variability by controlling calibration as well as sample analysis but require careful attention to function appropriately.

Two methods of quality control for blood gas analysis are used: tonometry and commercially prepared controls. Interpretation of blood gas quality control (QC) is the same for either method.

TONOMETRY

A **tonometer** is a device that allows precision gas mixtures to be equilibrated with either whole blood or a buffer solution. One type of tonometer creates a thin film of blood or buffer by spinning it in a chamber flooded with precision gas. A second type bubbles gas through the blood or buffer; the bubbles create a large surface for gas exchange. In both types the tonometer is maintained at 37° C and the gas is humidified. The time equilibration takes is determined by gas flow and volume of control material. A portion of the blood or buffer is then injected into the blood gas analyzer. The expected gas tensions are calculated from fractional concentrations of the precision gas, as described for calibration. If whole blood is used as the control material, only P_{O_2} and P_{CO_2} can be checked. Blood is ideal for quality control of the gas electrodes because its viscosity and gas exchange properties are the same as patient samples. No other control material provides the oxygen-carrying capacity of whole blood. For the most precise control of the Po_2 electrode, tonometry is the method of choice. However, pH cannot be accurately calculated for whole blood because its buffering capacity is usually unknown. Tonometry of a bicarbonate-based buffer using a known fractional concentration of CO_2 does allow both gas and pH electrodes to be quality controlled. The gas exchange characteristics of this type of buffer make it less useful than whole blood for quality control of Po_2 and Pco_2.

Tonometry can be performed inexpensively using pooled waste blood and small amounts of precision gas. Using pooled blood requires special care. All blood specimens must be handled using **universal precautions** (see "Infection Control and Safety," p. 316). Quality control of the pH electrode requires additional tonometry of a buffer. Three levels of control materials spanning the measuring range of the electrode are recommended. Three precision gas mixtures are therefore required.

Accuracy of tonometry is highly dependent on a standardized technique. Sampling syringes should be lubricated and then flushed with the precision gas. Careful attention to the preparation and sampling from the tonometer is required to obtain reproducible results. The values obtained using tonometry may depend on individual technique. Problems that occur with tonometry include contamination of the precision gas resulting from leaky connections, improper temperature control of the chamber, or inadequate gas flow to achieve equilibrium.

COMMERCIALLY PREPARED CONTROLS

There are three types of commercially prepared controls: blood-based, aqueous, or fluorocarbon-based. The blood-based matrix consists of a solution containing buffered human red cells. The aqueous material is usually a bicarbonate buffer. The fluorocarbon-based control material is a perfluorinated compound that has enhanced oxygen-dissolving characteristics. Multiple levels (i.e., acidosis, alkalosis, normal) of these materials provide control over the range of blood gases seen clinically.

All three types of controls are packaged in sealed glass ampules of 2- to 3-ml volume. They require minimum preparation for use. Blood-based material must be refrigerated, then warmed to 37° C and agitated before use. Aqueous- and fluorocarbon-based controls can be stored under refrigeration for long periods or at room temperature for day-to-day use. Most aqueous- and fluorocarbon-based controls have shelf lives of 1 year. Each requires agitation for 10 to 15 seconds before use. Commercially prepared controls may cost more than samples prepared using tonometry. They are convenient to use, however, and may be less susceptible to handling errors than tonometered materials.

One problem with aqueous controls (and to a lesser extent with fluorocarbon solutions) is poor precision of Po_2. The oxygen-carrying capacity of these materials is much lower than that of whole blood. As a result the Po_2 in the control changes rapidly on exposure to air. Controls with low Po_2 values become quickly "contaminated" after opening. Aqueous or fluorocarbon controls may produce such a wide range of "expected" values that their value as controls is limited. Some of these difficulties may be overcome by careful statistical evaluation of Po_2 control data as described in this section.

A sound statistical method of interpreting "control runs" is necessary to detect blood gas analyzer malfunctions (Box 10-5). A common method for detecting **"out-of-control"** situations is to calculate the control mean ±2 SD. A series of runs of the same control material are performed. Twenty to 30 runs provide an adequate base for calculation of the mean and SD (see Appendix F for a sample calculation). One SD on either side of the mean in a **normal distribution** includes approximately 67% of the data points. Two SDs include 95% of the data points in a normal distribution. Ninety-nine percent of the data points in a normal series fall within 3 SDs of the mean. A quality control value that falls within ±2 SDs of the mean can be considered in control. If the control value falls between 2 and 3 SDs from the mean, there is only a 5% chance that the run is in control. This normal variability that occurs when multiple measurements are performed is called **random error.** One of 20 control runs (i.e., 5%) can be expected to produce a result in the 2- to 3-SD range and still be acceptable.

To distinguish true out-of-control situations from random errors, more complex sets of rules have been developed. The most widely used rules are those proposed by Westgard et al (see bibliography). The rules are selected to provide the greatest probability for detecting real errors and rejecting false errors. This approach to quality control is termed the multiple-rule method. The

---

BOX 10-5
COMMON BLOOD GAS ANALYZER PROBLEMS

Some problems encountered in the blood gas laboratory that are detected by QC or proficiency testing
are as follows:

- *Electrode malfunction.* Protein deposited on membranes or electrodes is common and can usually be
  remedied by cleaning. Leaks in membranes and electrolyte depletion cause electrode drift or shifts
  in performance.
- *Temperature control.* Failure to maintain 37° C water or air bath or thermometer inaccuracy causes
  QC results to be out-of-control.
- *Improper calibration.* Problems during calibration almost always relate to inadequate or contaminated
  buffer or calibration gas. QC data consistently high or low may indicate a problem with reagents.
- *Mechanical problems.* Leaks in pump tubing, or poorly functioning pumps, allow calibrating solutions, controls, and patient samples to be contaminated. Air bubbles introduced during analysis
  cause gas tensions to be in error. Inadequate rinsing may also occur with pump problems or improperly functioning valves. This usually results in blood clotting in the transport tubing or measuring chamber.
- *Improper sampling technique.* Failure to anaerobically collect arterial specimens, to properly store
  samples in ice water, excessive heparin, or bubbles in the specimen all may result in questionable results. Another common problem related to sampling is inadvertently obtaining a venous specimen.
  Adequately functioning electrodes, as demonstrated by good QC, can distinguish poor sampling
  from actual clinical abnormalities.

---

multiple-rule method usually requires that two or more control levels be evaluated on the same
measurement device (electrode). The multiple-rule method may be applied as follows:

---

1. When one control observation exceeds the mean ±2 SDs, a "warning" condition exists.

2. When one control observation exceeds the mean ±3 SDs, an out-of-control condition exists.

3. When two consecutive control observations exceed the mean +2 SDs or the mean −2 SDs,
   an out-of-control condition exists.

4. When the range of differences between consecutive control runs exceeds 4 SDs, an
   out-of-control condition exists.

5. When four consecutive control observations exceed the mean +1 SD or the mean −1 SD,
   an out-of-control condition exists.

6. When 10 consecutive control observations fall on the same side of the mean (±), an
   out-of-control condition exists.

These are just some of the rules which may be applied; not all rules have to be used at all times.

Rules 1 and 2 detect marked changes in electrode performance, sometimes called a shift, by
examining how far from the mean a single control value falls. Rules 3 through 6 look for "trends"
in electrode response by evaluating the recent history of control runs. Similar rules may be applied
by linking multiple levels (i.e., high, low, normal) of control material. For example, if three levels
of controls are all greater than 2 SDs above their respective means, it is likely that the electrode is
out-of-control.

One problem with a strict statistical approach is that if outliers (i.e., values more than 2 SDs
from the mean) are always excluded, the SD itself becomes smaller with repeated calculation.
Eventually valid control data may be rejected. This situation can be managed by including data in
the calculations that are clinically acceptable, even though they may be more than 2 SDs above or
below the mean. When using the multiple-rule method, it is necessary not only to evaluate the
mean and SD of the current control run, but to keep a control history as well. This is often
accomplished by means of a control chart (Fig. 10-4). A graph for each control is created with the
mean ±2 SDs on the Y axis and control run number (or time) on the X axis. Individual controls are
then plotted as they are run to track electrode performance.

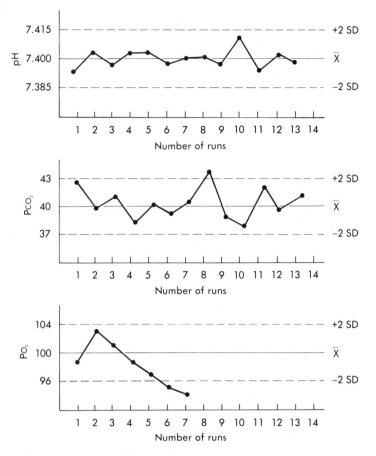

FIG. 10-4 *Blood gas quality control charts.* Three examples of Shewhart/Levey-Jennings charts for pH, P_{CO_2} and P_{O_2}. The mean for a specific control material is plotted as a *solid line* and the ±2 SDs lines are *dashed.* The left Y axis on each graph is labeled with the actual mean and 2 SD values. Consecutive control "runs" are plotted on the horizontal X axis. On the pH control chart *(top)* all of the values vary about the mean in a regular fashion—the electrode appears "in control" for the 13 measurements plotted. The P_{CO_2} chart *(middle)* shows somewhat more variability. Control run 8 shows a value outside of the ±2-SD range. This is probably a "random" error because it is the only control value outside the ±2-SD limits. Subsequent controls show normal variability about the mean, also suggesting that run 8 was a random error. The P_{O_2} chart *(bottom)* shows a "trend" of decreasing control values. Runs 6 and 7 both produce values more than −2 SDs below the mean. This pattern suggests that the electrode is malfunctioning and needs to be serviced. By applying multiple rules (see text) to the interpretation of consecutive control runs, with or without charts, most "out-of-control" situations can be detected.

To provide adequate quality control of a blood gas analyzer, three levels of control materials are normally used. Three levels of control for each of the three electrodes (i.e., pH, P_{CO_2}, and P_{O_2}) requires that 9 means and 9 SDs must be calculated for each instrument. When controls are run several times daily, tracking multiple runs can become complex. To simplify this task, computerized quality control programs are often used. Such programs are often included in the software for automated blood gas analyzers. Many laboratory computer systems also support statistical databases for control data. The chief advantages of computerized QC are simplified data storage and maintenance of necessary statistics. Multiple rules can be applied easily to each new control run to detect problems. Computerized records and control charts can be printed. These types of QC records are required by many accrediting agencies. (See Appendix D for a list of some regulatory agencies.)

Quality control of blood gas analyzers should be performed on a schedule appropriate for the number of specimens analyzed. In most laboratories, controls must be performed daily or more often. In busy laboratories, multiple levels of controls may be required on each shift. QC is also usually required after electrode maintenance is performed.

Routine QC establishes the precision of the electrodes. Instrument precision must be determined so that blood gas interpretation can be related to a range of values. For example, the variability of a Po_2 electrode may be determined to be ± 6 mm Hg (i.e., 2 SDs) around a mean of 50 mm Hg. Each Po_2 result (around 50 mm Hg) can then be interpreted within a range of 6 mm Hg above or below the reported value.

Several other techniques related to QC of blood gas analyzers are commonly used. Interlaboratory proficiency testing consists of comparing unknown control specimens from a single source in multiple laboratories. This allows an individual laboratory to compare its results with other laboratories. Results using different methodologies (i.e., analyzers) may also be compared. Results of proficiency testing are also reported as means and SDs for each instrument participating in the program. Proficiency testing does not measure precision as does daily quality control. It provides a measure of the absolute accuracy of the individual laboratory. A laboratory may have an acceptable level of precision as determined by daily QC but be inaccurate when compared with other laboratories. Proficiency testing often detects systematic errors that occur because of improper calibration, contaminated reagents, or procedural errors. Multiple levels of unknowns are usually provided to check the range of values seen in clinical practice. Proficiency testing programs are available from professional organizations such as the College of American Pathologists, as well as from commercial vendors. Satisfactory performance on interlaboratory proficiency testing has been mandated by the U.S. Department of Health and Human Services under the Clinical Laboratory Improvement Act of 1988 (see Appendix D).

Criteria for Acceptability of Pulmonary Function Studies

Quality assurance in the pulmonary function laboratory requires not only appropriate calibration and QC, but also careful attention to the testing technique. Testing technique may be compared with "sampling" technique in other laboratory sciences. In pulmonary function testing, sampling refers to procedures used to obtain patient data. These include eliciting maximal effort and cooperation from the patient, as well as the correct performance of the equipment. Applying objective criteria to determine the validity of data is one means of providing high-quality results.

USING CRITERIA FOR ACCEPTABILITY

Criteria for assessing the validity of each test have been described in Chapters 2 through 8. Standards for pulmonary function testing have been published by the ATS, European Respiratory Society, British Thoracic Society, and American Association for Respiratory Care. Criteria for acceptability have three primary uses:

1. To provide a basis for decision making during testing. Standards or guidelines can be used to decide whether equipment is functioning properly, whether the patient is giving maximal effort, or whether testing should be continued or repeated. Standardized criteria also help to characterize the types of problems known to occur during specific tests (e.g., leaks).

2. To evaluate validity of pulmonary function data from an individual patient. Criteria may be applied either by the technologist performing the test, by computer software, or by the clinician responsible for interpretation.

3. To score or evaluate the performance of the technologist. Many pulmonary function tests, especially spirometry, depend on the interaction between technologist and patient. Criteria for acceptability can be used to gauge the performance of individual technologists and to provide objective feedback.

Implementation of a quality assurance program in the pulmonary function laboratory should use acceptability criteria during testing, both to evaluate individual tests and to rate technologists. For each of these, certain procedures will be similar:

1. *Examine printed tracings or displayed graphics* whenever available. Compare the observed tracing with the characteristics of an acceptable curve. Either direct recording, such as a kymograph tracing, or computer-generated graphics may be used. Graphics may be super-

imposed or displayed side-by-side to assess patient effort and cooperation. The user should be able to modify the graphic display (e.g., change graphing scale) to allow for extremes such as very low flows or volumes. During testing graphs of multiple efforts should be available. Storage of graphic data (all acceptable maneuvers) may be useful for assessing data quality later.

2. *Look at numerical data.* Are the highest values of multiple efforts within the accepted range of reproducibility? The decision to perform additional maneuvers is usually based on reproducibility. Data from multiple efforts should be maintained during testing to allow selection of appropriate results for the final report. Storage of all data may be necessary for subsequent review or editing.

3. *Evaluate key indicators.* Most pulmonary function tests have one or two features that determine whether the test was performed acceptably. For spirometry, the start of test and duration of effort are key indicators. For gas dilution lung volumes, absence of leaks and test duration are key indicators. For $DL_{CO}SB$, inspired volume and breath-hold time are important. Key indicators vary with the methodology used for specific tests. In each instance the key indicator should be assessed in relation to an accepted standard. During testing, these indicators help to determine whether additional instruction or tests are needed.

4. *Check for consistent results.* The results of different test categories should be consistent with the clinical history and presentation of the patient. Spirometry, lung volumes, DL_{CO}, and blood gas values should all suggest a similar interpretation for a specific diagnosis. Discrepancies among tests may indicate a technical problem rather than a clinical condition.

TECHNOLOGIST'S COMMENTS

Scoring or grading the quality of individual patients' tests is an essential component of quality assurance for pulmonary function testing. This may be accomplished by notes added by the technologist administering the test. Some automated spirometers use software that grades test performance. Evaluation of all aspects of the test (i.e., spirometry, lung volumes, DL_{CO}) should be included.

The technologist's comments or notes can usually be added to the test results. The commentary should be based on standardized criteria. If a particular test meets all criteria, that fact should be stated. Failure to meet any of the laboratory's criteria should be documented as well. The reason why the patient was unable to perform the test acceptably should be explained whenever possible. Failure to meet criteria for acceptability does not necessarily invalidate a test. For some subjects, their best performance may fail one or more of the criteria. Table 10-6 lists examples of statements which might be used to document test quality.

The technologist's comments may be added to the final report. Many automated systems provide for "free text" comments to be included with tabular data. Some software supports **"canned text"** functions that allow predetermined statements (see Table 10-6) to be entered with a single keystroke. The technologist's name or initials should be included.

Some computerized spirometer systems automatically score FVC maneuvers. The score may be indicated by a letter or numeric code that is attached to each maneuver. For example, an FVC maneuver that meets all criteria (e.g., start-of-test) might be scored with an "A." Other systems allow the technologist to select a user-defined code to attach to individual maneuvers. Both of these techniques can be used to provide feedback that enhances quality assurance.

TECHNOLOGIST FEEDBACK

A well-trained and highly motivated technologist is a key component for obtaining valid data, particularly in tests that require patient instruction and encouragement. A QC program based on established criteria for acceptability can be used to provide feedback on test performance to individual technologists.

Routine review of tests performed by each technologist is recommended. If criteria for acceptability have been recorded (as described in this section), these can be evaluated against raw data to determine the accuracy of results. This information forms the basis for reinforcing superior performance or correcting identified problems. Feedback should include the type and extent of unacceptable or nonreproducible tests. Feedback should also include what corrective action can be taken to improve performance.

TABLE 10-6	Technologist's Comments*
Test	**Comments**
Spirometry	Meets all ATS recommendations.
	Poor start of test or patient effort.
	Expiration did not last 6 seconds or there was no obvious plateau.
	Back-extrapolated volume was >5% of FVC.
	Patient was unable to continue to exhale because of _____.
	Two best FVC maneuvers were not within 200 ml.
	Two best FEV_1 maneuvers were not within 200 ml.
	MVV does not correlate with FEV_1.
Lung volumes (gas dilution)	Lung volumes by _____ (method) _____ were performed acceptably.
	Lung volumes reported were the average of _____ (n) _____ FRC determinations.
	Slow VC was (greater/less) than FVC (_____ %).
	Lung volumes by gas dilution were unacceptable because of a leak.
	Equilibration not reached within 7 minutes—He dilution.
	Alveolar N_2 >1.5% after 7 minutes—N_2 washout.
Plethysmography	All plethysmographic measurements were performed acceptably.
	V_{TG} tangents were variable.
	Raw tangents were variable.
	Patient was unable to pant at the correct frequency.
$DL_{CO}SB$	Meets all ATS recommendations.
	DL_{CO} reported is average of _____ (n) _____ maneuvers.
	DL_{CO} corrected for an Hb of _____.
	Inspired volume <90% of best vital capacity (_____ %).
	Breath-hold time not within 9 to 11 seconds (_____ seconds).
	DL_{CO} values not within 3 ml CO/min/mm Hg or 10%.
	DL_{CO} not corrected for Hb or COHb.

*Values in parentheses may be filled in with appropriate values from the patient's data.

Infection Control and Safety

Pulmonary function tests, including blood gas analysis, often involve patients with blood-borne or respiratory pathogens. Reasonable precautions applied to testing techniques and equipment handling can prevent cross-contamination between patients. Similar techniques can prevent infection of the technologist performing the tests.

POLICIES AND PROCEDURES

Each laboratory should have written guidelines concerning safety and infection control. The guidelines should be part of a policy and procedure manual (see Table 10-1). Procedures should include but not be limited to hand-washing techniques, use of protective equipment such as laboratory coats and gloves, and guidelines for equipment cleaning. The handling of contaminated materials (e.g., waste blood) should be clearly described. Policies and procedures should include education of technologists regarding proper handling of biologic hazards. Most accrediting agencies require written plans for safety, waste management, and chemical hygiene. In the United States, the Occupational Safety and Health Administration **(OSHA)** has published strict guidelines regarding handling of blood and other medical waste (see Appendix D).

PULMONARY FUNCTION TESTS

Pulmonary function testing does not present a significant risk of infection for patients or technologists. However, some potential hazards are involved. Most respiratory pathogens are spread by either direct contact with contaminated equipment or an airborne route. Airborne organisms may be contained in **droplet nuclei,** on epithelial cells that have been shed, or in dust particles. The following guidelines can help reduce the possibility of cross-contamination or infection:

1. Disposable mouthpieces and nose clips should be used for spirometry. Reusable mouthpieces should be disinfected or sterilized after each use. Proper hand washing should be done immediately after direct contact with mouthpieces or valves. Gloves should be worn when handling potentially contaminated equipment. Hands should always be washed between patients.

2. Tubing or valves through which subjects rebreathe should be changed after each test. Any equipment that shows visual condensation from expired gas should be disinfected before reuse. This is particularly important for maneuvers such as the FVC where there is a potential for mucus, saliva, or droplet nuclei to contaminate the device. Breathing circuit components should be stored in sealed plastic bags after disinfection.

3. Spirometers should be cleaned according to the manufacturer's recommendations. The frequency of cleaning should be appropriate for the number of tests performed. For open-circuit systems, only that part of the circuit through which air is rebreathed needs to be decontaminated between patients. Some flow-based systems offer pneumotachometers that can be changed between subjects. These may be advantageous if patients with known respiratory infections must be tested. Pneumotachometers not located proximal to the patient are less likely to be contaminated by mucus, saliva, or droplet nuclei. Disposable flow sensors should not be reused. Volume-displacement spirometers should be flushed using their full volume at least five times between patients. Flushing with room air helps clear droplet nuclei or similar airborne particulates. Water-sealed spirometers should be drained at least weekly, allowed to dry completely, and refilled only with distilled water. Bellows and rolling-seal spirometers may be more difficult to disassemble but should be disinfected on a routine basis. After disassembly and disinfection, the spirometer may require recalibration.

4. Bacteria filters may be used in some circuits to prevent equipment contamination. Systems used for spirometry, lung volumes, and diffusing capacity tests often use breathing manifolds that are susceptible to contamination. Bacteria filters may be used to prevent contamination of these devices. Filters may impose increased resistance, thus affecting measurement of maximal flows. Some types of filters show increased resistance after continued use in expired gas. Spirometers fitted with filters should be calibrated with the filter in line, and should meet the minimal recommendations in Table 10-2. If filters are used for procedures such as lung volume determinations, their volume must be included in the calculations. Filters may be useful in protecting equipment from contamination when patients with known respiratory pathogens must be tested.

5. Small-volume nebulizers, such as those used for bronchodilators or bronchial challenge, offer the greatest potential for cross-contamination. These devices, if reused, should be sterilized to destroy vegetative microorganisms, fungal spores, tubercle bacilli, and some viruses. Preferably, disposable single-use nebulizers should be used. Metered-dose devices may be used for bronchodilator studies by using disposable mouthpieces or "spacers" to prevent colonization of the device.

6. Gloves or other barrier devices minimize the risk of infection for the technologist who must handle mouthpieces, tubing, or valves. The risk of transmission from subjects with hepatitis B, human immunodeficiency virus (HIV), or acquired immunodeficiency syndrome (AIDS) through respiratory secretions is slight. Special precautions should be taken whenever there is evidence of blood on mouthpieces or tubing. There is a risk of acquiring infections such as tuberculosis or pneumonia caused by *Pneumocystis carinii* from infected patients. A mask should be worn by the technologist when testing subjects who have active tuberculosis or other diseases that can be transmitted by coughing. Masks may be required for "**reverse isolation**" when testing immunocompromised patients.

7. Patients with respiratory diseases such as tuberculosis may warrant specially ventilated rooms, particularly if many individuals need testing. Risk of cross-contamination or infection can be greatly reduced by filtering and increasing the exchange rate of air in the testing room. Equipment can be reserved for testing only infected patients. Patients with known pathogens

can also be tested in their own room or at the end of the day (to facilitate equipment decontamination).

8. Surveillance should include routine cultures of reusable components, such as mouthpieces, tubing, and valves, after disinfection.

BLOOD GASES

The Centers for Disease Control and Prevention (CDC) have established universal precautions that apply to personnel handling blood or other body fluids containing blood. Universal precautions apply to blood, semen, vaginal secretions, cerebrospinal fluid, synovial fluid, pleural fluid, pericardial fluid, and amniotic fluid. Some of these fluids are commonly encountered in the blood gas laboratory. These fluids present a significant risk to the health care worker. Hepatitis B, HIV, and other blood-borne pathogens must be assumed to be present in these fluids.

Body fluids to which the universal precautions do not apply include feces, nasal secretions, sputum, sweat, tears, urine, and vomitus, unless they contain visible blood. Some of these fluids may be encountered in the pulmonary function laboratory. These fluids present an extremely low or nonexistent risk for HIV or hepatitis B. However, they are potential sources for nosocomial infections from other nonblood-borne pathogens. Universal precautions do not apply to saliva, but infection control practices such as use of gloves and hand washing further minimize the risk involved in contact with mucous membranes of the mouth.

These universal precautions should be applied in the pulmonary function or blood gas laboratory:

1. Treat *all* blood and body fluid specimens as potentially contaminated.

2. Exercise care to prevent injuries from needles, scalpels, or other sharp instruments. Do not resheath used needles by hand. If a needle must be resheathed, use a one-handed technique or a device that holds the sheath. Do not remove used needles from disposable syringes by hand. Do not bend, break, or otherwise manipulate used needles by hand. Use a rubber block or cork to obstruct used needles after arterial punctures. Place used syringes and needles, scalpel blades, and other sharp items in puncture-resistant containers. Locate the containers as close as possible to the area of use.

3. Use protective barriers to prevent exposure to blood, body fluids containing visible blood, and other fluids to which universal precautions apply. Examples of protective barriers include gloves, gowns, laboratory coats, masks, and protective eye wear. Gloves should be worn when drawing blood samples. Gloves cannot prevent penetrating injuries caused by needles or sharp objects. Gloves are also indicated if the technologist has cuts, scratches, or other breaks in the skin. Protective barriers should be used in situations where contamination with blood may occur. These situations include obtaining blood samples from an uncooperative patient, performing finger-heel sticks on infants, or receiving training in blood drawing. Examination gloves should be worn for procedures involving contact with mucous membranes. Masks, gowns, and protective goggles may be indicated for procedures that present a possibility of blood splashing. Blood splashing may occur during arterial line placement or when drawing samples from arterial catheters.

4. Wear gloves while performing blood gas analysis. Laboratory coats or aprons that are resistant to liquids should also be worn. Protective eye wear may be necessary if there is risk of blood splashing during specimen handling. Maintenance of blood gas analyzers, such as repair of electrodes and emptying of waste containers, should be performed wearing similar protective gear. Laboratory coats or aprons should be left in the specimen handling area. Blood waste products (e.g., blood gas syringes) should be discarded in clearly marked biohazard containers.

5. Immediately and thoroughly wash hands and other skin surfaces that are contaminated with blood or other fluids to which the universal precautions apply. Hands should be washed after removing gloves. Blood spills should be cleaned up using a solution of 1 part 5% sodium hypochlorite (bleach) in 9 parts of water. Bleach should also be used to rinse sinks used for blood disposal.

CASE 10A

This case concerns the use of blood gas QC to detect analytical errors.

Background

F.F. is a 30-year-old fireman referred for pulmonary function testing and arterial blood gas analysis as part of a 5-year physical exam required by his fire district. He has no extraordinary symptoms or history suggestive of pulmonary disease. He has never smoked. He performed all portions of the spirometry, lung volumes, and DL_{CO} maneuvers acceptably. All results were within normal limits for his age and height. Arterial blood gases were drawn for analysis.

Blood gases	(F_{IO_2} 0.21)
pH	7.41
Pa_{CO_2} (mm Hg)	39
Pa_{O_2} (mm Hg)	54
Sa_{O_2} (%)	96.0
COHb (%)	1.2
HCO_3^- (mEq/L)	24.1

Because of the low Pa_{O_2} in an otherwise normal subject and because the Sa_{O_2} measured independently by co-oximetry showed normal saturation, the P_{O_2} electrode of the automated blood gas analyzer was questioned.

A review of the two most recent automatic calibrations revealed the following:

	Calibration	Expected	Drift
9 AM			
pH	7.387	7.384	0.003
P_{CO_2} (mm Hg)	39.1	38.6	0.5
P_{O_2} (mm Hg)	132	140.1	−8.1
10 AM			
pH	7.383	7.384	−0.001
P_{CO_2} (mm Hg)	38.4	38.6	−0.2
P_{O_2} (mm Hg)	151.2	140.1	11.1

For each automatic calibration, the instrument analyzes a calibration gas or buffer and compares the measured value to an expected value. Drift is the amount of adjustment applied to a particular electrode to bring it within calibration limits. The excessive drift exhibited by the P_{O_2} electrode prompted a review of the most recent QC runs performed on the analyzer.

Blood gas quality control (five most recent runs)

Control	Mean (mm Hg)	SD	Runs* 1	2	3	4	5
Level A	45	±2.1	46	47	49	42	50
Level B	100	±2.0	101	99	97	96	105
Level C	150	±3.1	147	151	151	149	143

*Control runs performed every 8 hours.

Questions

1. Why is the patient's P_{O_2} so low?
2. What is the interpretation of the 9 AM and 10 AM automated calibrations for the blood gas analyzer?
3. What do the routine quality control runs show?
4. What corrective action, if any, is necessary?

Discussion

1   Cause of the low P_{O_2}

The findings in this case regarding O_2-electrode function are not unusual. An abnormally low Pa_{O_2} in an otherwise healthy person with normal lung function suggested that an analytical error had occurred. If the subject had presented with evidence of lung disease or abnormalities in his pulmonary function test, the inaccuracy of the Pa_{O_2} might have gone unnoticed or led to inappropriate therapy.

2   Automatic blood gas analyzer calibrations

Excessive drift of the oxygen electrode should have prompted the immediate attention of the technologist performing the blood gas analyses. A common problem with automated analyzers is their apparent simplicity. Because calibrations are performed automatically, there is a tendency to overlook the corrections which the analyzer makes. Automated analyzers adjust the zero and gain of each electrode to correct for small changes that occur in electrode performance. These small changes may be caused by a buildup of protein at the tip, electrolyte exhaustion, or slight temperature alterations. If there is a large change in electrode performance, the instrument attempts to correct the electrode's output just as it would for small changes that occur normally. Some automated analyzers flag a large drift in electrode performance as an error, whereas others simply report the drift. In this case, the reported drifts signaled that the P_{O_2} electrode was fluctuating markedly. One calibration reading was high and the next one read lower than the expected value.

3   Quality controls

The change in electrode performance should have been detected by the routine QC run before the excessive drift was observed during automatic calibration. Blood gas QC used in this laboratory consisted of multiple levels of control materials. Means and SDs had been determined for each level.

Examination of control runs 1 through 4 reveal acceptable electrode performance. All values are within ±2 SDs of the mean. Run 5 (the most recent run) shows values that are all 2 SDs or more away from the mean. These control results might be expected to occur 5% of the time simply because of the random error associated with sampling. If run 5 is compared with the previous 4 runs and multiple rules (see "Calibration and Quality Control of Blood Gas Analyzers," p. 309) are applied, the electrode is clearly out-of-control. When multiple levels of controls are evaluated, more than one control value outside of the 2-SD limit suggests an out-of-control situation. For both level A and level B, there is a change of 4 SDs from run 4 to run 5. Changes of this magnitude are not consistent with random error and are detected only when a control history is kept. Similarly, there are inconsistencies within run 5 across the three levels of controls. Levels A and B both show control values that are more than 2 SDs *above* their respective means, whereas level C shows a value that is more than 2 SDs *below* its mean. This pattern suggests fluctuating electrode performance, as displayed during the automatic calibrations that followed.

4   Corrective action

The P_{O_2} electrode was removed from the instrument. A new membrane was installed after the tip was polished with an abrasive to expose the platinum cathode. The electrode was refilled with fresh electrolyte. The instrument was recalibrated and multiple levels of controls were repeated. All P_{O_2} values fell within 2 SDs of the established mean. The subject's blood, which had been kept in an ice-water bath, was reanalyzed and a Pa_{O_2} value of 89 mm Hg was obtained.

SUMMARY

THIS CHAPTER HAS FOCUSED on various elements of quality assurance as applied to pulmonary function testing. Calibration of spirometers, gas analyzers, and body plethysmographs have been discussed. Special emphasis has been placed on techniques to ensure that pulmonary function equipment meets established standards of accuracy. QC methods have been reviewed, including the use of large-volume syringes and biologic controls.

Calibration and QC of blood gas analyzers have been discussed, as well as advantages and disadvantages of automated calibration. Basic statistical concepts commonly used in laboratory situations have been covered, including the application of multiple control rules.

Testing technique is a key element in ensuring the validity of pulmonary function data. Some guidelines for applying acceptability criteria (as listed throughout the text) have been given. These included decision making during testing, assessing test quality for interpretive purposes, and providing feedback on technologist performance.

Infection control and safety issues have been presented. Cleaning of spirometers and related equipment, along with techniques to avoid cross-contamination, have been listed. Universal precautions applicable to blood gas analysis and pulmonary function testing have been reviewed. As for other chapters, a case study and self-assessment questions have been included.

SELF-ASSESSMENT QUESTIONS

1 *Multiple injections by a 3-L syringe into a bellows spirometer produce the following results:*

First injection:	3.03 L
Second injection:	2.99 L
Third injection:	2.96 L

Which of the following best describes these results?
a. The spirometer shows excessive drift.
b. The volume is being inappropriately corrected to BTPS.
c. The spirometer bellows are sticking.
d. Spirometer performance is acceptable.

2 *A 3-L syringe is used to calibrate a flow-sensing spirometer; the spirometer reads a volume of 3.04 L. The software correction factor for this system would be which of the following:*
a. 0.95
b. 0.99
c. 1.01
d. Outside of acceptable limits

3 *According to ATS recommendations, the range and accuracy for a diagnostic spirometer should be which of the following:*
a. 0 to 14 L with less than 1.5 cm $H_2O/L/sec$
b. 0.5 to 8 L ±3% of reading or ±0.05 L, whichever is greater
c. 0.5 to 6 L ±5% of reading or ±0.1 L, whichever is greater
d. 0.1 to 5 L ±3% of reading or ±0.05 L, whichever is greater

4 *A biologic control subject has an established FVC of 5.00 L with an SD of 0.20 L. After spirometer maintenance, the following values are obtained from the biologic control:*

Effort 1:	5.70 L
Effort 2:	5.75 L
Effort 3:	5.67 L

Based on these findings, the pulmonary function technologist should conclude what?
a. Spirometer performance is within acceptable statistical limits.
b. Spirometer performance is questionable.
c. The control subject's efforts were greater than normal.
d. The control subject's efforts were not temperature corrected to BTPS.

5 *A CO_2 analyzer is calibrated using a 5% CO_2 mixture with a water vapor absorber in the sample line. If the barometric pressure is 747 mm Hg and the analyzer is set up to read partial pressure, the analyzer should be adjusted to read which of the following?*
a. 40 mm Hg
b. 37 mm Hg
c. 35 mm Hg
d. 31 mm Hg

6 *Quality control of an automated $D_{L_{CO}}$ system is performed using a 3-L syringe. The syringe is filled to 1.5 L with room air, then connected to the system. A simulated $D_{L_{CO}}SB$ maneuver is performed with 1.5 L of test gas drawn into the syringe. Acceptable performance of the gas analyzers should produce a $D_{L_{CO}}$ of which of the following:*
a. 0 ml CO/min/mm Hg
b. 25 ml CO/min/mm Hg
c. 50 ml CO/min/mm Hg
d. 100 ml CO/min/mm Hg

7 *Quality control of a body plethysmograph is performed using an isothermal lung analog and a biologic control subject with the following results:*

	Expected Result	Quality Control Result
Lung simulator	4.00	3.91
Biologic control	3.44	3.54

Based on these findings, the pulmonary function technologist should conclude what?

a. There is a leak in the door seal.
b. Box pressure calibration was performed incorrectly.
c. Mouth pressure calibration was performed incorrectly.
d. The box is functioning within acceptable limits.

8 *An automated blood gas analyzer performs regularly scheduled calibrations and no electrode drift is noted. Multiple-level QC shows values for P_{CO_2} and P_{O_2} that are within 2 SDs of the mean, but all pH values are more than 3 SDs above the mean. Which of the following is most likely the cause?*

a. Contaminated buffers
b. Contaminated calibration gas
c. Analyzer temperature is not 37° C
d. Gas-liquid correction factor set too low

9 *Tonometry of whole blood may be used to provide QC for which of the following?*

a. P_{O_2} and P_{CO_2} electrodes
b. P_{CO_2} and pH electrodes
c. P_{O_2} electrode only
d. pH electrode only

10 *Quality control runs on a P_{O_2} electrode show the following results when plotted on a QC chart:[69]*

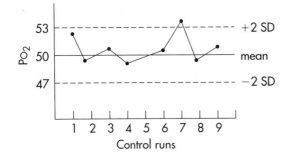

Which of the following best describes the result of run 7?

a. An out-of-control situation
b. A shift
c. A trend
d. A random error

11 *A patient who is short of breath performs eight FVC maneuvers, and these results are recorded from the three best efforts:*

	Trial 5	Trial 6	Trial 8
FVC (L)	4.8	4.4	4.7
FEV_1 (L)	1.9	1.6	1.6
$FEF_{50\%}$ (L/sec)	0.7	0.5	0.6

Which of the following are appropriate to report in the technologist's comments?

a. "Spirometry meets all ATS criteria."
b. "FVC is not reproducible."
c. "FEV_1 is not reproducible."
d. "$FEF_{50\%}$ shows poor patient effort."

12 *A patient whose VC is 3.5 L performs two $DL_{CO}SB$ maneuvers with the following results:*

	Trial 1	Trial 2
DL_{CO} (ml CO/min/mm Hg)	20.3	19.0
V_I (L)	3.5	3.0
Breath-hold time (sec)	10.9	11.7

The pulmonary function technologist should do which of the following?

a. Perform at least one additional maneuver
b. Report the average of trials 1 and 2
c. Report the $DL_{CO}SB$ as 20.3 ml CO/min/mm Hg
d. Report the $DL_{CO}SB$ as 19.0 ml CO/min/mm Hg

13 *Which of the following are true regarding infection control of pulmonary function equipment?*

I.   Disposable mouthpieces and nose clips should be used.
II. Tubing or valves through which the patient rebreathes should be changed at least weekly.
III. Volume-displacement spirometers should be flushed five times between patients.
IV. Spirometers should be calibrated with bacteria filters in place.

a. I and II only
b. III and IV only
c. I, II, and III
d. I, III, and IV

14 *The pulmonary function technologist should observe which of the following precautions in drawing an arterial blood sample for analysis?*

a. Determine whether gloves are needed by checking the patient's history
b. Carefully resheath used needles using the original protective covering
c. Dispose of used needles in red plastic bags marked "biohazard"
d. Use protective barriers if there is danger of blood splashing

SELECTED BIBLIOGRAPHY

General References

Clausen JL, ed: *Pulmonary function testing guidelines and controversies,* New York, 1982, Academic Press.

Morris AH, Kanner RE, Crapo RO, et al: *Clinical pulmonary function testing,* ed 2, Salt Lake City, 1984, Intermountain Thoracic Society.

Calibration and Quality Control

Clausen JL, Hansen JE, Misuraca L, et al: Interlaboratory comparisons of blood gas measurements, *Am Rev Respir Dis* 123(suppl):104, 1981.

Gardner RM, Crapo RO, Billings RG, et al: Spirometry: what paper speed? *Chest* 84:161, 1983.

Hankinson JL, Gardner RM: Standard waveforms for spirometer testing, *Am Rev Respir Dis* 126:362, 1982.

Hankinson JL: Pulmonary function testing in the screening of workers: guidelines for instrumentation, performance, and interpretation, *J Occup Med* 28:1081, 1986.

Leary ET, Graham G, Kenny MA: Commercially available blood-gas quality controls compared with tonometered blood, *Clin Chem* 26:1309, 1980.

Leith DE, Mead J: *Principles of body plethysmography,* National Heart, Lung, and Blood Institute, Division of Lung Diseases, 1974.

Nelson SB, Gardner RM, Crapo RO, et al: Performance evaluation of contemporary spirometers, *Chest* 97:288-297, 1990.

Shigeoka JW: Calibration and quality control of spirometer systems, *Respir Care* 28:747, 1983.

Westgard JO, Groth T, Aronsson T, et al: Performance characteristics of rules for internal quality control: probabilities for false rejection and error detection, *Clin Chem* 23:1857, 1977.

Criteria for Acceptability of Pulmonary Function Studies

Enright PL, Johnson LJ, Connett JE, et al: Spirometry in the Lung Health Study: methods and quality control, *Am Rev Respir Dis* 143:1215-1223, 1991.

Ferris BG, ed: Epidemiology standardization project: recommended standardized procedures for pulmonary function testing, *Am Rev Respir Dis* 118(suppl 2):55, 1978.

Gardner RM, Clausen JL, Epler GR, et al: Pulmonary function laboratory personnel qualifications, *Am Rev Respir Dis* 134:623-624, 1986.

Gardner RM, Clausen JL, Crapo RO, et al: Quality assurance in pulmonary function laboratories, *Am Rev Respir Dis* 134:626-627, 1986.

Nathan SP, Lebowitz MD, Knudson RJ: Spirometric testing: number of tests required and selection of data, *Chest* 76:384, 1979.

Snow M: Determination of functional residual capacity, *Respir Care* 34:586, 1989.

Infection Control

Centers for Disease Control and Prevention: Guidelines for preventing the transmission of *Mycobacterium tuberculosis* in health care facilities, *MMWR Morb Mortal Wkly Rep* 43:1-132, 1994.

Centers for Disease Control and Prevention: Update: universal precautions for prevention of transmission of human immunodeficiency virus, hepatitis B virus, and other bloodborne pathogens in healthcare settings, *MMWR Morb Mortal Wkly Rep* 37:377, 1988.

Centers for Disease Control and Prevention: Recommendations for prevention of HIV transmission in healthcare settings, *MMWR Morb Mortal Wkly Rep* 36:3S, 1987.

Garner JS, Favero MS: CDC guidelines for the prevention and control of nosocomial infections: guideline for handwashing and hospital environmental control, *Am J Infect Control* 14:110, 1986.

Johns DP, Ingram C, Booth H, et al: Effect of a microaerosol barrier filter on the measurement of lung function, *Chest* 107:1045-1048, 1995.

Kirk YL, Kenday K, Ashworth HA, et al: Laboratory evaluation of a filter for the control of cross-infection during pulmonary function testing, *J Hosp Infect* 20:193-198, 1992.

Rutala DR, Rutala WA, Weber DR, et al: Infection risks associated with spirometry, *Infect Control Hospital Epidemiol* 12:89-92, 1991.

Simmons BP, Wong ES: Guidelines for prevention of nosocomial pneumonia, *Am J Infect Control* 11:230, 1983.

Tablan OC, Williams WW, Martone WJ: Infection control in pulmonary function laboratories, *Infect Control* 6:442, 1985.

Zibrak JD, O'Donnell CR, Wissler J, et al: Infection control in the respiratory management of patients with HIV-related disorders, *Respir Care* 34:734, 1989.

Standards and Guidelines

American Association for Respiratory Care: Clinical practice guideline: spirometry, 1996 update, *Respir Care* 41:629-636, 1996.

American Association for Respiratory Care: Clinical practice guideline: body plethysmography, *Respir Care* 39:1184-1190, 1994.

American Association for Respiratory Care: Clinical practice guideline: static lung volumes, *Respir Care* 39:830-836, 1994.

American Association for Respiratory Care: Clinical practice guideline: in-vitro pH and blood gas analysis and hemoximetry, *Respir Care* 38:505-510, 1993.

American Association for Respiratory Care: Clinical practice guideline: sampling for arterial blood gas analysis, *Respir Care* 37:913-917, 1992.

American Thoracic Society: Single-breath carbon monoxide diffusing capacity (transfer factor); recommendations for a standard technique—1995 update, *Am J Respir Crit Care Med* 152:2185-2198, 1995.

American Thoracic Society: Standardization of spirometry—1994 update, *Am J Respir Crit Care Med* 152:1107-1136, 1995.

British Thoracic Society and Association of Respiratory Technicians and Physiologists: Topical review: guidelines for the measurement of respiratory function, *Respir Med* 88:165-194, 1994.

National Committee for Clinical Laboratory Standards (NCCLS): *Protection of laboratory workers from infectious disease transmitted by blood, body fluids, and tissue,* ed 2, Publication M29-T2, 1992.

Quanjer PH, Tammeling GJ, Cotes JE, et al: Lung volumes and forced ventilatory flows: report of the working party, standardization of lung function tests; European Community for Steel and Coal—official statement of the European Respiratory Society, *Eur Respir J* 6(suppl 16):5-40, 1993.

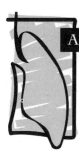

Answers to Self-Assessment Questions

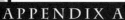

CHAPTER 1
1. d
2. c
3. a
4. b
5. d
6. c
7. b
8. a
9. a
10. b
11. b
12. b

CHAPTER 2
1. c
2. b
3. d
4. a
5. b
6. c
7. b
8. b
9. d
10. b
11. d
12. b

CHAPTER 3
1. d
2. a
3. b
4. a
5. a
6. c
7. d
8. d
9. a
10. b
11. b
12. a

CHAPTER 4
1. c
2. b
3. c
4. c
5. a
6. b
7. d
8. c
9. c
10. a

CHAPTER 5
1. a
2. a
3. b
4. c
5. a
6. c
7. c
8. a
9. b
10. b

CHAPTER 6
1. b
2. b
3. b
4. b
5. b
6. d
7. b
8. a
9. a
10. a

CHAPTER 7
1. b
2. c
3. a
4. d
5. d
6. a
7. b
8. c
9. d
10. b
11. b
12. a

CHAPTER 8
1. a
2. b
3. b
4. c
5. d
6. a
7. d
8. c
9. a
10. a

CHAPTER 9
1. d
2. b
3. c
4. c
5. d
6. a
7. b
8. a
9. b
10. a
11. a
12. d
13. b
14. a
15. c
16. a
17. d
18. a
19. d
20. a

CHAPTER 10
1. d
2. b
3. b
4. b
5. c
6. a
7. d
8. a
9. a
10. d
11. c
12. a
13. d
14. d

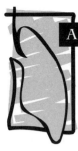

Reference Values

Typical Values for Pulmonary Function Tests

Values are for a healthy young man, 1.7 M² body surface area.

Test	Value
Lung volumes (BTPS)	
IC	3.60 L
ERV	1.20 L
VC	4.80 L
RV	1.20 L
FRC	2.40 L
V_{TG}	2.40 L
TLC	6.00 L
(RV/TLC) × 100	20%
Ventilation (BTPS)	
V_T	0.50 L
f	12 breaths/min
$\dot{V}_E$	6.00 L/min
V_D	0.15 L
$\dot{V}_A$	4.20 L/min
V_D/V_T	0.30
Pulmonary mechanics	
FVC	4.80 L
FEV_1	4.00 L
$FEV_{1\%}$	83%
$FEF_{25\%-75\%}$	4.7 L/sec
$\dot{V}max_{50}$	5.0 L/sec
PEF	10.0 L/sec
MVV	160 L/min
C_L	0.2 L/cm H_2O
C_{LT}	0.1 L/cm H_2O
Raw	1.5 cm H_2O/L/sec
SGaw	0.25 L/sec/cm H_2O
MIP	130 cm H_2O
MEP	250 cm H_2O
Gas distribution	
$\Delta N_{2\ 750-1250}$	<1.5% N_2
7-minute N_2	<2.5% N_2
Diffusion	
$D_{L_{CO}}SB$	25 ml CO/min/mm Hg
$D_L/\dot{V}_A$	4.2 ml CO/min/mm Hg/L
Blood gases and related tests	
pH	7.40
Pa_{CO_2}	40 mm Hg
HCO_3^-	24.0 mEq/L
Pa_{O_2}	95 mm Hg
Sa_{O_2}	97%
COHb	<1.5%
MetHb	<1.5%
$\dot{Q}s/\dot{Q}_T$	<7%

Selecting and Using Reference Values

Reference values for pulmonary function tests are derived by statistical analysis of a group of "normal" subjects. These subjects are classified as normal (i.e., healthy) because they have no history of lung disease in themselves or their families. Minimal exposure to risk factors, such as smoking or environmental pollution, is usually considered in selecting normals.

All pulmonary function measurements vary in healthy subjects. Some tests vary much more than others. Arterial pH and Pa_{CO_2} have a very narrow range in healthy subjects. However, $FEF_{25\%-75\%}$ may vary by almost ±2 L/sec. This variability becomes important when measured values are compared with reference values. Most measurements regress; that is, they vary in a predictable way in relation to one or more physical factors. The physical characteristics that most influence pulmonary function are as follows:

- Age
- Sex
- Height (standing/sitting)
- Race or ethnic origin
- Weight or body surface area

The altitude at which subjects reside may also influence their lung function. By analyzing each variable in regard to the subject's physical characteristics, regression equations can be generated to predict the expected value. Most regression analyses presume that lung function changes are linearly related to physical characteristics such as age and height. This may not be true in subjects who are very old or young, or very tall or short.

Race or ethnic origin influences stature and body proportions. Lung function, particularly lung volumes and diffusing capacity ($D_{L_{CO}}$), differs significantly among races. Some computerized pulmonary function systems apply a "correction factor" to reference values for Caucasians to adjust expected values for a different race. Although differences in lung function among races is well documented, no single correction factor is applicable to all measurements. Some laboratories reduce reference values for volumes (e.g., forced vital capacity [FVC], total lung capacity [TLC]) by factors of 10% to 15% for African-Americans. Ideally, separate regression equations derived from healthy subjects of each race tested should be available. Race-specific reference values should be used if they are representative of the population the laboratory tests.

Several methods for applying reference values are used:

- Tables
- Nomograms
- Graphs
- Regression equations

When a computer is unavailable, tables, nomograms, or graphs may be used. Figs. B-1 and B-2 are examples of nomograms used to obtain a reference value. A ruler is placed so that it intersects the height and age scales for the subject. The expected values can then be read from points where the ruler crosses the other scales. Figs. B-3, B-4, and B-5 are graphs that may be used to obtain reference values for children. In these figures, lung function is graphed against height. The use of computers (or calculators) allows regression equations to be available in software. In most automated systems the user selects sets of prediction equations best suited to the population being tested. Some software allows the user to enter or modify prediction equations. This provides a means of using new reference equations as they become available.

Establishing a lower limit of normal is done in one of several ways. Some clinicians use a fixed percentage of the reference value to determine the degree of abnormality. The measured value is divided by the reference

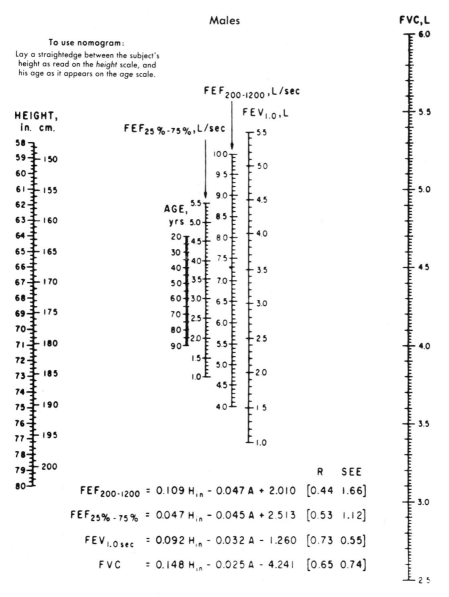

$$FEF_{200-1200} = 0.109\,H_{in} - 0.047\,A + 2.010 \quad [0.44 \quad 1.66]$$

$$FEF_{25\%-75\%} = 0.047\,H_{in} - 0.045\,A + 2.513 \quad [0.53 \quad 1.12]$$

$$FEV_{1.0\,sec} = 0.092\,H_{in} - 0.032\,A - 1.260 \quad [0.73 \quad 0.55]$$

$$FVC = 0.148\,H_{in} - 0.025\,A - 4.241 \quad [0.65 \quad 0.74]$$

FIG. B-1 *Prediction nomograms (BTPS), spirometric values in normal men.* (From Morris JF, Koski WA, Johnson LD: *Am Rev Respir Dis* 103[1]:57, 1971.)

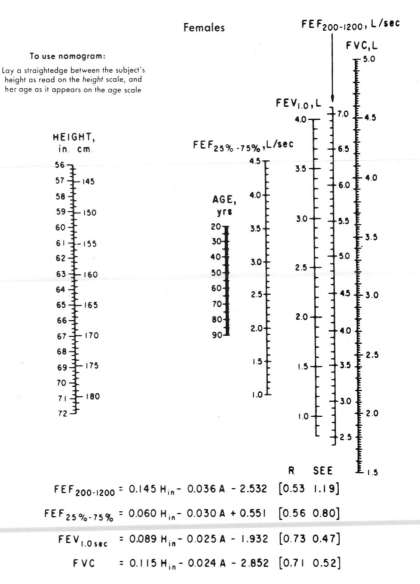

To use nomogram:
Lay a straightedge between the subject's height as read on the *height* scale, and her age as it appears on the age scale

$$FEF_{200-1200} = 0.145\,H_{in} - 0.036\,A - 2.532 \quad [0.53 \ 1.19]$$

$$FEF_{25\%-75\%} = 0.060\,H_{in} - 0.030\,A + 0.551 \quad [0.56 \ 0.80]$$

$$FEV_{1.0sec} = 0.089\,H_{in} - 0.025\,A - 1.932 \quad [0.73 \ 0.47]$$

$$FVC = 0.115\,H_{in} - 0.024\,A - 2.852 \quad [0.71 \ 0.52]$$

FIG. B-2 *Prediction nomograms (BTPS), spirometric values in normal women.* (From Morris JF, Koski WA, Johnson LD: *Am Rev Respir Dis* 103[1]:57, 1971.)

value and multiplied by 100. Plus or minus 20% is often used as the limit of normal. This method is simple. It approximates lower limits of normal for adults of average age and height for FVC and FEV_1. Eighty percent of predicted is close to the fifth percentile in these subjects. Using a fixed percentage results in shorter, older subjects being classified as abnormal. Tall, younger subjects may be erroneously classified as normal, even though they have disease. Using a fixed percentage of reference produces erroneous lower limits for $FEF_{25\%-75\%}$ and for instantaneous flows ($\dot{V}_{max}$). The lower limit of normal for these flow measurements is approximately 50% of the predicted value. Fixed percentages may be acceptable in children if the variability is proportional to the predicted "mean" value.

A more precise approach bases the lower limit on the reference value and its variability. If lung function varies in normal fashion (a Gaussian or bell-shaped distribution curve), the mean ±1.96 standard deviations (SDs) defines the 95% confidence limits. Statistically, 95% of the healthy population falls within approximately 2 SDs of the mean. If a subject's measured value is outside of the range defined by his mean ±1.96 SDs, there is only a 5% chance that the test is normal. For some pulmonary function variables, only the lower limit of normal (i.e., below the mean) is significant. For example, it is not usually clinically significant if the FVC is greater than predicted, only if it is lower. For such variables, 1.65 SDs may be used to define the lower limit of normal. Variables that can be abnormally high or low (e.g., residual volume [RV], TLC, $Paco_2$) must use the 1.96 SD method.

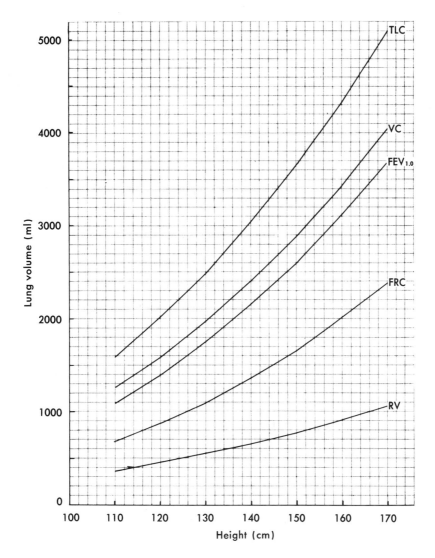

FIG. B-3 *Summary curves for lung volumes and FEV₁ in milliliters, for boys, as a function of height in centimeters.* Summary curves are derived from regression equations from several different studies. (From Polgar G, Promadhat V: *Pulmonary function testing in children,* Philadelphia, 1971, WB Saunders.)

Abnormality may also be expressed as the difference between the subject's reference and measured values in terms of confidence intervals (CI). The difference between the reference and measured values is divided by one CI (either 1.96 or 1.65 SDs). The result is expressed as a ratio:

$$\frac{\text{Reference} - \text{Measured}}{\text{CI}}$$

Using this method, a normal value is always less than or equal to 1.00, whereas abnormal values are greater. The extent of abnormality (obstruction or restriction) can also be described using the CI ratio. For example, $FEV_{1\%}$ may be evaluated as follows:

$FEV_{1\%}$	(CI)
Normal	<1 CI
Mild obstruction	>1 <2 CI
Moderate obstruction	>2 <4 CI
Severe obstruction	>4 CI

Each pulmonary function variable can be assessed using this method as long as its CI has been determined. Tests that are quite variable (e.g., $FEF_{25\%-75\%}$) have large CIs. In some instances the CI may be larger than the expected value. As a result, the lower limit of normal may be zero or even a negative value. Although statistically valid, the use of the CI may not be applicable in every situation.

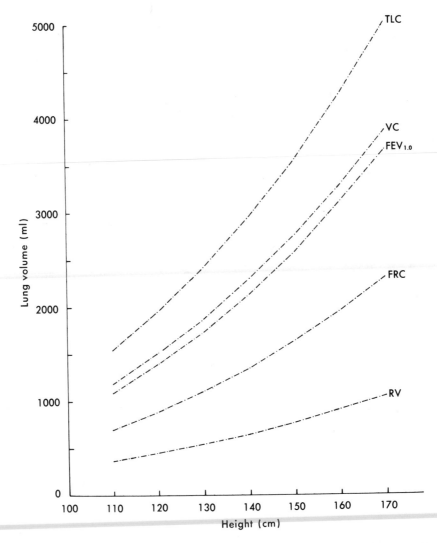

FIG. B-4 *Summary curves for lung values and FEV₁ in milliliters, for girls, as a function of height in centimeters.* Summary curves are derived from regression equations from several different studies. (From Polgar G, Promadhat V: *Pulmonary function testing in children,* Philadelphia, 1971, WB Saunders.)

A third method for determining lower limits of normal uses the fifth percentile. The fifth percentile is the percent of the reference value above which 95% of the healthy population falls. The fifth percentile method requires a large sample population. However, it does not require the pulmonary function variable to be normally distributed in the population. Lower limits of normal using the fifth percentile are usually defined for specific age groupings. Both the CI and fifth percentile methods yield similar results for lower limits of normal, for variables that are normally distributed in the population.

Individual laboratories should try to choose reference studies from a population similar to that to be tested. The following factors may be considerations in selecting reference values:

1. *Type of equipment used for the reference study:* Does it comply with the most recent recommendations (1994) of the American Thoracic Society? (See Chapter 10.)

2. *Methodologies:* Were procedures used in the reference study similar to those to be used, particularly for spirometry, lung volumes, and DL_{CO}?

3. *Sample population:* What were the age ranges of the subjects? Did the study generate different regressions for different ethnic origins? Did the study include smokers or other "at-risk" individuals as normals?

4. *Statistical data:* Are lower limits of normal defined? Are adequate data available (SD, CI) so that lower limits of normal can be calculated?

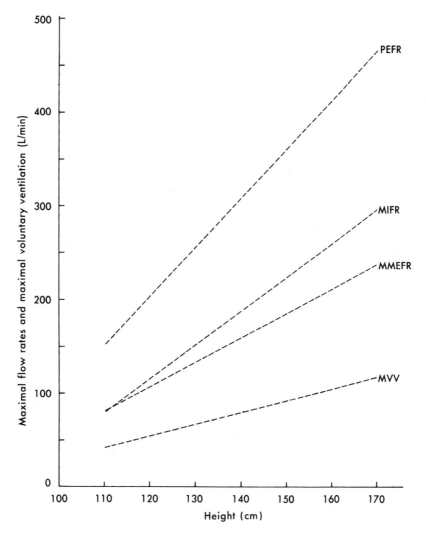

FIG. B-5 *Summary curves for maximal midexpiratory flow rate (FEF$_{25\%-75\%}$), peak expiratory flow (PEF), maximal voluntary ventilation (MVV), and maximal inspiratory flow rate (MIFR) in liters per minute, as a function of height for boys and girls.* Summary curves are derived from regression equations from several different studies. (From Polgar G, Promadhat V: *Pulmonary function testing in children,* Philadelphia, 1971, WB Saunders.)

5. *Conditions of the study:* Was the study performed at a different altitude or under different environmental conditions?

6. *Published reference equations:* Do reference values generated using the study's regressions differ markedly from other published references?

Each laboratory should perform measurements on 20 to 40 subjects who represent a healthy cross-section of the population that the laboratory usually tests. Measured values from these subjects should be compared with expected values using various reference equations. Equations that produce the smallest average differences should be selected. Evaluation of a small number of subjects may not show much difference between equa-

tions for FVC and FEV$_1$. There may, however, be noticeable discrepancies for DL_{co} or maximal flows. Equations for spirometry, lung volumes, and DL_{co} should all be taken from a single reference, if possible. If healthy subjects fall outside the limits of normal, the laboratory should examine its test methods, how the normal subjects were selected, or the prediction equations themselves.

There are no universally accepted reference values. Several excellent studies are available that address most of the considerations listed previously. The reference equations included here are widely used and compare favorably with other published studies. Other acceptable studies are included in the references. Laboratories are encouraged to evaluate these and other equations in selecting references.

Prediction Regressions for Pulmonary Function Tests

All values BTPS unless otherwise stated.

Test	Regression equation	SD	Source
VC (L)			
Males	$0.148H - 0.025A - 4.25$	0.58	1
Females	$0.115H - 0.024A - 2.85$	0.52	1
FRC (L)			
Males	$0.130H - 5.16$	—	2
Females	$0.119H - 4.85$	—	2
RV (L)			
Males	$0.069H + 0.017A - 3.45$	—	3
Females	$0.081H + 0.009A - 3.90$	—	3
Derived Lung Volumes			
	TLC (L) = VC + RV		
or	TLC (L) = FRC + IC		

Test	Regression equation	SD	Source
FVC (L)			
Males	Same as VC		1
Females	Same as VC		1
$FEV_{0.5}$ (L)			
Males	$0.24 + 0.02H - 0.024A$	0.51	4
FEV_1 (L)			
Males	$0.092H - 0.032A - 1.260$	0.55	1
Females	$0.089H - 0.024A - 1.93$	0.47	1
$FEF_{25\%-75\%}$ (L/sec)			
Males	$0.047H - 0.045A + 2.513$	1.12	1
Females	$0.060H - 0.030A + 0.551$	0.80	1

Test	Regression equation	SD	Source
PEF (L/sec)			
Males	$0.144H - 0.024A + 0.225$	—	5
Females	$0.090H - 0.018A + 1.130$	—	5
$\dot{V}max_{75}$ (L/sec)			
Males	$0.090H - 0.020A + 2.726$	—	5
Females	$0.069H - 0.019A + 2.147$	—	5
$\dot{V}max_{50}$ (L/sec)			
Males	$0.065H - 0.030A + 2.403$	—	5
Females	$0.062H - 0.035A + 1.426$	—	5
$\dot{V}max_{25}$ (L/sec)			
Males	$0.036H - 0.041A + 1.984$	—	5
Females	$0.023H - 0.035A + 2.216$	—	5
MVV (L/min)			
Males	$3.03H - 0.816A - 37.9$	—	5
Females	$2.14H - 0.685A - 4.87$	—	5
CV/VC (%)			
Males	$0.357A + 0.562$	4.15	6
Females	$0.293A + 2.812$	4.90	6

Test	Regression equation	SD	Source
CC/TLC (%)			
Males	$0.496A + 14.878$	4.09	6
Females	$0.536A + 14.420$	4.43	6
$D_{L_{CO}}SB$ (ml CO/min/mm Hg STPD)			
Males	$0.250H - 0.177A + 19.93$	—	8
Females	$0.284H - 0.177A + 7.72$	—	8
Maximal Expiratory Pressure (cm H_2O)			
Males	$268 - 1.03A$	—	9
Females	$170 - 0.53A$	—	9
Maximal Inspiratory Pressure (cm H_2O)			
Males	$143 - 0.55A$	—	9
Females	$104 - 0.51A$	—	9
$\dot{V}O_{2\,max}$ (L/min STPD)			
Males	$4.2 - 0.032A$	0.4	10
Females	$2.6 - 0.014A$	0.4	10
HR_{max} (beats/min)			
Males and females	$210 - 0.65A$	10-15	10
Pa_{O_2} (mm Hg)			
Males and females	$-0.279A + 0.113P_B + 14.632$	—	11

SOURCES FOR PREDICTION REGRESSIONS

1. Morris JF, Koski A, Johnson LC: Spirometric standards for healthy nonsmoking adults, *Am Rev Respir Dis* 103:57, 1971.
2. Bates DV, Macklem PT, Christie RV: *Respiratory function in diseases*, ed 2, Philadelphia, 1971, WB Saunders.
3. Goldman HI, Becklake MR: Respiratory function tests: normal values at median altitudes and the prediction of normal results, *Am Rev Tuberculosis* 79:457, 1959.
4. Kory RC, Callahan R, Syner JC: The veterans administration–army cooperative study of pulmonary function: I. Clinical spirometry in normal men, *Am J Med* 30:243, 1961.
5. Cherniack RM, Raber MD: Normal standards for ventilatory function using an automated wedge spirometer, *Am Rev Respir Dis* 106:38, 1972.
6. Buist SA, Ross BB: Predicted values for closing volumes using a modified single-breath nitrogen test, *Am Rev Respir Dis* 111:405, 1975.
7. Gelb AF, Maloney PA, Klein E, et al: Sensitivity of volume of isoflow in the detection of mild airway obstruction, *Am Rev Respir Dis* 112:401, 1975.
8. Gaensler EA, Wright GW: Evaluation of respiratory impairment, *Arch Environ Health* 12:146, 1966.
9. Black LF, Hyatt RE: Maximal respiratory pressures: normal values and relationships to age and sex, *Am Rev Respir Dis* 99:696, 1969.
10. Jones NL, Campbell EJM, Edwards RHT, et al: *Clinical exercise testing*, ed 2, Philadelphia, 1983, WB Saunders.
11. Morris AH, Kanner RE, Crapo RO, et al: *Clinical pulmonary function testing*, ed 2, Salt Lake City, 1984, Intermountain Thoracic Society.

ADDITIONAL RECOMMENDED SOURCES FOR PULMONARY FUNCTION PREDICTED VALUES

General

American Thoracic Society: Lung function testing: selection of reference values and interpretive strategies, *Am Rev Respir Dis* 144:1202, 1991.

Spirometry

Crapo RO, Morris AH, Gardner RM: Reference spirometric values using techniques and equipment that meet ATS recommendations, *Am Rev Respir Dis* 123:659, 1981.

Knudson RJ, Slatin RC, Lebowitz MD: The maximal expiratory flow-volume curve. Normal standards, variability, and effects of age, *Am Rev Respir Dis* 113:587, 1976.

Quanjer PH, ed: Report of working party—European community for coal and steel. Standardized lung function testing, *Bull Eur Physiopathol Respir* 19(suppl 5):7, 1983.

Schoenberg JB, Beck GJ, Bouhuys A: Growth and decay of pulmonary function in healthy blacks and whites, *Respir Physiol* 33:367, 1978.

Lung Volumes

Crapo RO, Morris AH, Clayton PD, et al: Lung volumes in healthy nonsmoking adults, *Bull Europ Physiopath Respir* 18:419, 1982.

Grimby G, Soderholm B: Spirometric studies in normal subjects: III. Static lung volumes and maximum voluntary ventilation in adults with a note on physical fitness, *Acta Med Scand* 173:199, 1963.

Diffusing Capacity

Bates DV, Macklem PT, Christie RV: *Respiratory function in disease,* Philadelphia, 1971, WB Saunders.

Crapo RO, Morris AH: Standardized single-breath normal values for carbon monoxide diffusing capacity, *Am Rev Respir Dis* 123:185, 1981.

Additional Recommended Sources for Pulmonary Function Predicted Values

Hsu KHK, Bartholomew PH, Thompson V, et al: Ventilatory functions of normal children and young adults—Mexican-American, white, and black. I. Spirometry, *J Pediatr* 95:14, 1979.

Polgar G, Promadhat V: *Pulmonary function testing in children: techniques and standards,* Philadelphia, 1971, WB Saunders.

Reference Values for Pulmonary Function Studies in Children

All values BTPS unless otherwise noted.

Test	Regression equation	SD	Source
Children 42-59 inches, 5-17 years old			
FVC (L)			
Males	$0.094H - 3.04$	0.176	1
Females	$0.077H - 2.37$	0.171	1
FEV_1 (L)			
Males	$0.085H - 2.86$	0.159	1
Females	$0.074H - 2.48$	0.166	1
$FEF_{25\%-75\%}$ (L)			
Males	$0.094H - 2.61$	0.388	1
Females	$0.087H - 2.39$	0.347	1
PEF (L/sec)			
Males	$0.161H - 5.88$	0.451	1
Females	$0.130H - 4.51$	0.487	1
MVV (L/min)			
Males and females	$3.81H - 134$	—	1
Children 60-78 inches, 5-17 years old			
FVC (L)			
Males	$0.174A + 0.164H - 9.43$	0.354	1
Females	$0.102A + 0.117H - 5.87$	0.287	1
FEV_1 (L/sec)			
Males	$0.126A + 0.143H - 7.86$	0.303	1
Females	$0.085A + 0.0100H - 4.94$	0.290	1
$FEF_{25\%-75\%}$ (L/sec)			
Males	$0.126A + 0.135H - 6.50$	0.612	1
Females	$0.083A + 0.093H - 3.50$	0.621	1
PEF (L/sec)			
Males	$0.205A + 0.181H - 9.54$	0.780	1
Females	$0.139A + 0.0100H - 4.12$	0.798	1
MVV (L/min)			
Males and females	$3.81H - 134$	—	1
VC (L)			
Males	Same as FVC		1
Females	Same as FVC		1
FRC (L)			
Males and females	$0.067 \times e^{0.05334H}$	—	2
RV (L)			
Males and females	$0.033 \times e^{0.05334H}$	—	2
Derived Lung Volumes (L)			
	$TLC = VC + RV$		
or	$TLC = FRC + IC$		
$DL_{CO}SB$ (ml CO/min/mm Hg STPD)			
Males and females	$0.693H - 20.13$	—	3

SOURCES FOR NORMAL VALUES—CHILDREN*

1. Dickman ML, Schmidt CD, Gardner RM: Spirometric standards for normal children and adolescent (ages 5 years through 18 years), *Am Rev Respir Dis* 104:680, 1971.

2. Weng TR, Levison H: Standards of pulmonary function in children, *Am Rev Respir Dis* 99:879, 1969.

3. Gaensler EA, Wright GW: Evaluation of respiratory impairment, *Arch Environ Health* 12:146, 1966.

*See also "Additional Recommended Sources for Pediatric Pulmonary Function."

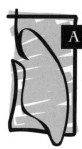

Conversion and Correction Factors

Conversion and Correction Factors
Converting Gas Volumes from ATPS to BTPS

$$\text{Volume (BTPS)} = \text{Volume (ATPS)} \times \frac{P_B - P_{H_2O}}{P_B - 47} \times \frac{310}{273 + T}$$

where:

$\quad\quad\quad P_B$ = barometric pressure, mm Hg

$\quad\quad P_{H_2O}$ = vapor pressure of water at spirometer temperature

$\quad\quad\quad\quad T$ = temperature in °C

$\quad\quad\quad\quad 47$ = vapor pressure of water at 37° C

$\quad\quad 310$ = absolute body temperature

Most of the factors of this equation can be combined into a single conversion factor. Local barometric pressure changes cause slight differences. The most significant differences occur with temperature changes.

Conversion factor	Gas temperature (°C)	P_{H_2O} (mm Hg)
1.112	18	15.6
1.107	19	16.5
1.102	20	17.5
1.096	21	18.7
1.091	22	19.8
1.085	23	21.1
1.080	24	22.4
1.075	25	23.8
1.068	26	23.8
1.063	27	26.7
1.057	28	28.3
1.051	29	30.0
1.045	30	31.8
1.039	31	31.8
1.032	32	35.7
1.026	33	35.7
1.020	34	35.7
1.014	35	42.2
1.007	36	44.6
1.000	37	47.0

Converting Gas Volumes from ATPS to STPD

$$\text{Volume (STPD)} = \text{Volume (ATPS)} \times \frac{P_B - P_{H_2O}}{760} \times \frac{273}{273 + T}$$

where:

P_B = barometric pressure

P_{H_2O} = water vapor pressure at spirometer temperature

T = temperature of the spirometer

760 = standard barometric pressure at sea level

273 = absolute temperature equal to 0° C

Calculating Water Vapor Pressure

$$P_{H_2O} = 47.07 \times 10^{\left[\frac{6.36(T - 37)}{232 + T}\right]}$$

where:

P_{H_2O} = water vapor pressure in mm Hg

T = temperature, from 0° to 40° C

Calculating Barometric Pressure at Altitude

$$P_B = 760 \times [1 - (6.873 \times 10^{-6} \times \text{Altitude})]^{5.256}$$

where:

P_B = barometric pressure in mm Hg

Altitude = altitude in feet above sea level

SI (Système International) Units

Conversion factors for units of measurement commonly used in pulmonary function testing. (Except for temperature, to convert a value expressed in conventional units to its equivalent in SI units, *multiply* the conventional units by the conversion factor. To convert from SI to conventional units, *divide* by the factor.)

Measurement	Conventional unit	SI unit	Conversion factor
Temperature	°C	K	°C + 273.15
Length	inch (in)	meter (m)	0.0254
	foot (ft)	m	0.3048
Area	in^2	cm^2	6.452
	ft^2	0	0.0929
Volume	ft^3	L	28.32
Pressure	cm H$_2$O	kilopascal (kPa)	0.09806
	mm Hg (torr)	kPa	0.1333
	pounds/in^2 (psi)	kPa	6.895
Work	kilogram meter (kg m)	joule (J)	9.807
Power	kg m/min	(J)	0.1634
Energy	kilocalorie (kcal)	(J)	4185
Compliance	L/cm H$_2$O	L/k/Pa	10.2
Resistance	cm H$_2$O/L/sec	kPa/L/sec	0.09806

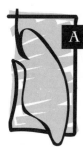

Regulations and Regulatory Agencies

Regulations and Regulatory Agencies

Several agencies regulate operations in pulmonary function and/or blood gas laboratories. These regulations concern laboratory procedures, infection control, safety, and reimbursement.

Occupational Safety and Health Administration

The Occupational Safety and Health Administration (OSHA) is an agency of the U.S. Government charged with developing and implementing policies to address hazards in the workplace. OSHA regulations apply to two main areas in pulmonary function and blood gas laboratories:

---

1. *Hazard communication* relates to all chemicals or substances used in the laboratory. Laboratories are required to maintain lists of hazardous substances. In addition, Material Safety Data Sheets (MSDS) must be kept. Employees must be trained regarding, and kept informed of, hazardous chemicals in their workplace.
2. Training regarding *blood-borne pathogens* is mandated. Employees who may be exposed to blood or blood products must receive training regarding the transmission of blood-borne pathogens. Methods of preventing exposure, identification of tasks that cause risk of exposure, and actions to be taken must be documented. Plans for removal of blood and blood products are necessary, as are explanations of personal protective equipment, such as gloves and gowns.

Regulations mandated by OSHA are published in the Federal Register and are continually updated.

National Institute for Occupational Safety and Health

The National Institute for Occupational Safety and Health (NIOSH) is an agency of the U.S. Government that enforces standards set by OSHA. NIOSH regulations concerning pulmonary function measurements are related to the "Cotton Dust Standard." The federal regulations (29 CFR: 1910.1043) describe how spirometry is to be performed in the examination of individuals exposed to cotton dust. The appendix to this statute lists standards for spirometers and recorders used, measurement techniques, interpretation of spirometry, and qualifications for personnel performing spirometry. Guidelines for minimal spirometry training are included. These NIOSH regulations regarding spirometry are often applied in areas of occupational exposure other than cotton dust, making them de facto standards.

Updates to NIOSH regulations are published in the Federal Register.

Health and Human Services

Health and Human Services (HHS) is a department of the U.S. Government. Programs impacting pulmonary function and blood gas laboratories are administered by the Health Care Financing Administration (HCFA).

Clinical Laboratory Improvement Amendments of 1988 (CLIA 88). CLIA 88 (42 CFR: 405, et al) consists of a series of rules regarding laboratory practices. These rules include blood gas laboratories, and may have ramifications for pulmonary function testing as well. Under CLIA 88 rules:

---

1. Laboratories must register and apply for certification. Level of certification depends on the complexity of tests performed.
2. Three categories of testing based on complexity of the testing method have been established:

    Waived tests: Waived tests include simple nonautomated tests such as pH measurement by dipstick method.

    Tests of moderate complexity: Tests of moderate complexity include automated tests or manual procedures with limited steps. Automated blood gas analyses that do not require operator intervention during the analytic process are included in the moderate complexity group.

    Tests of high complexity: Tests of high complexity include semiautomated or manual procedures that require multiple steps, preparation of complex reagents, and operator intervention in the analytic process.
3. Personnel requirements are linked to the complexity model for testing. For moderately complex tests, standards for laboratory directors, technical consultants, clinical consultants, and testing personnel are defined. For high-complexity tests, standards for technical and general supervisors are added to the list. The regulations list specific functions and qualifications for each position. Qualified individuals can fill more than

one position in either moderate or high-complexity testing.

4. Proficiency testing is required to externally evaluate each laboratory's performance. Each laboratory performing moderate or high-complexity tests must participate in proficiency testing. Proficiency tests must be performed for each regulated analyte for which the laboratory reports results. Proficiency testing samples must include five samples for each analyte or test. The laboratory must participate in the program at least three times per year. A separate grading formula is established for each analyte. For most analytes or tests, a score of 80% (i.e., acceptable measurement on four of five samples) is required. Laboratories that are unsuccessful (i.e., score less than 80%) on two out of three tests will be subject to sanctions for the involved test.

5. Each laboratory must establish a quality control program. Rules require that for tests of moderate complexity (e.g., blood gases) manufacturer's instructions be followed, a procedure manual be available, and calibrations be performed. Quality control runs with at least two levels must be performed daily. Instruments and test systems will be evaluated by the Food and Drug Administration (FDA) to determine the applicable levels of quality control required.

In addition to the laboratory regulations defined by CLIA 88, HHS sets standards for reimbursement under the DRG (Diagnosis Related Groups) system for Medicare patients. Reimbursement requires that charges for procedures performed be correctly classified using Current Procedural Terminology (CPT) codes. HHS also lists requirements for disability according to the Social Security Administration (SSA). These regulations specify levels of pulmonary function impairment which qualify candidates for disability reimbursement (see Chapter 8).

Updates to CLIA 88 regulations are published in the Federal Register. Regulations related to reimbursement under HCFA or SSA are published by those agencies respectively.

Joint Committee on Accreditation of Healthcare Organizations

The Joint Committee on Accreditation of Healthcare Organizations (JCAHO) is a voluntary accrediting agency that develops standards of quality for health care organizations. The JCAHO has published standards for all areas of the health care environment. The standards which affect pulmonary function laboratories are listed primarily under Respiratory Care Services. JCAHO standards require the following:

---

1. Pulmonary function and blood gas analysis capability should be appropriate for the level of respiratory care services provided, and should be readily available to meet the needs of patients. Blood gases should be available 24 hours/day.

2. The scope of diagnostic services must be defined in writing and must be related to other hospital departments by an organizational plan.

3. Services provided from outside of the hospital must meet all necessary requirements.

4. Medical direction should be provided by a physician qualified by special training or interest in respiratory problems and should be readily available for consultation.

5. Trained personnel should be available to meet the needs of the patients served. Hazardous procedures (e.g., arterial puncture) must be authorized in writing according to medical staff policy.

6. There must be written policies and procedures for pulmonary function testing and for obtaining and analyzing blood samples. The policies and procedures should address equipment maintenance, safety, infection control, and administration of medications.

7. There must be sufficient facilities (equipment, space) for performing pulmonary function studies and blood gas analysis. Requirements regarding performance of pulmonary function or blood gas studies must be met regardless of which hospital department performs them. Equipment must be calibrated and maintained according to the manufacturer's specifications.

Standards developed by the JCAHO are published annually in their document entitled *Accreditation Manual for Hospitals*.

Certifying and Standards Organizations

The following organizations offer certification or publish standards related to pulmonary function testing and/or blood gas analysis:

Organization	Certification/standards
American College of Sports Medicine (ACSM)	Provides training courses and certification for exercise technologists; publishes guidelines for exercise testing and training
American Thoracic Society (ATS)	Publishes standards for spirometry, single-breath $D_{L_{CO}}$, pulmonary function personnel qualifications, use of computers in pulmonary function testing, guidelines for quality assurance, and interpretive strategies; Standards published in the *American Review of Respiratory Disease*
Center for Disease Control and Prevention (CDC)	Promulgates standards related to infection control and disease prevention; regulations published in *Morbidity and Mortality Weekly Report*
College of American Pathologists (CAP)	Accredits clinical and research laboratories, including blood gas laboratories; provides quality control programs and proficiency testing survey materials

Organization	Certification/standards
National Board for Respiratory Care (NBRC)	Provides national certification for respiratory care practitioners, including pulmonary function technologists; offers credentials of Certified Pulmonary Function Technologist (CPFT) for entry level and Registered Pulmonary Function Technologist (RPFT) for advanced level practitioners
National Committee for Clinical Laboratory Standards (NCCLS)	Publishes standards for all areas of laboratory medicine, including blood gas laboratories

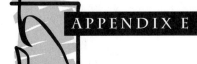

Equations

Some Useful Equations

Alveolar Air Equation

It is often necessary to determine the partial pressure of O_2 in alveolar gas. One practical application of the alveolar air equation is determination of P_{AO_2} for calculation of the present shunt. The alveolar air equation is as follows:

$$P_{AO_2} = (F_{IO_2} \times (P_B - 47)) - P_{ACO_2}\left(F_{IO_2} + \frac{1 - F_{IO_2}}{R}\right)$$

where:

F_{IO_2} = fractional concentration of inspired O_2

P_B = barometric pressure

47 = partial pressure of water vapor at 37° C

P_{ACO_2} = arterial CO_2 tension, presumed equal to alveolar CO_2 tension

R = respiratory exchange ratio ($\dot{V}_{CO_2}/\dot{V}_{O_2}$)

If the fraction of inspired O_2 is 1.0, the factor in the right-hand parentheses equals one and can be deleted. R varies, especially during exercise; it is often assumed to be 0.80.

Poiseuille's Law

Poiseuille's law relates variables that affect gas flow through a tube. The law has many applications in pulmonary physiology. It describes laminar gas flow through the conducting airways. It is also used in pneumotachography to relate flow and pressure changes within a tube. The law is stated as follows:

$$\Delta P = \frac{\dot{V}8\eta l}{\pi r^4}$$

where:

ΔP = change in pressure from one end of the tube to the other

$\dot{V}$ = flow through the tube

η = coefficient of viscosity of the gas

l = length of the tube

r = radius of the tube

The equation can be rearranged as follows:

$$\frac{\Delta P}{\dot{V}} = \frac{8\eta l}{\pi r^4}$$

The ratio of pressure differences at the end of the tube (ΔP) to flow through the tube ($\dot{V}$), defines *resistance*. Resistance varies directly with the length of the conducting tube. It varies inversely with the fourth power of the radius. A twofold increase in length of the tube doubles resistance. A reduction of the radius by half increases the pressure difference 16 times. In the airways, narrowing caused by secretions or other lesions can significantly increase airway resistance. Poiseuille's law applies to any round tube in which laminar flow is possible. Pneumotachography is based directly on this law (see "Pressure Differential Flow Sensors," Chapter 9). The length and radius of a pressure differential flow sensor remain constant. The viscosity of respiratory gases varies only slightly. The variables in Poiseuille's equation, except for ΔP and $\dot{V}$, can be reduced to a single constant. Flow can then be defined as follows:

$$\dot{V} = \frac{\Delta P}{K_R}$$

where:

K_R = a resistance constant determined by length and radius of the flow tube

Using this equation, $\dot{V}$ can be measured by determining the pressure differential. This is easily accomplished by means of pressure transducers.

Thoracic Gas Volume Equation

Measurement of the V_{TG} with the body plethysmograph is based on Boyle's law:

$$P_1V_1 = P_2V_2$$

or by expanding:

$$P_1V_1 = (P_1 + \Delta P)(V_1 + \Delta V)$$

where:

P_1 = initial dry pressure in the lungs (713 mm Hg or 970 cm H_2O)

V_1 = V_{TG} or volume of gas in the thorax

ΔV = change in lung volume

ΔP = change in lung pressure

Then by rearranging:

$$P_1\Delta V + V_1\Delta P + \Delta V\Delta P = 0$$

Solving for V_1:

$$V_1 = -\frac{\Delta V}{\Delta P}(P_1 + \Delta P)$$

Because ΔP is small compared with P_1, $P_1 + \Delta P \approx P_1$, therefore:

$$V_1 = -\frac{P_1(\Delta V)}{\Delta P}$$

In terms of the plethysmographic method (and disregarding the sign):

$$V_{TG} = 970\frac{(\Delta V)}{(\Delta P)}$$

A sloping line is recorded on a computer screen or an oscilloscope. The slope represents the change in mouth pressure per unit change in box volume ($\Delta P/\Delta V$) or λV_{TG}, as the subject pants against an occluded airway. The equation then becomes:

$$V_{TG} = \frac{970}{\lambda V_{TG}}$$

This is the working form of the equation. Box pressure and mouth pressure calibration factors are also required to complete the calculation (see Appendix F). Measurement of the slope of the tracing allows rapid calculation of V_{TG}.

Fick's Law of Diffusion (Modified)

In reference to gas exchange across a membrane, Fick's law states that:

$$\dot{V}_{gas} = \frac{A}{T} \times D \times (P_1 - P_2)$$

where:

A = area of the membrane

T = thickness of the membrane

$P_1 - P_2$ = pressure gradient across the membrane

D = diffusion constant for a specific gas

D is related to the molecular weight and solubility of the gas to which it refers by:

$$D \propto \frac{\text{Solubility}}{\sqrt{\text{Molecular weight}}}$$

Because A and T remain relatively constant in the lungs:

$$D_L \propto \frac{\dot{V}_{gas}}{P_A - P_C}$$

where:

D_L = diffusion constant for the lung

P_A = alveolar gas pressure

P_C = capillary gas pressure

When D_L is measured with carbon monoxide (CO), the capillary partial pressure is assumed to be zero, thus:

$$D_L = \frac{\dot{V}_{CO}}{P_{ACO}}$$

All CO methods of measuring D_L use this basic equation. The single-breath and steady-state methods differ in that the former measures $\dot{V}_{CO}$ during breath holding, whereas the latter measures it during normal breathing. The steady-state methods vary by the way in which they measure P_{ACO}.

Fick Principle (Cardiac Output Determination)

The Fick principle relates $\dot{V}_{O_2}$ to arterial-mixed venous O_2 content difference ($C[a - \bar{v}]O_2$) to determine cardiac output ($\dot{Q}$):

$$\dot{Q}_T = \frac{\dot{V}_{O_2}}{C_{aO_2} - C\bar{v}_{O_2}}$$

This equation forms the basis for determining various fractions of the cardiac output, namely, the shunt fraction ($\dot{Q}_S$) and the fraction participating in ideal gas exchange ($\dot{Q}_C$). The relationship between $\dot{Q}_S$ and the total cardiac output $\dot{Q}_T$ can be expressed as a ratio using the concept of O_2 content differences:

$$\frac{\dot{Q}_S}{\dot{Q}_T} = \frac{C_{cO_2} - C_{aO_2}}{C_{cO_2} - C\bar{v}_{O_2}}$$

where:

$C_{cO_2} - C_{aO_2}$ = content difference between pulmonary end capillary blood, C_{cO_2}, and arterial blood, C_{aO_2}, which increases when blood passes through the pulmonary system without coming into contact with alveolar gas (a shunt)

$C_{cO_2} - C\bar{v}_{O_2}$ = content difference between blood returning to the lungs by way of the pulmonary artery and the pulmonary end-capillary blood; the total change reflects the arterialization of mixed venous blood.

If all pulmonary capillary blood equilibrates with alveolar gas, C_{cO_2} and C_{aO_2} become identical, no matter what the value of the denominator, so the ratio becomes zero and the shunt must be zero. If some blood does not equilibrate, the numerator becomes larger in relation to the denominator and an increased $\dot{Q}_S/\dot{Q}_T$ results.

Pulmonary end-capillary O_2 content (C_{cO_2}) is impossible to sample and represents a mathematical entity rather than an actual phenomenon. A modified form of the equation is used clinically (as described in Chapter 6):

$$\frac{\dot{Q}_S}{\dot{Q}_T} = \frac{(P_{AO_2} - P_{aO_2})(0.0031)}{(C[a - \bar{v}]O_2) + (P_{AO_2} - P_{aO_2})(0.0031)}$$

where:

$P_{AO_2} - P_{aO_2}$ = difference in O_2 tension between the alveoli and arterial blood

0.0031 = solubility factor to convert O_2 tension to volume percent

The equation is applied after the subject has breathed 100% O_2 long enough to completely saturate the Hb (P_{aO_2} greater than 150 mm Hg). The only difference between pulmonary end-capillary blood (assumed to be in equilibrium with the P_{AO_2}) and arterial blood exists in the difference in O_2 content in the dissolved form. This difference is related to the normal a-$\bar{v}$ content difference ($C[a-\bar{v}]O_2$) plus the actual dissolved content difference, denoted by the same term in both numerator and denominator. A ratio between the content difference of shunted blood and the total difference is derived using dissolved O_2 differences. P_{AO_2} is determined by the alveolar air equation outlined previously in this Appendix.

Calculated Bicarbonate (HCO_3^-)

The bicarbonate concentration in plasma can be calculated using the Henderson-Hasselbalch equation if pH and P_{CO_2} are known:

$$pH = pK + \log\frac{(HCO_3^-)}{(H_2CO_3)}$$

The working form of the equation becomes as follows:

$$(HCO_3^-) = 0.0306 \times P_{CO_2} \times 10^{((pH - 6.161)/(0.9524))}$$

where:

HCO_3^- = bicarbonate concentration, in mEq/L

0.0306 = solubility coefficient for CO_2

6.161 = the pK of carbonic acid

0.9524 = an empirically determined constant

The total CO_2 concentration can then be determined by summing the HCO_3^- and the dissolved CO_2:

$$T_{CO_2} = 0.0306 \times P_{CO_2} + (HCO_3^-)$$

Calculated Oxygen Saturation

Although it is preferable to measure oxygen saturation (see Chapter 6), saturation of Hb with O_2 can be calculated if the pH and P_{O_2} are known. Assuming that the Hb is normal (i.e., having a P_{50} of 26.6), saturation may be calculated as follows:

$$Hbo_2 = \frac{Z^{2.60}}{(26.6)^{2.60} + Z^{2.60}} \times 100$$

where:

$$Z = P_{O_2} \times 10^{(-0.48(7.40 - pH))}$$

where:

P_{O_2} = partial pressure of O_2 in the sample

pH = negative log of the hydrogen ion concentration in the sample

−0.48 = the Bohr factor (normal blood)

Because the Hb is assumed to be normal, calculated saturation may be in error if the O_2 binding capacity of the Hb is altered (see Chapter 6).

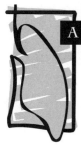

Sample Calculations

Sample Calculations

Open-circuit FRC Determination (N_2 Washout) (see Chapter 3)

FRC	Unknown
FEN_{2final}	0.06
$FAN_{2alveolar1}$	0.76
$FAN_{2alveolar2}$	0.01
Volume expired (VE)	27.5 L
Test time (T)	7 minutes
N_{2tiss}	0.04 L/min (correction factor)
Spirometer temperature:	24° C

1. $FRC = \dfrac{[FEN_{2final} \times (VE + VD)] - (T \times N_{2tiss})}{FAN_{2alveolar1} - FAN_{2alveolar2}}$

2. $= \dfrac{[0.06 \times (27.5 + 1.0 \text{ L}) - (7.0 \text{ min} \times 0.04 \text{ L/min})}{0.76 - 0.01}$

3. $= \dfrac{(0.06 \times 28.5) - (0.28 \text{ L})}{0.75}$

4. $= \dfrac{1.71 \text{ L} - 0.28 \text{ L}}{0.75}$

5. $= \dfrac{1.43}{0.75}$

6. FRC = 1.91 L (ATPS)

This value is ATPS and must be corrected to BTPS. The spirometer temperature was 24° C. Using the appropriate correction factor from p. 335.

7. FRC (BTPS) = 1.91×1.08

8. FRC (BTPS) = 2.06

Closed-circuit FRC Determination (Helium Dilution) (see Chapter 3)

FRC	Unknown
He added	0.5 L
$\%He_{initial}$	9.5% (0.095 as a fraction)
$\%He_{final}$	5.5% (0.055 as a fraction)
He absorption correction:	0.1 L
Spirometer temperature:	24° C

1. $FRC = \left[\dfrac{(\%He_{initial} - \%He_{final})}{\%He_{final}} \times \text{System volume} \right] - \text{He correction}$

2. System volume $= \dfrac{He_{added}}{\%He_{initial}}$

$= \dfrac{0.5\ L}{0.095}$

$= 5.26\ L$

3. $FRC = \left[\dfrac{(0.095 - 0.055)}{0.055} \times 5.26\ L \right] - 0.1\ L$

4. $\qquad = (0.73 \times 5.25\ L) - 0.1\ L$

5. $\qquad = 3.84\ L - 0.1\ L$

6. $FRC = 3.74\ L\ (ATPS)$

Correcting to BTPS with appropriate correction factor from p. 335:

7. $FRC\ (BTPS) = 3.74 \times 1.08$

8. $FRC\ (BTPS) = 4.04\ L$

Single-breath $D_{L_{co}}$ (see Chapter 5)

Volume inspired (V_I):	4.0 L
F_{ICO}	0.003
$F_{ACO_{T2}}$:	0.00125
F_IHe:	0.10
F_EHe	0.075
P_B:	760 mm Hg
Breath-hold time ($T_2 - T_1$):	10.0 sec
Spirometer temperature:	25° C
Hb:	10.0 g/dl
COHb:	5.5%

1. $D_{L_{co}}SB = \dfrac{V_A \times 60}{(P_B - 47)(T_2 - T_1)} \times Ln\left(\dfrac{F_{ACO_{T1}}}{F_{ACO_{T2}}}\right)$

2. $V_A = \dfrac{V_I}{F_EHe/F_IHe}$

$= \dfrac{4.0\ L}{0.075/0.10}$

$= 5.33\ L\ (5333\ ml)$

3. $F_{ACO_{T1}} = F_{ICO} \times F_EHe/F_IHe$

$= 0.003 \times \dfrac{0.075}{0.10}$

$= 0.0025$

4. $D_{L_{co}}SB = \dfrac{5333\ ml \times 60\ sec}{(713\ mm\ Hg) \times (10.0\ sec)} \times Ln\left(\dfrac{0.0025}{0.00125}\right)$

5. $\qquad = \dfrac{319980}{7130} \times Ln\ (1.8)$

6. $\qquad = 44.9\ ml/min/mm\ Hg \times (0.5878)$

7. $D_{L_{co}}SB = 26.38\ ml\ CO/min/mm\ Hg\ (ATPS)$

This value is ATPS and is normally converted to STPD (0° C, 760 mm Hg, dry). The correction factor can be calculated as follows:

8. STPD correction factor $= \dfrac{273}{273 + T\ °C} \times \dfrac{P_B - P_{H_2O}\ T\ °C}{760}$

where:

T °C = spirometer temperature

P_{H_2O} T °C = partial pressure of water vapor at the spirometer temperature
(in this case: 24 mm Hg at 25° C)

9. STPD Correction factor $= \dfrac{273}{273 + 25} \times \dfrac{760 - 24}{760}$

10. $\qquad\qquad = 0.916 \times 0.968 = 0.887$

$\qquad\qquad = 0.887$

11. $D_{L_{CO}}SB = (26.38$ ml CO/min/mm Hg$) \times (0.887)$

$\qquad\qquad = 23.4$ ml CO/min/mm Hg (STPD)

This value should also be corrected for the Hb, in this case 10 g/dl:

12. Hb correction $= \dfrac{10.22 + Hb}{1.7 \times Hb}$

$\qquad = \dfrac{10.22 + 10.0}{1.7 \times 10.0}$

$\qquad = 1.19$

13. $D_{L_{CO}}SB$ (corrected) $= (1.19) \times (23.4)$

$\qquad\qquad = 27.9$ ml CO/min/mm Hg (STPD)

If the COHb level is known, the $D_{L_{CO}}SB$ can be corrected for the back pressure of CO:

14. COHb adjusted $D_{L_{CO}} =$ Measured $D_{L_{CO}} \times \left(1.00 + \dfrac{\%COHb}{100}\right)$

15. $\qquad\qquad = 27.9 \times \left(1.00 + \dfrac{5.5}{100}\right)$

16. COHb adjusted $D_{L_{CO}} = 29.4$ ml CO/min/mm Hg (STPD)

Thoracic Gas Volume (V_{TG}) (see Chapter 3)

Data for V_{TG} and Raw are from the same subject.

V_{TG}	Unknown
V_{TG} tangents	0.71 (angle 35.4)
	0.73 (angle 36.1)
	0.73 (angle 36.1)
P_B	755 mm Hg
Subject weight	71 Kg
P_{MOUTH} calibration	10 cm H_2O/cm
P_{BOX} calibration	30 ml/cm
Deadspace correction	100 ml
Plethysmograph volume	530 L

1. Average V_{TG} tangent (TAN) $= \dfrac{(0.71 + 0.73 + 0.73)}{3}$

$\qquad\qquad = 0.72$

The barometric pressure correction is calculated as follows:

2. $P_{B_{corr}} = (P_B - 47) \times 1.36$

$\qquad = (755$ mm Hg $- 47$ mm Hg$) \times 1.36$

$\qquad = 963$ cm H_2O

The subject volume correction (K) is calculated as follows:

3. $K = \dfrac{[\text{Pleth volume} - (\text{Subject weight}/1.07)]}{\text{Pleth volume}}$

$\quad = \dfrac{[530\ L - (71\ kg/1.07)]}{530\ L}$

$\quad = 0.874$

4. $V_{TG} = \left(\dfrac{P_{B_{corr}}}{TAN} \times \dfrac{P_{boxcal}}{P_{MOUTHcal}} \times K \right) - \text{Dead space}$

5. $= \left(\dfrac{963 \text{ cm H}_2\text{O}}{0.72} \times \dfrac{30 \text{ ml/cm}}{10 \text{ cm H}_2\text{O/cm}} \times 0.874 \right) - 100 \text{ ml}$

After cancelling like terms in the numerator and denominator (cm, cm H$_2$O):

6. $= (1338 \times 3 \text{ ml} \times 0.874) - 100 \text{ ml}$

$V_{TG} = 3408 \text{ ml } (3.41\text{L})$

Airway Resistance (Raw) and Conductance (SGaw) (see Chapter 2)

Raw:	Unknown
P_m/P_{BOX} TAN:	0.61 (angle = 31)
$\dot{V}/P_{BOX}$ TAN:	3.0 (angle = 72)
P_{MOUTH} calibration:	10 cm H$_2$O/cm
P_{BOX} calibration:	30 ml/cm
$\dot{V}$ calibration:	1.0 L/sec/cm
R_{sys}:	0.25 cm H$_2$O/L/sec

1. $\text{Raw} = \left(\dfrac{P_{MOUTH}/P_{BOX} TAN}{\dot{V}/P_{BOX} TAN} \times \dfrac{P_{MOUTHcal}}{\dot{V}_{cal}} \right) - R_{sys}$

2. $= \left(\dfrac{0.61}{3.0} \times \dfrac{10 \text{ cm H}_2\text{O/cm}}{1.0 \text{ L/sec/cm}} \right) - 0.25$

3. $= (0.203 \times 10) - 0.25$

4. $\text{Raw} = 1.78 \text{ cm H}_2\text{O/L/sec}$

Several repetitions of the panting maneuver are usually performed. Unlike the V_{TG} maneuver, however, tangents are not averaged. Because flow and volume tangents influence each other, Raw is calculated and then averaged. To calculate SGaw (specific airway conductance), the volume at which each Raw maneuver was performed is calculated as for V_{TG}, using the P_{MOUTH}/P_{BOX} tangent from the specific maneuver. In this example:

1. $\text{SGaw} = (1/\text{Raw})/V_{TG}$

2. $V_{TG} = \left(\dfrac{963 \text{ cm H}_2\text{O}}{0.61} \times \dfrac{30 \text{ ml/cm}}{10 \text{ cm H}_2\text{O/cm}} \times 0.874 \right) - 100$

3. $= (1579 \times 3 \text{ ml} \times 0.874) - 100$

4. $= 4040 \text{ ml } (4.04\text{L})$

Calculating the SGaw:

5. $\text{SGaw} = (1/1.78 \text{ cm H}_2\text{O/L/sec})/4.04 \text{ L}$

6. $= 0.14 \text{ cm H}_2\text{O/L/sec/L}$

The average of three to five maneuvers is usually reported, after the SGaw for individual efforts has been calculated.

Exercise Study (see Chapter 7)

Volume exhaled (V)	20.0 L (ATPS)
Collection time (sec)	60 sec
Temperature (T)	24° C
F_{EO_2}	0.17
F_{ECO_2}	0.03
f_b	25/min
HR	100/min
Pa_{O_2}	95 mm Hg
Pa_{CO_2}	35 mm Hg
P_B	750 mm Hg
Mechanical V_D	18 ml (0.018 L)
Subject's weight	55 kg

The first step is to calculate conversion factors to correct ventilation and gas exchange measurements to BTPS and STPD, respectively. This STPD factor is for conversion from BTPS:

$$1. \ \text{BTPS factor} = \frac{P_B - P_{H_2O}}{P_B - 47} \times \frac{273 + 37}{273 + T}$$

$$= \frac{721}{703} \times \frac{310}{297}$$

$$= 1.07$$

$$2. \ \text{STPD factor} = \frac{P_B - 47}{760} \times \frac{273}{273 + 37}$$

$$= \frac{703}{760} \times 0.881$$

$$= 0.815$$

Next, parameters of ventilation may be calculated as follows:

$$3. \ \dot{V}_E \ (\text{BTPS}) = \frac{V_{exhaled} \times 60}{\text{Collection time in seconds}} \times \text{BTPS factor}$$

$$= \frac{20.0 \ \text{L} \times 60}{60} \times 1.07$$

$$= 21.4 \ \text{L (BTPS)}$$

$$4. \ V_T \ (\text{BTPS}) = \frac{\dot{V}_E \ (\text{BTPS})}{f_b}$$

$$= \frac{21.4}{25}$$

$$= 0.856 \ \text{L (BTPS)}$$

$$5. \ V_D \ (\text{BTPS}) = V_T \ (\text{BTPS}) \times \left[1 - \frac{F_{ECO_2} \times (P_B - 47)}{Pa_{CO_2}} \right] - V_{D_{mech}}$$

$$= 0.856 \times \left[1 - \frac{0.03 \times 703}{35} \right] - 0.018$$

$$= 0.856 \times [1 - 0.603] - 0.018$$

$$= (0.856 \times 0.397) - 0.018$$

$$= 0.340 - 0.018$$

$$= 0.322 \ \text{L}$$

$$6. \ \dot{V}_A \ (\text{BTPS}) = \dot{V}_E \ (\text{BTPS}) - [f_b \times V_D \ (\text{BTPS})]$$

$$= 21.4 - [25 \times 0.322]$$

$$= 21.4 - 8.05$$

$$= 13.4 \ \text{L}$$

$$7. \ V_D/V_T = \frac{0.322}{0.856}$$

$$= 0.38$$

Next, gas exchange parameters are computed as follows:

$$8. \ \dot{V}_E \ (\text{STPD}) = \dot{V}_E \ (\text{BTPS}) \times \text{STPD factor}$$

$$= 21.4 \times 0.815$$

$$= 17.4 \ \text{L}$$

9.

$$\dot{V}_{O_2} \text{ (STPD)} = \left[\left(\frac{1 - F_{EO_2} - F_{ECO_2}}{1 - F_{IO_2}} \times F_{IO_2}\right) - F_{EO_2}\right] \times \dot{V}_E \text{ (STPD)}$$

$$= \left[\left(\frac{1 - 0.17 - 0.03}{1 - 0.2093} \times 0.2093\right) - 0.17\right] \times 17.4$$

$$= \left[\left(\frac{0.80}{0.79} \times 0.2093\right) - 0.17\right] \times 17.4$$

$$= [(1.01 \times 0.2093) - 0.17] \times 17.4$$

$$= [0.212 - 0.17] \times 17.4$$

$$= 0.042 \times 17.4$$

$$\dot{V}_{O_2} \text{ (STPD)} = 0.731 \text{ L}$$

10.

$$\dot{V}_{CO_2} \text{ (STPD)} = (F_{ECO_2} - 0.0003) \times \dot{V}_E \text{ (STPD)}$$

$$= (0.03 - 0.0003) \times 17.4$$

$$= 0.297 \times 17.4$$

$$= 0.517 \text{ L}$$

11.

$$R = \frac{\dot{V}_{CO_2} \text{ (STPD)}}{\dot{V}_{O_2} \text{ (STPD)}}$$

$$= \frac{0.517}{0.731}$$

$$= 0.71$$

12.

$$\dot{V}_E/\dot{V}_{O_2} = \frac{\dot{V}_E \text{ (BTPS)}}{\dot{V}_{O_2} \text{ (STPD)}}$$

$$= \frac{21.4}{0.731}$$

$$= 29.3 \text{ L/L } \dot{V}_{O_2}$$

13.

$$\dot{V}_{O_2}/HR = \frac{\dot{V}_{O_2} \text{ (STPD)}}{HR} \times 1000$$

$$= \frac{0.731 \text{ L/min}}{100 \text{ beats/min}} \times 1000$$

$$= 7.31 \text{ ml } O_2/\text{beat}$$

The calculation of energy expenditure at any particular workload is described by the term *METS*, for multiples of the resting $\dot{V}_{O_2}$. The MET level for any workload can be calculated by one of two methods. In each method:

14.

$$METS = \frac{\dot{V}_{O_2} \text{ (STPD) exercise}}{\dot{V}_{O_2} \text{ (STPD) rest}}$$

but the means of estimating $\dot{V}_{O_2}$ (STPD) at rest differs. $\dot{V}_{O_2}$ (STPD) at rest can be measured, or it may be estimated as 0.0035 L/min/kg (3.5 ml/kg). Using the second method in this example:

$$METS = \frac{0.731 \text{ L/min}}{0.0035 \text{ L/min/kg} \times 55 \text{ kg}}$$

$$= 3.80$$

If the subject's measured $\dot{V}_{O_2}$ at rest had been 0.225 L/min (STPD) then:

$$METS = \frac{0.731 \text{ L/min}}{0.225 \text{ L/min}}$$

$$= 3.25$$

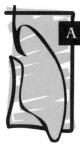

The Mean and the Standard Deviation

Calculation of the Mean and the Standard Deviation

The mean ($\overline{X}$) and standard deviation (SD) are computed to determine the variability of a series of values. The SD is affected by every value in the series, especially extreme values. If the values are normally distributed, that is, each value has an equal chance of appearing, the SD may be used to relate any subsequent value to the population of values already obtained. In the laboratory setting, this concept is often applied to determine the variability of blood gas electrodes or spirometers. Performing multiple measurements of the same quantity (i.e., the "control"), allows the mean to be determined and precision to be expressed by the SD of the measurements. Assuming that all of the values sampled are normally distributed, 68.3% of them will be within ±1 SD of the mean, 95.5% will be within ±2 SDs, and 99.7% within ±3 SDs. When the mean and standard deviation have been determined for a series of measurements, subsequent values may be checked to see if they are "in control." Values between ±2 and ±3 SDs from the mean should occur only 5% of the time, and values more than ±3 SDs from the mean should occur less than 1% of the time.

The mean ($\overline{X}$) is calculated as follows:

$$\overline{X} = \frac{\Sigma\,(X)}{N}$$

where:

Σ = a symbol meaning "the sum of"

X = individual data values

N = number of items sampled

The SD is calculated as follows:

$$SD = \sqrt{\frac{\Sigma\,(X^2)}{N}}$$

where:

X^2 = deviations from the mean (X − $\overline{X}$) squared

N = number of items sampled

If the SD is computed from a sample of 30 items or less, N-1 is substituted for N.

Example calculation of the mean and SD for a series of P_{CO_2} values:

Sample #	P_{CO_2} (mm Hg)	Deviation from mean (X)	Deviation squared (X^2)
1	39	−0.9	0.81
2	40	0.1	0.01
3	43	3.1	9.61
4	42	2.1	4.41
5	39	−0.9	0.81
6	38	−1.9	3.61
7	40	0.1	0.01
8	41	1.1	1.21
9	38	−1.9	3.61
10	39	−0.9	0.81
Total	399		24.90
Mean	39.9		2.49

$$SD = \sqrt{\frac{24.9}{(10-1)}}$$
$$= \sqrt{2.77}$$
$$= 1.66$$

The range of P_{CO_2} values (in this example) within 2 SDs of the mean is 39.9 ± (2 × 1.66) or from 36.6 to 43.2 mm Hg.

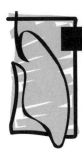

Glossary of Important Terms

(See also Pulmonary Terms and Symbols)

α₁-Antitrypsin An antienzyme that inhibits proteases in the blood; a genetically inherited deficiency can lead to emphysema

A/D converter Analog to digital converter

A-a gradient Difference in partial pressure of oxygen between the alveoli (A) and arterial blood (a)

absorbance The process of taking up or receiving

absorption To take up without reflecting (light or sound)

accuracy The extent to which a measurement is close to the true value

acidemia An increase in hydrogen ion concentration in the blood

acidosis An increase in the hydrogen ion concentration in the body

aerobic Referring to the production of energy by oxidative phosporylation

afterload The back pressure and/or volume of blood leaving the atrium or ventricle

agonist An agent which opposes or competes against another force

airway resistance (Raw) The pressure drop across the airways related to flow at the mouth (see Chapter 2)

airway obstruction Any process or disease that interferes with air flow into or out of the lungs

algorithm Rule of procedure for solving a mathematical problem that frequently involves repetition of an operation

alkalemia A decrease in hydrogen ion concentration in the blood

alkalosis A decrease in the hydrogen ion concentration in the body

Allen's test Momentary occlusion of the radial and ulnar arteries to establish adequacy of collateral circulation

ALS Amyotrophic lateral sclerosis; disease of the anterior horn cells of the spinal cord

alveolar ventilation That part of the total ventilation that participates in gas exchange at the alveolar level

alveolar Referring to the gas exchange units (alveoli) of the lung

alveolitis Inflammation of the alveoli, often allergic in origin

alveolocapillary Referring to the membrane of the lung which separate the gas exchange units (alveoli) from the pulmonary capillaries

amiodarone An antiarrhythmic agent used in the treatment of ventricular arrhythmias

anaerobic Without oxygen; in metabolism, the production of energy without oxidative phosphorylation

analog signal A signal which is proportionate to something else; a measurable quantity

anatomic dead space That part of the lung volume which is not part of the gas exchange units; the upper airway, trachea, and bronchi down to the level of respiratory bronchioles

anemia A lack of hemoglobin and/or red blood cells

aneurysm Localized abnormal dilatation of a blood vessel

angina Chest pain, usually associated with myocardial ischemia

antiarrhythmic A drug that corrects abnormal heart rhythms

anticholinergic Opposing or annulling the physiologic action of acetylcholine; inhibiting the parasympathetic nervous system

anticoagulated The property of blood that has been treated with a chemical that interferes with clotting

antihistamines Any of various compounds used for treating allergic reactions and cold symptoms by inactivating histamine

aortic stenosis Constriction of the aortic orifice at the cardiac base or narrowing of the aorta

apices Plural of apex; referring to the upper upper lobes and/or segments of the lungs in an upright subject

apnea Absence of breathing

arm span The distance from finger-tip to finger-tip with arms outstretched

arrhythmia A disordered cardiac rhythm

asbestosis Fibrotic lung disease caused by inhalation of asbestos fibers

asthma Obstructive airway disease characterized by reversible airway narrowing, mucus hypersecretion, inflammation, and episodic shortness of breath

atelectasis A state of fluid filled or collapsed alveoli

ATPS Ambient temperature, pressure, and saturation (water vapor)

β-Adrenergic Stimulating the sympathetic nervous system β-receptors

β-Blocker A drug that blocks or inhibits the β-receptors in the sympathetic nervous system

back pressure Pressure caused by resistance to flow in a tube or vessel

balance To bring into equilibrium; in reference to an instrument, to adjust the starting point or "zero"

berylliosis Fibrotic lung disease produced by inhalation of dust from beryllium

bias In statistics, the systematic distortion of a measurement caused by the sampling process; also error

bicarbonate A buffer present in blood and other body solutions

biologic control Use of healthy human subjects as a standard for measuring actual performance of an instrument or procedure

black lung Legal term describing chronic respiratory disease in a coal miner

bleomycin A potent chemotherapeutic agent used in the management of lung cancer

BMR Basal metabolic rate; the metabolic rate (i.e., oxygen consumption) of a healthy subject at rest

bolus A large mass or amount

brachial Refers to the brachial artery, a site for arterial puncture

breath-by-breath Refers to measurement of respiratory variables on each breathing cycle

bronchiectasis A pulmonary obstructive disease characterized by destruction of the bronchial walls

bronchiolitis obliterans An obstructive lung disease in which small airways are almost completely destroyed

bronchochallenge Any pulmonary function study that attempts to induce constriction of the airways, usually to demonstrate the presence of asthma

bronchoconstriction Spasm of the airways causing a narrowing of the lumen

bronchodilator Any drug or agent that opens the airways to promote increased airflow

bronchoscopy Visualization of the airways via a tube or optical fibers

bronchospasm Constriction of the smooth muscle surrounding the airways resulting in obstruction

BSA Body surface area, usually measured in square meters

buffer A solution that will maintain a given pH despite addition of small amounts of base or acid

bullectomy Excision of large dilated air sacs (bullae) from the lungs

bullous Having bullae or large air sacs; refers to a type of emphysema in which the alveoli are very large and overdistended

bundle branch block Interruption of electrical conduction in one of the bundle branches of the cardiac system

calorimetry Measurement of the heat produced by an object

canned text In computing, a phrase or statement generated automatically upon request

capnography The measurement and/or recording of the exhaled carbon dioxide (CO_2)

carbon monoxide An odorless, tasteless, colorless gas capable of combining chemically with hemoglobin approximately 210 times more readily than oxygen; CO

carbonic acid Acid produced by the hydration of carbon dioxide

carboxyhemoglobin Compound resulting from the combination of carbon monoxide (CO) gas and hemoglobin (Hb)

cardiac output The volume of blood pumped by the heart per minute

cardiomyopathy Chronic disease of the heart muscle that may involve hypertrophy and obstructive disease of the heart

cathode The negative pole of an electrolytic cell

chemotherapy The use of chemical agents in the treatment or control of disease, usually cancer

CHF Congestive heart failure

chronic bronchitis Obstructive lung disease characterized by chronic cough and mucus production on most days for at least three months for two consecutive years

claustrophobia Fear of being in a small enclosed space or area

closing capacity The volume (as a portion of total lung capacity) remaining in the lungs when airways begin to close

co-oximeter A spectrophotometer designed for analyzing the various forms of hemoglobin

CO_2 narcosis Sleepiness or somnolence caused by high levels of carbon dioxide in the blood

CO_2 absorber A device for removing carbon dioxide from a breathing circuit; usually a chemical absorber

CO_2 production Measurement of the volume of carbon dioxide excreted by the tissues per minute; usually measured during exercise or metabolic studies (see Chapters 7 and 8)

COHb Carboxyhemoglobin; the fraction of Hb bound by carbon monoxide

compliance The distensibility of the lungs; volume change per unit of pressure change (see Chapter 2)

control A system or device for establishing standards and measuring actual performance or comparing results

COPD Chronic obstructive pulmonary disease

cor pulmonale Right-sided heart failure caused by lung disease

corticosteroids Any of various adrenal cortex steroids

couplet Two premature ventricular contractions in a row

cromolyn sodium A drug that prevents bronchospasm, presumably by stabilizing Mast cells in the airways, preventing release of inflammatory agents

C_{rs} Respiratory system compliance

CV In statistics, coefficient of variation; the standard deviation divided by the mean for a sample measurement

cyanosis Bluish coloration of the nailbeds or skin associated with hypoxemia; caused by elevated levels of reduced hemoglobin

cycle ergometer A stationary bicycle designed specifically for exercise testing; ergometers allow work to be estimated

cyclosporine A potent drug used to suppress tissue rejection in organ transplantation

cystic fibrosis A hereditary disorder of the exocrine glands characterized by deficiency in pancreatic enzymes and respiratory symptoms

$\Delta\%N_{2\ 750-1250}$ Delta percent change in nitrogen from the 750 to 1250 ml points of the SBN_2 test

damping Attenuation of a signal such that it no longer accurately represents a phenomenon

dead space The volume of the lung that is ventilated but not perfused by pulmonary capillary blood flow

debilitated Weakened or having impaired strength

deconditioning The effects of lack of exercise, usually including elevated heart rate and blood pressure and muscular inefficiency

defibrillator A device used to shock the heart when fibrillation is present

demand valve A device which opens in response to volume, flow, or pressure changes

denervated Having the nerves to a specific organ disabled or cut

desaturation Reduction of oxygen level caused by dissociation of O_2 from Hb

desiccant A drying agent

dessicator A device for chemically removing water vapor from a gas

diaphragmatic Related to the diaphragm

diastolic Referring to blood pressure while the ventricle is filling (diastole)

diffusing capacity ($D_{L_{CO}}$) The capacity of the lungs to transfer carbon monoxide in ml/min/mm Hg (see Chapter 5)

diffusion Movement of a gas through a gaseous or liquid medium, dependent on the molecular weight and solubility of the gas

diluent A diluting agent

diuretics A class of drugs that promote fluid excretion

dosimeter A device for delivering a precise dosage of a drug

drift In electronics, to vary or deviate from a set adjustment; variation in the output of an instrument

droplet nuclei Aerosol particles containing viral, bacterial, or myocbacterial pathogens

dynamic hyperinflation Increased lung volume that occurs during breathing or forced breathing, as with exercise

dynamic compression The collapse of airways caused by a pressure gradient that occurs with breathing or forced breathing

dysfunction Improper or incorrect action

dyspnea Shortness of breath; difficult or labored respiration

dyspnea index Minute ventilation during exercise expressed as a fraction of the MVV

ECG Electrocardiogram; a recording of the heart's electrical activity

echocardiography The use of high-frequency sound waves to image the heart

ectopic Misplaced or unusual; in the heart, any beat not originating from the S-A node

edema Leakage of fluids from blood vessels caused by imbalance in pressures

EELV End-expiratory lung volume; the volume in the lungs at the end of a breath, usually the FRC; denotes a dynamic lung volume which may change with the level of activity (exercise)

effusion A leakage of fluid into a body space or tissue

EIA Exercise-induced asthma

EIB Exercise-induced bronchospasm

Eisenmenger's syndrome A congenital abnormality involving the heart and great vessels; pulmonary hypertension is usually severe

ejection fraction The portion of the ventricular volume ejected during systole

electrode A device used to establish electrical contact with a nonmetallic part of a circuit; in electrochemistry, a device to measure current or voltage during chemical analysis

electrolyte Any nonmetallic substance that when dissolved in a suitable solvent allows current to flow by movement of ions

emboli Multiple blood clots that travel from their site of origin to lodge in another blood vessel

emphysema Obstructive airway disease characterized by destruction of alveolar walls and collapse of small airways; may be accompanied by air trapping and hyperinflation of the lungs

end-tidal Referring to gas collected at the end of a quiet breath, usually assumed to represent alveolar gas

enteral Passing through the stomach and intestines

eucapnic Maintaining a normal level of carbon dioxide in the lungs and blood

explosive decompression A process or device that uses rapid expansion of gas to generate a known flow

exponential A number placed to the right of and above another number denoting the power to which that number is to be raised

exudate A fluid accumulation caused by infection or inflammation

false negative The result of a test or examination in which a diagnosis is incorrectly overlooked

false positive The result of a test or examination in which the diagnosis is incorrectly supported

febrile Having a fever

fibrillation Rapid, tremulous contractions of muscles; often used to describe a serious cardiac arrhythmia

fibrosis Scarring of tissue caused by chemical or biological agents, repeated infection or inflammation, as in pulmonary fibrosis

fibrotic Referring to the presence of scar tissue or fibrous changes related to inflammation and healing

Fick method A means of determining cardiac output by measuring oxygen consumption and arteriovenous oxygen content difference

F_{IO_2} Fractional concentration of inspired oxygen

flow-volume loop A plot of maximal inspiratory and expiratory flows versus FVC and FIVC on a single graph or display

fractional Used to describe the concentration of one or more gases in a mixture, expressed as a decimal fraction

frequency response The ability of an instrument to detect a changing signal, dependent on the signal's frequency

full scale Referring to entire range over which an instrument is capable of measuring

gain The amplification of a signal from an instrument

glottis Elongated space between the vocal cords; also the structure surrounding this space

goiter Enlargement of the thyroid gland

gradient Change in the value of a quantity with change in a given variable

Guillain-Barré A progressive disease of the peripheral nerves

half-life The time required for half of a substance to deteriorate

Hb Hemoglobin concentration, usually expressed in ml/dl

hematocrit Ratio of volume of packed red cells to volume of whole blood

hemoglobin An iron-containing conjugated protein respiratory pigment occurring in the red blood cells of vertebrates

hemolysis The process or condition in which red blood cells are broken open

hemoptysis Coughing up of blood

hemorrhage Copious discharge of blood from blood vessels

heparin A substance that inhibits blood clotting, commonly used to preserve blood specimens

hilar Related to the hilum, or roots of the lungs

histamine Chemical compound ($C_5H_9N_3$) that causes dilatation and increased permeability of blood vessels which play a role in allergic reactions

honeycombing Resembling or having a honeycomb pattern; usually seen on chest x-ray examination

hypercapnia Higher than normal level of carbon dioxide; usually greater than 45 mm Hg in arterial blood

hyperinflation Overinflation of the lungs; usually denoted by an increased total lung capacity above the upper limit of normal (120%)

hyperpnea Rapid breathing

hyperreactive Excessively responsive to stimulation

hyperventilation Ventilation in excess of CO_2 production resulting in respiratory alkalosis

hypocapnia A low level of carbon dioxide in arterial blood

hypotension Low blood pressure, usually less than 90/50

hypothermic Having a temperature below normal; usually below 37° C

hypoventilation Inadequate ventilation to remove CO_2 resulting in respiratory acidosis

hypoxemia Abnormally low level of oxygen in the blood

hypoxia Inadequate oxygen to meet tissue demands

idiopathic Describing a finding or syndrome that is self-originated or arising spontaneously from an unknown cause

in vivo Referring to measurements or observations made in the living organism

incremental Referring to exercise tests that increase the workload by fixed amounts over given intervals

infiltrates Abnormal fluid filling tissues or spaces

infrared Lying outside the visible spectrum at its red end

integration The operation of solving a differential equation; specifically to find the area under a curve

interstitial lung disease A group of lung disorders characterized by infiltrates, inflammation of the alveolar walls, loss of lung volume, and exertional dyspnea

ischemic Having decreased blood flow

isocapnia A normal level of carbon dioxide, usually in the blood

isothermal lung analog A glass jar or container filled with copper or steel wool, used for quality control of a body plethysmograph

Kb Kilobyte; 1024 bytes

ketosis The presence or process of ketones in the body or blood

kilopascal Unit of pressure measurement in the International System; 1 mm Hg = 0.133 kilopascals

kinetics The activity of some object; in exercise testing refers to gas exchange patterns (oxygen uptake, CO_2 production)

kpm Kilopond-meters; the work of moving a 1 kg mass 1 meter vertically against the force of gravity

kymograph A recording device, usually a rotating drum, on which a graph of motion or pressure may be traced

kyphoscoliosis A combination of anterior-posterior and lateral curvature of the spine

kyphosis Abnormal curvature of the spine anteriorly

lactate See **lactic acid**

lactic acid An acid produced by anaerobic metabolism at high levels of work

laminar flow Streamline flow in a viscous fluid or gas near a solid boundary

large airway obstruction Any process or disease that limits flow in the upper airway, trachea, or mainstem bronchi

laryngoscope A device used to visualize the larynx and vocal cords, specifically for intubating the trachea

LED A light-emitting diode

linear Referring to a system in which a given input produces a consistent output

linear regression A statistical procedure in which a straight line is established through a data set that best represents a relationship between two subsets or methods

linearity The ability to produce a proportional output for a given input across a fixed range

lipogenesis Formation of fat, usually from carbohydrate

lobectomy Surgical excision of the lobe of an organ such as the lung

logarithm The exponent that indicates the power to which a number is raised to produce a given number

luminescence An emission of light produced by physiologic or chemical processes

lung reduction A surgical procedure in which poorly perfused lung tissue is removed

lung transplantation Removal of one or both native lungs and replacement with lungs from a donor

lupus erythematosus Slowly progressive systemic disease characterized by degenerative changes of the collagenous tissues

manometer A device for measuring pressure using a tube marked with a scale and containing a fluid (mercury or water); level of the fluid varies with the pressure applied above it

maximal expiration The point at which no further air can be exhaled from the lungs

maximal inspiration The point at which the lungs are completely filled

Mb Megabytes; 1024 kilobytes

MDI Metered-dose inhaler; a small canister containing a propellent gas to deliver bronchodilator medication

mediastinal Located in or near the mediastinum

medullary centers Those areas of the medulla oblongata that are responsible for controlling the rate and depth of breathing

metabolic acidosis An acid-base imbalance characterized by a pH less than 7.35 resulting from accumulation of acid other than that produced by carbon dioxide

metabolic alkalosis An acid-base imbalance characterized by a pH greater than 7.45 resulting from a loss of acid (other than that caused by CO_2) or to an accumulation of bases

metabolism The process of breaking down food substrates to produce energy

methacholine A potent chemical which increases parasympathetic muscle tone in the airways when inhaled; used to induce bronchoconstriction to test for hyperreactivity of the airways

MetHb Methemoglobin; the fraction of Hb in which the iron atoms have been oxidized to the Fe^{+++} state

METS Metabolic equivalents based on a multiple of resting oxygen consumption; usually equal to an oxygen consumption of 3.5 ml/min/kg of body weight

microprocessor An integrated circuit capable of performing logical and mathematical calculations; the primary component of a computer

minute ventilation The total volume of gas moved in and out of the lungs each minute; also called the minute volume

mixed expired Referring to gas collected that includes dead space and alveolar gas; usually collected in a bag, balloon, or spirometer

mixing chamber A container with baffles for collecting expired gas for analysis

molar Units of measure for concentration of solute in a solvent based on the number of moles (gram molecular weight) of solute

morbidity The state or quality of being affected by disease

mouthpiece A device that connects a subject to the breathing circuit for pulmonary function tests

MRI Magnetic resonance imaging; a type of scan that evaluates structures subjected to strong magnetic fields

Müller's maneuver Production of negative intrathoracic pressure by closing the glottis and making a forced inspiratory effort

multifocal Refers to ectopic beats of the heart arising from different locations (foci)

myasthenia gravis A disease of the neuromuscular system characterized by progressive weakness, often episodic; neck, throat, and facial muscles may be primarily affected

myocardial Related to the heart muscle

myxedema A dry, waxy swelling of the skin or other tissues associated with hypothyroidism

natural logarithm A logarithm with e (2.71828) as its base

neoplasm Cancer, usually a tumor

neuromuscular Related to the nerves, muscles, or the junction of the two

nodal Referring to cardiac rhythms originating in the A-V node

normal distribution In statistics, the even distribution of data points on either side of the mean; a Gaussian distribution

normoxia An adequate level of oxygen, usually an F_{IO_2} of 0.21

nose clips A spring-like device used to compress the nose and prevent nasal breathing during pulmonary function testing

O_2 consumption Measurement of the volume of oxygen used by the tissues per minute; usually measured during exercise or metabolic studies (see Chapters 7 and 8)

O_2 pulse The volume of oxygen (ml) consumed per heartbeat

O_2Hb Oxyhemoglobin saturation; the fraction of Hb bound with oxygen

obesity-hypoventilation A syndrome characterized by chronic respiratory acidosis in a subject who is overweight

obstruction Any process that interferes with air flow into or out of the lungs

obstructive sleep apnea (OSA) A syndrome in which the subject experiences cessation of airflow caused by blockage of the upper airway during sleep

occlusion pressure The pressure generated during the first 100 msec of a breath against an occluded airway; also called P_{100} or $P_{0.1}$

occupational lung disease Pulmonary disease related to exposure in the workplace

optode An optical electrode

orthopnea Difficulty breathing related to body position; especially, shortness of breath while lying supine

oscilloscope An instrument in which variations in a fluctuating electrical signal appear as a wave on a fluorescent screen; used to display electrical signals analogous to physiologic waveforms

OSHA Occupational Safety and Health Administration

out-of-control The state or condition when an instrument does not perform measurements accurately or precisely

oxidation-reduction A chemical process in which one element gives up electrons (oxidation) while another element receives them (reduction)

oximetry The measurement, either directly or indirectly, of the oxygen saturation of the blood

oxygen uptake $\dot{V}_{O_2}$ or the volume of oxygen consumed per minute

pallor Lack of color, paleness

parallel port A computer connection in which data words are transmitted, rather than individual bits of data

parasympathetic Relating to that part of the autonomic nervous system that contains chiefly cholinergic fibers and increases the tone/contractility of smooth muscle

parenchyma The essential and distinctive tissue of an organ such as the lung

parenteral Nourishment occurring outside of the stomach and intestines

pathogen Any microorganism capable of producing disease

PD_{20} Provocative dose of a drug which causes a 20% change in a specified variable

peak flow meter Any device that can register PEF

pectus excavatum An abnormal depression of the sternum

percent grade Referring to a treadmill or similar device; describes the slope of the walking surface

percutaneously Through the skin

pericarditis Inflammation of the pericardium

PET Positron emission tomography; a type of scan capable of imaging metabolically active organ structures

pH Negative logarithm of the hydrogen ion concentration used as a positive number

phase delay The time interval between when an event occurs and when it is registered by an instrument or analyzer; also, the delay between the response times of two separate instruments

phlegm Mucus that is coughed up

Pitot tube A tube that has a short, right-angled bend placed vertically in a moving body of air; the mouth of the bent part is directed upstream and uses a manometer to measure velocity of flow (Henri Pitot, 1771)

plethysmograph From the Greek "plethys" for pressure; any device for recording pressure. In pulmonary function testing, a boxlike device in which the patient sits to measure pressure and volume changes in the lung (see Chapters 2 and 3)

pleura The lining of the lungs and thoracic cavity

pleurisy Inflammation of the pleural surfaces

pneumoconiosis Lung disease related to inhalation of dust

Pneumocystis carinii A microorganism that causes pneumocystosis, a type of interstitial cell pneumonitis

pneumonectomy Surgical excision of a lung

pneumonitis Inflammation of airways and alveoli caused by irritants or infection

pneumotachometer Any device used to measure gas flow; in pulmonary function testing, a device used to measure flow and its integral volume

pneumothorax A partial or total collapse of the lung caused by entry of air into the pleural space

polarographic Referring to an electrode that is polarized by applying a voltage between an anode and cathode in order to make a measurement

potentiometer An instrument for measuring electromotive forces

precision The extent to which an instrument measures a known value repeatedly; reproducibility

precordial Refers to the position of ECG leads on the patient's chest over the heart

predicted value The expected or reference value for a lung function test; usually derived from studying a large population of healthy subjects

preload The pressure and/or volume of blood entering the atrium or ventricle

proficiency testing The process of comparing measurements of a known value from different sources to establish a level of accuracy

pulmonary hypertension Elevated blood pressure in the pulmonary vascular system; usually a mean pulmonary artery pressure greater than 35 mm Hg

pulmonary embolism A blood clot arising in the venous system that breaks loose and then lodges in the pulmonary vascular system

pulse oximetry Estimation of arterial saturation by analysis of light absorption of blood pulsing through a capillary bed (finger or ear lobe)

PVC Premature ventricular contraction

Qc Pulmonary capillary blood volume

quality control The process of establishing the accuracy, precision, or other desired output of a procedure or measurement

RR interval The distance or time between successive R waves on the ECG; used to calculate heart rate

radiation therapy The use of radioactive substances to treat disease, often used in cancer therapy

RAM Random access memory; must be periodically refreshed or data are lost

ramp test An exercise test in which the workload is increased continuously rather than incrementally

random error Variability of a measurement outside of accepted limits that occurs in a nonreproducible fashion

rebreathing Referring to or describing a system which allows the subject to breathe continuously while measurements are made

REE Resting energy expenditure; the caloric needs of the body estimated from oxygen consumption and carbon dioxide production usually expressed in kcal/24 hours (see Chapter 8)

reference equation An equation used to predict an expected value for a particular test parameter

refractory period An interval that is resistant to treatment or change

regression A statistical method for estimating one variable based on the progression of another variable

RER Respiratory exchange ratio; the ratio of carbon dioxide produced to oxygen consumed per minute

resection Surgical removal of part of an organ or structure

respiratory acidosis An acid-base imbalance characterized by a pH less than 7.35 because of an increased level of carbon dioxide in the blood

respiratory alkalosis An acid-base imbalance characterized by a pH greater than 7.45 because of excessive ventilation

respirometer A device for measuring breathing

restriction Any process that interferes with the bellows action of the lungs or chest, usually with a loss of lung volume

restrictive disease Any process or disease that interferes with the bellows action of the lungs, the chest wall, or both

reverse isolation Isolation procedures designed to protect the patient from infectious organisms carried by staff or visitors

ROM Read only memory; data are stored even when power to the device is suspended

RQ Respiratory quotient; the ratio of carbon dioxide produced to oxygen consumed at the cell level

RQnp Nonprotein RQ; the respiratory quotient produced by metabolism of fats and carbohydrates

Rrs Respiratory system resistance (infants)

RTC Rapid thoracoabdominal compression; use of a squeeze jacket to cause forced expiration in infants

ST segment A portion of the electrical conduction pattern of the ECG; used to assess cardiac ischemia

sarcoidosis Chronic disease of unknown origin characterized by formation of nodules resembling true tubercles, especially in lymph nodes, lungs, bones, and skin

scleroderma A disease primarily of the skin, characterized by thickening and hardening of subcutaneous tissues

scoliosis Abnormal curvature of the spine laterally

scrubber See CO_2 absorber

SD Standard deviation; in statistics, a mathematical statement of dispersion of a set of values from the mean

semilog Semilogarithmic; referring to a graph or display on which one axis is represented by a logarithmic scale while the other axis is arithmetic

sensitivity In medicine, the ability of a test or examination to detect the presence of disease

serial port A computer connection in which data are transmitted one bit at a time at a rapid rate

shunt A bypass; in the lungs, an area in which blood flows through the lungs without coming into contact with alveolar gas

silicosis Fibrotic lung disease caused by inhalation of silica dust

sine-wave pump A pump that uses a circular motion, such as a flywheel, to produce output that varies above and below a set level in a regular fashion

slope To adjust the output or gain of an instrument

small airways In the lungs, airways less than 2 mm in diameter; these airways are supported by surrounding alveolar structures

solenoids A cylinder containing a wire coil with a movable core; the core moves when an electrical current is applied

solubility coefficient A number that describes the volume of one substance that will dissolve in another substance under given conditions

span To adjust or confirm the measuring range of an instrument

specificity In medicine, the ability of a test or examination to exclude those who do not have a specific disease or disorder

spectrophotometer A device for analyzing chemical composition by measuring light intensity at various wavelengths

spirometer Any device used to measure lung volumes and flows

spreadsheet In computing, a program that allows entry of data and formulas to provide calculations

steady-state test In exercise testing, refers to tests conducted long enough for cardiopulmonary variables to reach a state of equilibrium

sternotomy A surgical procedure which involves opening the chest cavity through the sternum

STPD Standard temperature (0° C), pressure (760 mm Hg), dry

stridor High-pitched noise from the upper airway, usually on inspiration

suppurative To form or discharge mucus or pus

SV Stroke volume

Swan-Ganz catheter A balloon-tipped catheter which can be floated through the right atrium and ventricle into the pulmonary artery

systolic Referring to the blood pressure during ventricular contraction (systole)

tangent A number which describes the slope of a line

tension pneumothorax A pneumothorax in which the pressure within the chest exceeds atmospheric pressure

theophylline A drug related to caffeine and theobromine that promotes bronchodilatation

thermistor A resistor that is sensitive to temperature changes; used for measurement of gas or blood flow

thermodilution Refers to a method of determining cardiac output by measuring temperature change of a solution injected into the right atrium and passing into the pulmonary artery

thoracotomy A surgical procedure in which the thorax is opened

thrombophlebitis Inflammation of a vein, developing before the formation of a thrombus

thrombi Formation of a blood clot

tidal volume The volume of gas moved in and out of the lung with each breath

tonometer An instrument used to measure or establish pressure of a gas in a liquid

tonometering The process of equilibrating a gas dissolved in a solution

tracer Referring to an element used to track or measure another element, as in a tracer gas

transcutaneous Referring to a measurement made through the skin

transducer Any device that produces a signal (electrical voltage or current) in response to a physiologic phenomenon such as pressure or sound

transudate A fluid accumulation caused by pressure imbalance

treadmill A device that incorporates a motor-driven belt on which walking, jogging, or running can be performed

trigger Something that sets another thing in motion; in asthma, the agent that causes the reaction to begin

tuberculosis A chronic granulomatous infection caused by an acid-fast bacillus *Mycobacterium tuberculosis*; usually affecting the lungs and transmitted by droplet nuclei

universal precautions Standards for handling blood or specimens containing blood when there is possibility of infection

upgrade In computing, the process of changing software or hardware to a newer version to provide enhancements or corrections

UUN Urinary urea nitrogen; the amount of nitrogen excreted in the urine over a 24-hour period

Valsalva maneuver High intrathoracic pressure caused by closing the glottis and constricting the abdominal and chest muscles

valvular insufficiency Inadequate function of one or more of the valves of the heart, allowing backward flow or leakage

vasoconstriction A reduction in the lumen of a blood vessel

VCD Vocal cord dysfunction

ventilatory reserve The difference between maximal exercise ventilation and the MVV, sometimes expressed as a ratio or percentage

ventilatory threshold The workload at which ventilation and $\dot{V}_{CO_2}$ increase at a more rapid rate, indicative of anaerobic metabolism

ventricular Referring to cardiac rhythms originating in the ventricles

watt A measure of power; 1 watt equals 6.12 kpm/min

Wheatstone bridge A bridge for measuring electrical resistances consisting of a conductor joining two branches of a circuit (Sir Charles Wheatstone, 1875)

wheezing High-pitched or musical breath sounds, usually on expiration; associated with airway narrowing

zirconium A tetravalent metallic element with a high melting point used in alloys and in ceramics

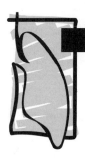

Index